Psychotropic Drug Directory 2001/02
The professionals' pocket handbook and aide memoire

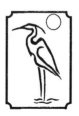

The views expressed in this book reflect the experience of the author and are not necessarily those of Lundbeck Ltd. Any products referred to by the author should only be used as recommended in the manufacturers' data sheets.

Psychotropic Drug Directory 2001/02
The professionals' pocket handbook and aide memoire

Stephen Bazire

Quay Books

Mark Allen Publishing Ltd

Quay Books Division
Mark Allen Publishing Ltd, Jesses Farm
Snow Hill, Dinton, Nr Salisbury, Wilts, SP3 5HN

British Library Cataloguing in Publication Data
A catalogue record for this book is available from the British Library

Printed in the UK by Bath Press, Bath

CONTENTS

Chapter 5 — Drug-induced psychiatric disorders

Chapter 6 — Miscellaneous information

Index and abbreviations used

FOREWORD

Before using this book...

Someone asked me recently 'why is it called the Drug Directory?' Well, when the book originally started, back in 1989, it was called the 'Psychotropic Aide Memoire', and an aide memoire it was. As the book got bigger, it ceased becoming an aide memoire to most people (except perhaps the David Taylors of this world) and a new title was devised (concocted while on a Morris tour in Norwich, with the help of several not entirely sober friends) to try to describe the contents, and how you should use them. The 'directory' part is because the book contains general principles, lists, issues, advice and references to help you make decisions but then directs you where to go to get the further information you might need, since it would be virtually impossible to convey all the subtleties of a research paper, case report or review in a couple of lines. I have, for instance, added about 700 new references to the text this year. If I spent a couple of hours thoroughly reading and analysing each and every paper, I'd never be able to finish the book and would have to give up the day job. So, you really should check papers before making important decisions.

I hope the book continues to provide a handy reference source and the sections are subsequently arranged in a problem-orientated manner and with a minimum level of knowledge assumed. Information given should be followed up in the appropriate sources when time allows. References, where quoted, are either of good recent review articles or of specific information. Further information can be obtained by referring to the main paper cited and also to the reference section of that main paper. Lists and references are as comprehensive as possible but could never claim to be fully complete, nor could this book ever be as comprehensive as a MedLine or PsychLit search on a chosen topic. The listing of a drug use in this book does not in any way imply that it is licensed or safe for this use and all information is presented in good faith. As ever, I am keen to receive constructive comments, advice about dodgy papers and stats etc.

Throughout I have tried to be as objective as possible. It must be up to the reader to make up his or her mind on a topic but I hope the statements and references will have pointed you in the right direction and the time saved in looking papers up will allow more thought. It is inevitable that some papers are from specialist journals but where possible I have always quoted more accessible journals in preference. If the only paper published on the use of a drug is from an obscure or ancient source this may well indicate the status of the paper.

CHANGES TO THIS EDITION

Major updates have been made to all chapters and, as a result of many requests, I have added an asterisk to those sections with new data. With ever more valproate salts commercially available, I am now referring to it as just valproate. The new drugs included are bupropion, galantamine, levetiracetam and oxcarbazepine.

Under an EC Directive, British Approved Names (BANs) were being phased out by December 1998, although at the time of writing completion of this appears further away than ever. I have continued the use of the new recommended International Non-proprietary Names (rINNs) for these drugs (*Pharm J* 1997, **259**, 668–69).

ACKNOWLEDGEMENTS

Writing and continually updating a book such as this is a tremendous challenge and indeed drain on my stamina and enthusiasm. Subsequently, the continued help, encouragement, constructive criticism and advice I have received from colleagues and correspondents has always been utterly invaluable and very rewarding. It is wonderful to know that the book has helped improve the pharmaceutical care of many people with mental health needs. I would thus like to thank all the people I have thanked in previous editions, the many members of the UK Psychiatric Pharmacy Group who have conveyed continued enthusiasm, encouragement and support, and all those people I have met at conferences and talks or who have written to me. I must continue to pay a special tribute to the staff (both clinical and managerial) of Norfolk Mental Health Care NHS Trust, for continuing to provide a caring, ethical and stimulating environment within which to work, including the support over recent years from Kevin Long. Thanks as ever must go to Peter Dingle from Grove Computers, Norwich, my pharmacy staff at Hellesdon for continuing to tolerate and humour me, particularly after my first year as UKPPG Chairman. I also wish to thank Tamzin Ewers and Binkie Mais from Quay Books, Jill Bloom (Drug Information Pharmacist from Moorfields Eye Hospital) for her expert help with the glaucoma section, Chris Wood and Andy Cutting, Vaughan Williams, Fairport Convention, Emmylou Harris, Richard Thompson and John Kirkpatrick for the company, Paul Woods, David Abrahamson, people who have fed back on the contents and/or spotted ambiguities (including John Todd, Niall Campbell, Jane Throssell, Jan van Laarhoven and Richard Morgan), Judy Cane, my parents and my godmother Kate Baxter for continuing to show interest, and finally Jill, Rosemary and Christopher for putting up with a study now overflowing with untidy bits of incomprehensible paper, only some of which is now mine.

Stephen Bazire *BPharm, MRPharmS, DipPsychPharm*
Pharmacy Services Director,
Norfolk Mental Health Care NHS Trust,
Hellesdon Hospital,
Norwich NR6 5BE
England
e-mail: steve.bazire@norfmhc-tr.anglox.nhs.uk
www.ukppg.org.uk
Declaration of interests: www.ukppg.org.uk/committee.html

December, 2000

CHAPTER ONE
DRUG TREATMENT OPTIONS in psychiatric illness

This chapter lists drugs which are indicated for, or have been tried in, the conditions listed. The conditions are those where pharmacotherapy has received attention in the medical press, and the author would welcome suggestions for inclusions here. References should be consulted for fuller details of non-Product Licence uses. Drugs are classified as follows:

BNF Listed — are drugs listed in the British National Formulary as indicated in the UK for that condition. See the appropriate section in the BNF for a review of a drug's role in therapy and its prescribing details. Information provided here is in addition to that in the standard texts and may prove useful. The current UK SPCs are available on-line by visiting www.emc.vhn.net.

+ Combinations — are those which have been used. They carry the risks of additive side-effects and interactions.

● **Unlicensed/Some efficacy** — are drugs of some clinical efficacy, or are strategies which can be employed but where no Product Licence exists in the UK.

○ **Unlicensed/Possible efficacy** — are drugs of minor or unproven importance or efficacy. Again, no Product Licence exists in the UK.

▼ **No efficacy** — are drugs not thought to be of clinical use.

Information in these last three categories is given to provide help once all recognised treatments have been tried. These classifications are to some extent arbitrary and the information is based on data presently available.

It is the prescribers responsibility to ensure all precautions are taken when prescribing drugs for non-Product Licence uses.

1.1 ACUTE PSYCHIATRIC EMERGENCY (APE)

Including rapid tranquillisation. See also aggression (*1.2*), mania/hypomania (*1.19*) and psychosis/schizophrenia (*1.26*)

Violent patients (usually either schizophrenic, manic or substance abusers) present a risk to themselves and others. Swift, safe and effective treatment is thus often needed. Rapid tranquillisation (RT) is defined as the procedure for giving varying amounts of antipsychotic medication over brief intervals of time to control agitated, threatening and potentially destructive patients. It should not be confused with rapid neuro-leptisation, which consists of giving high loading doses of antipsychotics in the first few days/weeks of hospitalisation to accelerate remission. The continued use of cocktails or obsolete/unlicensed drugs is unnecessary.

Routes: IV administration is generally quicker-acting than IM, which is often little quicker than oral drugs (especially if concentrated liquids are used) but allows physical restraint to be removed more quickly. IV drug use does, however, carry many additional dangers and IM use should generally be the preferred choice except in exceptional circumstances. IM absorption will be more rapid in an active patient than a quiet one. Parenteral (IV/IM) doses generally have a higher potency than oral doses, so 'when required' or regular doses prescribed as 'im/po' are entirely inappropriate. All 'when required' doses should be checked daily to ensure maximum doses are not being exceeded. Benzodiazepines are generally safe by (slow) injection, but antipsychotics can be fatal in moderate doses in drug-naive people.

Doses: The need for high doses of antipsychotics is unnecessary, as violent patients respond to standard doses and higher doses may in fact be less effective (eg. Baldessarini *et al, Arch Gen Psych* 1988, **45**, 79–91). Whilst high doses may be used to obtain a sedative effect, use of concommitant benzodiazepines is safer and more effective.

Time intervals: There is little published data on optimum times between doses but single stat dose use or doses given at 60 minute intervals (allowing reasonable assessment of the effects of previous doses) until the desired control is achieved is often used (Dubin, *J Clin Psych* 1988, **49**[Supp12], 5–11).

Conditions: Manic patients may respond well to benzodiazepines, with antipsychotics as adjuncts. Schizophrenic patients usually respond best to antipsychotics, with benzodiazepines as adjuncts. In substance misuse, benzodiazepines and antipsychotics may be effective, but more studies are needed (Dubin, *J Clin Psych* 1988, **49** [Suppl 12], 5–11).

General principles of rapid tranquillisation: (*B J Psych* 1992, **160**, 831)

1. Obtain a drug history and carry out a physical examination if possible. Unless known previous exposure to psychotropics, use doses at lower end of the ranges.
2. High potency antipsychotics are preferred, eg. haloperidol.
3. Parenteral administration is generally quickest and most reliable.
4. No anticholinergics should be used as this may confuse the clinical picture.
5. Swap to oral doses as soon as possible.
6. Check bp and temperature frequently.
7. Although rapid tranquillisation can be carried out in the community, great care is needed.

Complications of rapid tranquillisation at usual doses: (reviewed by Goldberg *et al* in *Clin Neuropharmacol* 1989, **4**, 233–48).

1. Cardiovascular complications (3%) – drugs causing QT prolongation are contraindicated in patients with pre-existing cardiac problems, and care is needed in adrenaline-driven excited patients. This may be the cause of sudden death, which may occur within 2–3 minutes of IV injection. In very many cases toxic blood concentrations are present.
2. Respiratory complications (2%).
3. Local bruising, pain or extravasation (common, in up to 30% patients).
4. Acute hypotension (minimised if the patient can lie down) – greater risk with phenothiazines and in the elderly, minimal risk with haloperidol.
5. Seizures, especially in non-compliant epileptics – avoid high dose chlorpromazine.
6. Mega-colon (rare), heatstroke and aspiration.
7. Neuroleptic malignant syndrome – see 1.22 for risk factors. Close observation of temperature should be carried out, especially in early stages. Check CPK.
8. A depot given inadvertently into a vein may be rapidly fatal.
9. Extrapyramidal symptoms, especially acute dystonia. This may occur in 10–30% of patients within the first 24 hours and later in up to 50% of young males. Akathisia should be considered if agitation occurs or recurs after antipsychotic loading has achieved adequate behavioural control.

Review*: 'ABC of mental health: Mental health emergencies', Atakan and Davies, *BMJ* 1997, **314**, 1740–42 (causes, safety, RT and aftercare), acute psychosis (Hilliard, *J Clin Psych* 1998, **59**[Suppl 1], 57–60).

BNF Listed

Drugs in this section are licensed for emergency, short-term or adjunct therapy of, eg. acute psychosis, mania, anxiety or exacerbations of chronic psychosis, violent or impulsive behaviour, psychomotor agitation and excitement or violent or dangerously impulsive behaviour (see SPCs for details).

Chlorpromazine

Chlorpromazine injection should be given by deep IM injection only, at 25–50mg every 6–8hrs, with a lower dose (up to 25mg 8 hrly) in the elderly. The IM injection is 2–4 times as potent, on a mg for mg basis, as oral chlorpromazine, and so prescriptions for '100mg po/im' are entirely inappropriate and potentially dangerous.

Diazepam (see also combinations)

The recommended dose of diazepam is 10mg IV or IM, repeated after not less than 4 hours. IV infusion is possible. IV diazepam is much more consistently absorbed than IM. If the IV route is used, it is strongly recommended to be into the large vein of the antecubital fossa, with the patient in a supine position, if possible, to minimise the incidence of hypotension. The maximum IV dose is 5mg per minute. Mechanical ventilation should be available at higher doses in case of respiratory depression as hypoxic drive can be affected. Diazepam has a long half-life and active metabolites and so accumulation and toxic delirium (especially in the elderly or liver-impaired) must be avoided by use of decreased doses later on.

Droperidol*
Droperidol was discontinued in 2001 due to QT concerns (review by Chambers and Druss, *J Clin Psych* 1999, **60**, 664–67).

Haloperidol (see also combinations)
Haloperidol can be used at BNF dose, eg. 10–20mg (review, n=136, Alinton *et al, Ann Emerg Med* 1987, **16**, 319–22). Some concerns about QT prolongation have been raised and the IV route is probably best avoided unless essential.

Levomepromazine (methotrimeprazine)
This highly sedative antipsychotic is licensed as an alternative to chlorpromazine, especially when sedation is needed. The injection should be diluted with an equal volume of sodium chloride before use.

Lorazepam (see also combinations)
Lorazepam is usually given by the IV route into a larger vein, as IM absorption is as slow as oral administration, but more rapid in an active patient and IM generally carries less risk than IV. Lorazepam injection may be diluted 50:50 with water or normal saline pre-injection. The dose in acute anxiety is 0.025–0.03mg/kg (1.75–2.1mg for a 70kg person), repeated 6-hourly. Many areas use 0.5–2mg po/im every 1–2 hours until symptoms are controlled, missing doses when excessive sedation occurs. This can be a highly effective therapy. Caution is needed in renal and hepatic impairment and in the elderly, where a lower dose may be needed. Lorazepam does not accumulate with repeated doses nor in hepatic impairment, distinct advantages over diazepam.

Trifluoperazine
This is licensed as an adjunct therapy.

Zuclopenthixol acetate *
'Clopixol Acuphase' can be given at a dose of 50–150mg stat, then repeated after 2–3 days (maximum every 1–2 days) after the first injection. The maximum cumulative dose is 400mg per 'course', ie. 4 injections or 2 weeks, whichever comes first. The maximum single dose in the elderly is 100mg.

While zuclopenthixol acetate appears as effective as haloperidol in APE, sedation at 4 hours may be greater and there is an advantage of the need for fewer injections (McNulty and Pelosi, *EBMH* 1998, **1**, 56). Several reviews have suggested that more data is needed to prove an advantage over standard therapies (Coutinho *et al, Schizophr Res* 2000, **46**, 111–18; Fenton *et al, CDSR* 2000, CD000525). Care is needed with Acuphase® to avoid it being given into a vein of a struggling or over-active patient.

+ Combinations
Combinations of drugs are highly effective and generally allow lower doses of both to be used. Patients receiving only a single drug in APE at first are more likely to need second injections (Pilowski *et al, BJPsych* 1992, **160**, 831–35). In the only major UK study, a combination of antipsychotic and sedative was favoured by staff as the most effective.

Antipsychotic + benzodiazepine (particularly haloperidol plus lorazepam or diazepam)
This combination is widely and strongly recommended (eg. extensive review by Dubin, *J Clin Psych* 1988, **49** [Suppl 12], 5–11; Goldberg *et al, Clin Neuropharmacol* 1989, **12**, 233–48) as the drugs act synergistically, reducing the amount of each drug (but particularly the antipsychotic) required. The effect of the combination is rapid and predictable and the patient less likely to require a second injection. 10mg IM/IV of both haloperidol and diazepam for a 'drug naive' patient is strongly recommended, with up to 20mg of each for previously antipsychotic-treated patients. Lorazepam (see separate entry) is a widely used alternative to diazepam, with 2mg IM plus haloperidol IM 5mg being significantly better than lorazepam alone after 60–180 minutes in one APE study (n=98, RCT, Battaglia *et al, Am J Emerg Med* 1997, **15**, 335–40). No serious adverse effects occurred in either treatment group, suggesting superior efficacy for haloperidol-lorazepam over lorazepam alone (n=20, d/b, Bieniek *et al, Pharmacotherapy* 1998, **18**, 57–62). See also next section.

O   Unlicensed/possible efficacy
Amylobarbital/amobarbital sodium
Great care is needed if used in APE. The IM route should be preferred. If IV must be used, the vial should be diluted and injected *slowly* (maximum 50mg/min) to prevent sudden respiratory depression. It is contraindicated in marked hepatic impairment.

Clomethiazole (chlormethiazole)
See SPC for doses for other indications.

Clonazepam
Clonazepam is licensed only for status epilepticus in all its clinical forms. The dose is 1mg (1ml) by slow (1mg per 30 seconds) IV injection, which is strongly recommended to be into the large vein of the antecubital fossa, with the patient in a supine position if possible, to minimise the incidence of hypotension. Care is needed in the elderly and caution in chronic pulmonary insufficiency.

Midazolam
2.5–10mg IV may be rapidly effective (6–20 minutes) in controlling acute agitation (eg. reports by Mendoza *et al, J Clin Psych* 1987, **48**, 291–92; Bond *et al, Am J Psych* 1989, **146**, 925–26). Great care is needed to avoid respiratory depression when given IV.

Paraldehyde
Infusion should be carried out in specialist centres ONLY, as it needs intensive care facilities.

Valproate
See entry under mania (*1.20*).

1.2 AGGRESSION
See also acute psychiatric emergency (*1.1*), borderline personality disorder (*1.11*) and self-injurious behaviour (SIB) (*1.29*)

Aggression is considered as behaviour with verbal or physical threats which, if carried out, would cause harm to others, self or property. It can include situational (provoked), non-situational (unprovoked), passive, physical or interictal (especially in temporal lobe epilepsy).

Aggression is not a diagnosis in itself, but as well as being potentially drug-induced (through either intoxication or withdrawal), can be considered a symptom of many conditions, including dementia, personality disorders, PTSD, PMS, trauma etc, or as an expression of a variety of emotional or behavioural motivations. Low GABA levels and low serotonin levels in various parts of the brain are associated with aggressive behaviour, and enhanced noradrenaline and dopamine levels in the brain are associated with increased aggression.

Role of drugs:
Drugs may be useful in helping control some cases where suppression of aggression is considered important on safety grounds.

Reviews*: pharmacotherapy (Fava, *Psychiatr Clin North Am* 1997, **20**, 427–51), non-antipsychotic drug treatments (Smith and Perry, *Ann Pharmacother* 1992, **26**, 1400–8), general (Hughes, *Psychiatr Serv* 1999, **50**, 1135–37).

BNF Listed
Lithium *
Most studies have involved aggression in patients with learning disabilities and a two-month trial at 0.6–1.0 mmol/l may be justified in patients unmanagable by environmental factors. Lithium has been shown to reduce aggression and the frequency of episodes in learning disabilities (eg. Langee, *Am J Ment Retard* 1990, **94**, 448–52), reducing impulsive aggression in patients with organic brain damage (Tyrer, *Eur Neuro-Psychopharmacol* 1994, **4**, 234–36), brain damaged individuals (Bellus *et al, Brain Inj* 1996, **10**, 849–60) and in two trials in children with aggression or conduct disorder, albeit poorly tolerated (n=50, RCT, Campbell *et al, J Am Acad Child Adolesc Psych* 1995, **34**, 445–53, 694; n=86, RCT, d/b, p/c, Malone *et al, Arch Gen Psych* 2000, **57**, 649–54). Lithium may exert an effect via several mechanisms, eg. enhancement of serotonin.

+   Combinations
Fluvoxamine + antipsychotics
An aggressive schizophrenic improved when fluvoxamine 100mg/d was added to risperidone 8mg/d (n=1, Silver and Kushnir, *Am J Psych* 1998, **155**, 1298).

●   Unlicensed/Some efficacy
Antipsychotics *
Evidence for the efficacy of anti-psychotics in aggression is suggestive

rather than conclusive as a clinical effect is difficult to quantify. It may be that raised dopamine levels are associated with aggression (Pabis and Stanislav, *Ann Pharmacother* 1996, **30**, 278–87), in which case dopamine-blocking drugs may have some rationale. Use of higher doses of antipsychotics are generally considered to be effective only via a sedating effect. A number of drugs have been used. Risperidone may have some role (De Deyn and Katz, *Int J Ger Psych* 2000, **15**[Suppl 1], S14–22), especially at a lower dose (eg. Buckley *et al, J Am Acad Psych Law* 1997, **25**, 173–81). A study of behavioural disturbances in learning disability showed zuclopenthixol (2–20mg/d) to be significantly superior to haloperidol (0.5–5mg/d) at notably modest doses (n=24, d/b, c/o, Malt *et al, B J Psych* 1995, **166**, 374–77). A trial showed pipo-thiazine to be superior to placebo in controlling aggression in learning disabilities (n=10, 13/52, Lynch *et al, B J Psych* 1985, **146**, 525–29). For their use in the elderly, see *1.13*.

○   Unlicensed/Possible efficacy
Benzodiazepines

These are reported to be effective in episodic behavioural disorders by aborting aggression in the prodromal stage. Lorazepam has been used in resistant aggression of dementia, with 1.5–3mg/d effective orally over several years in some patients (*Am J Psych* 1990, **147**, 1250), as has 1–2mg lorazepam IV (Salzman *et al, J Clin Psych* 1991, **52**, 177–80). Use should normally be limited to only a few weeks to minimise the incidence of disinhibition or paradoxical reactions (Dietch and Jennings, *J Clin Psych* 1988, **49**, 184–88, although the actual incidence may be as low as perhaps <1%) and the problems of dependence/withdrawal, sedation etc.

Beta-blockers*

Beta-blockers (principally propranolol) have been reported to help control aggression in learning disabilities (case report and review, *Am J Mental Retardation* 1990, **95**, 110–19), autism (120mg/d nadolol, Ratey *et al, J Clin Psychopharmacol* 1987, **7**, 35–41), schizophrenia (up to 120mg/d nadolol,

Clin Pharm 1989, **8**, 132–35) and in intermittent explosive disorders (80–300mg/d propranolol, Jenkins and Maruta, *Mayo Clin Proc* 1987, **62**, 204–14). Pindolol 40–60mg/d may be effective (d/b, c/o, 6/52, Greendyke and Kanter, *J Clin Psych* 1986, **47**, 423–26). More trials are needed to confirm these studies, and potential effects on bp and heart-rate will always limit their use (review by Haspel, *Harv Rev Psychiatry* 1995, **2**, 274–81).

Buspirone

Several studies (eg. Ratey *et al, J Clin Psych* 1991, **52**, 159–62) and case reports (eg. Quiason *et al, J Am Acad Child Adolesc Psych* 1991, **30**, 1026), have shown some beneficial effect. A three-month trial seems necessary, and a transient worsening may occur initially (Stanislav *et al, J Clin Psychopharmacol* 1994, **14**, 126–30).

Carbamazepine

Data for the use of carbamazepine in aggression is largely anecdotal, based on the proposed association between aggression and TLE or other EEG abnormalities but one trial showed 600mg/d to reduce aggressive behaviour with schizophrenia (RCT, Neepe, *J Clin Psych* 1983, **44**, 326–31). There are case reports of successful use in episodic dyscontrol/aggression (Lewin and Sumners, *B J Psych* 1992, **161**, 722, a link with TLE being considered), violent schizophrenics (Yassa and Dupont, *Can J Psych* 1983, **28**, 566–68) paroxysmal behaviour disorder (*Am J Psych* 1983, **140**, 1363–64) and the elderly demented (n=51, Tariot *et al, Am J Psych* 1998, **155**, 54–61).

Clonidine

In an open study, 150–400mcg/d reduced aggressiveness in 88% destructive children (n=17, Kemph *et al, J Am Acad Child Adolesc Psych* 1993, **32**, 577–81), who noted some increases in CSF GABA levels.

Cyproterone

200mg/d over one month has been successful in several cases (*B J Psych* 1991, **159**, 298–99; Thibaut and Colonna, *Am J Psych* 1992, **149**, 411) but the treatment is difficult to use and presents many problems (*B J Psych* 1992, **160**, 282–83).

Dexamfetamine (dexamphetamine)

Aggressive behaviour was reduced in two boys with ADHD given 15–30mg/d dexamfetamine over two weeks (Amery et al, J Am Acad Child Adolesc Psych 1984, **23**, 291–94), supported by another study (Cherek et al, Psychopharm 1986, **88**, 381–86).

Estrogens (oestrogens)

See dementia (*1.13*).

Gabapentin *

See dementia (*1.13*).

Lamotrigine *

See dementia (*1.13*).

Medroxyprogesterone

This synthetic progestogen (given monthly and alternating with placebo) reduced aggression in 2 of 3 antipsychotic-resistant schizophrenics (O'Connor and Baker, Acta Psych Scand 1983, **67**, 399–403).

Phenytoin

An inmate trial showed that 300mg/d phenytoin reduces impulsive aggressive acts but not premeditated attacks (n=60, d/b, p/c, Barratt et al, J Clin Psychopharmacol 1997, **17**, 341–49).

SSRIs

The use of SSRIs may be rational if low serotonin levels associated with aggression can be corrected. Aggression in learning disabilities may also be associated with unrecognised mood disorders, eg. depression. In a study with citalopram (20–60mg/d) for 24 weeks, aggressive incidents were significantly lower, with no deterioration nor significant side-effects (n=15, d/b, c/o, Vartiainen, Acta Psych Scand 1995, **91**, 348–61). A similar effect has been suggested with sertraline 50–200mg/d (open, Kavoussi et al, J Clin Psych 1994, **55**, 137–41; n=1, Campbell and Duffy, J Clin Psych 1994, **56**, 123–24). There is a case report and study of uncontrollable aggressive outbursts and anger attacks (secondary to stroke), unresponsive to other antidepressants and antipsychotics, responding rapidly to fluoxetine 20mg/d (Weinman and Ruskin, Am J Psych 1994, **151**, 1839; Fava et al, Am J Psych 1993, **150**, 1158–63).

Trazodone *

Reduced aggression has been reported (eg. n=1, Mashiko et al, Psychiatry Clin Neurosci 1996, **50**, 133–36; n=1, Bernstein, J Neuropsychiatry Clin Neurosci 1992, **4**, 348).

Tricyclics

Use is mentioned in Acta Psych Scand 1988, **78**, 188–90. See also SSRIs above.

Valproate *

Valproate may exert an effect by correcting any abnormally low GABA levels. Two open studies have shown valproate effective for impulsive aggressive behaviour in people with personality disorders (n=10, open, Kavoussi and Coccaro, J Clin Psych 1998, **59**, 676–80) and in adults with learning disabilities (n=28, Ruedrich et al, J Intellect Disabil Res 1999, **43**, 105–11), and case reports (eg. Mattes, J Nerv Ment Dis 1992, **180**, 601–2) where blood levels above 50mcg/ml seemed most effective.

Reviews * management of agitation and aggression in the elderly (Parks-Veal, Consultant Pharm 1999, **14**, 557–60) and review of 17 studies (none d/b, p/c) indicating valproate has a promising but unproven anti-aggressive effect (n=164, Lindenmayer and Kotsaftis, J Clin Psych 2000, **61**, 123–28).

1.3 AGORAPHOBIA

See also anxiety (*1.6*), panic disorder (*1.24*) and social phobia (*1.33*).

Agoraphobia, an anxiety disorder, is an overwhelming and disabling anxiety provoked by being alone or in public places. Panic attacks may accompany the phobia and depression may be present in up to a half of patients. A connection with serotonin deficiency has been shown.

Role of drugs:

Drug treatment may be effective in many patients and psychotherapy is considered an essential component of the treatment package. A meta-analysis of 54 published studies has shown that symptoms are improved by tricyclics, and high potency benzodiazepines, and although there may be a short-term deterioration, this usually turns to a longer-term improvement. The best long-term improvement is from exposure therapy, particularly combined with antidepressants, eg. imipramine (Mattick et al, J Nerv Ment

Dis 1990, **178**, 567–76). There is a weak but significant placebo response to drugs (Mavis-Sakalian *et al, Am J Psych* 1987, **144**, 785–87).

Reviews*: SSRIs in panic and agoraphobia (Bakker *et al, Int Clin Psychopharmacol* 2000, **15**[Suppl 2], S25–30).

BNF Listed

Citalopram

Citalopram is indicated in the UK for the symptoms of panic disorder, with or without agoraphobia. See also *1.24*.

Paroxetine *

Paroxetine may be less likely to produce 'jitteriness' than tricyclics (n=326, naturalistic, Toni *et al, Pharmaco-psychiatry* 2000, **33**, 121–31). See also *1.24*.

● **Unlicensed/Some efficacy**

Benzodiazepines

Alprazolam (Ballenger *et al, Arch Gen Psych* 1988, **45**, 413–22) and diazepam have been used and shown to help, particularly with anxiety symptoms.

MAOIs

Phenelzine has been studied in agoraphobia with panic attacks and shown to be highly effective at doses of up to 45mg/d (eg. Buigues and Vallejo, *J Clin Psych* 1987, **48**, 55–59).

Tricyclics

Up to 70% of cases may respond to tricyclics, but with 30% dropping out due to side-effects. 20% may worsen, with an increase in panic attacks. Clomipramine, at doses up to 300mg/d, has been shown to be effective (Johnson *et al, Arch Gen Psych* 1988, **45**, 453–59), with a continuous improvement shown over many weeks. Doses as low as 75mg/d may be effective (Gloger *et al, J Clin Psychopharmacol* 1989, **9**, 28–32). A relationship between plasma levels and response has been proposed. See also panic (*1.24*).

○ **Unlicensed/Possible efficacy**

Buspirone

Buspirone has been shown to be well-tolerated and enhance the effect of CBT in panic disorder with agoraphobia (n=41, 68/52, d/b, Cottraux *et al, B J Psych* 1995, **167**, 635–41), although a subsequent naturalistic study was

unable to replicate this long-term effect (Bouvard *et al, Psychother Psychsom* 1997, **66**, 27–32).

Trazodone

Trazodone, at up to 300mg/d, showed a significant effect, with improvement in anxiety, panic and phobia (n=11, Mavissakalian *et al, Am J Psych* 1987, **144**, 785–87).

Valproate

It has been suggested that valproate may have an effect (Roy-Byrne *et al, J Clin Psych* 1989, **50**[Suppl], 44–48).

▼ **No efficacy**

Moclobemide

The efficacy of moclobemide monotherapy in panic disorder with agoraphobia was unable to be shown in one study, although the long-term effects of CBT were enhanced with concomitant moclobemide (n=55, RCT, Loerch *et al, B J Psych* 1999, **174**, 205–12).

1.4 ALCOHOL DEPENDENCE and ALCOHOL ABUSE

See also alcohol withdrawal syndrome (*1.5*)

Symptoms:

The main diagnostic symptoms of alcohol dependence are of primacy of drinking over other activities, increased tolerance of alcohol, symptoms of repeated withdrawal, stereotyped pattern of drinking, compulsion to drink and relief drinking.

Risk factors: *

Some risk factors for alcohol abuse or being an alcohol-dependent drinker include:
1. Occupation, eg. brewers, reps, doctors, alcohol retailers.
2. Genetics (up to 30–40% influence).
3. Marital/social problems, eg. work.
4. Personality, eg. anxiety.
5. Psychopaths and criminals, eg. taking alcohol before criminal events.
6. Psychiatric illness, eg. depression, anxiety, phobia etc.
7. Use for hypnotic or analgesic purposes.
8. Adverse childhood or adolescent experiences.

The body metabolises one unit of alcohol per hour and peak levels occur one hour after the drink is consumed. One unit gives a man an alcohol blood level of about 15mg/100ml and a woman about 20mg/100ml. Absorption is rapid with low volume drinks, eg. spirits and slower with higher volumes, eg. beer. Alcohol consumption of 7.7–12.9 units per week is associated with the lowest mortality in men (White, *J Clin Epidemiol* 1999, **52**, 967–75, review by Caan, *EBMH* 2000, **3**, 61), an oft-quoted finding in bars throughout the world.

Role of drugs:

Pharmacological treatment can play its part in an overall plan. Vitamin deficiency occurs and can lead to Wernicke-Korsakoff syndrome, needing high dose vitamins by injection (see AWS, *1.5*). Other drugs may be useful to treat associated psychiatric morbidity, such as withdrawal, affective disorders, suicide and hallucinations. In the longer term, disulfiram can have a role to play in experienced hands and selected patients. The role of acamprosate is being established and more experience will be necessary. A recent review of the evidence concluded that there is good evidence of efficacy for naltrexone and acamprosate, but not for serotonergic agents or lithium and controlled trials of disulfiram indicate limited efficacy (Garbutt *et al, JAMA* 1999, **281**, 1318–25, 61 refs; reviewed in *EBMH* 2000, **3**, 15). In a review of acamprosate (n=3338) versus naltrexone (n=200) for relapse prevention in alcoholics, the authors conclude that both drugs were superior to placebo, drop-out rates were comparable, naltrexone caused more adverse effects and that acamprosate may be preferred because of its proven long-term effectiveness with carry-over (review of d/b, p/c studies, Hoes, *Clin Drug Invest* 1999, **17**, 211–16; see also Cornish and O'Brien, *Medicine* 1999, **27**, 26–29).

Other reviews*: management of Korsakoffs (Smith and Hillman, *Adv Psych Treat* 1999, **5**, 271–78), recent advances (Swift, *NEJM* 1999, **340**, 1482–90, 99 refs; Garbutt *et al, JAMA* 1999, **281**, 1318–25), haematological changes in alcohol dependence (Drummond and Ghodse, *Adv Psych Treat* 1999, **5**, 366–75, 30 refs), GP review and options (Feeney and Nutt, *Prescriber* 2000, **11**, 21–30; *Drug & Ther Bull* 2000, **38**, 60–64, 31 refs).

BNF Listed

Acamprosate

Acamprosate is licensed in the UK for abstinence maintenance therapy for up to one year in motivated alcohol-dependent patients. Acamprosate is a GABA analogue and may act to reduce the severity and frequency of relapse by enhancing GABA inhibitory neurotransmission and antagonising glutamate excitation (glutamate receptors increase in chronic alcohol dependency), reducing intake via reduced reward, a possible anti-craving effect. It takes about 7 days to reach therapeutic levels and so should be started soon after detoxification. Continued alcohol consumption negates the therapeutic effect, but occasional lapses do not necessarily do this. Many RCTs have shown some clinical effectiveness; one showed a 50% increase in days of continuous abstinence (n=538, Paille *et al, Alcohol and Alcoholism* 1995, **30**, 239–47), another small, but significant, improvement in abstinence rates in the first 60 days (67% *vs* 50%) and at 48 weeks (43% *vs* 21%) (n=272, Sass *et al, Arch Gen Psych* 1996, **53**, 673–80) and another showed acamprosate to be a valuable adjunct to psychosocial and behavioural treatment of episodic or chronic alcoholism (n=455, d/b, p/c, Whitworth *et al, Lancet* 1996, **347**, 1438–42, 29 refs). One review concluded that acamprosate is well-tolerated, its efficacy may be enhanced by the addition of disulfiram, as an adjunct to psychosocial and behavioural therapies (including counselling) and can be considered a promising first-line pharmacological therapy for the maintenance of abstinence in detoxified alcohol-dependent patients (Wilde and Goa, *Disease Management & Health Outcomes* 1998, **3**, 35–46). It is certainly not a miracle 'cure' for repeatedly failed detoxification patients and should be combined with continued counselling.

Reviews: mode of action (Littleton, *Addiction* 1995, **90**, 1179–88), general (*Drug & Ther Bull* 1997, **35**, 70–72), extensive review of its pharmacology and clinical potential, effect is dose dependent, may be enhanced by disulfiram, well tolerated (Wilde and Wagstaff, *Drugs* 1997, **53**, 1038–53, 62 refs), clinical pharmacokinetics (Siavin *et al, Clin Pharmacokinet* 1998, **35**, 331–45, 44 refs).

Disulfiram

Irreversible inhibition of ALDH (Hepatic Aldehyde-NAD reductase) by disulfiram leads to accumulation of acetaldehyde from incomplete alcohol metabolism (*Acta Psych Scand* 1992, **86**, 7–13, see also *4.7.1*). Disulfiram acts as a negative reinforcer for abstinence via the potential for an adversive disulfiram-alcohol interaction, ie. an adversive/conditioning and maintenance therapy in alcoholics (*B J Psych* 1984, **144**, 200–2). A review of 24 studies published from 1967–1995 implied that while disulfiram can reduce total alcohol consumption, studies are poor, patient selection variable and compliance low. Maximum benefit occurs with supervised treatment (Hughes and Cook, *Addiction* 1997, **92**, 381–95). The BNF tends to underestimate doses needed so it is suggested to start with a loading dose of 400mg/d (*B J Psych* 1984, **144**, 200–2) with 365mg/d the average dose used. 'Antabuse®' tablets are dispersable and so can be given as a liquid in a supervised setting (eg. with relatives, neighbours, clinics etc, *Alcohol & Alcoholism* 1986, **21**, 385–88). It can also be given as a

Disulfiram Test Dose

A test dose is now considered less necessary due to the risks involved and that the mode of action is via a conditioning process.

If considered necessary, wait 5 days after commencement of treatment for full enzyme block to occur.
1. Give 10–15ml of 95% alcohol (or 15–25ml spirits).
2. Reaction should start in 5–15 minutes.
3. Repeat in 30 minutes if no reaction. Reaction shows as flushed face, tachycardia, nausea, vomiting, fall in blood pressure. (Have crash box plus personnel available.) Usual cause of no reaction is too low a dose of disulfiram. Bronchospasm has also been reported (Beri *et al, BMJ* 1993, **306**, 396). .

twice-a-week dose (ie. daily dose x 7 divided by 2) as the enzyme block is irreversible and the clinical effect lasts about 7–10 days.

Reviews: general (*Acta Psych Scand* 1992, **86**[Suppl 369], studies (*B J Psych* 1992, **161**, 84–89; *Acta Psych Scand* 1992, **86**[Suppl 369] and compliance improvement, eg. implants, incentives, contracts, patient information etc, *Alcohol Clin Exp Res* 1992, **16**, 1035–41), efficacy (Hughes and Cook, *Addiction* 1997, **92**, 381–95).

B Vitamins

Vitamin deficiency is due to inadequate diet, impaired absorption, increased metabolic demand and impaired utilisation. Thiamine (B1) is thus primary and priority treatment (but probably underprescribed) to reverse the mental confusion secondary to thiamine deficiency (Wernicke's syndrome) (*Lancet* 1990, **ii**, 912–13) but only about 5-10mg is absorbed from each oral dose, via a saturable mechanism. The CSM advice on allergic reactions is in the BNF. **Review**: Cook and Thomson (*Br J Hosp Med* 1997, **57**, 461–65).

+ Combinations

Acamprosate + disulfiram

In one study, alcoholics were randomised over one year to placebo or acamprosate, and could request additional disulfiram. Disulfiram improved the effectiveness of acamprosate, but a high dropout did not allow full analysis (RCT, n=118, Besson *et al, Alcohol Clin Exp Res* 1998, **22**, 573–79).

● Unlicensed/Some efficacy

Naltrexone *

Naltrexone has been well studied and may have significant efficacy in alcohol dependence. Several double-blind trials have shown the effectiveness of 50mg/d, eg. less craving, more alcohol-free days and only 23% relapse (n=70, Volpicelli *et al, Arch Gen Psych* 1992, **49**, 876–80; n=97, O'Malley *et al, Arch Gen Psych* 1992, **49**, 881–89; 19 non-alcoholic drinkers, Swift *et al, Am J Psych* 1994, **151**, 1463–67). Naltrexone seems to have little effect on reducing alcohol sampling by abstinent alcoholics but has a significant effect on reducing subsequent drinking by somehow breaking the desire for the next drink, a view consistent with Volpicelli's findings above. Finally, one trial came to the stunning conclusion that, while naltrexone is moderately effective in reducing alcohol intake, its efficacy is far greater in people who comply with treatment (n=97, p/c, Volpicelli *et al, Arch Gen Psych* 1997, **54**, 737–42). The effect may be due to naltrexone blocking the pleasure (or 'high') caused by alcohol and reducing alcohol-seeking behaviour (Volpicelli *et al, Am J Psych* 1995, **152**, 613–15) or reduced craving for alcohol (n=43, O'Malley *et al, Am J Psych* 1996, **153**, 281–83), supporting the hypothesis that a central effect on modification of alcohol-induced craving is naltrexones mode of action. Naltrexone 50mg/d has also been shown to augment the effect of CBT in moderate alcohol dependence in socially stable individuals and may be synergistic with CBT. Naltrexone itself was slightly superior to placebo (n=131, RCT, Anton *et al, Am J Psych* 1999, **156**, 1758–64; reviewed by Chick, *EBMH* 2000, **3**, 75).

Review*: editorial (Volpicelli, *Lancet* 1995, **346**, 456; *Prescrire International* 1999, **8**, 9–11, 12 refs).

○   **Unlicensed/Possible efficacy**

Benzodiazepines

Although not recommended in alcoholics for the very real fear of addiction, benzodiazepines have been advocated if they are able to reduce alcohol dependence (as a 'lesser of two evils' strategy). Any use should be well-documented in the patient's notes.

Buspirone *

Two trials in anxious alcoholics have shown reduced anxiety, alcohol consumption and drinking days (n=61, 12/52, Kranzer *et al, Arch Gen Psych* 1994, **51**, 720–31) and to significantly reduce alcohol craving and consumption in motivated patients (n=50, d/b, p/c, Bruno, *Psychopathology* 1989, **22**[Suppl 1], 49–59), but no effect on drinking nor anxiety has been noted in two other studies (n=66, *Alcohol Clin Exp Res* 1992, **16**, 1007–13; n=156, RCT, Fawcett *et al, Alcohol Clin Exp Res* 2000, **24**, 666–74).

Review: general (Malec *et al, Alcohol Clin Exp Res* 1996, **20**, 853–58).

Carbamazepine *

One trial has shown a significant long-term effect on time to first drink and survival (n=29, 12/12, RCT, Mueller *et al, Alcohol Clin Exp Res* 1997, **21**, 86–92).

Imipramine

A study of alcoholics with co-morbid depression showed 45% to improve in mood and drinking behaviour on imipramine (n=60, *Am J Psych* 1993, **150**, 963–65).

Methylphenidate

Advocated by a small uncontrolled study (*Clin Neuropharmacol* 1986, **9**, 65–70).

Nalmefene *

Nalmefene 20mg/d reduced relapse to heavy drinking in alcohol dependence, supporting the view that opioid antagonists are effective (n=105, RCT, Mason *et al, Arch Gen Psych* 1999, **56**, 719–24).

Ondansetron *

Ondansetron, a 5-HT3 antagonist, at 8mcg/kg/d was superior to placebo in increasing drink-free days, especially for early-onset (pre-25yo) alcoholism (RCT, n=271, Johnson *et al, JAMA* 2000, **284**, 963–71).

Piracetam

Modest degrees of improvement of alcohol-related cognitive impairment have been seen with oral piracetam (Barnas *et al, Psychopharmacology* 1990, **100**, 361–65).

SSRIs

Citalopram has produced a modest (16–17%) but significant reduction in alcoholic drink intake and increase in drink-free days in studies of alcoholics (eg. Naranjo *et al, Clin Pharmacol Ther* 1992, **51**, 729–39), possibly by decreasing desire or reducing the reward (see also n=62, d/b, p/c, Tiihonen *et al, Pharmacopsychiatry* 1996, **29**, 27–29). 60mg/d fluoxetine reduced alcoholic and total drink intake compared to placebo and to fluoxetine 40mg/d (n=29, Naranjo *et al, Clin Pharmacol & Ther* 1990, **47**, 490–98), as has fluoxetine 20–40mg/d in alcoholics with co-morbid depression (RCT, n=51, Cornelius *et al, Arch Gen Psych* 1997, **54**, 700–5; review by Haslam, *EBMH* 1998, **1**, 41). However, a larger study failed to reproduce these effects (RCT, n=101, Kranzler *et al, Am J Psych* 1995, **152**, 391–97).

Trazodone

Low dose trazodone decreased craving, depressive and anxious symptoms in detoxified alcohol-dependent patients (open, n=25, Janiri *et al, Alcohol Alcoholism* 1998, **33**, 362–65).

▼ **No efficacy**

Lithium *

Three trials have shown lack of advantage over placebo (n=22, 3/12, d/b, Olbrich *et al, Nervenarzt* 1991, **62**, 182–86; n=53, 6/12, d/b, de la Fuente *et al, Mayo Clin Proc* 1989, **64**, 177–80; n=156, RCT, Fawcett *et al, Alcohol Clin Exp Res* 2000, **24**, 666–74).

Lithium + tryptophan

No effect on alcohol craving, consumption nor mental state cf. placebo (Malec *et al, Lithium* 1994, **5**, 23–27).

1.5 ALCOHOL WITHDRAWAL SYNDROME (AWS)

See also alcohol dependence and abuse (*1.4*)

Symptoms:

The presentation of alcohol withdrawal includes psychological symptoms (eg. anxiety and restlessness), psychotic symptoms (eg. hallucinations), tremor, sweating, tachycardia, gastrointestinal symptoms, fits, illusions, clouding of consciousness and delirium tremens (DT), Wernicke's Encephalopathy (Wernicke-Korsakoff syndrome). These last for about 48 hours after the last drink. Fits may first occur within 24 hours. AWS may be self-limiting or progress to delirium tremens. In DT, fits may occur (either primary or secondary to hypoglycaemia, hypomagnesaemia or hyponatraemia) as may suicidal ideation, gross disorientation, delusions, violence, marked tremor etc. DT peaks on the 3rd or 4th day, and physical complications are common, eg. pulmonary infection and hepatic encephalopathy.

Role of drugs:

Seizures and psychiatric disturbances are serious problems and treatment of severe AWS is essential. Withdrawal symptoms in hospital may be underestimated and this may lead to under-treatment. A meta-analysis and practice guideline (Mayo-Smith, *JAMA* 1997, **278**, 144–51, 175 refs; comments in *JAMA* 1997, **278**, 1317–18) concludes that:

● benzodiazepines are suitable agents for alcohol withdrawal

● dosage should be individualised according to withdrawal severity, co-morbidity and history of withdrawal seizures

● beta-blockers, clonidine, carbamazepine ameliorate withdrawal severity but evidence of their effect on delirium and seizures is lacking

● phenothiazines ameliorate withdrawal but are less effective than benzodiazepines in reducing delirium or seizures

● thiamine (IM or IV) should be an additional first-line treatment.

Reviews*: general (Hall and Zador, *Lancet* 1997, **349**, 1897–900), management of alcohol Korsakoff syndrome (Smith and Hillman, *Adv Psych Treat* 1999, **5**, 271–78), management of acute alcohol withdrawal (Williams and McBridie, *Alcohol Alcohol* 1998, **33**, 103–15; Holbrook *et al, Can Med Ass J* 1999, **160**, 675–80, 42 refs; Claassen and Adinoff, *CNS Drugs* 1999, **12**, 279–91) and in the elderly (Kraemer *et al, Drugs & Aging* 1999, **14**, 409–25).

BNF Listed

Benzodiazepines *

Benzodiazepines are the drugs of choice for treating acute alcohol withdrawal (meta-analysis of 11 RCTs, n=1286, Holbrook *et al, Can Med Ass J* 1999, **160**, 649–55). Chlordiazepoxide and diazepam are the established treatments in the UK, with lorazepam also used, as it has an intermediate half-life and no active metabolites, both particularly useful in the elderly or those with hepatic damage. Lorazepam 2mg IV was more effective than placebo (3% lorazepam *vs* 24% placebo recurrence) in the prevention of recurrent generalised, alcohol-related seizures (n=186, p/c, D'Onofrio *et al, NEJM* 1999, **340**, 915–19; reviewed in *EBMH* 1999, **2**, 107; plus correspondence from Sosis, Matz, D'Onofrio *et al, NEJM* 1999, **341**, 609–10). A longer acting benzodiazepine allows a smoother withdrawal, and might be preferred (review comparing benzodiazepines in AWS by Bird and Makela, *Ann Pharmacother* 1994, **28**, 67–71). Doses may also be adjusted in a more refined, symptom-triggered way, with adequate monitoring of symptoms, in patients with particular needs (Saitz *et al, JAMA* 1994, **272**, 519–23 plus editorial 557–58; see also symptom-triggered out-patient detoxification with variable dose chlordiazepoxide, n=108, Wiseman *et al, J Clin Psych* 1998, **59**, 289–93). Withdrawal symptoms may be underestimated and hence under- treated. Beware of an extended metabolism in liver damage (see *3.6*) and of respiratory depression.

Reviews*: chlordiazepoxide withdrawal regimens (Chick, *Adv Psych Treat* 1996, **2**, 249–57), chlordiazepoxide *vs* clomethiazole (Duncan and Taylor, *Psych Bull* 1996, **20**, 601–3), general (Peppers, *Pharmacotherapy* 1996, **16**, 49–58).

Clomethiazole (chlormethiazole)

Regarded as safe and effective treatment of AWS at up to 16 capsules/d, reducing over 5 to 9 days, it has a low addictive potential (Schied *et al, Acta Psych Scand* 1986, **73**[Suppl 329], 136–39) but dependence (mainly psychological) can be seen in some patients on longer-term therapy (*BMJ* 1987, **294**, 592). The dangers of toxicity may have been exaggerated.

Reviews *: clomethiazole home detoxification schedules and counter to the argument that clomethiazole is highly toxic (Sowerby and Hunter, *J Substance Misuse* 1997, **2**, 62–63, 114–17), general (Duncan and Taylor, *Psych Bull* 1996, **20**, 601–3; Morgan, *Alcohol Alcohol* 1995, **30**, 771–74).

Vitamin B supplementation

B vitamins act as co-enzymes for essential carbohydrate metabolism. Deficiency of nicotinamide, riboflavine (B_2) and pyridoxine (B_6) can cause neuropathies. Thiamine (B_1) must be primary and priority treatment to reverse the mental confusion secondary to thiamine deficency (Wernicke's Encephalopathy) (*Lancet* 1990, **ii**, 912–13). A reasonable strategy on the

use of Pabrinex (IV, HP), is 2 ampoule pairs tds for 2 days, then 1 pair daily until oral thiamine can be tolerated (Chataway and Hardman *Postgrad Med J* 1995, **71**, 249). Be aware that oral thiamine has a saturable absorption mechanism which allows only about 5–10mg/d to be absorbed. It may be necessary to administer glucose *after* thiamine when administering thiamine to prevent Wernicke Encephalopathy (Chataway and Hardman, *Postgrad Med J* 1995, **71**, 249–53).

● **Unlicensed/Some efficacy**

Alcohol IV

IV alcohol can be used if aggressive therapy is needed (*Drug Intell Clin Pharm* 1990, **24**, 1120–22; Janda *et al, DICP Ann Pharmacother* 1990, **24**, 545).

Carbamazepine

An effective and useful treatment, carbamazepine is probably active via an anti-kindling effect. It is non-addictive and its metabolism is generally little affected by liver dysfunction but may be inhibited by higher doses of alcohol. Higher blood levels would thus occur in the same person than if abstinent, so beware of enhanced side-effects (Sternebring *et al, Eur J Clin Pharmacol* 1992, **43**, 393–97). It can be useful also for outpatient detoxifications due to its safety and lack of abuse potential (*Am J Psych* 1991, **158**, 133).

○ **Unlicensed/Possible efficacy**

Antipsychotics

Decreased dopamine activity may occur in DT (*Postgrad Med J* 1990, **66**, 1005–9) so care is needed with anti-dopaminergic drugs, as this may aggravate symptoms and lower the seizure threshold. NMS may also occur and not be recognised (*Acta Psych Scand* 1986, **73**[Suppl 329], 120–23). Temperature regulation and liver function pose further difficulties (*Postgrad Med J* 1990, **66**, 1005–9).

Beta-blockers

Beta-blockers such as atenolol (Kraus *et al, NEJM* 1985, **313**, 905–9) and propranolol may be useful in treating some symptoms of mild to moderate AWS, eg. tachycardia and tremor, as adjuncts (*Pharmacotherapy* 1989, **9**, 131–43) and to reduce craving (*Arch Int Med* 1989, **149**, 1089–93) but are not recommended by all (*Drug Intell Clin Pharm* 1991, **25**, 31–32). The variable kinetics of propranolol in cirrhosis and portal hypertension must be considered (Cales *et al, B J Clin Pharmacol* 1989, **27**, 763–70; comparison with diazepam, Worner, *Am J Drug Alcohol Abuse* 1994, **20**, 115–24).

Buprenorphine
Once daily and alternate daily dosing has been used to treat abrupt withdrawal (Fudala *et al, Clin Pharmacol & Ther* 1990, **47**, 525–34).

Clonidine
Clonidine may help to alleviate tremor, tachycardia and hypertension in AWS but not reduce the incidence of fits or DT (*J Stud Alcohol* 1987, **48**, 356–70).

Dexamethasone
4–7 injections of 4mg were shown to be fully effective in reducing symptoms (n=110, *Arch Int Med* 1991, **114**, 705–6) and 3mg 12hrly was successful in a single case (Fischer, *Lancet* 1988, **i**, 1340–41).

Flumazenil
Flumazenil (0.5mg IV 6 hourly for 48 hours) was shown to be superior to placebo in reducing symptoms of acute alcohol withdrawal (n=20, RCT, s/b, Gerra *et al, Curr Ther Res* 1991, **50**, 62–66), but an earlier study found no effect (Adinoff *et al, Biol Psych* 1986, **21**, 643–49).

Gabapentin *
A gabapentin reduction regimen has been used in out-patient detoxifications, with minimal abuse potential and lack of cognitive impairment (n=6, 5/7, Myrick *et al, Am J Psych* 1998, **155**, 1632) and as add-on to clomethiazole (n=4, Bonnet *et al, Pharmacopsychiatry* 1999, **32**, 107–9).

Hydroxyzine
100mg IM every six hours has been shown to reduce alcohol withdrawal effects but is less effective than the benzodiazepines (eg. clorazepate, Dilts *et al, Am J Psych* 1977, **134**, 92).

Lithium
One study showed lithium may decrease withdrawal symptoms, 300mg tds for 6–9 days (n=12, Sellers *et al, Clin Pharmacol Ther* 1976, **19**, 199) although it would obviously have no effect on seizure prevention.

Lofexidine
Several studies have shown lofexidine (eg. 0.4mg qds for 2–3 days) to be superior to placebo in controlling withdrawal symptoms (n=63, Cushman *et al, Alcoholism: Clin and Experimental Res* 1985, **9**, 103–8; n=23, Cushman and Sowers, *Alcohol: Clin Exp Res* 1989, **13**, 361–64; n=28, Brunning *et al, Alcohol Alcohol* 1986, **21**, 167–70).

Magnesium sulphate
Magnesium deficiency is known to occur in DT but one review does not recommend routine use (*Ann Pharmacother* 1992, **26**, 650–52).

Nitrous oxide (analgesic)
Analgesic nitrous oxide showed a rapid and effective relief of AWS symptoms in a controlled study (n=104, *B J Psych* 1991, **159**, 672–75).

Phenobarbital (phenobarbitone) *
Phenobarbital is an anticonvulsant and may help reduce withdrawal tremors (*NEJM* 1988, **319**, 715–16; see also Rodgers and Crouch, *Am J Health-Sys Pharm* 1999, **56**, 175–78).

Phenytoin
300mg/d may be useful as a prophylactic anticonvulsant in patients with pre-existing epilepsy but does not prevent other withdrawal symptoms (*NEJM* 1988, **319**, 715–16).

Propofol *
Benzodiazepine treatment-refractory AWS has been successfully treated with propofol infusion (n=4, McCowan and Marik, *Critical Care Med* 2000, **28**, 1781–84).

▼ No efficacy

Fluvoxamine
A trial of fluvoxamine in alcoholic Korsakoff syndrome showed no therapeutic role and included 2 apparently fluvoxamine-induced episodes of depression (n=8, O'Carroll *et al, Psychopharmacol* 1994, **116**, 85–88).

ALZHEIMER'S DISEASE
See Dementia (*1.13*).

ANOREXIA and BULIMIA NERVOSA
See Eating disorders (*1.16*).

1.6 ANXIETY DISORDER (generalised)

Generalised Anxiety Disorder (GAD) includes also panic disorder (*1.24*) with or without agoraphobia (*1.3*), OCD (*1.23*), social phobia (*1.32*), PTSD (*1.25*).

Symptoms:

There are numerous symptoms of generalised anxiety disorder (although anxiety can in itself be a symptom of many conditions) but can be classified into two main groups:
Psychological symptoms include fearful anticipation, irritability, poor concentration, restlessness, sensitivity to noise, disturbed sleep (lying awake worrying, waking intermittently, unpleasant dreams, but not usually early morning waking) and poor memory (due to poor concentration).
Physical symptoms are mainly due to overactivity of the sympathetic system or increased muscle tension, eg. gastrointestinal (dry mouth, difficulty swallowing, wind, loose motions etc), CNS (tinnitus, blurred vision, dizziness), respiratory (constricted chest, difficulty inhaling, overbreathing), cardiovascular (palpitations, heart pain, missed beats, neck throbbing), genitourinary (increased micturition, lack of libido and impotence), muscular tension (tension headache, tremor) and panic attacks (sudden episodes of extreme anxiety or apprehension).

Anxiety must be differentiated from depression, early schizophrenia, dementia, drugs/alcohol abuse including withdrawal and physical illness.

Role of drugs:

Anxiolytics used as a 'first-aid' measure are quite rational but it is difficult to assess the longer-term effectiveness of these drugs as anxiety tends to vary for reasons other than drug treatment. The decision for longer-term treatment must be considered on an individual basis, with the risk:benefit analysis varying with the disability caused by the symptoms, age of the person etc. Psychological interventions include explanations, reassurance, support and, in more persistent conditions, cognitive and behavioural therapy (Hoehn-Saric, *CNS Drugs* 1998, **9**, 85–98).

Reviews *: general (Roerig, *J Am Pharm Ass* 1999, **39**, 811–21; Hallström, *Hosp Med* 2000, **61**, 8–9; Feeney and Nutt, *Prescriber* 1999, **10**, 69–85; Bell and Wilson, *Prescriber* 2000, **11**, 46–48; Argyropoulos and Nutt, *Eur Neuropsychopharmacol* 1999, **9**[Suppl 6], S407–S412), optimum use (Tyrer, *Adv Psych Treat* 1997, **3**, 72–78), practical advice on diagnosis and treatment (Nutt and Bell, *Adv Psych Treat* 1997, **3**, 79–85), anxiety in the elderly (Krasucki, *Prescriber* 1998, **9**, 21–31), GAD and treatment options (*Drugs & Ther Perspect* 1998, **12**, 10–14).

BNF Listed

Benzodiazepines *

Benzodiazepines may be extremely useful for chronic anxiety and should not be overlooked (rational defence of BDZ prescribing, Williams and McBride, *B J Psych* 1998, **173**, 361–62). Use of benzodiazepines can be restricted to short-term (up to 4-weeks) or intermittent courses, as prior benzodiazepine exposure does not predispose patients to more severe discontinuation symptoms in subsequent courses (review, Rickels and Freeman, *J Clin Psych* 2000, **61**, 409–13).

Chronic users of benzodiazepines who seek help in reducing or discontinuing tend to have important previous and current psychiatric problems. They are usually taking relatively low doses but should not necessarily be considered as being 'addicted' or 'dependent' as a large proportion may be taking the drug appropriately for a chronic psychiatric condition (n=34, Romach *et al, Am J Psych* 1995, **152**, 1161–67).

Although the benzodiazepines have a relative lack of toxicity in overdose, there is some difference between different drugs, eg. temazepam (with rapid absorption and high sedative effect) and possibly flurazepam have a greater toxicity in overdose than other benzodiazepines, eg. diazepam, clonazepam, nitrazepam and oxazepam (303 overdose study by Buckley *et al, BMJ* 1995, **310**, 219–21). All are capable of being fatal in overdose (especially combined with alcohol) and should not be prescribed for patients at high risk of overdose. Users of benzodiazepines are also at greater risk of road-traffic accidents, especially if combined with alcohol (involved in accidents, n=19,386 over 3 years, Barbone *et al, Lancet* 1998, **352**, 1331–36).

Reviews*: avoidance of dependence (Marriot and Tyrer, *Drug Safety* 1993, **9**, 93–103), extensive review of the use of benzodiazepines (Shader and Greenblatt (*NEJM* 1993, **328**, 1398–405), guidelines for the clinical use of benzodiazepines (Nelson and Chouinard, *Can J Clin Pharmacol* 1999, **6**, 69–83), advantages and disadvantages, mode of action (Argyropoulos and Nutt, *Eur Neuropsychopharmacol* 1999, **9**[Suppl 6], S407–S412; Lader, *Eur Neuropsychopharmacol* 1999, **9**[Suppl 6], S399–405), CSM warning about driving (*Curr Prob Pharmacovig* 1999, **25**, 17).

Alprazolam

A black-listed benzodiazepine once claimed to have some antidepressant activity, probably due to inadequate trial design (*JAMA* 1983, **251**, 215; review by Greenblatt and Wright, *Clin Pharmacokinetics* 1993, **24**, 453–71).

Bromazepam

UK black-listed benzodiazepine.

Chlordiazepoxide

Chlordiazepoxide has a slower onset of action and many active metabolites.

Clobazam

See entry under epilepsy (*1.17.1*).

Clorazepate (dipotassium clorazepate)

Black-listed pro-drug to desmethyl-diazepam, there is little to distinguish it from other benzodiazepines.

Diazepam

Diazepam is the standard longer-acting benzodiazepine, with sedative, anxiolytic and muscle relaxant properties (amongst others). It has a long half-life and many active metabolites.

Benzodiazepines are indicated for short-term relief of severe anxiety. Other treatment methods should then be started, eg. relaxation, psychotherapy, treating any underlying depression etc. The BNF (*Sec 4.1.2*) sets out cautious advice for the use of benzodiazepines, eg. for short-term use, not used in depression or personality disorder etc.

Lorazepam

A shorter-acting benzodiazepine with potent receptor-binding properties. Dependence seems to have been a particular problem with this drug and it has received a bad press because of this.

Oxazepam

A shorter-acting benzodiazepine, the ultimate metabolite of diazepam and some other benzodiazepines and with no active metabolites.

Others

Beta-blockers

Propranolol, oxprenolol etc at 20–60mg/d may be useful for somatic anxiety symptoms such as tachycardia, sweating, tremor etc and for short-term problems. Studies have shown propranolol less effective than diazepam (n=26, d/b, p/c, c/o, Hallström *et al, B J Psych* 1981, **139**, 417–21) and more effective than placebo (n=57, p/c, Hudson, *B J Clin Pract* 1988, **42**, 419–26). 80–120mg/d may be too high a dose in many patients and can lead to cardiac symptoms. The best response appears to be in doses sufficient to reduce resting pulse by 7bpm (Hallström *et al, B J Psych* 1981, **139**, 417–21) and in patients presenting with autonomic complaints, eg. palpitations, shortness of breath, sweating, rapid ventilation etc.

Buspirone *

Buspirone is a non-benzodiazepine anxiolytic with negligible sedative, hypnotic, anticonvulsant and muscle relaxant properties. In general, it is considered as effective as the benzodiazepines in GAD, with a lower incidence of dependence, a better side-effect profile and less memory and cognitive impairment (Pecknold, *Drug Safety* 1997, **16**, 118–32), although it has been noted that the efficacy studies were not performed in patients diagnosed with GAD using current criteria (review, Roerig, *J Am Pharm Ass* 1999, **39**, 811–21). It has a slow onset of action and is as effective as benzodiazepines at four weeks (*J Clin Psych* 1982, **43**, 103–7), but may need four weeks at 30mg/d to start working optimally. Buspirone possibly acts on 5-HT$_{1A}$ receptors and has no effect on withdrawal in benzodiazepine-dependent persons (*J Clin Psychopharmacol,* 1987, **43**,

34–37). Indeed, patients with GAD who have recently discontinued BDZs may suffer more ADRs and respond slower to buspirone than those who have neither had BDZs or discontinued more than a month before (n=735, DeMartinis *et al*, *J Clin Psych* 2000, **61**, 91–94). It has a low 'peak' effect and so the abuse potential is low and abrupt withdrawal has not been shown to produce withdrawal symptoms (*Arch Gen Psych* 1988, **45**, 444–50).
Reviews*: general (Pecknold, *Drug Safety* 1997, **16**, 118–32, 241 refs; Apter and Allen, *J Clin Psychopharmacol* 1999, **19**, 86–93), clinical pharmacology and therapeutic applications (Fulton and Brogden, *CNS Drugs* 1997, **7**, 68–88), pharmacokinetics (Mahmood and Sahajwalla, *Clin Pharmacokinet* 1999, **36**, 277–87, 48 refs).

Hydroxyzine

A poorly studied antihistamine related to the phenothiazines which may be mildly useful in some cases.

● **Unlicensed/Some efficacy**

Antipsychotics *

All have low efficacy and marked side-effects. Loxapine, haloperidol (superior to diazepam, s/b, n=60, Budden, *Curr Med Res Opin* 1979, **5**, 759–65), flupentixol and chlorpromazine have been used. Thioridazine was formerly widely used but is now only licensed for schizophrenia. The use of PRN antipsychotics makes assessment of the underlying causes of agitation more difficult. Such doses should be used carefully and only for infrequent, sustained agitation (Druckenbrod *et al*, *Ann Pharmacother* 1993, **27**, 645–48).

Mirtazapine

Mirtazapine (15–45mg/d) has been shown to be effective within a week for the symptoms of GAD with comorbid depression (open, n=10, 8/52, Goodnick *et al*, *J Clin Psych* 1999, **60**, 446–48). 15mg/d may be as effective as diazepam 10mg/d in reducing insomnia and anxiety when given the night before surgery (Sorensen *et al*, *Acta Psych Scand* 1985, **71**, 339–46; see also an outpatient study (n=40, d/b, p/c, Sitsen and Moors, *Drug Invest* 1994, **8**, 339–44). More data is awaited on this potentially useful action.

SSRIs

SSRIs may have some efficacy in anxiety. Lower doses may be needed initially, as drugs such as fluoxetine, may increase symptoms over the first 1–2 weeks of treatment. Up to 300mg/d of fluvoxamine may be equipotent with lorazepam in mixed anxiety and depression (Laws *et al*, *Acta Psych Scand* 1990, **81**, 185–89). The UK SPCs for paroxetine and fluoxetine include depression with anxiety, and one study suggested paroxetine may be effective for GAD (Rocca *et al*, *Acta Psych Scand* 1997, **95**, 444–50).

Trazodone

Trazodone has been claimed to be equipotent with some benzodiazepines, eg. a trial showed trazodone to be at least as effective as diazepam and imipramine in generalised anxiety, although the antidepressants had more side-effects (n=230, d/b, p/c, 8/52, Rickels *et al*, *Arch Gen Psych* 1993, **50**, 884–95).

Tricyclic antidepressants

Tricyclics may be useful for persistent or disabling anxiety not part of an adjustment/stress reaction. They may take several weeks to act but may be very potent (*Arch Gen Psych* 1986, **43**, 79–85). A trial showed imipramine to be at least as effective as diazepam and trazodone in generalised anxiety, although the antidepressants had more side-effects such as akathisia (n=230, d/b, p/c, 8/52, Rickels *et al*, *Arch Gen Psych* 1993, **50**, 884–95).

Venlafaxine *

Licensed in the US for anxiety, venlafaxine is effective for depression with anxiety (compared with fluoxetine, n=359, RCT, Silverstone and Ravindran, *J Clin Psych* 1999, **60**, 22–28; case series, n=11, Johnson *et al, J Clin Psychopharmacol* 1998, **18**, 419). Venlafaxine up to 225mg/day was superior to placebo in non-depressed outpatients with generalized anxiety disorder (n=251, RCT, 6/52, Gelenberg *et al, JAMA* 2000, **283**, 3082–88), and the XL formulation once-daily was effective and well-tolerated in the short-term for GAD in non-depressed out-patients (n=377, RCT, 8/52, Rickels *et al, Am J Psych* 2000, **157**, 968–74; see also

Feighner *et al*, *J Aff Dis* 1998, **47**, 55–52). A Wyeth meta-analysis of venlafaxine for depression and anxiety indicated that venlafaxine is more effective than placebo (6 short-term trials, Rudolph *et al*, *J Clin Psychopharmacol* 1998, **18**, 136–44; see also Sheehan, *J Clin Psych* 1999, **60**[Suppl 22], 23–28).

○ **Unlicensed/Possible efficacy**

Amylobarbital/amobarbital

45–120mg/d has been used for short-term, treatment-resistant acute anxiety states where other, safer, drugs are insufficient.

Gabapentin

In patients with a history of alcohol dependency or abuse, gabapentin 100–900mg/d may produce sustained clinical improvement in symptoms of anxiety (n=4, Pollack *et al*, *Am J Psych* 1998, **155**, 992–93).

Haloperidol

Severe agitation in critically ill people has been treated successfully with IV haloperidol (Fraser and Riker, *Hosp Pharm* 1994, **29**, 689–91, 695).

Mianserin

Mianserin may be equipotent with chlordiazepoxide in anxiety (n=106, d/b, 6/52, Bjertnaes *et al*, *Acta Psych Scand* 1982, **66**, 199–207) and against diazepam (Murphy, *B J Clin Pharmacol* 1978, **5**, 81S–85S).

Nabilone *

Two studies have shown 1–8mg/d nabilone to significantly improved anxiety (n=5, open, Fabre *et al*, *Curr Ther Res* 1978, **24**, 161–69; n=8, RCT, Glass *et al*, *J Clin Pharmacol* 1981, **21**[Suppl 8–9], 383S–96S).

Valproate

There has been some speculation that valproate may have anxiolytic actions (*Am J Psych* 1990, **147**, 950–51) via an effect of enhancing GABA.

St. John's wort

A short study showed hypericum plus valerian to be as effective as diazepam in anxiety (n=100, d/b, 2/52, Panijel, *Therapiewoche* 1985, **41**, 4659–68).

▼ **No efficacy**

Caffeine *

Caffeine consumption should be calculated (see caffeinism *1.35*) in anxiety as higher intakes can cause nervousness, anxiety, restlessness, irritability, palpitations etc, probably by an abnormal sensitivity to caffeine (*Arch Gen Psych* 1992, **49**, 867–69) via antagonism of adenosine receptors (*Arch Gen Psych* 1985, **42**, 233–43). One study, however, of chronic schizophrenic in-patients showed no change in anxiety when caffeine was removed from the diet (n=26, Mayo *et al*, *B J Psych* 1993, **162**, 543–45).

Review: anxiogenic effects of caffeine (Bruce, *Postgrad Med J* 1990, **66**[Suppl 2], S18–24).

Ondansetron *

One study showed 4mg/d to be no better than placebo, although placebo response rates were high (n=97, RCT, Romach *et al*, *J Clin Psychopharmacol* 1998, **18**, 121–31).

1.7 ATTENTION DEFICIT HYPERACTIVITY DISORDER (ADHD) — including hyperkinetic disorder

Symptoms: *

Attention deficit disorder has 'hyperactivity' (ADHD) as a subclassification. ADHD is characterised by a developmentally inappropriate degree of gross motor activity, impulsivity, inattention and temper outbursts. Children with ADHD have extreme and persistent restlessness, sustained and prolonged motor activity and difficulty in maintaining attention. They are impulsive, reckless, prone to accidents, have learning difficulties (partly due to poor concentration) and often have antisocial behaviour and a fluctuating mood. Onset is before 7 years of age. Symptoms usually fade out by puberty but learning disability and antisocial behaviour may persist into adult life and may, but not always, lead to poor achievement (views on ADHD in *JAMA* 1992, **268**, 1004–7; *JAMA* 1993, **269**, 2368). A variety of transmitter dysfunctions have been proposed, eg. 5-HT, GABA etc. D4 receptor gene and dopamine transporter abnormalities have been implicated, so dopaminergic drugs may be useful (Spencer *et al*, *J Am Acad Chil Adolesc Psych* 1996, **35**, 409–32).

Role of drugs: *

Drugs are useful for the treatment of

severe hyperkinesis or in those resistant to non-drug measures. Drug therapy may be a useful adjunct to other therapies, as 73–94% may respond to stimulants and 68–83% to tricyclics. A recent robust study of medication and/or behavioural therapy in children (7–10yrs) with ADHD indicated strongly that careful medication management was effective in reducing core ADHD symptoms, superior to behavioural therapy and with some limited evidence that the combination was more effective than either alone on some indirect outcome measures (n=579, NTA-CG, *Arch Gen Psych* 2000, **56**, 1073–86; review by Sawyer and Graetz, *EBMH* 2000, **3**, 82). A review of 25 studies of the pharmacotherapy of ADHD in adults concluded that stimulants are the most effective agents, and these drugs remain the treatment of choice (Wilens *et al, CNS Drugs* 1998, **9**, 347–56). Lack of response to one stimulant does not necessarily predict lack of response to a different one (eg. Elia *et al, Psychiatry Res* 1991, **36**, 141–55). There is a natural reluctance by many prescribers to use stimulants in younger children and so mild symptoms should be treated with environmental changes. Moderate to severe symptoms may require drug therapy. Dietary restrictions have been reported to help a small number of children (*Ann Pharmacother* 1992, **26**, 565–66) but additive-free diets (eg. the Feingold diet) have not been shown to be effective.

Reviews*: extensive overviews (meta-analysis, Klassen *et al, Can J Psych* 1999, **44**, 1007–16; various, *J Clin Psych* 1998 [Suppl 7], 3–79), general (Williams *et al, B J Gen Pract* 1999, **49**, 563–71, 167 refs; McNicholas and Gringras, *Prescriber* 2000, **5**, 19–29), basic bibliography (Anderson, *Hosp Pharm* 1997, **32**, 273, 20 refs), ADHD in adults (Toone and van der Linden, *B J Psych* 1997, **170**, 489–91, 25 refs), treatment strategies (Hill, *Arch Dis Childhood* 1998, **79**, 381–84; editorial, Elia *et al, NEJM* 1999, **340**, 780–88, 84 refs), problems in the management of ADHD (Zametkin and Ernst, *NEJM* 1999, **340**, 40–47, 39 refs). **NB**. Drug trials need to be interpreted carefully as different diagnostic criteria have been used in different studies.

BNF listed
Dexamfetamine (dexamphetamine) *
Amfetamine is clearly superior to placebo on a variety of key measures, remaining effective over the 15 months in one trial (n=62, RCT, Gillberg *et al, Arch Gen Psych* 1997, **54**, 857–64; reviewed by Hall, *EBMH* 1998, **1**, 86). Children with ADHD and chronic tic disorder who had received methylphenidate or dexamfetamine for at least 1 year showed no evidence of tic exacerbation while receiving medication or after placebo substitution (n=19, d/b, p/c, Nolan *et al, Pediatrics* 1999, **103**, 730–37). A trial of dexamfetamine in adults with ADHD showed a significant effect in the short-term, with more data needed to justify long-term therapy (n=68, RCT, Paterson *et al, Aus NZ J Psych* 1999, **33**, 494–502).

Methylphenidate *
At appropriate doses of methylphenidate (10–80mg/d), a large proportion of children with ADHD obtain remission of symptoms (Klein and Wender, *Arch Gen Psych* 1995, **52**, 429–33). It can also be useful in adults (Spencer *et al, Arch Gen Psych* 1995, **52**, 434–43). Predictors of a positive response include younger age, demonstrable inattention, normal or near normal IQ and low anxiety (Buitelaar *et al, J Am Acad Child Adolesc Psych* 1995, **34**, 1025–32). Methylphenidate was highly effective in boys with ADHD, with high levels of hyperactivity at school and relatively low age being reasonable predictors of response (n=36, RCT, Zeiner *et al, Acta Paediatr* 1999, **88**, 298–303). An additional 10mg dose at 4pm may markedly improve late afternoon/evening behaviour without delaying sleep onset or reducing sleep quality (n=12, Kent *et al, Pediatrics* 1995, **96**, 320–25). Use only on school days has been suggested (Cameron and Hill, *Adv Psych Treat* 1996, **2**, 94–102). The response to methylphenidate in ADHD does not appear to be moderated by co-morbid anxiety (n=91, RCT, 4/12, Diamond *et al, J Am Acad Chold Adolesc Psych* 1999, **38**, 402–9; reviewed in *EBMH* 1999, **2**, 108). Although some tics are significantly worse with methylphenidate, this is generally not to the

extent of contraindicating a trial (Gadow *et al, Arch Gen Psych* 1995, **52**, 444–55) and another study showed that in children with ADHD, normal doses of methylphenidate did not cause nor exacerbate tics (n=91, p/c, d/b, Law and Schachar, *J Am Acad Child Adolesc Psych* 1999, **38**, 944–51; reviewed in *EBMH* 2000, **3**, 31). Methylphenidate's mode of action may be blockade of central dopamine transporters (Volkow *et al, Am J Psych* 1998, **155**, 1325–31). **Review***: pharmacokinetics and efficacy (Kimko *et al, Clin Pharmacokinet* 1999, **37**, 457–70, 75 refs).

Pemoline *
In the UK, pemoline is available on a named-patient basis only due to serious hepatic toxicity (*Curr Prob* 1997, **23**, 10; Wilens *et al, J Clin Psychopharmacol* 1999, **19**, 257–64).

● **Unlicensed/Some efficacy**

Bupropion *
Bupropion (mean 3.3mg/kg/d) and methylphenidate (mean 0.7mg/kg/d) were equipotent in children with ADHD in one trial (RCT, n=15, 6/52, Barrickman *et al, J Am Acad Child Adolesc Psych* 1995, **34**, 649–57), and in adolescents with substance misuse disorders (n=13, open, 5/52, Riggs *et al, J Am Acad Child Adolesc Psych* 1998, **37**, 1271–78) and thus provides a pharmacological alternative to stimulants in ADHD (review, Popper, *Child Adolesc Psychiatr Clin N Am* 2000, **9**, 605–46).

Clonidine *
Clonidine is widely used for ADHD. In a trial of clonidine (up to 0.2mg/d) and desipramine (up to 100mg/d) in children with both ADHD and Tourette's syndrome, desipramine was superior to clonidine in reducing ADHD and tic symptoms (d/b, p/c, c/o, Singer *et al, Pediatrics* 1995, **95**, 74–81). Other limited studies have shown clonidine (orally or as a patch, which is usually better tolerated) as a viable alternative to stimulants but without stimulant side-effects (full review in *Ann Pharmacother* 1992, **26**, 37–39). Overall, most studies are small and a large RCT is needed to identify its role (review, Chafin *et al, J Ped Pharm Pract* 1999, **4**, 308–15, 32 refs). A thorough meta-analysis of 11 studies indicated that clonidine 0.1–0.3mg/d has a moderate effect in reducing core ADHD symptoms (better in those without comorbid disorders), which is less than with stimulants, and associated with many side-effects. Parents' efficacy ratings correlated negatively with sedation caused by clonidine (n=150, Connor *et al, J Am Acad Child Adolesc Psych* 1999, **38**, 1551–59; reviewed by Greenhill, *EBMH* 2000, **3**, 74).

MAOIs
MAOIs are not considered generally as effective as stimulants but may help some non-responders (*Clin Pharm* 1990, **9**, 632–42), eg. tranylcypromine has been considered as effective as stimulants but the dietary restrictions proved too difficult to manage (*Arch Gen Psych* 1985, **42**, 962–66).

Tricyclics
Tricyclics are considered useful in patients non-responsive or intolerant of stimulants. Imipramine, clomipramine, nortriptyline and desipramine have been used, in doses of 10–150mg/d (mean 80mg). In a retrospective, naturalistic study, tricyclics were shown to be effective at antidepressant doses (n=37, Wilens *et al, J Nerv Ment Dis* 1995, **183**, 48–49), although other authors have suggested that lower doses (eg. 25–50mg/d) are effective (Ratey *et al, J Child Adolesc Psychopharmacol* 1992, **2**, 267–75). They produce drowsiness, sadness and irritability, but are less likely to cause insomnia than stimulants (*Med Lett Drugs Ther* 1990, **32**, 53). Sudden death, including cardiac arrest, has been reported with relatively low plasma levels (*J Am Acad Child Adolesc Psych* 1991, **30**, 104–8) and so close monitoring is warranted.

○ **Unlicensed/Possible efficacy**

Antipsychotics
Some antipsychotics have been used for uncontrollable and explosive behaviour but their side-effect profile makes them unsatisfactory and potentially dangerous. This potential for long-term side-effects and worsening cognitive learning function usually outweigh their potential advantages. Some ADHD patients were included in a study by

Hardan *et al* (*J Am Acad Child Adolesc Psych* 1996, **35**, 1551–56) on the use of risperidone.

Fluoxetine

Serotonin function may be abnormal in ADHD (Fargason and Ford, *South Med J* 1994, **87**, 302–9) and fluoxetine 20–60mg/d may produce some statistical improvements in some rating scales (n=22, open, Barrickman *et al, J Am Acad Child Adolesc Psych* 1991, **30**, 762–67).

Gabapentin

Aggression, temper and violence responded almost completely ('a miracle') to gabapentin 900mg/d in a 15-year-old boy with ADHD (among other diagnoses) resistant to other therapies (n=1, Ryback and Ryback, *Am J Psych* 1995, **152**, 1399).

Levodopa/carbidopa

The combination has been shown to be superior to placebo but not stimulants (*Pediatr Ann* 1985, **14**, 383–400).

Thyroid

Generalised resistance to thyroid hormone occurred in one patient with ADHD, suggesting thyroid replacement may help (*NEJM* 1993, **328**, 997–1001) but this has caused some controversy (*NEJM* 1993, **329**, 966–67).

Venlafaxine

There has been a trial (n=10, open, Findling *et al, J Clin Psych* 1996, **57**, 184-89) and case reports (Peak and Gormly, Willens *et al, Am J Psych* 1995, **152**, 1099–100) of response to 56.25–300mg/d.

▼ No efficacy

Barbiturates

These have been tried but excitation and agitation may result in a negative effect.

Benzodiazepines

As for barbiturates.

Caffeine

Caffeine has not proven effective as a minor stimulant (Dulcan, *Pediatr Ann* 1985, **14**, 383–400).

1.8 AUTISTIC DISORDER

Symptoms: *

Autism is a neurodevelopmental disorder, characterised by an excessive or morbid dislike of others or society, not respond-ing with normal human emotions towards other people, a morbid self-centred attitude and with major impairments or abnormalities in language, communication, social interactions, imagination and behaviour. The main features include 'autistic aloneness', poor speech and language disorder development, an obsessive desire for sameness, bizarre behaviour or mannerisms, a restricted repertoire of activities and interests, rituals and compulsive behaviour. Onset is not later than 3 years of age, the incidence 4 in 10,000, or up to 20 in 10,000 if including associated conditions (Gillberg and Wing, *Acta Psych Scand* 1999, **99**, 399–406). Up to 25% develop seizures in adolescence and 75% have an IQ in the retarded range. 60+% need long-term residential care. Links with gluten allergy are emerging.

Role of drugs:

Drugs may be of limited use in treating some of the more severe behavioural symptoms. SIB is common (see *1.30*) and may be helped by low dose antipsychotics; autistic individuals seem to be very sensitive to antipsychotics and so lower doses may be needed and a therapeutic window may exist with higher doses counter-productive. Family support, education, skills training, behavioural therapy and social support can be significant aspects of the overall managment.

Reviews*: general (*Drugs & Therapy Perspectives* 1998, **12**, 5–8), drug therapy (Harteveld and Buitelaar, *CNS Drugs* 1997, **8**, 227–36, 67 refs; King, *J Autism Dev Disord* 2000, **30**, 439–45), ADHD in autism (Aman and Langworthy, *J Autism Dev Disord* 2000, **30**, 451–59).

● Unlicensed/Some efficacy

Haloperidol

There is a good body of evidence supporting the use of this drug. 0.5–3mg/d in 40 autistic children (2–7 years old) reduced behavioural symptoms (eg. aggression and SIB) and improved learning, with excessive sedation, irritability and dystonic reactions noted. It may be effective over six months, even if non-continuous therapy is used (n=60, Perry *et al, J Am Acad Child Adoles Psych* 1989, **28**,

87–92) and was considered powerfully effective in one controlled study (n=45, p/c, d/b, Anderson *et al, J Autism Dev Dis* 1989, **19**, 227–39). The Perry paper is the only study of long-term efficacy. As adverse reactions can be significant, a 'start low and go slow' routine is recommended.

○ Unlicensed/Possible efficacy

Antidepressants *

Serotonin reuptake inhibitors may have a role to play, particularly in adults with strong behavioural rigidity. Children and adolescents may be more sensitive to SSRIs and so once again 'start low and go slow' is the advice. One trial showed clomipramine to be superior to placebo and desipramine in autistic symptoms, anger and ritualism (n=12, d/b, c/o, 10/52, *Arch Gen Psych* 1993, **50**, 441–47). In a second study in autism and severe mental retardation, clomipramine reduced compulsions and adventitious movements (n=5, open, Brasic *et al, Neurology* 1994, **44**, 1309–12). Fluvoxamine has been shown superior to placebo (n=30, 12/52, d/b, p/c, McDougle *et al, Arch Gen Psych* 1996, **53**, 1001–8). There are two cases of dramatic response of OCD-like behavioural symptoms in autistic adults to fluoxetine 20mg/d (Koshes, *Am J Psych* 1997, **154**, 578).

Antipsychotics, other * (see also haloperidol)

As haloperidol has significant side-effects, other antipsychotics are usually preferred and can also be used for the treatment of the marked tension and agitation which often occurs in autism (mentioned in *B J Hosp Med* 1990, **43**, 448–52), particularly in low dose. **Risperidone** may be particularly useful in view of its low EPS profile. Two open trials have shown a rapid and significant improvement in explosive aggressive autism (n=11, Horrigan and Barnhill, *J Autism Dev Disorder* 1997, **27**, 313–23), some improvement in severe behavioural symptoms in young autistics (12/52, open, n=10, Nicolson *et al, J Am Acad Adolesc Psychiatry* 1998, **37**, 372–76) and was more effective than placebo in a 12-week trial (n=31, d/b, p/c, McDougle *et al, Arch Gen Psych* 1998, **55**,

633–41). In an open trial in three autistic children (8–12 years old), **clozapine** markedly improved SIB, hyperactivity and aggressiveness, with two remaining on the drug long-term (Zuddas *et al, Am J Psych* 1996, **153**, 738).

Buspirone

Small open studies suggest some effect from reduced anxiety (eg. n=14, open, Ratey *et al, J Clin Psych* 1989, **50**, 382–84) and two of four autistic children responded given buspirone 15mg/d (n=4, Realmuto *et al, J Clin Psychopharmacol* 1989, **9**, 122–25).

Carbamazepine

There are some reports of a useful effect (eg. Gillberg, *J Autism Dev Disord* 1991, **21**, 61–77).

Clonidine

Two controlled studies have indicated a modest effect on reduced hyperactivity, impulsivity and irritability (n=9, d/b, p/c, Fankhauser *et al, J Clin Psych* 1992, **53**, 77–82; n=8, p/c, d/b, c/o, Jaselskis *et al, J Clin Psychopharmacol* 1992, **12**, 322–27) but many seem to develop tolerance and adverse effects can be significant.

Lithium

Use of lithium when a cyclical pattern of symptom exacerbation is noted has been tried (eg. n=2, Kerbeshian *et al, J Clin Psychopharmacol* 1987, **7**, 401–5).

Methylphenidate *

The considerable negative effects on tantrums and moods may sometimes be outweighed by the positive effects on attention and stereotype behaviour (Strayhorn *et al, J Am Acad Child Adoles Psych* 1988, **27**, 244–47). Two studies have shown a significant reduction in hyperactivity in autism (n=10, d/b, p/c, c/o, Quintana *et al, J Autism Dev Disord* 1995, **25**, 283–94; n=13, d/b, p/c, c/o, Handen *et al, J Autism Dev Disord* 2000, **30**, 245–55), with 10–50mg/d significantly improving rating scales (n=9, *J Am Acad Child Adoles Psych* 1988, **27**, 248–51).

Naltrexone *

Three controlled studies have shown disappointing results (eg. n=13, d/b, p/c, c/o, Kolmen *et al, J Am Acad Child Adolesc Psych* 1995, 34, 223–31; n=23, 4/52, d/b, p/c, c/o, Willemsen-Swinkels *et al, Biol Psych* 1996, **39**, 1023–31). Although 1mg/kg/d may reduce withdrawal, hyperactivity and SIB, with sedation the only major side-effect (*J Am Acad Child Adoles Psych* 1989, **28**, 200–6), most other measures do not improve. There may be a therapeutic window with doses of 10–25mg/d optimal in some people.

Valproate

Some improvement in behavioural symptoms associated with autism has been reported (open, Plioplys, *Arch Pediatr Adolesc Med* 1994, **148**, 220–22).

Vitamins

High dose pyridoxine, with magnesium, has been claimed to produce moderate benefits, although the risks seem considerable.

▼ No efficacy
Secretin *

Despite much interest, complete lack of significant effect has been demonstrated (eg. n=95, RCT, Dunn-Geier *et al, Dev Med Child Neurol* 2000, **42**, 796–802; n=20, RCT, Owley *et al, MedGenMed* 1999, **6**, E2; n=56, open, Chez *et al, J Autism Dev Disord* 2000, **30**, 87–94), and it remains an almost completely unproven therapy.

1.9 BENZODIAZEPINE DEPENDENCE and WITHDRAWAL

Although short-term benzodiazepine use at standard doses is usually without substantial risk of toxicity and dependence, higher dose and longer-term use is not without risk (*Am J Psych* 1991, **148**, 151–52). Lorazepam, diazepam and flunitrazepam may be more liable to abuse than chlordiazepoxide, nitrazepam and oxazepam (*J Clin Psychopharmacol* 1990, **10**, 237–43), probably due to the more rapid absorption and higher receptor potency.

Reviews*: withdrawal syndrome (Petursson, *Addiction* 1994, **89**, 11455–59), general (Hallström, *Int J Psych Clin Pract* 1998, **2**, 31–34; Ferguson, *Prescriber* 1999, **10**, 118–21; Rickels *et al, J Clin Psychopharmacol* 1999, **19**[Suppl 2], 12S–6S), abuse (history, nature and extent, Robertson and Treasure, *CNS Drugs* 1996, **5**, 137–46, 59 refs), techniques and outcomes of BDZ detoxifications (n=82, Charney *et al, J Clin Psych* 2000, **61**, 190–95).

Patients where withdrawal should not be attempted:

Elderly maintained symptom-free by low and unchanging doses
Chronic physical disorders controlled by BDZs (eg. epilepsy)
Where quality of life is so improved by BDZs that long-term use, preferably with intermittent/variable doses, is justified (eg. chronic or severe anxiety or insomnia and an inadequate personality, people who relapse to alcohol and other more dangerous substances when BDZ-free)

Characteristics of benzodiazepine users:

1. Older medically ill or with spasticity or epilepsy:
Benzodiazepine ususally prescribed by a non-psychiatrist. Seldom abused, doses non-escalated, effective long-term. Care with subtle cognitive changes which can occur.

2. Psychiatric patients with panic or agoraphobic disorders:
Seldom abused, doses not escalated, necessary long-term.

3. Psychiatric patients with recurrent dysphoria:
Long-term indications for use less clear. Abuse of other drugs often occurs.

4. Chronic sleep disordered patients:
Drug may be active or preventing a rebound syndrome.

How to minimise the risk of dependence:
(*Postgrad Med J* 1984, **60** [Suppl 2] , 41–6, Darke *et al, Addiction* 1994, **89**, 1683–90)

Carefully select patients (eg. avoid especially dependence prone, lower education, multiple drug users, criminal background)
Keep the dose low
Stop where possible eg. use shorter courses
Use intermittent or variable doses
Use antidepressants if depression mixed with anxiety is present

Withdrawal symptoms in the dependent patient: (*Med Tox* 1988, **3**, 324–33)

1° Psychological: Tension (to above pre-treatment levels), restlessness, agitation, panic attacks
Physical — Dry mouth, sweating, tremor, sleep disturbance, lethargy, headache, nausea, palpitations
Mental — Impaired memory and concentration, confusion
2° Moderate — Perceptual changes (ie. hypersensitivy to light/sound), dysphoria, flu-like symptoms, anorexia, sore eyes, depersonalisation, depression, abnormal sensations of movement, rebound insomnia
Severe (rare)
Convulsions, psychoses (eg. visual hallucinations, paranoia), delusions

Risk factors for poor withdrawal (need to seek specialist advice):

Previous severe withdrawal (including history of seizures) or post-withdrawal reaction
Lack of adequate social support
Elderly or infirm
History of abuse of alcohol/other drugs (*J Psychoact Drug* 1983, **18**, 85–96)
Concomitant severe medical or psychiatric illness (including personality problems)
High dose/longer-term use (eg. >30mg/d diazepam equiv. >1yr)

BNF Listed

Antidepressants
The BNF recommends the use of antidepressants if clinical depression is present, although many antidepressants may be anxiolytic in their own right.

Diazepam
Transferring from the current benzodiazepine to diazepam (if necessary) is a common strategy, as diazepam is a longer-acting benzodiazepine and possibly easier to withdraw from.

● Unlicensed/Some efficacy

Buspirone
The BNF cautions against use as it may aggravate withdrawal symptoms (see also buspirone, section *1.6*). Patients stabilised on lorazepam changed to buspirone 15mg/d or placebo for 6 weeks (lorazepam tapered over first two weeks), then all given placebo for two weeks, showed buspirone to relieve benzodiazepine withdrawal symptoms and have no rebound anxiety on withdrawal (n=44, RCT, Delle Chiaie *et al, J Clin Psychopharmacol* 1995, **15**, 12–19).

Carbamazepine
Carbamazepine is thought to block the development of drug-induced kindling and hence block the development of withdrawal symptoms. Kindling is the term for prior intermittent low intensity electrical or chemical stimulation which lowers the threshold of response to future low-intensity stimulation (Gorelick, *Curr Opin Psych* 1992, **5**, 430–35). 600–800mg/d has been shown to be effective in benzodiazepine withdrawal in several studies (eg. Ries *et al, J Psychoactive Drugs* 1991, **23**, 73–76), including high dose (up to 300mg/d) diazepam (Neppe and Sindorf, *J Nerv Ment Dis* 1991, **179**, 234–35) and in people with panic disorder (Klein *et al, Am J Psych* 1994, **151**, 1760–66). Up to 800mg/d also reduces the chance of withdrawal convulsions and can minimise withdrawal symptoms (eg. emotional lability), especially if withdrawal is abrupt (*Am J Psych* 1989, **146** 536–37). It may also reduce the incidence of relapse (n=40, RCT, 12/52, Schweizer *et al, Arch Gen Psych* 1991, **48**, 448–52).

Clonazepam
This may be useful as an anticonvulsant benzodiazepine during withdrawal (*Southern Med J* 1988, **81**, 830–36).

Clonidine
This may be a helpful adjunct in withdrawal (*BMJ* 1984, **288**, 1135–40, 1101–2), especially at relatively high dose.

Valproate
900–1200mg/d may reduce the intensity of symptoms in protracted withdrawal as well as acting as an anticonvulsant (Apelt and Emrich, *Am J Psych* 1990, **147**, 950–51). Doses of 150–1200mg/d were effective in relieving withdrawal symptoms in a report of four patients (Apelt and Emrich, *Am J Psych* 1994, **147**, 1990).

○ Unlicensed/Possible efficacy

Antihistamines
These may be useful as non-benzodiazepine hypnotics where insomnia is a problem.

Dothiepin (dosulepin)

Up to 150mg/d of dothiepin may slightly reduce benzodiazepine withdrawal symptoms but did not aid drug withdrawal overall and so appears to have limited use (n=87, d/b, Tyrer *et al*, *B J Psych* 1996, **168**, 457–61).

Melatonin *

Controlled-release melatonin has been successfully used to facilitate discontinuation of benzodiazepines (n=34, d/b, 6/52, Garfinkel *et al, Arch Inter Med* 1999, **159**, 2456–60).

Phenobarbital (phenobarbitone)

The anticonvulsant properties are useful and can help avoid giving an alternative benzodiazepine during withdrawal (*J Psychoact Drugs* 1983, **15**, 85–95, 99–104).

Propranolol

Use only if other measures have failed (*Postgrad Med J* 1988, **64**[Suppl], 40–44).

▼ No efficacy

Antipsychotics

Low dose anxiolytic use may be useful but may make withdrawal symptoms worse (*Lancet* 1987, **i**, 78–79).

Flumazenil

Flumazenil may be useful only in overdose where respiratory depression occurs (*Lancet* 1987, **ii**, 463). The BNF states caution in BDZ dependence.

1.10   BIPOLAR MOOD DISORDER (prophylaxis thereof)

See also depression (*1.14*) and mania (*1.19*) for treatment of a particular episode, plus rapid-cycling mood disorder (*1.28*)

Bipolar disorder is a fluctuating, chronic illness with a variety of presentations and sub-divisions. DSM-IV divides the condition into bipolar I (one or more manic or mixed episodes, wide mood swings), bipolar II (the most common form, one or more episodes of depression with at least one hypomanic but no manic episode) and bipolar III (pseudobipolar, often triggered by antidepressants, and which may present as a mixed state).

Bipolar disorder is often unrecognised, misdiagnosed and under-treated or inadequately treated: One investigator showed that 23% bipolars consult a professional within 6 months of symptom onset, but 48% consult 3 or more professionals before receiving a correct diagnosis (10% saw 7 or more) and 34% wait 10 or more years for diagnosis (Lish *et al, J Aff Dis* 1994, **31**, 281–94). The average time from onset of symptoms to starting maintenance therapy is 8.3 years (Baldessarini *et al, Am J Psych* 1999, **156**, 811). Sadly, many suicide attempts are made during this 8-year latency period before lithium is started, the only proven anti-suicide drug. There is an overlap with personality disorder, eg. labile affect, irritability, mood instability, stress, low mood/dysphoria, so some have warned of over-diagnosing BPD and under-diagnosing bipolar disorder. Poor outcome is associated with anxiety (n=124, Feske *et al, Am J Psych* 2000, **157**, 956–62) and concurrent personality disorders (n=59, Dunayevich *et al, J Clin Psych* 2000, **61**, 134–39).

It is also clear that well-being and functioning is inversely proportional to the number of bipolar episodes and so strategies to reduce relapse must be rigorously followed, especially minimising difficult-to-treat bipolar depression (n=64, retrospective, MacQueen *et al, Acta Psych Scand* 2000, **101**, 374–81).

Role of drugs: *

Lithium, carbamazepine and valproate are widely used for the prophylaxis of bipolar disorder, although the evidence for carbamazepine and valproate is not robust. A substantial proportion of patients still do not receive adequate TDM (no tests for 12 months in 37% lithium, 42% valproate and 42% carbamazepine users, n=718, Marcus *et al, Am J Psych* 1999, **156**, 1014–18). CBT can significantly help to reduce risk factors for relapse and produce better outcomes in combination with mood stabilisers (review of combination approaches, Rothbaum and Astin, *J Clin Psych* 2000, **61**[Suppl 9], 68–75).

Reviews*: APA Practice Guidelines (*Am J Psych* 1994, **151**[12]), suggested treatment algorithms (Calabrese and Woyshville, *J Clin Psych* 1995, **56**[Suppl 3], 11–18; Goodwin *et al, Int J Psych Clin*

Pract 1997, **1**, S9–12), consensus statement (Frances *et al, J Clin Psych* 1998, **59**[Suppl 4], 73–89), anticonvulsants and antipsychotics (Porter *et al, Adv Psych Treat* 1999, **5**, 96–103; Keck *et al, J Clin Psych* 1998, **59**[Suppl 6], 74–81, 114 refs), general (Shelton *et al, J Clin Psych* 1998, **59**, 484–95), reviews of mood stabilisers for bipolar, schizoaffective, depression, mania etc (various authors, *J Clin Psych* 1999, **60**[Suppl 5], 3–52; Bowden, *J Clin Psych* 2000, **61**[Suppl 9], 35-40), practical guide to drug treatment (Bauer and Ahrens, *CNS Drugs* 1996, **6**, 35–52), diagnosis and treatment in children and adolescents (Silva *et al, CNS Drugs* 1999, **12**, 437–50), genetics (Potash and DePaolo, *Bipolar Disord* 2000, **2**, 8–26), suicide and bipolar (Jamison, *J Clin Psych* 2000, **61**[Suppl 9], 47–51), longitudinal course (Suppes *et al, J Clin Psych* 2000, **61**[Suppl 9], 23–30, 134 refs), bipolar disorder in the elderly (Eastham *et al, Drugs & Aging* 1998, **12**, 205–24).

BNF Listed *

Several active comparisons between lithium, carbamazepine and valproate have been carried out, eg. lithium (0.63mmol/l) was shown to be superior to carbamazepine (mean 621mg/d) when comparing recurrences, hospitalisations, need for concurrent drugs and ADRs needing discontinuation (n=144, RCT, Greil *et al, J Aff Dis* 1997, **43**, 151–61). A complex one-year study comparing divalproex, lithium and placebo (2:1:1) failed to show divalproex to be superior to either of the others in time to any mood episode, but there was a trend for divalproex (40/52) over placebo (28/52) and lithium (24/52). Divalproex was slightly superior on a number of secondary measures. A high lithium drop-out rate and initial placebo-stable recruits sadly renders some of the data statistically weak (RCT, n=372, Bowden *et al, Arch Gen Psych* 2000, **57**, 481–89).

Carbamazepine *

Long-term therapy in affective disorders is well-established, either as an alternative to lithium or used in combination in treatment-resistant cases. However, six studies of maintenance carbamazepine in bipolar disorder show equivocal results, eg. incomplete protection, and some uncertainty remains (reviewed by Keck *et al, J Clin Psych* 1998, **59**[Suppl 6], 74–81, 114 refs; see also Dardennes *et al, B J Psych* 1995, **166**, 378–81, supported by Post *et al, B J Psych* 1997, **170**, 202–4). Indeed one study (Frankenburg *et al, J Clin Psychopharmacol* 1988, **8**, 130–32) showed that only 18% of carbamazepine-treated bipolars remained stable for 3–4 years and another showed a 50% relapse rate (Post *et al, J Clin Psychopharmacol* 1990, **10**, 318–27). Carbamazepine is reported to be better for early onset illness and with an alternating pattern of mood. Various studies have shown that low dose carbamazepine (15–25 micromol/l) is as effective as high dose carbamazepine (28–40 micromols/l) and lithium (0.6–0.8micromol/l) in bipolar patients, but in unipolar patients, low dose was less effective than the other two (n=58, *J Aff Dis* 1993, **28**, 221–31). A comparison of 10 studies of carbamazepine against lithium shows a roughly similar efficacy (n=572, table in Davis *et al, Acta Psych Scand* 1999, 406–17). A thorough review of the available trials implies that trough carbamazepine levels of 7mg/l or above are strongly associated with therapeutic response in bipolar patients (Taylor and Duncan, *Psych Bull* 1997, **21**, 221–23) and thus may require higher doses (eg. 600mg/d) than are currently recommended. There is little evidence yet for a rebound mania on discontinuation (eg. n=6, Macritchie and Hunt, *J Psychopharmacol* 2000, **14**, 266–68).

Lithium *

Lithium is widely used for the treatment and prophylaxis of bipolar illnesses and with care can be successful and safe. It is effective in Bipolar I and II, by reducing relapses and increasing interepisode intervals (Tondo *et al, Am J Psych* 1998, **155**, 638–45). Although the nine major placebo-controlled trials of lithium as prophylaxis of bipolar disorder have methodological flaws (eg. most used an abrupt lithium-withdrawal control group, which Baldessarini has now shown increases relapse in its own right, detailed discussion of these shortcomings by Moncrieff, *B J Psych* 1995,

167, 569–74), their findings, however, are of great importance (reply to Moncrieff by Goodwin, *B J Psych* 1995, **167**, 573–74). One might also ask of the doubters that if lithium doesn't work, how come there's a known dose-response curve, and withdrawal of something that doesn't work produces relapse? (19 RCTs, n=865, Davis *et al, Acta Psych Scand* 1999, 406–17).

Prophylaxis*: Lithium appears highly effective as prophylactic therapy. Meta-analysis of all comparative studies shows lithium to have a highly significant reduction in relapse (19 RCTs, n=865, Davis *et al, Acta Psych Scand* 1999, 406–17), provided it is taken regularly, monitored regularly and the dose and therapy reviewed regularly to minimise side-effects, especially those of weight gain and cognitive dulling. Commencing lithium within the first ten years of illness predicts better preventative outcomes than beginning prophylaxis later, both in major depression, recurrent and bipolar patients (n=270, Franchini *et al, Eur Arch Psychiatry Clin Neurosci* 1999, **249**, 227–30). The prophylactic efficacy is probably maintained for at least ten years (Berghofer *et al, Acta Psych Scand* 1996, **93**, 349–54). Data is accumulating that long-term lithium markedly reduces the excess mortality of people with recurrent affective disorders (retrospective study, n=273, Müller-Oerlinghausen *et al, Acta Psych Scand* 1996, **94**, 344–47), probably, at least in part, by (see below) reducing suicide (Gershon and Soares, *Arch Gen Psych* 1997, **54**, 16–20). Lithium maintenance yields striking long-term reductions of depressive as well as manic morbidity in both bipolar disorder subtypes, with greater overall benefits in Bipolar II patients and with earlier treatment (n=317, retrospective, Tondo *et al, Am J Psych* 1998, **155**, 638–45). Regular lithium use over 5 years has been shown to produce a drastic reduction in time in hospital as 'almost the rule', but irregular use leads to a much poorer outcome (n=402, Maj *et al, Am J Psych* 1998, **155**, 30–35).

The main problems appear to be when therapy is given to carelessly selected patients given insufficient support (see compliance), education and supervision, illustrated by naturalistic studies, which have shown a poorer outcome than controlled trials. Goodwin argues strongly that treatment with lithium should be for at least two years (and more probably three years at the minimum) and that up to two years it may have at best no beneficial effect (premature stopping resulting in premature recurrence of mania).

Suicide reduction*: Reduced suicide rates have been strongly suggested by studies, something unique in bipolar to lithium (Baldessarini and Jamison, *J Clin Psych* 1999, **60**[Suppl 2], 117–22). Suicide rates with lithium, carba-mazepine and amitriptyline have been compared and support the view that lithium has a specific antisuicide effect (RCT, 2.5 years, n=378, Theis-Flechtner *et al, Pharmacopsychiatry* 1996, **29**, 103–7). Although suicide protection may be incomplete, it is 7-fold lower than in non-lithium treated patients (review of 22 studies, Tondo and Baldessarini, *J Clin Psych* 2000, **61**[Suppl 9], 97–104). It should be noted that excess mortality has also been reported with lithium (n=133, retrospective over 16 years, Brodersen *et al, B J Psych* 2000, **176**, 429–33).

Dosing*: Once-daily lithium reduces side-effects, simplifies dosage requirements (review by Hammond, *Ann Pharmacother* 1994, **28**, 472–73) and may reduce renal damage, but probably not effect 24-hr urine volume (*Acta Psych Scand* 1993, **87**, 92–95) nor renal function (Abraham *et al, Acta Psych Scand* 1995, **92**, 115–18). Alternate daily lithium has been advocated but has not been shown to significantly reduce side-effects although polyuria/polydipsia may be slightly reduced (n=50, d/b, Jensen *et al, J Aff Dis* 1996, **36**, 89–93) and higher relapse rates (factor of three) have been reported, and disputed (Jensen *et al, Acta Psych Scand* 1995, **92**, 69–74; Andrade, *Acta Psych Scand* 1996, **94**, 281; Jensen *et al, Acta Psych Scand* 1996, **94**, 281–82).

A simple and accurate equation to predict daily lithium dose has been proposed, which is better than the Zetin method (n=100, Terao *et al, J Clin Psychopharmacol* 1999, **19**, 336–40):

Daily lithium carbonate dose (in milligrams) = 100.5 + (752.7 x expected lithium concentration in millimoles per litre) – (3.6 x age in years) + (7.2 x weight in kilograms) – (13.7 x blood urea nitrogen [BUN] in milligrams per deciliter).

Plasma levels*: Plasma levels of 0.4–0.8mmol/L are generally considered safe and effective as prophylaxis, and below 0.4–0.6mEq/L may be less protective against relapse (eg. Gelenberg *et al, NEJM* 1989, **321**, 1489–93). There was no difference in the protection against affective disorder relapse between high (0.8–1.0mmol/L) and low (0.5–0.8mmol/L) serum lithium levels (naturalistic, n=91, Vestergaard *et al, Acta Psych Scand* 1998, **98**, 310–15), but only a third completed two years lithium prophylaxis successfully, and alcohol or other medication abuse was associated with poor outcome. In acute mania, 1.3–1.5mmol/l, with care, may be appropriate (Thau *et al, Lithium* 1993, **4**, 149–59). In the elderly, a third to half less lithium may be needed due to reduced clearance (*J Clin Psychopharmacol* 1987, **7**, 153–58). Plasma monitoring is often poor, but even distribution of clinical guidelines in Aberdeen in 1996 resulted in only transient improved renal and thyroid monitoring and of plasma levels (Eagles *et al, Acta Psych Scand* 2000, **101**, 349–53).

Predictive methods of estimating the final lithium dose in hospitalised manic in-patients may allow therapeutic levels to be reached quicker and lengths of stay can be reduced (Marken *et al, Ann Pharmacother* 1994, **28**, 1148–52). The brain:plasma ratio is usually considered a relatively constant 1:1 but can vary widely (reported cases of 100:1), which may explain why some people get side-effects on low doses and also means that plasma levels have to be interpreted carefully.

Mode of action*: Lithium may exert its effect via G proteins, and down-regulates intracellular protein kinase C levels (Manji *et al, J Clin Psych* 1996, **57**[Suppl 13], 34–46), as does valproate and tamoxifen. Another possible action by up-regulation of the neuroprotective protein Bcl-2 in the CNS (Manji *et al, J Clin Psych* 2000, **61**[Suppl 9], 82–96) with speculated rebound reduction in Bcl-2 production on lithium withdrawal.

Compliance or concordance: The main reason for lithium failure is non-compliance (either complete or erratic) and the patient (and any partner or carer) needs to be aware of the long-term commitment needed. Naturalistic studies have indicated that its effectiveness in clinical practice can be significantly compromised by poor compliance and poor monitoring. It has been suggested that specialised care, eg. via lithium or mood clinics, to improve patient and professional compliance with lithium use, would improve this (Guscott and Taylor, *B J Psych* 1994, **164**, 741–46).

Future compliance to lithium after discharge from hospital (and hence likelihood of readmission within one year) has been predicted by measuring pre- and post-leave levels, the so-called lithium level-to-dose ratio (LDR) (Terao and Terao, *Lithium* 1994, **5**, 115–16). For a general review of strategies to improve compliance, see Schou (*Acta Psych Scand* 1997, **95**, 361–63).

Discontinuation: Early (particularly manic) relapse in bipolar illness following lithium discontinuation is now well accepted. Two important studies have proven an effect. Firstly, bipolar illness relapse rates were very high (median 50% risk of relapse within 4 months, 100% over 3.5 years) when lithium was stopped abruptly, ie. over 1–14 days, than when stopped slowly, ie. over 15–30 days, with a significant excess over the first six months (Baldessarini *et al, J Clin Psych* 1996, **57**, 441–48). A second study showed a mean time to recurrence (14 months) of 5.6 times as long for gradual discontinuation as for rapid discontinuation (2.5 months to relapse). (Baldessarini *et al, Am J Psych* 1997, **154**, 551–53). Both these papers are essential reading for anyone prescribing and/or discontinuing lithium therapy. Discontinuation has been shown to be associated with elevated rates of psychiatric hospitalisation and use of emergency services (Johnson and McFarland, *Am J Psych* 1996, **153**, 993–1000). Since lithium has been shown to reduce mortality, discontinuation is also likely to be associated with increased mortality.

Lithium refractoriness: lithium discontinuation in stable patients, despite adequate lithium levels, has been reported to induce a refractory state (eg. Bauer, *Am J Psych* 1994, **151**, 1522). However, a two-year study of lithium maintenance treatment periods (mean 4 years) was unable to show this (n=86, Tondo *et al, Am J Psych* 1997, **154**, 548–50) and another was also unable to show any evidence that lithium discontinuation results in treatment resistance when lithium is resumed (n=28, Coryell *et al, Am J Psych* 1998, **155**, 895–98), although this study has been criticised as being underpowered (Maj, *Am J Psych* 1999, **156**, 1130, plus reply). There are many unreported cases where apparent lack of efficacy on re-exposure has occurred (study and review by Maj *et al, Am J Psych* 1995, **152**, 1810–11).

Withdrawal: A short-term withdrawal syndrome may occur on abrupt discontinuation, showing as changes in talkativeness, self-confidence, motor performance and sleep (*Irish J Psychol Med* 1990, **7**, 42–44) but a distinct withdrawal syndrome is not established (review of evidence by Schou, *B J Psych* 1993, **163**, 514–18; discussion by Thalayasingan *et al, B J Psych* 1994, **164**, 417–19; reviewed in detail by Goodwin, *B J Psych* 1994, **164**, 149–52). See also discontinuation above for discussion of relapse.

Reviews*: general (*Drug and Ther Bull* 1999, **37**, 22–24; Baldessarini and Tondo, *Arch Gen Psych* 2000, **57**, 187–90; Friedrich, *JAMA* 1999, **281**, 2271–73; Cookson, *B J Psych* 1997, **171**, 120–24; Schou, Goodwin and Johnson, *Bipolar Disord* 1999, **1**, 5–16), plasma monitoring (Aronson and Reynolds, *BMJ* 1992, **305**, 1273), proposed guidelines on good practice in lithium prophylaxis (Birch *et al, Lithium* 1993, **4**, 225–30), neurobiology and mode of action (Lenox and Hahn, *J Clin Psych* 2000, **61**[Suppl 9], 5–15,

123 refs), historical perspectives (Soares and Gershon, *J Clin Psych* 2000, **61**[Suppl 9], 16–22, Nemeroff, *J Clin Psych* 2000, **61**[Suppl 9], 3–4), pharmacokinetics and pharmacodynamics (Kilts, *J Clin Psych* 2000, **61**[Suppl 9], 41–46), prophylaxis (editorial review, Vestergaard, *Acta Psych Scand* 2000, **101**, 341–42),

+ **Combinations**

A retrospective review indicated an increased use of polypharmacy in refractory bipolar over recent decades (n=178, Frye *et al, J Clin Psych* 2000, **61**, 9–15). For a review of mood stabiliser combinations, see Freeman and Stoll, *Am J Psych* 1998, **155**, 12–21.

Lithium + antipsychotics

Lithium is frequently used with antipsychotics in maintenance therapy, although only two controlled studies exist. One study showed improved efficacy in mania compared to lithium monotherapy, although poorly tolerated (n=33, 8/52, Small *et al, Psychopharmacol Bull* 1995, **31**, 265–72). A two-year study showed no improved prophylactic effect from flupentixol depot and lithium compared to lithium monotherapy (d/b, n=11, Esparon *et al, B J Psych* 1986, **148**, 723–25). Anecdotal reports indicate an additive effect, eg. with clozapine, risperidone, olanzapine etc (reviewed by Freeman and Stoll, *Am J Psych* 1998, **155**, 12–21).

Lithium+calcium-channel blockers

Although there are some reports of efficacy, potential drug interactions make this combination hazardous (reviewed by Freeman and Stoll, *Am J Psych* 1998, **155**, 12–21).

Lithium + carbamazepine

This combination is widely used, and seems safe and effective, especially for rapid-cycling. A variety of retrospective and prospective studies have shown a well-tolerated and improved prophylactic effect compared to lithium monotherapy (eg. n=33, Small *et al, Psychopharmacol Bull* 1995, **31**, 265–72). Occasional neurotoxic reactions have been reported, but mostly in patients with pre-existing brain damage (Shukla *et al, Am J Psych* 1984, **141**,

1604–6). An additive anti-thyroid effect may occur, lowering T4 and free T4 levels (*Am J Psych* 1990, **147**, 615–20) although the addition of carbamazepine to lithium has also been claimed help to counteract lithium-induced sub-clinical hypothyroidism, possibly improving efficacy (Bocchetta *et al, Acta Psych Scand* 1996, **94**, 45–48).

Lithium + fluoxetine
Fluoxetine-augmentation of lithium in bipolar mood disorder can help prevent breakthrough depression (n=26, open, 3-year, Tondo *et al, Int J Psych Clin Pract* 1997, **1**, 203–6).

Lithium + lamotrigine
Case reports indicate this may be a useful combination (eg. Calabrese *et al, Am J Psych* 1996, **153**, 1236).

Valproate + antipsychotics
Many combinations are used, although there is little data to show a proven efficacy. Reports of valproate used effectively with clozapine and risperidone have appeared (reviewed by Freeman and Stoll, *Am J Psych* 1998, **155**, 12–21).

Valproate + carbamazepine
There have been several reports of efficacy, eg. when valproate was added to carbamazepine non-responders, 69% responded (n=29, Schaff *et al, J Clin Psych* 1993, **54**, 380–84), and a case report in rapid-cycling (Ketter *et al, J Clin Psychopharmacol* 1992, **12**, 276–81). Plasma level monitoring is needed as both drugs can interact (see *4.5.1*).

Valproate + lamotrigine
An open study has indicated some efficacy (reviewed by Freeman and Stoll, *Am J Psych* 1998, **155**, 12–21), although the incidence of rash appears higher and valproate increases lamotrigine levels (see *4.5.4*).

Valproate + lithium
This combination appears safe and effective in resistant bipolar disorder. A one-year pilot study showed that bipolar I patients taking divalproex plus lithium were significantly less likely to relapse than those taking lithium monotherapy (n=12, Solomon *et al, J Clin Psych* 1997, **58**, 95–99), although side-effects were more common. Other case reports suggest a synergistic effect.

● **Unlicensed/Some efficacy**
Antipsychotics *
The main roles of antipsychotics in bipolar disorder are:
1. Adjunctive to mood stabilisers for management of acute mania or psychotic depression.
2. Adjunctive maintenance in treatment-resistance.

There is no compelling evidence that antipsychotics are effective as maintenance therapy alone in bipolar disorder. There are no RCTs comparing antipsychotics with mood stabilisers in bipolar disorder, although they are prescribed for up to 84% of bipolars (84%, Tohen and Zarate, *J Clin Psych* 1998, **59**[Suppl 1], 38–49; 39%, n=88, 6/12, open, Soares *et al, J Aff Dis* 1999, **56**, 1–8), and six months after an acute episode, up to 95% may still be taking them, at an average of 634mg/d CPZ equivalents (n=40, Sernyak *et al, Am J Psych* 1994, **151**, 133–35). Most patients (even treatment resistant) can and should be stabilised without the need for chronic antipsychotics (retrospective, n=133, Brotman *et al, J Clin Psych* 2000, **61**, 68–72). Although it is unproven that bipolar disorder is a hyper-dopaminergic state, it has been shown that in antipsychotic-naive or antipsychotic-free (for 6 months) psychotic bipolars, there is an increase in D_2 receptor density (Pearlson *et al, Arch Gen Psych* 1995, **52**, 471–77) and so dopamine-blocking drugs may have some rationale. Five open trials have shown reduced manic episodes and reduced time acutely ill (reviewed by Keck *et al, J Clin Psych* 1998, **59**[Suppl 6], 74–81). Depot antipsychotics may be useful in some patients as prophylaxis of bipolar mood disorder, by reducing relapses and time in hospital (18 out-patient audit and review by Littlejohn *et al, B J Psych* 1995, **166**, 827–29), although flupentixol depot appeared to have no prophylactic effect as lithium augmentation (d/b, c/o, Esparon *et al, B J Psych* 1986, **148**, 723–25).

Clozapine, risperidone and olanzapine may be of equivalent efficacy as adjuncts to mood stabilisers in bipolar disorder (retrospective, n=42, Guille *et al, J Clin Psych* 2000, **61**, 638–42).

Several studies have shown **risperidone** to be useful in mania and bipolar disorder (eg. n=14, open out-patient study where 64% improved, Ghaemi *et al, Can J Psych* 1997, **42**, 196–99; n=12, open, Ghaemi and Sachs, *Int Clin Psychopharmacol* 1997, **12**, 333–38). A one-year trial of **clozapine** in treatment-resistant bipolar or schizo-effective patients showed clozapine to have significant mood-stabilising properties compared to placebo (n=38, RCT, Suppes *et al, Am J Psych* 1999, **156**, 1164–69; see also n=193, Banov *et al, J Clin Psych* 1994, **55**, 295–300; n=34/91, open, Ciapparelli *et al, J Clin Psych* 2000, **61**, 329–34). **Quetiapine** may have some applications as an alternative or adjunct in bipolar or schizo-affective disorders (n=145, open, Zarate *et al, J Clin Psych* 2000, **61**, 185–89). **Review***: atypicals in bipolar and schizoaffective disorders (Ghaemi and Goodwin, *J Clin Psychopharmacol* 1999, **19**, 354–61).

Valproate *

Whilst now licensed for mania, valproate is not yet actually licensed as a mood stabiliser, albeit widely used for this (review, Davis *et al, Acta Psych Scand* 1999, **100**, 406–17). A one-year study comparing divalproex, lithium and placebo (2:1:1) failed to show divalproex to be superior to lithium or placebo in the time to any mood episode, but there was a noticeable trend for divalproex (40/52) over placebo (28/52) and lithium (24/52), and it was slightly superior on a number of secondary measures (RCT, n=372, Bowden *et al, Arch Gen Psych* 2000, **57**, 481–89). Case studies and open trials (eg. Calabrese *et al, J Clin Psychopharmacol* 1992, **12**[Suppl 1], 53S–56S) suggest a therapeutic effect, particularly in prevention of mania or mixed episodes. Valproate may be highly effective in some patients with bipolar disorder refractory to lithium and carbamazepine (n=24, Denicoff *et al, Am J Psych* 1997, **154**, 1456–58).

A thorough review of the available trials implies that trough valproate levels of 50mg/l are strongly associated with therapeutic response in bipolar and manic patients (Taylor and Duncan, *Psych Bull* 1997, **21**, 221–23) and thus, may require higher doses (eg. 1000mg/d) than currently recommended. There is also some preliminary data that valproate may allow reduction in the doses of antipsychotics needed in bipolar disorder with psychosis, or even replace them (Reutens and Castle, *B J Psych* 1997, **170**, 484–85). It may be possible to predict response (Bowden, *J Clin Psych* 1995, **56** [Suppl 3], 25–30). See also entry under mania/hypomania (*1.19*).

○ Unlicensed/Possible efficacy

Calcium-channel blockers *

Verapamil 120–450mg/d (mean 200–450mg/d) has shown promise as a mood stabiliser (*Biol Psych* 1989, **25**, 128–40), even in the elderly (*Int J Ger Psych* 1992, **7**, 913–15). **Nimodipine** has been effective in some trials (eg. Pazzaglia *et al, Psychiatr Res* 1993, **49**, 257–72; Goodnick, *J Clin Psych* 1995, **56**, 330) and is highly lipophilic, allowing adequate CNS concentrations and minimal peripheral effects, an advantage over verapamil. **Diltiazem** has also been suggested as effective (n=8, 12/12, open, Silverstone and Birkett, *J Psychiatry Neurosci* 2000, **25**, 276–80) They may have some role as add-on therapy in resistant cases.

Fatty acids (omega 3)

In a not very stringent 4-month trial, omega-3 fatty acids produced a significantly longer remission than placebo, as well as scoring higher on most other outcome measures (d/b, n=30, Stoll *et al, Arch Gen Psych* 1999, **56**, 407–12; general review by Greener, *Prog Neurol Psych* 1999, **3**, 26–27).

Gabapentin *

A naturalistic study of resistant bipolar illness produced 18 positive responses with **gabapentin** (average 539mg/d, range 33–2700mg/d, n=28, Schaffer and Schaffer, *Am J Psych* 1997, **154**, 291–92) and gabapentin was considered moderately to markedly effective in 30% patients with bipolar or unipolar depression mood disorders (retrospective, open, n=50, Ghaemi *et al, J Clin Psych* 1998, **59**, 426–29). However, see also the entry under mania/hypomania (*1.19*), where it appears of little efficacy in mania/hypomania.

Review*: Letterman and Markowitz, *Pharmacotherapy* 1999, **19**, 565–72.

Lamotrigine *
More RCTs are awaited but there is growing evidence of efficacy. In an open study (monotherapy and adjunctive) in treatment-resistant bipolar disorder, lamotrigine showed a marked reduction in manic symptoms over 8 weeks, sustained for 48 weeks, and reduced depressive symptoms, suggesting a useful potential effect (open, n=75, Calabrese *et al*, *Am J Psych* 1999, **156**, 1019–23). Lamotrigine 50–200mg/d monotherapy was significantly more effective than placebo in bipolar I depression, the effect being seen as early as the third week (n=195, RCT, Calabrese *et al*, *J Clin Psych* 1999, **60**, 79–88), and a comparison with a mood stabiliser or antidepressant would now be appropriate (reviewed by Haslam, *EBMH* 1999, **2**, 75).
Reviews: general (Keck *et al*, *J Clin Psych* 1998, **59**[Suppl 6], 74–81, 114 refs; Duncan *et al*, *Psych Bull* 1998, **22**, 630–32; Maidment, *Ann Pharmacother* 1999, **33**, 864-67, 18 refs; Engle and Heck, *Ann Pharmacother* 2000, **34**, 258–62, 28 refs).

Methylphenidate *
Methylphenidate was effective and tolerable in 78% depressed bipolars (open, 12/52, n=14, El-Mallakh, *Bipolar Disord* 2000, **2**, 56–59).

Omega 3 fatty acids
See Fatty acids (omega 3)

Pramipexole
There are reports of treatment-resistant bipolar depression, where the D3 agonist pramipexole augmentation produced improvement (n=2 Goldberg *et al*, *Am J Psych* 1999, **156**, 798).

Spironolactone
A case report exists of positive effects in combination with lithium (*BMJ* 1986, **292**, 661–62) and 100mg/d improved behaviour in a 6-patient study (*J Nerv Ment Dis* 1978, **166**, 517–20).

Tamoxifen
There is some interest in tamoxifen as mood stabiliser, as it shares some intracellular properties with lithium (see lithium in this section).

Tiagabine *
Tiagabine 4mg/d was successful as adjunctive therapy in multiple drug-resistant bipolar disorder, continuing to be effective over several months (n=2, Schaffer and Schaffer, *Am J Psych* 1999, **156**, 2014–15).

1.11 BORDERLINE PERSONALITY DISORDER

See also aggression (*1.2*)

There are a large number of personality disorders, of which borderline personality disorder is but one. Treating personality disorders (and hence personality itself) is obviously somewhat controversial. Patients with BPD more often present for treatment than schizoid, paranoid and avoidant personality types. Research is now often directed towards treating symptom clusters rather than the underlying personality disorder, eg. anxiety, aggression, impulsiveness, etc.

Symptoms:
The main symptoms of BPD are of a deeply ingrained maladaptive pattern of behaviour, recognisable from adolescence and continuing through most of adult life. Such people show continued boredom, anger, unstable relationships, impulsive self-harmful behaviour (eg. gambling, stealing, binge-eating, or drinking), variable moods, recurrent suicide threats or behaviour and uncertainty about their personal identity.

Role of drugs:
BPD may account for up to 7.5% of psychiatric admissions, with a raised incidence of psychiatric morbidity and mortality. Drug use in some people with BPD is supported by the literature. The drugs will not alter ingrained character traits or the effects of abuse, but they may produce modest benefits, with the occasional striking result and be more effective if combined with psychotherapy. Drug therapy, however, is fraught with problems. Side-effects may be grossly exaggerated to avoid treatment and patients may be actively anti-medication (see Sweeney, *J Clin Psych* 1987, **48**[Suppl 8], 32–35 for strategies to minimise this). Therapeutic alliances (eg. giving a drug a 'trial'), and not abandoning the patient if the drugs work, may help. Care in patients with suicidal

tendencies is necessary.

In a critical review of this topic, Tyrer concludes that 'the null hypothesis that drug treatment of personality disorder is inappropriate has not yet been disproved', and that 'our current drug treatment of personality disorder is like following a badly marked track through a dense fog — you can see only a very short distance ahead but are grateful for any guidance going' (Tyrer, *Psych Bull* 1998, **22**, 242–44, 25 refs).

Reviews*: general (Hori, *Psychiatry Clin Neurosci* 1998, **52**, 13–19; Soloff, *Psychiatr Clin North Am* 2000, **23**, 169–92), classification, epidemiology, diagnosis and assessment, intervention and management (Marlowe and Sugarman, *BMJ* 1997, **315**, 176–79).

● **Unlicensed/Some potency**

Antipsychotics

It has been generally accepted that patients with DSM-IV borderline or schizotypical personality disorders may gain significant benefit from psychotherapy and small doses of antipsychotics (Goldberg *et al, Arch Gen Psych* 1986, **43**, 680–86). Haloperidol (mean dose 7.24mg/d, Soloff *et al, Arch Gen Psych* 1986, **43**, 691–70), and trifluoperazine (mean dose 7.8mg/d, Cowdrey and Gardner, *Arch Gen Psych* 1988, **45**, 111–19) may improve anger, hostility and behavioural symptoms. Low dose risperidone may be effective but better tolerated (eg. n=1, Szigethy and Schulz, *J Clin Psychopharmacol* 1997, **17**, 326–27). Two studies have, however, challenged this view. **Haloperidol** at 4mg/d was no better than placebo in BPD except for a minor effect on behaviour dyscontrol and anger in one study (Soloff *et al, Arch Gen Psych* 1993, **150**, 377–85) and a follow-up study of 54 haloperidol responders who were allowed to continue for a further 16 weeks at up to 6mg/d showed the drug poorly tolerated, and having only a mild effect on irritability (Cornelius *et al, Am J Psych* 1993, **150**, 1843–48). Generally, high-potency drugs in low dose were preferred by patients (due to lack of the abhorred sedative effects). Finally, two open trials of **clozapine** (25–100mg/d)

in severe BPD patients produced a general improvement in symptoms in one (n=12, Benedetti *et al, J Clin Psych* 1998, **59**, 13–107) and significantly reduced SIB, aggression, seclusion and violence in the other (n=7, Chengappa *et al, J Clin Psych* 1999, **60**, 477–84). More studies are thus needed.

○ **Unlicensed/Possible efficacy**

Antidepressants

Some symptoms of BPD are shared with depression, eg. self-condemnation, emptiness, hopelessness, boredom and somatic complaints (Rogers *et al, Am J Psych* 1995, **152**, 268–70) and so the use of antidepressants may have some logic. See tricyclics, SSRIs, MAOIs etc in this section.

Benzodiazepines

Benzodiazepines are generally considered as contraindicated in BPD due to the tendency to disinhibit and induce rage reactions and dependence, eg. alprazolam was shown to be significantly worse than placebo for behavioural control (Cowdrey and Gardner, *Arch Gen Psych* 1988, **45**, 111–19) and the only double-blind study showed alprazolam to be no better than placebo in children with anxious or avoidant disorders (Simeon *et al, J Am Acad Adolesc Psych* 1993, **13**, 29–33). The use of rapidly absorbed short-acting drugs (eg. lorazepam) may have some limited use in patients with intermittent explosive disorders, where intermittent use can help abort episodes of dyscontrol.

Carbamazepine *

Carbamazepine may be useful for episodic dyscontrol and aggression. Although episodic dyscontrol is not epileptic, there are some common precipitating factors (eg. prodromal symptoms, severe disturbance and post-episode relief of tension), hence the use of anticonvulsants. Carbamazepine was superior to placebo for behaviour control but not for dysphoria in one study of prison inmates, anecdotally producing a state of 'reflective delay' (Cowdrey and Gardner, *Arch Gen Psych* 1988, **45**, 111–19, see also lithium) and with 600mg/d, aggressive outbursts were dramatically reduced (in intensity and frequency) compared to placebo (n=14,

Gardner and Cowdrey, *Am J Psych* 1986, **143**, 519–22). However, an RCT failed to show any effects (n=20, RCT, 30/7, de al Fuente and Lotstra, *Eur Neuropsychopharmacol* 1994, **4**, 479–86).

Lithium

Lithium has been reported to be useful for episodic dyscontrol and aggression, affective disorder in BPD, emotionally unstable adolescents and alcoholics with a PD. Anecdotally, it produced a state of 'reflective delay' ('Now I can think whether to hit him or not' as one inmate put it).

MAOIs

There was some evidence that MAOIs are effective in depression associated with BPD, eg. tranylcypromine (Cowdrey and Gardner, *Arch Gen Psych* 1988, **45**, 111–19) and phenelzine. However, two studies have shown phenelzine at 60mg/d to be no better than placebo except for a minor effect on hostility and anger (Soloff *et al, Arch Gen Psych* 1993, **150**, 377–85) and in a 16-week 90mg/d follow-up of phenelzine responders found it to be poorly tolerated and having only a mild effect on irritability and depressive symptoms (Cornelius *et al, Am J Psych* 1993, **150**, 1843–48).

Methylphenidate

There is one case where methylphenidate was thought to have been effective in a patient with both ADHD and BPD (Van Reekum and Links, *Can J Psych* 1994, **39**, 186–87), although this is open to debate (see amfetamines in this section).

SSRIs

Some studies indicate that SSRIs may have a role, eg. irritability and aggression improved in the 44% completers in a trial of 50–200mg/d sertraline (n=16, 8/52, Kavoussi *et al, J Clin Psych* 1994, **55**, 137–41). Another study showed that 20–60mg/d fluoxetine significantly reduced anger and distress, with a significant placebo effect also being detectable (n=22, p/c, Selzman *et al, J Clin Psychopharmacol* 1995, **15**, 23–29). Fluoxetine was partially effective in reduced impulsive aggressive behaviour in another study, but with high drop-out rates (n=40, RCT, Coccaro and Kavoussi, *Arch Gen Psych* 1997, **54**, 1081–88,

review by Hawton, *EBMH* 1998, **1**, 79). Two earlier open trials had suggested some efficacy (n=12, Norden, *Prog Neuro-Psychopharmacol & Biol Psych* 1989, **13**, 885–93; n=22, 12/52, Markovitz *et al, Am J Psych* 1991, **148**, 1064–67). Careful dose titration was needed to minimise agitation.

Tricyclics

Generally tricyclics are not considered effective in depression associated with BPD (eg. Black *et al, J Aff Dis* 1988, **14**, 115–22) although they may help, particularly in females and those with a history of depression, hypersomnia, with unstable or drug abusing males more likely to be non-responders (Akiskal *et al Arch Gen Psych* 1980, **37**, 777–83). Tricyclics may even cause deterioration compared to placebo (Soloff *et al, Am J Psych* 1986, **143**, 1603–5).

Valproate

A small study indicated that valproate was an effective treatment for impulsive aggressive behaviour in people with personality disorders who had not responded to SSRIs (n=10, open, Kavoussi and Coccaro, *J Clin Psych* 1998, **59**, 676–80).

▼ **No efficacy**

Amfetamines

Dexamfetamine has been used but with the exception of the occasional patient has proved ineffective. It may be possible to test for amfetamine responsiveness (reviewed by Stein in *B J Psych* 1992, **161**, 167–84).

Phenytoin

Two studies have failed to show a consistent beneficial effect and often showed a negative effect (eg. Rosenblatt *et al, Curr Ther Res* 1976, **19**, 332–36).

1.12 CATATONIA

See also schizophrenia (*1.26*)

Symptoms:

Catatonia is usually a rare and potentially lethal type of schizophrenia, dominated by psychosis, stupor, negativism, resistant rigidity, hyperpyrexia, excitement or posturing. It has been linked with Neuroleptic Malignant Syndrome (*1.22*), (eg. Fink, *Biol Psych* 1996, **39**, 1–4).

Role of drugs:

ECT is generally considered the treatment of choice. The APA Task Force endorsed ECT as effective for catatonic schizophrenia (*Am J Psych* 1992, **149**, 144–5), organic catatonia (*Am J Med* 1990, **88**, 442–43) and lethal catatonia (*Acta Psych Scand* 1990, **82**, 90–92). Organic catatonia can respond to treatment of the underlying cause, eg. drug withdrawal etc. Antipsychotics are generally unhelpful. Antipsychotic-induced catatonia is also potentially fatal and must be treated symptomatically. A careful history may elicit a drug-symptom association and the potentially offending drug(s) stopped.

Reviews*: general (Fink, *Biol Psychiatry* 1994, **36**, 431–33; Singerman and Raheja, *Ann Clin Psychiatry* 1994, **6**, 259–66; Philbrick and Rummans, *J Neuropsychiatry Clin Neurosci* 1994, **6**, 1–13), clinical features, diagnosis, management and prognosis (Clark and Rickards, *Hosp Med* 1999, **60**, 740–43 and 812–15)

+ Combinations

Lorazepam + dexamfetamine

See separate drugs/groups.

Lorazepam + ECT

Concurrent or sequential use may be successful (n=5, Petrides *et al, Biol Psych* 1997, **42**, 375–81).

Thyroid hormone + reserpine

There is a case report of the combination successfully abolishing periodic catatonia (n=1, Komori *et al, Acta Psych Scand* 1997, **96**, 155–56).

● Unlicensed/Some efficacy

Benzodiazepines

There are many reports of successful benzodiazepine use in catatonia. 1.5–2mg IV lorazepam improved 4 patients with antipsychotic-induced catatonia (*J Clin Psychopharmacol* 1983, **3**, 338–42). In an open study comparing lorazepam and ECT, 76% responded to lorazepam (IV and/or oral) within five days and most who failed responded promptly to ECT. A positive response to initial parenteral challenge with lorazepam predicted a positive outcome (n=28, Bush *et al, Acta Psych Scand* 1996, **93**, 137–43). In another open study, short-term benzodiazepine

administration (oral lorazepam 2mg or diazepam 10mg IM followed, if needed, by 2–18mg oral lorazepam over 48 hours) was successful in 88% showing catatonic symptoms (n=18m Ungvari *et al, Acta Psych Scand* 1994, **89**, 285–88), although the effect may only be short-term (n=18, RCT, Ungvari *et al, Psychopharmacology* [*Berl*] 1999, **142**, 393–98). Clonazepam at 2.5mg/d orally or 1mg IV (n=3, *Am J Psych* 1989, **146**, 1230) and 10mg of diazepam IV (n=2, *Am J Psych* 1984, **141**, 284–85) and midazolam (mentioned in *Am J Psych* 1991, **148**, 809) have been used.

○ Unlicensed/Possible efficacy

Antipsychotics

These have been used (referred to in *Am J Psych* 1992, **149**, 144–45) but are generally considered unhelpful. There is, however, a remarkable case of almost complete recovery from multiple drug-resistant long-standing catatonia with risperidone up to 8mg/d (Cook *et al, Arch Gen Psych* 1996, **53**, 82–83).

Barbiturates

Thiopental and amobarbital have been used (referred to in *Am J Psych* 1992, **149**, 144–45).

Bromocriptine

5mg/d was successful in a single case (*B J Psych* 1991, **158**, 437–38).

Dantrolene

75mg IV stat successfully treated two cases of lethal catatonia (*Am J Psych* 1991, **148**, 268).

Dexamfetamine (dexamphetamine)

20mg/d was found to be synergistic with lorazepam in one catatonic schizophrenic (see lorazepam) with no evidence of tolerance (*Am J Psych* 1991, **148**, 1265).

Lithium

There have been some isolated case reports of lithium-responsive catatonia (Pheterson *et al, J Am Acad Child Psych* 1985, **24**, 235–37) with some speculation of an affective component to the condition.

Zolpidem

There have been a number of reports of dramatic improvement in catatonia with zolpidem (eg. Mastain *et al, Rev Neurol* 1995, **151**, 52–56). Zolpidem has been used as a diagnostic tool for catatonia, eg. by inducing resolution in people thought to have schizophrenia and allowing interviews to take place (cases by Thomas *et al, Lancet* 1997, **349**, 702, and Zaw and Bates, *Lancet* 1997, **349**, 1914).

1.13 DEMENTIA including Alzheimer's, Lewy Body Dementia etc

Symptoms:

Dementia: is an acquired progressive and irreversible reduction in the level of previously attained intellectual, memory and personality/emotional functioning. The main clinical features include disturbed behaviour (disorganised, inappropriate, distracted, restless, antisocial behaviour), lack of insight, impaired thinking (slow, impoverished, incoherent, rigid), poverty of speech, low mood, poor cognitive function (forgetfulness, poor attention, disorientation in time and later place), and impaired memory. Some dementias can be treated, eg. vitamin depletion (eg. B_{12}, folic acid, thiamine), infections (encephalitis, neurosyphilis) and drug toxicity.

Alzheimer's disease: * is a form of dementia characterised by senile plaques and neurofibrillary tangles present, with reduced levels of acetylcholine and other transmitters in the brain. The degree of dementia is clearly associated more with the degree of neurofibrillary pathology than with the amyloid plaque burden. It usually presents as a steady deterioration. The main features of its insidious onset are forgetfulness, lack of spontaneity, disorientation, depressed mood, decline in self-care, poor sleep (waking disorientated and perplexed) and intellectual impairment (dysphasia, dyspraxia, language decline).

Lewy Body dementia: * is a variant of Alzheimer's disease, more common in men. The key features include early-onset, persistent, well-formed, visual hallucinations and motor features of Parkinsonism. Patients may be extremely sensitive to antipsychotics which may result in a sudden onset of EPSEs, profound confusion and deterioration, and can lead to death (McKeith *et al, BMJ* 1992, **305**, 673–78; CSM warning in *Curr Problems* 1994, **20**, 6).

Role of drugs: *

Although drugs acting via transmitters do not affect the basic neurological decline,

loss of cholinergic function is still the most consistent change (Francis *et al, J Neurol Neurosurg & Psych* 1999, **66**, 137–47), behaviour disturbances may be transmitter based and well-controlled trials have shown more encouraging results.

Reviews*: general (Mayeux and Sano, *NEJM* 1999, **341**, 1670–79, 111 refs; Hachinski *et al, Arch Neurol* 1999, **56**, 735–39; Richards and Hendrie, *Arch Int Med* 1999, **159**, 789–98, 64 refs; Fairbairn, *Prescribers' J* 2000, **40**, 77–85; Hughes and Livingstone, *Prescriber* 2000, 85–95; Dooley and Lamb, *Drugs & Aging* 2000, **16**, 199–226), drug treatment (Sramek and Cutler, *Drugs & Aging* 1999, **14**, 359–73; McGleenon *et al, B J Clin Pharmacol* 1999, **48**, 471–80), guidelines for the appropriate use of cholinesterase inhibitors (Schachter and Davis, *CNS Drugs* 1999, II, 281–88; see also *ibid* 1999, **12**, 214; Van Den Berg *et al, Drugs & Aging* 2000, **16**, 123–38), selectivity of cholinesterase inhibition (Weinstock, *CNS Drugs* 1999, **12**, 307–23), role of atypical antipsychotics (Madhusoodanan *et al, CNS Drugs* 1999, **12**, 135–50), biochemistry of Alzheimer's disease (Stege and Bosman, *Drugs & Aging* 1999, **14**, 437–46), delirium management (Flacker and Marcantonio, *Drugs & Aging* 1998, **13**, 119–30).

BNF Listed

Co-dergocrine ('Hydergine'®) *

The Cochrane review of the 19 adequate trials suggests that co-dergocrine shows significant benefits on most rating scales but that the data is limited (Olin *et al, CDSR* 2000, CD000359; see also Bullock, *EBMH* 1999, **2**, 15).

Donepezil *

Donepezil is an acetylcholinesterase inhibitor licensed for the symptomatic treatment of mild or moderate Alzheimer's disease. Results from a multinational trial show that the response is dose-related (10mg/d> 5mg/d) with all measured scales improving (n=818, p/c, 30/52, Burns *et al, Demen & Ger Cog Dis* 1999, **10**, 237–44). In a trial of donepezil in patients with Alzheimer's disease, 5mg (n=154) and 10mg (n=157) improved cognitive function and global functioning (RCT, 24/52, Rogers *et al,*

Neurology 1998, **50**, 136–45; review by Warner, *EBMH* 1998, **1**, 88). Donepezil may also have potential mildly positive effects on emotional and behavioural symptoms in AD as well as cognitive function (n=25, open, Weiner *et al, J Clin Psych* 2000, **61**, 487–92). No withdrawal effects have been seen, probably as its half-life is 70 hours. Several studies have indicated donepezil may be cost-effective (Neumann *et al, Neurology* 1999, **52**, 1138–46; Foster and Plosker, *PharmacoEconomics* 1999, **16**, 99–114). The Cochrane Review concludes that donepezil produces modest improvements in cognitive function (Birks *et al, CDSR* 2000, CD001190).

Reviews*: Barner and Gray (*Ann Pharmacother* 1998, **32**, 70–77, 25 refs; Shintani and Uchida, *Am J Health-Sys Pharm* 1997, **54**, 2805–10; Dooley and Lamb, *Drugs Aging* 2000, **16**, 199–226).

Galantamine *
Galantamine, derived from snowdrop bulbs, is indicated for mild to moderate Alzheimer's disease. It is a competitive reversible inhibition of acetylcholinesterase, but also stimulates pre- and postsynaptic nicotinic receptors. Doses should be twice a day, preferably with morning and evening meals to minimise cholinergic side-effects. Gradual introduction is recommended, starting at 4mg bd for 4/52, then 8mg bd for 4/52, increasing to 12mg bd if appropriate. Galantamine has been shown at 16–24mg/d to be significantly superior to placebo (n=978, 5/12, RCT, Tariot *et al, Neurology* 2000, **54**, 2269–76), with the benefit sustained over 12 months with the 24mg/d dose (n=636, 6/12 plus 6/12 extension, RCT, Raskind *et al, Neurology* 2000, **54**, 2261–68). A review of 5 RCT phase III trials showed galantamine to be significantly superior to placebo (n=3,000, Lilienfeld and Parys, *Dement Geriatr Cogn Disord* 2000, **11** [Suppl 1], 19–27). There appears to be no rebound from abrupt discontinuation.

Reviews: general (Sramek *et al, Expert Opin Investig Drugs* 2000, **9**, 2393–402; Blesa, *Dement Geriatr Cogn Disord* 2000, **11**[Suppl 1], 28–34).

Rivastigmine *
Rivastigmine is a carbamate-derived acetylcholinesterase inhibitor licensed for the treatment of mild to moderately severe Alzheimer's disease. 6–12mg/d in divided doses has shown a modest effect in delaying cognitive decline, with 20% of patients showing some significant benefit. The dose must be titrated at weekly intervals to reduce side-effects. In a recent trial, rivastigmine improved global functioning and cognition, particularly in daily living activities (n=725, RCT, 26/52, Rosler *et al, BMJ* 1999, **318**, 633–38). Another trial comparing low-dose rivastigmine (1–4mg/d), high-dose rivastigmine (6–12mg/d) and placebo showed a dose-dependent clinically and statistically significant improvement in cognitive and global assessments, and in activities of daily living. (RCT, n=725, Rosler *et al, B303 Exelon Study Group, BMJ* 1999, **318**, 633–40; see also editorial by Flicker, *BMJ* 1999, **318**, 515–16 editorial, who concluded the effect appears modest, but may be more prominent in some patients than others). A Cochrane Review of 7 trials concluded that rivastigmine was beneficial at 6–12mg/d in mild to moderate Alzheimer's (n=3370, Birks *et al, CDSR* 2000, CD001191; review in *EBMH* 2000, **3**, 10).

Reviews*: general (Jones, *Prescriber* 1999, **10**, 133–36; Sim, *Hosp Med* 1999, **60**, 731–35; *Drug & Ther Bull* 2000, **38**, 15–16, 13 refs; Anon, *Formulary Monograph Service* Jul 2000, 279–86; *Prescrire International* 1999, **8**, 47–48; Jann, *Pharmacotherapy* 2000, **20**, 1–12, 50 refs; Gottwald and Rozanski, *Expert Opin Investig Drugs* 1999, **8**, 1673–82).

Tacrine *
Tacrine is licensed in the UK, but not marketed. It is a longer-acting, competitive, reversible cholineresterase inhibitor that produces moderate symptomatic benefit in some people with Alzheimer's disease. About 15% can tolerate the drug and derive clinical improvement and a further 15% will tolerate the drug and show no worsening of cognitive symptoms, although the overall course of the disease is not detectably altered. A review of 49 trials (inc. 21 RCTs), showed modest efficacy in some patients with mild to moderate

AD, but the long-term effects unknown (Arrieta and Artalejo, *Age & Ageing* 1998, **27**[Suppl1], 161–79). A Cochrane Review concludes that the evidence for tacrine is unconvincing, but sparse (Qizilbash *et al, CDSR* 2000, CD000202). Raised liver enzymes are the major problem.

+   **Combinations**
Donepezil + gabapentin *
Behavioural control from gabapentin may augment the cognitive improvement from donepezil (n=2, Dallocchio *et al, J Clin Psych* 2000, **61**, 64).

○   **Unlicensed/Possible efficacy**
Amantadine
In a study cerebral infarction presenting as dementia, some improved significantly on doses of up to 100–150mg/d (n=33, Jibiki *et al, Acta Therapeutica* 1993, **19**, 389–96).

Antidepressants
Lower doses can be used to treat depression although side-effects can be a problem. Increasing the trial treatment period from 4 to 8 weeks increases the 'response' rate from 54% to 70% (*Int J Geriatr Psych* 1989, **4**, 191–95) and so longer trials may be justified. Drugs with no anticholinergic effect should be preferred.

Antipsychotics *
Antipsychotics are widely used as symptomatic treatments of aggressive, agitated behaviour and as sedatives. With the availability of newer agents, the use of traditional agents such as phenothiazines may be unnecessary clinically, although not without significant financial implications. An in-depth review of clinical data concluded that conventional anti-psychotics appear to be only modestly effective for behavioural problems associated with dementia, and their short-term benefit is outweighed by the dramatically increased risk of TD among the elderly (Pollock *et al, Consultant Pharm* 1999, **14**, 1251–58). Antipsychotics should not be used as substitutes for poor standards of care, must be adjuncts to other interventions, must be monitored and reviewed regularly. They increase the rates of falls, sedation, EPSEs and rate of decline in cognitive function,

irrespective of initial severity (McShane *et al, BMJ* 1997, **314**, 266–70). A meta-analysis of the 16 RCTs published between 1966 and 1997, showed that antipsychotics have an inconsistent and small but significant effect compared to placebo, but with the drugs having similar efficacy, side-effects and drop-out rates (Lanctôt *et al, J Clin Psych* 1998, **59**, 55–61). Haloperidol 2–3mg/d decreased psychosis and disruptive behaviour, although 20% developed moderate to severe EPSEs (Knable, *EBMH* 1999, **2**, 47–48).

Of the newer agents, **risperidone** seems effective at an optimum dose of 1mg/d in this population, eg. for persistent, purposelessness vocalisations (eg. n=2, Kopala and Honer, *Int J Ger Psychiatry* 1997, **12**, 73–77) and for aggression and behavioural disturbances (n=344, 13/52, d/b, De Deyn *et al, Neurology* 1999, **53**, 946–55). Maximum benefit may occur after 7–10 days with minimal sedation (n=5, Jeanblanc and Davis, *Am J Psych* 1995, **152**, 1239). In patients with Lewy Body dementia, psychotic and behavioural symptoms may respond well to low dose risperidone (n=3, Allen *et al, Lancet* 1995, **346**, 185), although even then severe EPSEs (especially rigidity) have occurred at 1mg/d (n=3, McKeith *et al, Lancet* 1995, **346**, 699). In an open-label study extension, patients with dementia receiving risperidone (optimal range 0.75–1.5mg/d) had a very low incidence of TD compared to that expected with typical antipsychotics (n=330, open, Jeste *et al, Am J Psych* 2000, **157**, 1150–55). 1mg/d was shown to be the optimum dose of risperidone for improving psychotic and aggressive behaviour in institutionalised elderly patients with severe dementia (RCT, n=625, Katz *et al, J Clin Psych* 1999, **60**, 107–15). Starting at very low doses (eg. 0.25mg/d) using the syrup formulation improves tolerability. In a trial of **olanzapine** 2.5–7.5mg/d in Lewy Body Dementia, only 2 tolerated the drug with clear improvement, and 5 could not tolerate it or gained no benefit (n=8, open, Walker *et al, Int J Ger Psych* 1999, **14**, 459–66).

Reviews*: general plus algorithm (Defilippi and Crismon, *Pharmacotherapy* 2000, **20**, 23–33, 43 refs).

Buspirone *

There have been reports of vocal grunts, rocking, difficult behaviour and choreaothetoid movements improving with buspirone (eg. n=1, *Lancet* 1988, **i**, 1169; n=1, Hamner *et al, J Clin Psychopharmacol* 1996, **16**, 261–62).

Carbamazepine

A study of nursing home patients with agitation and dementia comparing individualised doses of carbamazepine with placebo showed significant short-term efficacy with generally good safety and tolerability (6/52, 51 sites, randomised, Tariot *et al, Am J Psych* 1998, **155**, 54–61).

Cycloserine

Cycloserine 5–50mg/d (a partial agonist acting at the NMDA glycine receptor complex) has been shown to enhance implicit memory in Alzheimer patients, supporting the development of NMDA receptor-mediated glutamatergic interventions for the treatment of Alzheimer-related memory disorders (n=108, p/c, d/b, 10/52, Schwartz *et al, Neurology* 1996, **46**, 420–24). 100mg/d cycloserine produced a significant improvement in cognitive scores in a short trial (n=17, RCT, Tsai *et al, Am J Psych* 1999, **156**, 467–69).

Estrogen (oestrogen) *

Estrogen is a potent factor that prevents vascular disease and improves blood flow in diseased vessels, including blood flow in regions of the brain affected by AD. Estrogen also has direct effects on neuronal function that may play an important role not only in the preservation of neurons, but in the repair of neurons damaged by disease processes. It has been suggested that the effects of estrogen on the CNS may be effective in the treatment and prevention (review, Birge, *Neurology* 1997, **48** [Suppl 7], S36–41), as endogenous estrogen levels may decline in post-menopausal women in whom Alzheimer's disease develops (n=143, Manly *et al, Neurology* 2000, **54**, 833–38). A meta-analysis of 7 randomised and 1 non-randomised studies indicates that estrogen therapy may reduce the risk of developing dementia in post-menopausal women (Yaffe *et al, JAMA* 1998, **279**, 688–95; review by Whalley, *EBMH* 1998, **1**, 119). However, a series of recent trials have failed to show an effect from Premarin 0.625mg/d or 1.25mg/d (RCT, n=120, 12/12, Mulnard *et al, JAMA* 2000, **283**, 1007–15; Shaywitz and Shaywitz, *JAMA* 2000, **283**, 1055–56; editorial, review by Hogervorst and McShane, *EBMH* 2000, **3**, 83) short-term estrogen (RCT, n=42 women, 16/52, Henderson *et al, Neurology* 2000, **54**, 295–302) and conjugated estrogens 12.5mg/d (n=50, d/b, 12/52, Wang *et al, Neurology* 2000, **54**, 2061–66).

Reviews*: use in elderly men (review and n=2, Shelton and Brooks, *Ann Pharmacother* 1999, **33**, 808–12), general (Monk and Brodaty, *Demen & Ger Cog Disord* 2000, **11**, 1–10).

Gabapentin *

Gabapentin has been used for behavioural agitation in Alzheimer's (Regan and Gordon, *J Clin Psychopharmacol* 1997, **17**, 59–60; n=1, Goldenberg *et al, Drugs & Aging* 1998, **13**, 183–84), and in aggressive and agitated demented elderly patients, 70% were much or greatly improved with gabapentin (n=24, case series, Hawkins *et al, Am J Ger Psych* 2000, **8**, 221–25; see also n=1, Ryback and Ryback, *Am J Psych* 1995, **152**, 1399).

Ginkgo biloba *

Ginkgo biloba 120mg/d stabilised and, in some patients improved, cognitive function for 6–12 months in mild-to-moderate Alzheimer's and multi-infarct dementia (n=155) compared to placebo (n=154), (RCT, Le Bars *et al, JAMA* 1997, **278**, 1327–32). It must be given for 1–3 months before the full therapeutic effect is seen (review in *Medical Letter* 1998, **40**, 63–64). In a trial of mild to severe Alzheimer's, the placebo group showed a significant decline in all measures (ADAS-cog, GERRI and CGI) whilst the GB group were considered to have at least slightly improved on some scales (n=309, d/b, p/c, 26/52, Le Bars *et al, Dement & Ger Cog Disord* 2000, **11**, 230–37). A rigorous meta-analysis by Oken *et al* (*Arch Neurol* 1998, **55**, 1409–15, reviewed by Bernabei, *EBMH*

1999, **2**, 82), concluded that GB was effective in mild-to-moderate Alzheimer's, and only slightly inferior to donepezil and rivastigmine.

Insulin *

Elevating insulin levels (with or without hyperglycaemia) improves memory in people with Alzheimer's (n=23 + 14 controls, Craft *et al, Arch Gen Psych* 1999, **56**, 1135–40).

Lamotrigine *

There is a case of frontal lobe dementia responding well to lamotrigine up to 100mg/d, but not to other treatments (n=1, 6/12, Devarajan *et al, Am J Psych* 2000, **157**, 1178, letter).

Naftidrofuryl *

This is a cerebral vasodilator with some limited effect on cognitive and global functioning (eg. n=84, RCT, Emeriau *et al, Clin Ther* 2000, **22**, 834–44; Goldline, *Clin Ther* 2000, **22**, 1251–52).

Naltrexone and naloxone

The opioid system may play a role in memory storage. Small scale studies showed some clinical efficacy, but these have not been replicated (review in *Ann Pharmacother* 1993, **27**, 447–80).

Nicotine *

Studies have shown reduced nicotinic cholinergic receptors in the frontal cortex. Nicotine may stimulate the release of acetylcholine in this area. Nicotine is known to improve attention, memory, vigilance and information processing in (so far) healthy humans, but transdermal nicotine (up to 21mg/d) had no significant effect on cognitive functions in patients with Alzheimer's disease (n=18, p/c, d/b, c/o, Snaedal *et al, Dementia* 1996, **7**, 47–52). A Cochrane Review concludes that there is no reliable evidence for a beneficial effect (Lopez-Arrieta *et al, CDSR* 2000, CD00149).

NSAIDs *

There is some evidence that NSAIDs might prevent or delay the onset of Alzheimer's and Pick's diseases. A retrospective study in probable Alzheimer's showed that the NSAID group showed less decline in verbal fluency, orientation and spatial recognition (n=210, Rich *et al, Neurology* 1995, **45**, 51–55) and a population-based study suggested a possible protective effect of NSAIDs on the risk of AD (Andersen *et al,*

Neurology 1995, **45**, 1441–45). A further study showed that people who took NSAIDs (other than aspirin) on more than an occasional basis were 30–60% less likely to develop Alzheimer's disease than those who did not, with some evidence of a dose-dependent effect (Stewart *et al, Neurology* 1997, **48**, 626–32). However, a trial of diclofenac + misoprostol in Alzheimer's disease showed no significant differences, but with a trend towards NSAID having some positive effects (n=41, RCT, 25/52, Scharf *et al, Neurology* 1999, **53**, 197–201). A 5-year case-control study of post-mortem brain tissue, showed no significant differences in the amount of inflammatory glia, plaques, or tangles in either diagnostic group, and so long-term NSAIDs in people with Alzheimer's disease may enhanced cognitive performance but not alleviate the progression of the pathological changes (n=22, Halliday *et al, Arch Neurol* 2000, **57**, 831–36; see also postmortem study, Mackenzie, *Neurology* 2000, **54**, 732–35).

Reviews: general (Lucca, *CNS Drugs* 1999, **11**, 207–24 and 372; Flynn and Theesen, *Ann Pharmacother* 1999, **33**, 840–49).

Piracetam *

Piracetam stimulates ACh release. Mild effects may occur when used alone or with an ACh precursor, although a Cochrane Review concludes that the evidence is not robust enough to prove an effect (Flicker *et al, CDSR* 2000, CD001011).

Selegiline *

Selegiline may improve MMSE scores, but with no apparent effect on brain lesions or degenerative changes in brain tissue (n=17, Alafuzoff *et al, Eur J Clin Pharmacol* 2000, **55**, 815–19), although one trial (with questionable method-ology) of 10mg/d indicated some slowing of the disease (n=341, RCT, Sano *et al, NEJM* 1997, **336**, 1216–22). A Cochrane Review concludes that the evidence is promising but not yet conclusive to recommend routine use (Birks and Flicker, *CDSR* 2000, CD000442).

SSRIs *

Two studies have shown a potential effect with **citalopram**. Improved confusion, mood, restlessness and irritability was noted with citalopram in one study in Alzheimer's, but not vascular dementia (n=98, *B J Psych* 1990, **157**, 894–901) and improved cognitive and emotional functioning has been reported with citalopram in patients with dementia (eg. Nyth *et al*, *Acta Psych Scand* 1992, **86**, 138–45; review by Pollock *et al*, *Consultant Pharm* 1999, **14**, 1251–58). A trial showed slight improvement in confusion/anxiety with fluvoxamine, but not cognition or behaviour (n=46, *Acta Psych Scand* 1992, **85**, 453–56).

Testosterone *

Testosterone supplements have been reported to prevent Alzheimer's disease in both men and women (Anon, *Pharm J* 2000, **264**, 205).

Trazodone *

Some improvements in agitated behaviours in dementia have been shown, (comparison with haloperidol, n=28, RCT, *Am J Geriatr Psychiatry* 1997, **5**, 60–69).

Valproate

In a prospective study in 16 patients (68–95yr) unresponsive to other pharmacotherapy, divalproex sodium 750–2500mg/d for 5 to 34 weeks was generally well tolerated and was moderately effective in decreasing physical agitation and aggression. Delusions and hallucinations did not appear to improve markedly (n=16, open, Herrmann, *Can J Psych* 1998, **43**, 69–72). Delirium and aggression may improve in demented patients (n=13, open, Horiguchi *et al*, *Int J Psych Clin Pract* 1998, **2**, 35–39).

Vitamins *

A study in Hawaii suggested that vitamin E and C supplements may protect against vascular dementia and may improve cognitive function in later life in men (n=3385, Masaki *et al*, *Neurology* 2000, **54**, 1265–72).

Zolpidem

This has been used for dementia-related insomnia and night-time wandering (Shelton and Hocking, *Ann Pharmacother* 1997, **31**, 319–22).

▼ No efficacy

Prednisone *

Prednisone 10-20mg/d has been shown to be ineffective (RCT, n=138, 56/52, Aisen *et al, Neurology* 2000, **54**, 588–93), despite initial enthusiasm from a pilot study, where 20mg/d showed some short-term effect in suppressing acute phase proteins, which have a role in plaque formation (n=20, open, Aisen *et al, Dementia* 1996, **7**, 201–6).

Thiamine

No effect was noted in a one year trial (n=15, *Arch Neurol* 1991, **48**, 81–83).

1.14 DEPRESSION

See also bipolar mood disorder (*1.10*), dysthymia (*1.15*), rapid cycling mood disorder (*1.27*) and mania/hypomania (*1.19*)

Depression is a common illness, affecting 3% of the population per year, 25% of whom do not see their GP and in 50% of those that do, it is not detected. Sadly, depression remains under-diagnosed, under-treated (especially in men and under 30s) and antidepressants appear under-represented in suicides (n=5281 suicides, Isacsson *et al, B J Psych* 1999, **174**, 259–65). The overall cost of depression (eg. work, family, other illnesses) is very high for an eminently treatable condition.

Symptoms:

People with depression usually show a mixture of biological symptoms (insomnia or hypersomnia, diurnal variation in mood, low appetite, fatigue or loss of energy, constipation, loss of libido, weight loss or gain) and psychiatric symptoms (depressed mood, loss of interest or pleasure, poor memory, psychomotor agitation or retardation, recurrent thoughts of death or suicide, anxiety, feelings of worthlessness or guilt, including delusions etc). Depression does not include the normal reaction to the death of a loved one.

Causes:

Precipitating factors can include, drugs and drug abuse, physical illness and stress, eg. bereavement, loss of job, birth of child, break-up of relationship, work stress, poor social background, time of year etc.

Role of drugs: *

Although most depressions will resolve

with time, antidepressants have a major role in hastening this recovery and reducing suffering. Antidepressants are effective, not addictive and do not generally lose efficacy with prolonged use. Adequate doses (see later) are needed for clinical effect, and continuation for an appropriate period (see later) will minimise relapse. Inadequate treatment and the use of toxic drugs is difficult to defend other than on acquisition cost grounds. Sadly, there still appears to be much sub-therapeutic dosing and duration in the UK, with paroxetine and fluoxetine most likely to be prescribed for a therapeutic period (151 GP practice study, Lawrenson *et al, J Aff Dis* 2000, **59**, 149–57). Drugs may also be effective in reducing medically unexplained physical symptoms, eg. headache, tinnitus etc in depression (review, O'Malley *et al, J Fam Pract* 1999, **48**, 980–90; reviewed by Price, *EBMH* 2000, **3**, 84).

A viable option is combining medicines with long-term maintenance CBT (Blackburn and Moore, *B J Psych* 1997, **171**, 328–34) or IPT (RCT, n=187, elderly, Reynolds *et al, JAMA* 1999, **281**, 39–45), where a combination is generally more effective than either individually (meta-analysis, DeRubeis *et al, Am J Psych* 1999, **156**, 1007–13; disputed by Taylor *et al, Am J Psych* 2000, **157**, 1025–26), including where CBT may reduce relapse rates in people on maintenance antidepressants with residual depressive symptoms (Paykel *et al, Arch Gen Psych* 1999, **56**, 829–35; review by McGinn, *EBMH* 2000, **3**, 48). In patients either randomised to counselling or antidepressants, or were allowed to choose between drugs and counselling, no differences were found either in the initial characteristics or in the outcomes and both were equally effective at 8 weeks, so expressing a preference had no apparent effect or benefit on outcomes (n=323, Bedi *et al, B J Psych* 2000, **177**, 312–18).

Treatment of depression*:

The general principles of treatment of depression (with antidepressants) can be summed up by the six D's: diagnosis, drug-related, drug, dose, duration and discontinuation:

1. Diagnosis – making or being able to make a diagnosis helps.

2. Drug-related causes eliminated, eg. excessive caffeine intake, other drugs liable to cause depression (see *5.5*), physical (eg. low folate levels) and environmental causes etc.

3. Drug and Dose

Acute therapy: Antidepressants must be increased to therapeutic doses, eg. standard dose SSRI, 125–150mg/d tricyclic, and maintained for an adequate duration. If depression remains completely unchanged at 4 weeks of therapeutic dosing, an alternate drug should be tried. Minimal improvement within the first 4 weeks should indicate a further 2-week trial, then change to an alternate drug if there is no further response (n=593, Quitkin *et al, Arch Gen Psych* 1996, **53**, 785–92). These times should probably be doubled in the elderly. It has been suggested that: (i) among responders, the onset of improvement occurs in more than 70% of cases within the first 3 weeks of treatment (ii) there is no evidence of a pronounced increase in improvement rates beyond this time point, and (iii) early improvement is highly predictive of better long-term outcomes (Stassen and Angst, *CNS Drugs* 1998, **9**, 177–84). NB. The now often quoted meta-analysis by Bollini *et al* (*B J Psych* 1999, **174**, 297–303, gently reviewed by Goodwin in *EBMH* 1999, **2**, 106) claims that 'sub-therapeutic' doses of antidepressants are effective. This paper is flawed regarding tricyclics and is only valid if fluoxetine 30mg/d is considered sub-therapeutic, plainly inaccurate as 5mg/d is the minimum effective dose. For advice on switching anti-depressants, see *2.2.2*.

4. Duration:

A. Continuation therapy*: Proper treatment of depression requires relief not just of acute symptoms but continued treatment while the person remains vulnerable. Inadequate or no treatment for six months post-response in controlled trials has resulted in relapse rates as high as 50% (cf. 20% with adequate treatment, although compliance was not certain in these cases). If depression remits in 12 weeks, continued treatment for 6 months minimises the risk of relapse, but longer therapy confers little additional benefit, except in people with additional relapse risk factors (n=395, RCT, 52/52, Reimherr *et al, Am J Psych* 1998, **155**, 1247–53). People who continue with their initial antidepressant (rather than need to switch or just discontinue) also have lower relapse/recurrence rates over two years (retrospective study, n=4052, Melfi *et al, Arch Gen Psych* 1998, **55**, 1128–32). Consistent antidepressant use (eg. 4/12 continuous therapy with an SSRI) is associated with lowest risk of relapse or recurrence (Claxton *et al, B J Psych* 2000, **177**, 1633–68). Continuation doses should be the **same or close to the therapeutic dose** (*J Aff Dis* 1993, **27**, 139–45). In the elderly, therapy for up to two years after recovery may be needed (*Int J Ger Psych* 1992, **7**, 617–19; *B J Psych* 1993, **162**, 175–82) although the need for such long-term therapy has been challenged (*Lancet* 1993, **341**, 1444). Patients should also be advised that anti-depressants are not 'addictive' as such.

B.   Prophylactic   therapy*: Maintenance therapy is indicated for many people. 25% people with depression only have one episode (Piccinelli and Wilkinson, *B J Psych* 1994, **164**, 297–304) so 75% have a further episode, usually within 2 to 3 years, if untreated. There is a 10-fold greater risk of recurrence of depression in a person with one previous episode of depression than with no previous episode of depression and a 14–18-fold greater risk with more than one previous episode (Thase and Sullivan, *CNS Drugs* 1995, **4**, 261–77). In a 10-year prospective study of multiple recurrences of major depression, the risk of recurrence increased by 16% with each successive episode, but the risk of recurrence progressively decreased as duration of recovery increased (n=318, Solomon *et al, Am J Psych* 2000, **157**, 229–33). Risk factors for relapse include recurrent dysthymia, concurrent non-affective psychiatric illness, chronic medical disorder and a

history of relapses. With episodes less than 2½ years apart, treatment for at least 5 years may be warranted (Kupfer *et al Arch Gen Psych* 1992, **49**, 769–73). Most antidepressants have been shown to be effective for continuation or maintenance therapy of unipolar depression (reviewed by Montgomery *et al, Int Clin Psychopharmacol* 1994, **9** [Suppl 1], 49–53; *B J Hosp Med* 1994, **52**, 5–6).

General minimum treatment: duration recommendations:

First episode — 6 months post-recovery (see 3 above)
Second episode — 2–3 years
Third episode — 5 years or longer.

5. **Discontinuation:** When discontinuing therapy is considered appropriate, slowly reduce doses over a minimum of four weeks. Discontinuation syndromes have been reported for nearly all antidepressants. Discontinuation symptoms usually appear within 1–3 days of stopping treatment and improve within a week, while recurrence of depression begins after 3 weeks and continues to worsen. See switching antidepressants in *2.2.2* for a further review, eg. symptoms and management.

Treatment-resistant depression: *
True 'treatment-resistant' depression often needs a systematic approach to solve. Remember also that resistant depression may also be undiagnosed bipolar (see next section):

1. **Escalate doses for an adequate duration,** an appropriate action for drugs with a dose-response curve, eg. up to 300mg/d or more of a tricyclic or other drug (eg. venlafaxine), or to tolerance (monitoring plasma levels carefully), remembering that a few people have multiple copies of, eg.CYP2D6 and may rapidly metabolise tricyclics. Treatment for up to 9–17 weeks may also be needed (Greenhouse *et al, J Aff Dis* 1987, **13**, 259–66). SSRIs tend to have a flat dose-response curve, so switching is probably the best ploy (Corruble and Guelfi, *Acta Psych Scand* 2000, **101**, 343–48).

2. **Check blood levels** – levels of 300–400mcg/l of tricyclics have been used by some in true refractory cases

(see Hodgkiss *et al, Hum Psycho-pharmacol* 1995, **10**, 407–15). Dothiepin, amitriptyline and clomipramine have been the tricyclics preferred for high dose therapy.

3. **Switch drugs** – ensure all drug classes have been tried optimally, eg. SSRIs, tricyclics, venlafaxine, mirtazapine, moclobemide (at much higher doses than are currently recommended, eg. over 600mg/d), MAOIs (although high dose moclobemide may be a suitable and safer alternative) etc.

4. **Augment or combine** – use logical combinations of antidepressants, (see later in this section), eg. mirtazapine (open, n=20, Carpenter, *J Clin Psych* 1999, **80**, 45–49), lithium, particularly with tricyclics and MAOIs, carbamazepine (but not with tricyclics, where it reduces plasma levels, see *4.5.1*), valproate, lithium/clomipramine/tryptophan, phenelzine/lithium/tryptophan and tricyclic/MAOI. SSRIs should not routinely be used with tricyclics unless with regular blood level testing or at all with MAOIs or tryptophan (see *4.3.4*). Use of logical augmentation is also possible, eg. levothyroxine, liothyronine, buspirone, pindolol, mirtazapine etc.

5. **Assure compliance**, eg. by plasma levels etc.

Reviews*: algorithm, the role of psychosurgery and ECT, and extensive review (Bridges *et al, B J Hosp Med* 1995, **54**, 501–6), drug treatments (O'Reardon *et al, Curr Opin Psych* 2000, **13**, 93–98).

Bipolar depression:

This tends to be much longer-lasting than unipolar depression (up to 50% may still be depressed at one year, Hlastala *et al, Depress Anxiety* 1997, **5**, 73–83), and much more difficult to treat. The general principles of management include:

1. Use of mood stabilisers in the initial acute stage, eg. lithium and valproate show good responses in open trials of bipolar depression (discussion by Sachs *et al, Psychiatr Clin North Am* 1996, **19**, 215–36), as does carbamazepine (open, Dilsaver *et al, Biol Psych* 1996, **40**, 935–37).

2. Add an antidepressant if necessary, starting with lowest switch risk drugs, eg. SSRIs, mirtazapine, bupropion.

3. Minimise antidepressant exposure by attempting gradual taper after a continuation phase, provided the patient is genuinely euthymic.

4. Offer ECT for patients at immediate risk of self-harm or unable to tolerate antidepressants. ECT may be better in older people.

5. Beware of inducing a mixed state in bipolar III, where the risk of self-harm is high.

The risk of switching to mania with antidepressants in bipolar depression varies from 31–70%. It usually occurs within the first 12 weeks, is lower if used with a mood stabiliser and, if it develops, the best plan is to reduce the antidepressant dose immediately and allow the mood to settle for a month or so. The switch rates in double-blind trials have been reported to be imipramine 9.5%, placebo 7% and fluoxetine 0–16% (n=89, Cohn *et al, Int Clin Psychopharmacol* 1989, **4**, 313–22), and tranylcypromine 24% and imipramine 28% (n=56, RCT, Himmelhoch *et al, Am J Psych* 1991, **148**, 910–16).

Loss of antidepressant efficacy:

This has been reported during long-term maintenance treatment (dubbed 'poop-out') in 9–33% patients with many drugs, eg. fluoxetine, sertraline, amoxapine, tricyclics, MAOIs etc. Reasons may include non-compliance, loss of initial placebo response, loss of true drug effect, pharmacological tolerance, accumulation of detrimental metabolites, change in illness pathology, unrecognised rapid cycling and a genuine lack of prophylactic efficacy. Strategies to overcome this include:

1. Increase the dose (logical, and works with, eg. fluoxetine, ie. Fava *et al, Am J Psych* 1994, **151**, 1372–74).

2. Decrease the dose (this may work if the dose has exceeded any 'therapeutic window', but this is poorly supported by published data).

3. Addition of dopamine antagonists, eg. bromocriptine (reviewed by Byrne and Rothschild, see below).

4. Augment with mood stabilisers, anticonvulsants, thyroid, another antidepressant etc.

5. Drug holiday (poorly supported by the literature).

6. Switch to a different drug or another similar drug.

7. Ensure compliance.

Reviews: study and review (Byrne and Rothschild, *J Clin Psych* 1998, **59**, 279–88), short section within review by Sechter and Lane (*J Serotonin Res*, 1997, 30–33).

Choice of drugs:

All the main drugs appear to have broadly similar efficacy and so antidepressant choice will be based upon the features of depression, suicide risk, concomitant therapy, concurrent illness, side-effect tolerability, time to reach therapeutic dose, cost and special considerations, eg. cognitive impairment, driving etc. As non-compliance or inadequate dosage are the main causes of drug failure, choice of drug should consider these factors. Nearly all antidepressants can be given once a day.

Suicidality:

The risk of suicide appears to be the same with tricyclics as with the newer drugs, but the rates of death are higher with tricyclics (study of USA national database, Kapur *et al, JAMA* 1992, **268**, 3441–45; Jick *et al, BMJ* 1995, **310**, 215–18). 81.6% of UK deaths from single antidepressant overdose from 1987–1992 (average 268, range 238–288pa) were due to amitriptyline and dothiepin and 97% of all single antidepressant overdose deaths were due to the tricyclics (Henry *et al, BMJ* 1995, **310**, 221–24). The SSRIs and other newer agents have low toxicity in overdose. Antidepressants have been alleged to be associated with the emergence of suicidal tendencies (review by Teicher *et al, Drug Safety* 1993, **8**, 186–212). In fact, fluoxetine shows a slight *reduction* in suicidal behaviour, rather than an increase (n=185, Leon *et al, Am J Psych* 1999, **156**, 195–201). In Sweden, a study of 5281 suicides from 1992–94 showed that antidepressants were detectable in only 12.4% of men and 26.2% of women but overdose by antidepressant was the probable cause of death in only 2.1% of men and 7.9% of women, indicating that underuse of anti-depressants was perhaps more relevant than absolute toxicity (n=5281, Isacsson *et al, B J Psych* 1999, **174**, 259–65).

Reviews: toxicity of newer anti-depressants (Henry, *Adv Psych Treat* 1997, **3**, 41–45), maintenance pharmaco-therapy in unipolar depression (Forshall and Nutt, *Psych Bull* 1999, **23**, 370–73),

prevention and relapse of depression (Edwards, *Adv Psych Treat* 1997, **3**, 52–57) and refractory depression in bipolars (Post *et al, Depress Anxiety* 1997, **5**, 175–89), rational drug use (Cohen, *Pharmacotherapy* 1997, **17**, 45–61), depression in late life consensus statement (Lebowitz *et al, JAMA* 1997, **278**, 1186–90), algorithm for pharmaco-therapy in unipolar depression (Kasper *et al, Int J Psych Clin Pract* 1997, **1**, S5–7), emergency treatment of depression (Porter and Ferrier, *Adv Psych Treat* 1999, **5**, 3–10), general (Hawley *et al, Prescriber* 1999, **10**, 69–88; Hale, *BMJ* 1997, **315**, 43–46, 6 refs; Spigset and Martensson, *BMJ* 1999, **318**, 1181–91; Doris *et al, Lancet* 1999, **354**, 1369–75, 85 refs), TDM of antidepressants (Burke and Preskorn, *Clin Pharmacokinet* 1999, **37**, 147–65, 87 refs), in primary care (Mulrow *et al, Am J Med* 2000, **108**, 54–64; Thornett, *Prescriber* 2000, **11**, 49–61), in children and adolescents (Emslie and Mayes, *CNS Drugs* 1999, **11**, 181–89) and in women (Desai and Jann, *J Am Pharm Assoc* 2000, **40**, 525–37).

Types of antidepressants:

There are many classifications of anti-depressants. It is important to remember that reuptake inhibition by anti-depressants is just the start of a cascade of events involving changes in the sensitivities of receptors at (somato-dendritic) sites, eg. $5HT_{1A}$ receptors, at pre- and post-synaptic sites, as well as changes in neuronal signal transduction beyond the receptor. All neurotransmitter systems seem interdependent. On a transmitter/probable mechanism basis, the following may, however, be useful:

1. Noradrenaline and serotonin reuptake inhibition, eg. tricyclics, venlafaxine (above 150mg/d).
2. Serotonin reuptake inhibition, eg. SSRIs, venlafaxine (lower dose).
3. Noradrenaline reuptake inhibition, eg. reboxetine.
4. $5\text{-}HT_2$ receptor blockade plus sero-tonin reuptake inhibition, eg. nefazo-done, trazodone.
5. Monoamine oxidase inhibition, eg. moclobemide, MAOIs.
6. Pre-synaptic alpha-2-autoreceptor and heteroceptor blockade, eg. mirtazapine.
7. Serotonin precursor, eg. tryptophan.

8. Dopamine reuptake blockers, eg. bupropion (only licensed in UK for smoking cessation).

BNF Listed

Selective Serotonin Reuptake Inhibitors (SSRIs)

The SSRIs are now first choice drugs in depression in most patients due to their low overdose risk, safety in heart disease and better side-effect profile (eg. lacking anticholinergic, sedation and weight gain effects).

Although chemically distinct, the SSRIs are essentially more similar than different, are all effective antidepressants but their ADR profiles and potential for interactions may help identify clinical differences. Discontinuation rates with SSRIs are probably lower than with the older TCAs (10% overall, 25% due to side-effects), but not *that* great (Anderson and Tomenson, *BMJ* 1995, **310**, 1433–38) and not significantly lower than with the newer tricyclics eg. lofepramine (meta-analysis and investigation of hetero-genicity, Hotopf *et al, B J Psych* 1997, **170**, 120–27).

Reviews*: differences in their pharmacological and clinical profiles (de Jonghe and Swinkels, *CNS Drugs* 1997, **7**, 452–67; Edwards and Anderson, *Drugs* 1999, **57**, 507–33, 118 refs).

Citalopram *

Citalopram is well-established across Europe and USA and has been shown to be effective and well-tolerated in studies against standard antidepressants. 10-20mg/d is significantly more effective than placebo, with particularly robust effects in melancholic depression seen at 40–60mg/d (n=650, RCT, Feighner and Overø, *J Clin Psych* 1999, **60**, 824–30). It has been shown to have superior tolerability to clomipramine and imipramine (two trial comparison by Fuglum *et al, Acta Psych Scand* 1996, **94**, 18–25), mianserin in the elderly (n=336, RCT, Karlsson *et al, Int J Geriatr Psych* 2000, **15**, 295–305), and possibly an earlier onset of recovery than fluoxetine (n=357, RCT, Patris *et al Int Clin Psychoharmacol* 1996, **11**, 129–36) and sertraline (n=323, RCT, Stahl *et al, Biol Psych* 2000, **48**, 894–901). In patients who had responded to citalopram 40mg/d

for four months, halving the dose to 20mg/d for a maintenance phase (2-yrs) resulted in a 50% relapse rate, reinforcing the view that full-dose maintenance therapy is required (n=50, Franchini *et al, J Clin Psych* 1999, **60**, 861–65). It has a very low incidence of interactions (*4.3.2.1*). The green and yellow 20mg pack in the UK has led to increased use among football supporters in the author's home city of Norwich.

Reviews*: general (Tan and Levin, *Pharmacotherapy* 1999, **19**, 675–89; Noble and Benfield, *CNS Drugs* 1997, **8**, 410–31, 103 refs; Thomas and Holimon, *Am J Health-Sys Pharm* 1999, **56**, 2242–44; Parker and Brown, *Ann Pharmacother* 2000, **34**, 761–71, 60 refs; Bezchlibnyk-Butler *et al, J Psychiatry Neurol* 2000, **25**, 241–54).

Fluoxetine *

Fluoxetine is licensed in the UK for depression, with or without anxiety. Fluoxetine has been shown to be clearly superior to placebo and slightly superior to tricyclics with significantly fewer drop-outs (rigorous meta-analysis, 30 trials, n=4120, Bech *et al, B J Psych* 2000, **176**, 421–28). People who take fluoxetine for depression are more likely to take it for six months than if given a tricyclic (n=536, randomised, unblinded, 2yr follow-up, Simon *et al, Arch Fam Med* 1999, **8**, 319–25; reviewed in *EBMH* 2000, **3**, 23). 20mg/d is the standard dose, and although early dose-finding studies showed 60mg/d to be less effective than 20–40mg/d and not statistically better than placebo, some resistant depressions may respond to 60–80mg/d (*J Aff Dis* 1992, **25**, 229–34). Complete lack of response at 2 weeks is a strong predictor of lack of response at 8 weeks (n=143, open, Nierenberg *et al, Am J Psych* 1995, **152**, 1500–3). Claims of suicidal ideation (*Am J Psych* 1990, **147**, 570–72), possibly associated with development of akathisia (*B J Psych* 1992, **161**, 735–41), have been disproven (*BMJ* 1991, **303**, 685–92). Fluoxetine shows a slight *reduction* in suicidal behaviour, rather than an increase (n=185, Leon *et al, Am J Psych* 1999, **156**, 195–201). A long half-life may prove a problem in the elderly, although missed doses become less important in continuation and prophylactic therapy and discontinuation symptoms are rare.

Review: actions, relative efficacy and side-effects (Gram, *NEJM* 1994, **331**, 1354–61), pharmacoeconomics (Wilde and Benfield, *PharmacoEconomics* 1998, **13**, 543–61).

Fluvoxamine

Fluvoxamine has been compared with, and shown to be as effective as, many standard tricyclics, eg. imipramine (*Int Clin Psychopharmacol* 1989, **4**, 239–44). One trial showed it to be effective as monotherapy in delusional depression (n=59, Gatti *et al, Am J Psych* 1996, **153**, 414–16). It may have a higher incidence of nausea and vomiting (*PEM News*, 1991, No 7) than other SSRIs. Most adverse effects occur in the first month and neuro-psychiatric symptoms are the most common, with headache (3.8%) and dizziness (3.3%) (Edwards *et al, B J Psych* 1994, **164**, 387–95).

Review: Levien and Baker, *Hospital Pharmacy* 1994, **29**, 608 (60 refs).

Paroxetine *

Paroxetine is licensed in the UK for depression, including that accompanied by anxiety. Several short-term trials comparing it with standard tricyclics have been published (see *Drugs* 1991, **41**, 225–53), eg. with imipramine and placebo (Fabre, *J Clin Psych* 1992, **53**[Suppl 1], 40–43) and it has been shown to be equipotent with fluoxetine at six weeks (De Wilde *et al, Acta Psych Scand* 1993, **87**, 141–45) but less effective than clomipramine (DUAG, *J Aff Dis* 1990, **18**, 289–99). It has a flat dose-response curve, with 20mg/d optimum and no significant advantage for escalating dosage to 40mg/d (n=544, RCT, Benkert *et al, Acta Psych Scand* 1997, **95**, 288–96). Paroxetine's half-life increases from 10 to 21 hours on chronic dosing, but reduces when this is stopped, which may in part explain the many reports of discontinuation effects (see *2.2.2*).

Reviews: general (Bell and Nutt, *Hosp Med* 1999, **5**, 353–61), in general practice (Christiansen *et al, Acta Psych Scand* 1996, **93**, 158–63), pharmacology and use in depression and other disorders (Gunasekara *et al, Drugs* 1998, **55**, 85–120, 157 refs).

Sertraline *

The pharmacological profile of sertraline is similar to fluoxetine, but with a shorter half-life. It has been shown to be effective when compared with amitriptyline (Doogan and Caillard, *J Clin Psych* 1988, **49** [Suppl 1], 46–51), with 50mg/d equivalent in efficacy and side-effects to fluoxetine 20mg/d (n=165, Van Moffaert *et al, Hum Psychopharmacol* 1995, **10**, 393–405). Sertraline may be highly effective also in delusional depression (comparison *vs* paroxetine, n=46, d/b, Zanardi *et al, Am J Psych* 1996, **153**, 1631–33) and in the elderly, where it was as effective as nortriptyline but better tolerated (RCT, n=210, over 60yo, 12/52, Bondareff *et al, Am J Psych* 2000, **157**, 729–36). After a 3-month acute phase, relapse prevention has been shown (RCT, n=161, 4/12, Keller *et al, JAMA* 1998, **280**, 1665–72; see also Baldessarini *et al, JAMA* 1999, **282**, 323–24; n=64, *J Clin Psych* 1997, **58**, 104–7). Efficacy in chronic major depression has been shown (n=635, RCT, Keller *et al, J Clin Psych* 1998, **59**, 598–607). Patients in a community nursing home stabilised on sertraline once-daily for 12 or more weeks were successfully changed to equivalent doses of sertraline three times a week (n=44, Karki *et al, J Pharm Technol* 2000, **16**, 43–46). Sertraline has a favourable drug interaction profile (*4.3.2.5*).

Reviews: general (Perry and Benfield, *CNS Drugs* 1997, **7**, 480–500, 123 refs), pharmacokinetic profile (*Clin Pharmacokinet* 1997, **32** [Suppl 1], 1–55).

Tricyclics

Doses of 125–150mg/d of tricyclics are effective in depression and there is NO evidence from controlled clinical trials that doses of 75mg or less are effective, the few who seem to respond to lower doses and relapse on withdrawal (Thompson and Thompson, *Human Psychopharmacol* 1989, **4**, 191–204) probably include the 5% of people with low CYP2D6 activity and the 30% of placebo-responders.

The tricyclics are rapidly moving from first to third-line in depression, which is good news because sub-therapeutic use is still widespread, eg. as many as 88% of prescriptions for older tricyclics were at doses lower than the accepted effective levels (Donoghue and Tylee, *B J Psych* 1996, **168**, 164–68). If the older tricyclics are used, it may be difficult to reach therapeutic doses due to side-effects. For a good review of the use of sub-therapeutic doses of TCAs, see Donoghue (*Acta Psych Scand* 1998, **98**, 429–31). It is not appropriate to rely upon the meta-analysis by Bollini *et al* (*B J Psych* 1999, **174**, 297–303), as the efficacy of 'sub-therapeutic' antidepressant doses is only justified by considering fluoxetine 30mg/d as sub-therapeutic, which it isn't.

Patients taking tricyclics are 5 times more likely to have road traffic accidents than untreated controls (*Curr Problems* 1995, **21**, 12; Edwards, editorial in *BMJ* 1995, **311**, 887–88).

Amitriptyline
A widely-used tricyclic with potent anti-cholinergic, sedative and weight gaining properties. It has a long half-life and so sustained-release preparations are unnecessary.

Amoxapine
Amoxapine is structurally similar to maprotiline (in that it has a classic tricyclic structure with a fourth ring as a side structure). The once claimed faster onset of action is probably due to the sedative and anxiolytic effects of its metabolites (eg. loxapine) which have mild antipsychotic/sedative effects. It has a high incidence of seizures (up to 36% in overdose) as well as renal failure, endocrine and extra-pyramidal side-effects.

Clomipramine
A potent tricyclic with an active metabolite, with a possible added advantage in treating depression with an obsessional component. On one measure, clomipramine has been shown to have superior efficacy to imipramine and citalopram (two trial comparison by Fuglum *et al, Acta Psych Scand* 1996, **94**, 18–25). Clomipramine doses of 25, 50, 75, 125 and 200mg/d all show improvement, with 125 and 200mg/d showing the greatest improvement, although there was no placebo control group (n=151, 6/52, d/b, DUAG, *Clin Pharmacol & Therapeut* 1999, **66**, 152–65). Once daily dosage can be appropriate.

Intravenous infusion has been used and may have a rapid onset of action.

Desipramine
Desipramine has a low sedative effect and is suitable for once daily administration. It was discontinued world-wide in 2001.

Dothiepin (dosulepin)
Dothiepin is an established tricyclic in the UK although severe toxicity in overdose and standard side-effect profile makes its UK popularity slightly surprising. It has significant sedative effects and impairment of concentration and memory (eg. compared with lofepramine, Allen *et al, J Psychopharmacol* 1993, **7**, 33–38) and has been shown to be more toxic than other tricyclics, particularly due to its pro-convulsive and cardiac arrhythmic effects (*Lancet* 1994, **343**, 159). Dothiepin should thus not be used in someone actively suicidal. It is frequently prescribed in the community at sub-therapeutic antidepressant doses (eg. 75mg/d) which must be a major cause of treatment failure.

Doxepin
A standard tricyclic with moderate sedation, which may have fewer anti-cholinergic and cardiac effects than older tricyclics. It has an active metabolite and is suitable for once or twice daily dosing.

Imipramine
An established standard tricyclic suitable for once daily administration. Stimulant side-effects may be troublesome as may the anticholinergic effects, especially in the elderly.

Lofepramine
This established UK tricyclic may have relatively fewer side-effects than other tricyclics, eg. it has minimal sedative effects and impairment of concentration and memory compared with dothiepin (Allen *et al J Psychopharmacol* 1993, **7**, 33–38). It is surprisingly safe in overdose (*Med Tox* 1986, **1**, 411–20), with lofepramine seeming to block the cardiotoxic effects of the main metabolite, desipramine (full review in *Drugs* 1989, **37**, 123–40).

Maprotiline

Although claimed to be a tetracyclic, maprotiline is more a tricyclic and should be considered such. Cardiac effects are similar to the older tricyclics. It has the greatest incidence of seizures in overdose (and even at standard doses), compounded by its unusually long half-life. Use should be restricted to patients where these risks are absolutely minimal.

Nortriptyline

A mildly sedative tricyclic with low cardiotoxic side-effects and suitable for once daily administration. A study of melancholic depression in elderly patients, it was shown to be significantly more effective than fluoxetine (n=22, Roose et al, Am J Psych 1994, **151**, 1735–39). A therapeutic window of 50–170mg/ml has been identified (eg. Am J Psych 1985, **142**, 155).

Protriptyline *

Protriptyline was withdrawn world-wide in 2001.

Trimipramine

Structurally related to methotrimeprazine/levomepromazine, trimipramine has significant sedative properties, which can be useful for hypnotic and anxiolytic purposes.

> **SWITCHING OR DISCONTINUING ANTIDEPRESSANTS**
>
> For a table on switching antidepressants and the gaps needed, or advice on the problems of discontinuing, see Chapter 2.2.5

Other antidepressants

Mirtazapine *

Mirtazapine is described as a NaSSA (Noradrenergic and Specific Serotonergic Antidepressant). It blocks pre-synaptic alpha-2 adreno-receptors (increasing noradrenaline transmission) and indirectly enhances serotoninergic transmission, with additional $5-HT_2$ and $5-HT_3$ receptor blockade minimising the incidence of serotoninergic side-effects, eg. nausea, headache and sexual dysfunction. In a number of double-blind trials, mirtazapine has been shown to be as effective over six weeks as amitriptyline (meta-analysis of eight RCTs, n=161 treated, n=132 placebo showing mirtazapine superior to placebo and comparable to amitriptyline for depression and anxiety/agitation, Fawcett and Barkin, J Clin Psych 1998, **59** 123–27), clomipramine (n=174, Richou et al, Hum Psychopharm 1995, **10**, 263–71), superior to trazodone (n=200, van Moffaert et al, Int Clin Psychopharm 1995, **10**, 3–9) and as well-tolerated as fluoxetine but significantly more effective at 3 and 4 weeks of therapy (RCT, n=135, Wheatley et al, J Clin Psych 1998, **59**, 306–12). Relapse prevention has been shown to be superior to placebo and amitriptyline over 20 weeks, where it was well-tolerated (d/b extension study, n=217, Montgomery et al, Int Clin Psychopharmacol 1998, **13**, 63–73). A meta-analysis of all 3 completed comparative studies of mirtazapine versus SSRIs (fluoxetine [Wheatley et al, J Clin Psych 1998, **59**, 306–12], paroxetine [Benkert et al, J Clin Psych 2000, **61**, 656–63] and citalopram [Leinonen et al, Int Clin Psychopharm 1999, **14**, 329–37]), showed a similar ADR profile, but hinted at superior efficacy and a robust faster onset of action, statistically significant in all three studies in the first few weeks (Thompson, J Clin Psych 1999, **60** [Suppl 17], 18–22; discussion 46–48). Equivalent efficacy and onset of action to venlafaxine in severely depressed patients with melancholic features has been shown (Guelfi et al, J Clin Psychopharmacol 2001, in press). An earlier onset of action is related to better overall outcomes. Improved sleep has been shown (Ruigt et al, Eur J Clin Pharmacol 1990, **38**, 551–54). Blood dyscrasias have been reported only very rarely with mirtazapine in the clinical trial programme but do not seem to be a problem in clinical practice. The dose range is 15–45mg/d and recent data shows the optimum starting dose of 30mg/d is well-tolerated. **Reviews***: general (Holm and Markham, Drugs 1999, **57**, 607–63; J Clin Psych 2000, **61**, 609–16; Anon, Drug & Therapeut Bull 1999, **37**, 1–3), meta-analysis of studies (Kasper et al, Eur Neuropsychopharmacol 1997, **7**, 115–24), pharmacology (Davis and Wilde, CNS Drugs 1996, **5**, 389–402), kinetics (Delbressine et al, Clin Drug Investigat 1998, **15**, 45–55; Timmer et al, Clin Pharmacokinet 2000, **38**, 461–74, 56 refs).

Mianserin

Mianserin is a tetracyclic with prominent $5HT_{2A}$ and $5HT_{2C}$ antagonist properties, a good safety profile in overdose, low cardiotoxicity and marked sedative properties. Mianserin has been shown to be effective at 20–60mg/d in prophylaxis of recurrent depression (18/12, n=22, Kishimoto *et al, Acta Psych Scand* 1994, **89**, 46–51).

Moclobemide

Moclobemide (a RIMA or reversible inhibitor of monoamine oxidase-A) inhibits only MAO-A and not MAO-B, so an excess of tyramine in the body will displace moclobemide from MAO-A, allowing tyramine metabolism to occur, MOA-B remaining free. This results in a 'cheese-reaction' usually only at amounts above 100–150mg of tyramine (see *4.3.3.3*), unlikely under normal conditions. A meta-analysis of 38 double-blind and 2 single-blind trials with moclobemide (n=2416) showed it to be about equipotent with imipramine or sedative tricyclic antidepressants in agitated-anxious depressive patients, and all were clearly superior to placebo (Delini-Stula *et al, J Aff Dis* 1995, **35**, 21–30). A review of studies indicates that moclobemide may be useful in typical severe depression with melancholia (Paykel, *Acta Psych Scand* 1995, **91**[Suppl 386], 22–27).

Reviews: *Drugs* 1992, **43**, 561–96; Baldwin and Rudge, *B J Hosp Med* 1993, **49**, 497–99; Norman and Burrows, *Drug Safety* 1995, **12**, 46–51, 40 refs.

Nefazodone

Nefazodone, a phenylpiperazine related to trazodone, has a double action on serotonin, ie. relatively weak 5-HT re-uptake inhibition and powerful 5-HT$_2$ blockade (Fontaine, *Clin Neuropharmacol* 1992, **13**[Suppl 1], 99A), which may be a combined effect from the drug and its two major metabolites. The 5-HT$_2$ blockade may be responsible for a positive effect on sleep, where an increase in REM sleep time has been reported in a study in healthy men (Sharpley *et al, Biol Psych* 1992, **31**, 1070–73), and two 8-week double-blind trials (both n=43) showed nefazodone may have an effect in improving sleep disturbances in depression (Gillin *et al,*

J Clin Psych 1997, **58**, 185–92; Armitage *et al, J Clin Psychopharmacol* 1997, **17**, 161–68). Nefazodone has been compared favourably with imipramine (eg. Fontaine *et al, J Clin Psych* 1994, **55**[6], 234–41) but studies against newer antidepressants are obviously needed. The optimum dose has not been established but meta-analysis of dose-finding studies suggests 300–600mg/d as optimal. Some studies have shown 100–200mg/d as effective but 300mg/d not effective (D'Amico *et al, Psychopharmacol Bull* 1990, **26**, 147–50), whereas others have needed 400mg/d or more for an effect (eg. Feighner *et al, Psychopharmacol Bull* 1989, **25**, 219–21).

Reviews: pharmacokinetics (Barbhaiya *et al, Eur J Clin Pharmacol* 1996, **50**, 101; Cyr and Brown, *Ann Pharmacother* 1996, **30**, 1006–12; Greene and Barbhaiya, *Clin Pharmacokinet* 1997, **33**, 260–75, 51 refs), pharmacology and clinical efficacy (Davis *et al, Drugs* 1997, **53**, 608–36, 110 refs).

Reboxetine *

Reboxetine is a selective noradrenaline reuptake inhibitor with no dopamine, histamine, adrenergic nor serotonin effects at 8mg/d, but a weak anticholinergic action. In short-term studies it appears as effective as imipramine (Berzewski *et al, Eur Neuropsychopharmacol* 1997[Suppl 1], S37–S47) and as fluoxetine 20-40mg/d, with possibly greater efficacy in severe depression and in terms of social functioning in those that responded (RCT, n=168, 8/52, Massana *et al, Int Clin Psychopharmacol* 1999, **14**, 73–80). A higher level of social functioning has been shown with reboxetine, using a validated scale (SASS) but equivalent assessment against other antidepressants is awaited. Relapse prevention has been shown against placebo (46/52, d/b, n=283, Versiani *et al, J Clin Psych* 1999, **60**, 400–6), with reboxetine being well tolerated. There is no effect on reaction time (Hindmarsh, *Eur Neuropsychopharmacol* 1997 [Suppl 1], S17–S21). Interest in use as an SSRI adjunct must be tempered by the lack of safety data.

Reviews*: general (Holm and Spencer, *CNS Drugs* 1999, **12**, 65–83; Anon, *Formulary Monograph Service* 1999, 315–21, 29 refs; Scates and Doraiswamy, *Ann Pharmacother* 2000, **34**, 1302–12; Schatzberg, *J Clin Psych* 2000, **61**[Suppl 10], 31–38), clinical experience (Baldwin *et al, Int J Psych Clin Pract* 1998, **2**, 195–201).

Trazodone

Trazodone increases NA and 5-HT turnover with low cardiotoxicity and anti-cholinergic side-effects but a higher incidence of drowsiness and nausea. It has been shown to be effective when compared with imipramine (Gershon and Newton, *J Clin Psych* 1980, **41**, 100–4; Gerner *et al, J Clin Psych* 1980, **41**, 216–20). It is best taken with food to reduce peak blood levels.

Venlafaxine *

Venlafaxine is described as an SNRI (combined 5-HT and NA reuptake blocker), with minimal effects on other transmitters (except dopamine, where it has a minor but not insignificant effect). There is evidence for a dose-response relationship (eg. RCT, n=147, Mehtonen *et al, J Clin Psych* 2000, **61**, 95–100), with 5-HT reuptake inhibition across the dosage range, NA reuptake inhibition becoming significant around the 200mg/d dose (n=32, Harvey *et al, Arch Gen Psych* 2000, **57**, 503–9) and dopamine reuptake inhibition above 225mg/d. It has been shown in trials to be an effective antidepressant in major depression and in resistant depression (Nierenberg *et al, Neuropsychopharmacol* 1994, **10**[35 part 2], 85S). There is some evidence that venlafaxine may be useful in non-chronic treatment-resistant depression, eg. it was shown to be slightly superior at 200–300mg/d to paroxetine 30–40mg/d in such a population (n=122, RCT, Poirier and Boyer, *B J Psych* 1999, **175**, 12–16; discussion of weaknesses in *B J Psych* 2000, **176**, 398; review by Martin, *EBMH* 2000, **3**, 51). The sustained release preparation (Efexor XL) probably gives a reduced incidence of initial nausea and has a once a day dosage. **Reviews***: general (Kienke and Rosenbaum, *Depress Anxiety* 2000, **12** [Suppl 1], 50–54).

SWITCHING OR DISCONTINUING ANTIDEPRESSANTS

For a table on switching antidepressants and the gaps needed, or advice on the problems of discontinuing, see *Chapter 2.2.5*

Mono-amine oxidase inhibitors (MAOIs)
Isocarboxazid *
A hydrazine derivative which irreversibly blocks the MAO enzyme (editorial by Shader and Greenblatt, *J Clin Psychopharmacol* 1999, **19**, 105).

Phenelzine
A hydrazine derivative which irreversibly blocks the MAO enzyme. Patients with chronic atypical depression are at high risk of relapse if phenelzine is withdrawn 6 months after the initial response (Stewart *et al, Am J Psych* 1997, **154**, 31–36). Phenelzine is as effective as CBT in atypical depression (n=108, RCT, 10/52, Jarrett *et al, Arch Gen Psych* 1999, **56**, 431–37) and imipramine in resistant depression (*Am J Psych* 1993, **150**, 118–23).

Tranylcypromine
A non-hydrazine amfetamine-related MAOI with stimulant effects and a greater incidence of adverse drug interactions. It has been shown to be effective in tricyclic-resistant and anergic bipolar depression in one study (d/b, c/o, *Am J Psych* 1992, **149**, 195–98).

Others
Flupentixol
In low dose, either orally or as a depot, flupentixol can have some mild anti-depressant properties and in some double-blind studies it has proved superior to placebo and amitriptyline. Its efficacy has been queried (*J Psychopharmacol* 1990, **4**, 152–67) as the speed of action is more in line with an anxiolytic effect and an equally good case can be put forward for other antipsychotics in low dose.

Lithium *
Use of lithium as monotherapy in the treatment and prophylaxis of unipolar (as well as bipolar) depression has been well established (eg. meta-analysis by Souza and Goodwin, *B J Psych* 1991, **158**, 666–75; Schou, *Arch Gen Psych* 1994, **51**, 502–3) and has been associated with low mortality (Müller-

Oerlinghausen *et al, Acta Psych Scand* 1992, **86**, 218–22). It has also been shown to be highly significantly effective as an adjunct to other antidepressants (see combinations later). Doses of at least 750mg may be needed for clinical response, with 250mg/d leading to relapse (*B J Psych* 1993, **162**, 634–40). A meta-analysis of placebo-controlled studies has shown that lithium augmentation (600–800mg/d) increases response in depression refractory to tricyclics (8 studies) or SSRIs (one study) (n=234, RCT=9, Bauer and Dopfmer, *J Clin Psychopharmacol* 1999, **19**, 427–34; review by Lam, *EBMH* 2000, **3**, 44; *Bandolier* 2000, **7**, 4–5). Much anti-depressant response to lithium is probably mood stabilisation in depressed (but undiagnosed) bipolars. **Reviews**: lithium augmentation in refractory depression (Heit and Nemeroff, *J Clin Psych* 1998, **59**[Suppl 6], 28–33, 36 refs), general review (Rouillon and Gorwood, *J Clin Psych* 1998, **59**[Suppl 5], 32–41). See main entry under bipolar mood disorder (*1.10*) and bipolar depression (introduction).

Tryptophan

A naturally occurring amino acid and precursor to serotonin, tryptophan is usually used in combination with tricyclic or other antidepressants. Tryptophan deficiency results in a rapid lowering of mood (eg. Benkelfat *et al, Arch Gen Psych* 1994, **51**, 687–97; Smith *et al, Lancet* 1997, **349**, 915–19) and tryptophan depletion has been shown to reverse antidepressant-induced remission from depression (eg. Delgado *et al, Arch Gen Psych* 1990, **47**, 411–18) and so tryptophan therapy might be expected to help anti-depressant response if low tryptophan levels have occurred.

Due to a previous association with eosinophilia-myalgia syndrome (EMS), it is now only licensed in the UK for resistant depression, by hospital specialists, in patients with severe depression continuously for more than two years, after adequate trials of standard drug treatments and as an adjunct to other treatments. Such restrictions still seem very harsh compared to the low risk involved and possible benefits (n=202, McKeon *et al, Acta Psych Scand* 1994, **90**, 451–54). Close monitoring of eosinophil levels is necessary and to the signs and symptoms of EMS (eg. muscle or joint pain, fever and rash). The doctor and patient must be registered with OPTICS (Optimax Information and Clinical Support), with progress reported at 3 and 6 months, then 6-monthly (*CSM Current Problems* 1994, **20**, 2). For a review of therapeutic uses, see Smith, *Pharm J* 1998, **261**, 819–21, 40 refs.

Augmentation strategies (drugs with no intrinsic antidepressant activity)

Reviews: risk of adverse events with the use of augmentation therapy (reviewed by Schweitzer and Tuckwell, *Drug Safety* 1998, **19**, 455–64), extensive review (*J Clin Psych* 1998, **59**[Suppl], 3–73), anxiolytic antidepressant augmentation (Sussman, *J Clin Psych* 1998, **59**[Suppl 5], 42–50), anticonvulsants as anti-depressant augmentation (Dietrich and Emrich, *J Clin Psych* 1998, **59**[Suppl 5], 51–59).

Levothyroxine (thyroxine)

Subclinical hypothyroidism may well predispose to depression (Haggerty *et al, Am J Psych* 1993, **150**, 508–10). Augmentation with high-dose 150–300mg/d thyroxine proved to have an antidepressant effect in more than 50% of the previously treatment-resistant patients with chronic depression and/or dysthymia (n=9, open, 8/52, Rudas *et al, Biol Psychiatry* 1999, **15**, 45, 229–33; review by Joffe, *J Clin Psych* 1998, **59**[Suppl 5], 26–31). See studies with tricyclics and SSRIs etc. For a review of thyroid hormones in depression, including the HPT-axis, see Kirkegaard and Faber (*Eur J Endocrinol* 1998, **138**, 1–9).

Liothyronine

A meta-analysis of the 8 controlled studies showed liothyronine aug-mentation to produce twice as many responses in refractory depression compared to controls, with moderately large improvements, although one RCT showed negative results (Aronson *et al, Arch Gen Psych* 1996, **53**, 842–48). Subtherapeutic doses of T_3 triiodothyronine 25–50mcg/d (*Am J Psych* 1990, **147**, 255) or T_4 levothyroxine up to 0.1mg/d have been used as augmentation to tricyclics etc. (Joffe *et al, Arch Gen Psych* 1993, **50**, 387–93) and phenelzine (*J Clin Psych* 1988, **49** [Suppl] 409). This may be effective particularly in rapid-cycling disorder (1.27).

Modafinil *

Augmentation in antidepressant partial or non-responders by modafinil 100–200mg/d produced a remarkable response over 1–2 weeks in all 7 patients (case series, Menza *et al, J Clin Psych* 2000, **61**, 378–81).

Pindolol *

Antidepressants, eg. SSRIs may act by inhibiting the 5-HT reuptake pump, increasing 5-HT availability at post-synaptic receptors. However, this also includes enhancing 5-HT at $5\text{-}HT_{1A}$ receptors situated on the cell body which operate a feedback loop. The initial net outcome is that these cancel each other out. Over a period of weeks, however, the pre-synaptic $5\text{-}HT_{1A}$ receptors become desensitised and the system corrects itself, which may explain the delay in antidepressant action from antidepressants. Pindolol relatively selectively blocks $5\text{-}HT_{1A}$ receptors, and may block this feedback loop to increase the speed of onset of action (Artigas, *Arch Gen Psych* 1995, **52**, 969–71). A number of trials have now shown a clinically important effect. Pindolol in combination with paroxetine (Tome *et al, J Aff Dis* 1997, **44**, 101–9), fluoxetine (RCT, n=11, Perez *et al, Lancet* 1997, **349**, 1594–97) and trazodone/fluoxetine (d/b, n=26, Maes *et al, J Aff Dis* 1996, **41**, 201–10) suggest a faster onset of action and higher response rates. A three-year follow-up showed use of pindolol was associated with a marked improvement in long-term outcomes (n=3,485, Rasanen *et al, J Clin Psychopharmacol* 1999, **19**, 297–302). Other trials, however, have not been able to show that pindolol hastens the response to SSRIs (eg. fluoxetine, n=43, RCT, Berman *et al, Am J Psych* 1997, **154**, 37–43; Perez *et al, Arch Gen Psych* 1999, **56**, 375–79). US studies may differ from UK due to UK pindolol being the isomer and US being a

mixture, and the $5HT_{1A}$ receptor may be receptive to only one isomer (Isaac and Tome, *Am J Psych* 1997, **154**, 1790–91). **Reviews**: McAskill *et al, B J Psych* 1998, **173**, 203–8, concluding that larger trials are needed to confirm the effect (discussion by McAllister-Williams and Young, *B J Psych* 1998, **173**, 536–39; Blier and Bergeron, *J Clin Psych* 1998, **59**[Suppl 5], 16–23).

+ Combinations

There is some evidence that combined NA and 5-HT reuptake blocking drugs can produce a quicker antidepressant effect (Nelson, *Arch Gen Psych* 1991, **48**, 303–7), although it could be that combined drug use produces higher success rates by treating different depressive subgroups.

Bupropion + tranylcypromine *

The cautious use of this combination has been successful in resolving multi-drug resistant depression (n=1, Pierre and Gitlin, *J Clin Psych* 2000, **61**, 450–51).

Bupropion + venlafaxine/SSRIs *

56% of venlafaxine/SSRI-resistant depressed patients responded when bupropion was added (n=25, Spier *et al, Depress Anxiety* 1998, **7**, 73–75), and in multi-drug resistant depression, bupropion 300mg/d successfully augmented venlafaxine 450mg/d (n=1, Fatemi *et al, Ann Pharmacother* 1999, **33**, 701–3).

Buspirone + SSRIs

In a study of SSRI-resistant depressed patients, addition of buspirone produced a significant response in 68% (n=25, open, Joffe and Schuller, *J Clin Psych* 1993, **54**, 269–71), confirming an earlier open study, where 7 of 8 people on fluoxetine (6) or imipramine (1) responded when buspirone was added (Jacobsen, *J Clin Psych* 1991, **52**, 217–20) and a case report (Veivia *et al, J Pharm Technology* 1995, **11**, 50–52). Buspirone shares some pharmaco-dynamic properties with pindolol. However, an RCT failed to show any advantage of adding buspirone to an SSRI in treatment-resistant depression (n=119, Landen *et al, J Clin Psych* 1998, **59**, 664–68), although both the placebo (47%) and buspirone (51%) response rates were high, and an open label extension produced a higher (70%) response rate.

Clonazepam + SSRIs *

Clonazepam (up to 1mg/d) improved the speed of onset of fluoxetine (cf fluoxetine alone), possibly partly by suppressing SSRI side-effects (n=80, RCT, 3/52, Smith *et al, Am J Psych* 1998, **155**, 1339–45). However, the literature on benzodiazepine augmentation is confusing, with studies showing variable effects (discussion by Furukawa, *Am J Psych* 1999, **156**, 1840).

Hydrocortisone + metyrapone

Eight patients given hydrocortisone 30mg/d plus metyrapone showed significant reductions in depression over two weeks (p/c, s/b, c/o, O'Dwyer *et al, J Aff Dis* 1995, **33**, 123–28).

Lithium + antidepressants *

There are many studies showing this to be an effective and useful combination. In a trial where lithium or placebo was added to **lofepramine** or **fluoxetine** and where the TCA/SSRI had been ineffective by itself, 50% responded to lithium augmentation whereas only 25% responded to addition of placebo (n=62, d/b, Katona *et al, B J Psych* 1995, **166**, 80–86). Adequate lithium levels (0.4mmol/l or more) were necessary. Other studies have shown an additive effect with **sertraline** (n=11, 7/7, Dinan, *Acta Psych Scand* 1993, **88**, 300–1), **tricyclics** (n=50, *Arch Gen Psych* 1993, **50**, 387–93), **citalopram** (n=69, RCT, Baumann *et al, J Clin Psychopharmacol* 1996, **16**, 307–14) and **venlafaxine** (n=23, open, Hoencamp *et al, J Clin Psychopharmacol* 2000, **20**, 538–43). Patients maintained on lithium, but with breakthrough depression, responded more quickly to paroxetine 20–40mg/d than amitriptyline 75–150mg/d augmentation (n=42, RCT, 6/52, Bauer *et al, J Clin Psychopharmacol* 1999, **19**, 164–71). There is a view that all resistant depressions are unrecognised bipolars and, hence, the use of lithium is logical.

Lithium + antidepressants (eg. clomipramine, SSRI or phenelzine) + tryptophan

Variously known as the MRC Cocktail, Triple Therapy, Newcastle Cocktail and the London Cocktail, unpublished reports of 50% remission rates led to further work (Hale *et al, B J Psych* 1987, **151**, 213–17):

Clomipramine (to 150mg/d or to tolerance eg. 300–400mg/d)
+ Tryptophan (2–4g/d)
+ Lithium (standard levels)
* Alternatives to clomipramine include phenelzine and the SSRIs (Barker *et al, Int Clin Psychopharmacol* 1987, **2**, 261–72). Tryptophan enhances the action of clomipramine on 5-HT sites and improves 5-HT absorption. Lithium also affects 5-HT and is an antidepressant in its own right. The combination is effective in severe resistant depression. (*B J Psych* 1988, **152**, 720 using imipramine, case studies in *Lancet* 1990, **336**, 380).

Lithium + valproate

A study of refractory depression indicated that sodium valproate (750–1500mg/d) augmentation of lithium (900–1500mg/d) was effective in the 8 patients who did not respond to lithium alone (n=10, Sharma *et al, Lithium* 1994, **5**, 99–103).

Methylphenidate + SSRIs

Findings from the first 9 patients in a discontinued RCT showed there to be no advantage in adding methylphenidate to sertraline, in terms of quicker or better response (Postolache *et al, J Clin Psych* 1999, **60**, 123–24).

Mianserin + fluoxetine *

Mianserin 30mg/d augmented the efficacy of fluoxetine, and may shorten the latency of onset in major and treatment-resistant depression (n=31, RCT, Maes *et al, J Clin Psychopharmacol* 1999, **19**, 177–82).

Reboxetine + SSRIs *

Successful use of citalopram and reboxetine for resistant depression has been reported (Devarajan and Dursun, *Can J Psych* 2000, **45**, 489–90).

Tricyclics + MAOIs

Although the BNF urges extreme caution, this combination is known to be effective in some resistant depressions, eg. a study with trimipramine and MAOIs (eg. *BMJ* 1979, **ii**, 1315–17; alternate study view by O'Brien *et al, B J Psych* 1993, **162**, 363–68). A 3-year open trial of an isocarboxazid and amitriptyline combination in 25 treatment-resistant depressives showed that 50% responded, and that most of those remained in remission for up to three years, with no adverse reactions and may thus be a useful and safe treatment for at least some forms of resistant-depression (Berlanga & Ortega-Soto, *J Aff Dis* 1995, **34**, 187–92). Tranylcypromine plus clomipramine is known to be dangerous (two deaths) but other combinations can be used with care in an inpatient setting. Most problems occur when a tricyclic is added to an MAOI. Fewer adverse events have been reported with the reverse. The main adverse events include hyperthermia, delirium, seizures, agitation etc. rather than hypertension. It is best to take great care, eg. separate the doses (eg. MAOI in the morning, tricyclic in the evening), add one to the other in low dose and build up slowly or stop all antidepressants, wait a week, and then start both together at low dose and build up again. The last mentioned seems to be the most widely favoured strategy.

Tricyclic + SSRIs *

Fluoxetine and a tricyclic were effective in a retrospective study of patients not responsive to either agent alone and for whom standard protocols had for some reason not been followed (n=30, open, Weilberg *et al, J Clin Psych* 1989, **50**, 447–49) and fluoxetine 20mg/d and desipramine produced a rapid and effective response in depression in an open study (n=14, Nelson *et al, Arch Gen Psych* 1991, **48**, 303–7). The report by Seth *et al* (*B J Psych* 1992, **161**, 562–5) was so remarkable its findings were contested (Cowen and Power, *B J Psych* 1993, **162**, 266–67). The only double-blind prospective study on the subject showed that high dose fluoxetine (60mg/d) was in fact more effective in partial or non-responders to 20mg/d than a fluoxetine/desipramine combination (Fava *et al, Am J Psych* 1994, **151**, 1372–74). The improved outcome with the combination in people who did not respond to either alone is, in most people, likely to be due to raised TCA levels (n=13, Levitt *et al, J Clin Psych* 1999, **60**, 613; critical review of the therapeutic combination by Taylor, *B J Psych* 1995, **167**, 575–80). The combination should generally be avoided due to the high risk of an adverse interaction (*4.3.2*).

● **Unlicensed/Some efficacy**
Bupropion (amfebutamone) *

Bupropion is approved in USA for the treatment of depression. In placebo-controlled studies in acute depression, bupropion has shown an average response rate of 55%, compared to 29% for placebo. The most likely mechanism of action is weak dopamine reuptake blockade. The drug does not share a lower cardiovascular and suicide safety profile with the SSRIs, but is non-sedating, causes no weight gain and appears to have a reduced rate of male and female sexual adverse effects. Bupropion appears to have a greater risk of causing seizures than do the other newer antidepressants, especially in patients with eating disorders (who have lower body weights). The maximum dosage of 450mg/d should be adhered to since the risk of seizures is dose related (see *3.2*).

Carbamazepine

Evidence for use as a pure antidepressant is poor but use with lithium or as prophylaxis in bipolar disorder is better established (*Psychological Med* 1989, **19**, 591–604). In one study, 44% of patients with resistant depression showed moderate or marked improvement with carbamazepine (*J Clin Psych* 1991, **52**, 472–76). See main entry under bipolar mood disorder (*1.10*).

Estradiol/estrogen *

Estradiol skin patches showed a striking improvement in two trials in severe **postnatal depression**. The first showed at 1 month and 3 months (n=37, d/b, p/c, Henderson *et al, Lancet* 1991, **338**, 816–17) and the second showed a sustained improvement over five months with 200mcg/d transdermal estrogen (n=61, d/b, p/c, Gregoire *et al, Lancet* 1996, **347**, 930, further support by Lopez-Jaramillo *et al, Lancet* 1996, **348**, 135–36). The sublingual route allows a rapid delivery of estradiol with short duration of action mimicking natural ovarian function, thus offering a useful and potent therapeutic option in postnatal depression (n=2, Ahokas *et al, Lancet* 1998, **351**, 109, letter). Although estrogen and progesterone levels are associated with the development of postpartum mood disorders (n=8, Bloch *et al, Am J Psych* 2000, **157**, 924–30), progestogens do not seem to help PND, and may even be detrimental (Lawrie *et al*, Cochrane review 1999, reviewed in *EBMH* 2000, **3**, 19). For a review of estrogen as an adjunct to anti-depressants, see Stahl (*J Clin Psych* 1998, **59**[Suppl 4], 15–24).

Levothyroxine (thyroxine)

See combinations.

Liothyronine

See combinations.

Methylphenidate

The use of methylphenidate in depression continues to be discussed (Klein and Wender, *Arch Gen Psych* 1995, **52**, 429–33), as it has a major advantage of a rapid action, often within 48 hours. It may be effective as augmentation where antidepressants do not work fully, and in the elderly where apathy and withdrawal (but not hopelessness) are prominent features (mentioned by Salzman, *Curr Affective Illness* 1995, **14**, 5–13) and, as such, may help where depression is preventing the rehabilitation processes. It is also useful in medically-ill depressed patients, eg. those with cancer (McDaniel *et al, Arch Gen Psych* 1995, **52**, 89–99; Fawzy *et al, Arch Gen Psych* 1995, **52**, 100–13). 59% showed marked or moderate improvement in a trial of elderly depressed patients (n=29, *J Clin Psych* 1991, **52**, 263–67).

Reviews: extensive (Emptage and Semla, *Ann Pharmacother* 1996, **30**, 151–57, 43 refs) and for depression in elderly, medically ill patients (Frye, *Am J Health-Sys Pharm* 1997, **54**, 2510–11).

St. John's wort *

SJW is available over-the-counter in most European countries in a variety of preparations. One major meta-analysis indicated that *hypericum perforatum* extracts were significantly superior to placebo and as effective in mild-to-moderate depression as standard antidepressants (imipramine 75mg/d, maprotiline 75mg/d, amitriptyline 75mg/d), albeit at sub-therapeutic doses (Linde *et al, BMJ* 1996, **313**, 253–58; comment *BMJ* 1996, **313**, 241–42).

Some caution is necessary as the trials included a variety of different *hypericum* preparations, and one trial was published five times with two different first authors (*Bandolier* 1996, **3**, 1–2). More impressively, 800mg/d *hypericum* was shown to be equivalent to fluoxetine 20mg/d in mild to moderate depression, with equivalent ADR drop-outs (n=149, 6/52, RCT, Harrer *et al, Arzneimittelforschung* 1999, **49**, 289–96). High dose SJW was as effective in the short-term as lower-dose imipramine (up to 100mg/d) and more effective than placebo in moderate depression (n=263, RCT, 8/52, Philipp *et al, BMJ* 1999, **319**, 1534–39; critically reviewed by Morriss, *EBMH* 2000, **3**, 85) and as effective as 150mg/d imipramine (n=320, RCT, Woelk, *BMJ* 2000, **321**, 536–39). The mode of action is not certain, but might include serotonin or noradrenaline reuptake inhibition (Neary and Bu, *Brain Res* 1999, **816**, 358–63), MAO-A and B inhibition and sigma receptor activity (neuropharmacology reviewed by Bennett *et al, Ann Pharmacother* 1998, **32**, 1201–8). All current studies are short-term (up to 6/52), and many have high (up to 50%) drop-out rates, indicating that transient mild depression may be common in studies. More studies against standard antidepressants at therapeutic dose and closely defined depression are awaited. In the interim, some use in mild to moderate non-chronic depression seems valid (Deltito and Beyer, *J Aff Dis* 1998, **51**, 345–51), but care is needed in adjunctive therapy (particularly if purchased OTC – see *4.3.9*).

Reviews*: general (Josey and Tackett, *Int J Clin Pharmacol Ther* 1999, **37**, 111–19; Wheatley, *CNS Drugs* 1998, **9**, 431–40; Hotopf, *EBMH* 1999, **2**, 49; Wong *et al, Arch Gen Psych* 1998, **55**, 1033–44; Cott and Fugh-Berman, *J Nerv Ment Dis* 1998, **186**, 500–1; Pepping, *Am J Health-System Pharm* 1999, **56**, 329–30; Maidment, *Psych Bull* 2000, **24**, 232–34), in the elderly (Vorbach *et al, Drugs & Aging* 2000, **16**, 189–97) and systematic review of 8 studies (Gaster and Holroyd, *Arch Int Med* 2000, **160**, 152–56).

O   Unlicensed/Possible efficacy
Amisulpride
Amisulpride 50mg/d has been shown to have an antidepressant activity comparable with fluoxetine 20mg/d, with similar incidences of side-effects (n=281, d/b, Smeraldi, *J Aff Dis* 1998, **48**, 47–56).

Ascorbic Acid
Vitamin C is thought to remove toxic vanadium from cells, an excess of which may cause depression. An unproven effect.

Bromocriptine
A dopamine receptor stimulant which in doses of 10–60mg/d may show some antidepressant effects, although side-effects may be marked. It may be useful in refractory depression and depressed Parkinsons' sufferers (*Drug Intell Clin Pharm* 1989, **23**, 600–2).

Buprenorphine
An open study showed some efficacy in the treatment of refractory, unipolar depression, with a striking response in four (Bodkin *et al, J Clin Psychopharmacol* 1995, **15**, 49–57; see also Callaway, *Biol Psych* 1996, **39**, 989–90).

Buspirone (see also combinations)
A meta-analysis of studies showed a minor but statistically significant effect at up to 90mg/d in depressed patients (review in *J Psychopharmacol* 1993, **7**, 283–89). One study showed buspirone to be more effective than placebo but less effective than imipramine in major depression in elderly patients (RCT, n=177, Schweizer *et al, J Clin Psych* 1998, **59**, 175–83). It is a partial agonist at $5-HT_{1A}$ receptors and has been implicated in mania (*Am J Psych* 1990, **147**, 125), having stimulant properties (*Am J Psych* 1991, **148**, 1213–17).

Captopril
A clinical response was seen in four out of nine patients given captopril 50–100mg/d in an open trial (*J Clin Psychopharmacol* 1991, **11**, 395–96).

Clozapine
Use in refractory psychotic depression has been reported (n=1, Dassa *et al, B J Psych* 1993, **163**, 822–24).

Cyproheptadine *
This may be useful and tolerable if a suppressible DST exists (n=6, RCT, Greenway *et al, Pharmacotherapy* 1995, **15**, 357–60).

Dexamethasone
A number of studies have shown a marked improvement within a week when given 3–8mg IV (n=5, 7/7, *Am J Psych* 1991, **148**, 1401–2; n=37, 4/7, Arana *et al, Am J Psych* 1995, **152**, 265–67), to 8mg IV twice, 4 days apart (n=7, Beale and Arana, *Am J Psych* 1995, **152**, 959–60) and to 3mg/d for 4 days (n=10, Dinan *et al, Acta Psych Scand* 1997, **95**, 58–61), although other reports indicate that only a minority of patients respond (letter by Wolkowitz *et al, Am J Psych* 1996, **153**, 1112–13). This interesting effect may be via upregulation of glucocorticoid receptors, something the SSRIs also do.

Dexamfetamine *
Dexamfetamine may be rapidly effective for depression and fatigue, with one successful trial in men with HIV (n=23, RCT, 2/52, Wagner and Rabkin, *J Clin Psych* 2000, **61**, 436–40).

Folate
15mg/d in addition to psychotropic drugs has significantly improved clinical response and recovery from acute psychiatric disorders (*B J Psych* 1992, **160**, 714–15). Low folate levels have been associated with melancholic depression and non-response to antidepressants (eg. fluoxetine, Fava *et al, Am J Psych* 1997, **154**, 426–28) and so folate levels should be included in the assessment of treatment-resistant depressives and perhaps a routine part of clinical assessment of all depressed people (*B J Psych* 1993, **162**, 572).

Inositol *
Inositol is a precursor of an intracellular secondary messenger system for numerous neurotransmitters, and in one trial was shown to improve depression, opening the door for some repeat and even more imaginative trials (n=28, p/c, Levine *et al, Am J Psych* 1995, **152**, 792–94; follow-up and relapse analysis by Levine *et al, Israel J Psych Related Sci* 1995, **32**, 14–21). Inositol may also be useful in bipolar depression (as well as unipolar), as shown in a trial where 50% responded to 12g/d inositol (cf 30% on placebo) (n=24, RCT, 6/52, Chengappa *et al, Bipolar Disord* 2000,

2, 47–55). However, no significant effect in SSRI augmentation was noted in one study (n=27, RCT, Levine *et al*, *Biol Psych* 1999, **45**, 270–73).

Ketoconazole *

Ketoconazole inhibits cortisol secretion, lowering cortisol levels. It may have a slow-onset antidepressant effect (n=17, study by Murphy *et al, Can J Psychiatry* 1998, **43**, 279–86), particularly in hypercortisolemic (but not normal) patients (n=20, RCT, Wolkowitz *et al, Biol Psychiatry* 1999, **45**, 1070–74). Limited efficacy in treatment-refractory major depression has been noted (n=16, RCT, Malison *et al, J Clin Psychopharmacol* 1999, **19**, 466–70).

Lamotrigine *

Although its primary action is on voltage-sensitive sodium channels, inhibiting pathological release of glutamate, lamotrigine may also have an antidepressant effect. 72% of treatment-refractory depressed bipolars responded (n=22, open, 5/52, Kusumakar and Yatham, *Psychiatry Res* 1997, **72**, 145–48) and lamotrigine 50–200mg/d monotherapy was significantly more effective than placebo in bipolar I depression, the effect being seen as early as the third week (n=195, RCT, Calabrese *et al, J Clin Psych* 1999, **60**, 79–88). Lamotrigine may also be useful as an adjunct for refractory major depression (n=2, Maltese, *Am J Psych* 1999, **156**, 1833).

Levodopa

Levodopa has an 'activating' effect in some cases of depression but is not acting as a pure antidepressant (*J Psychopharmacol* 1990, **4**, 152–67).

Olanzapine

Olanzapine may have a role in augmentation of antidepressant treatment of psychotic depression (n=2, Malhi and Checkley, *B J Psych* 1999, **174**, 460) and a retrospective study indicated olanzapine 10mg/d may have efficacy in psychotic depression, with or without antidepressants (n=30, Rothschild, *J Clin Psych* 1999, **60**, 116–18).

Opiates *

Oxycodone or oxymorphone may produce a sustained effect in refractory and chronic depression, as well as reduced psychogenic pain and distress (n=3, Stoll and Reuter, *Am J Psych* 1999, **156**, 2017).

Pergolide *

Pergolide (a dopamine agonist) has been tried with moderate success as an adjuvant to tricyclics and MAOIs, eg. 55% showed improvement within 7 days, with doses of 0.5–1mg/d (n=20, Bouckoms and Mangini, *Psychopharmacol Bull* 1993, **29**, 207–11) and to tricyclics (n=20, open, Izumi *et al, J Aff Dis* 2000, **61**, 127–32).

Primidone

There is a case of long-standing cyclic depression respondinng completely to primidone given for hand tremor (Brown *et al, Lancet* 1993, **342**, 925).

Progabide

A single successful case occurred in a TD study (*Arch Gen Psych* 1990, **47**, 287–78).

Protirelin (Thyrotropin-Releasing Hormone, TRH)

Five of eight depressed patients given 500mcg of protirelin intrathecally responded robustly and rapidly (mood and suicidality) but the effect was short-lived (Marangell *et al, Arch Gen Psych* 1997, **54**, 214–22). TRH may thus be involved in mood regulation.

Risperidone

Addition of low dose risperidone (up to 1mg/d) to existing SSRI therapy produced rapid responses in SSRI-resistant patients (n=8, open, Ostroff and Nelson, *J Clin Psych* 1999, **60**, 256–59), and of psychotic depression unresponsive to antidepressants responded to risperidone 4mg/d (n=1, Land and Chang, *J Clin Psych* 1998, **59**, 624).

Selegiline

Selegiline was superior to placebo at higher doses (30mg/d), with a low side-effect incidence (*Arch Gen Psych* 1989, **46**, 45–50). MAO-B selectivity is lost at these doses and so a cheese-reaction is possible.

Sulpiride *

Sulpiride (mean dose 181mg/d) may be effective and well-tolerated in mild to moderate depression (n=177, RCT, 6/52, Ruther *et al, Pharmacopsychiatry* 1999, **32**, 127–35).

Tetracycline antibiotics

Minocycline and demeclocycline have been reported in case studies to have a detectable antidepressant effect (Levine *et al, Am J Psych* 1996, **153**, 582).

Valproate

Valproate can be used to augment tricyclics and is probably only of minimum to moderate potency (*Am J Psych* 1990, **147**, 431–34) although response in resistant unipolar depression or dysthymia has been reported (n=1, *B J Psych* 1992, **160**, 121–23).

Verapamil

Dramatic response in an elderly lady has been reported (n=1, *B J Psych* 1991, **158**, 124–25) but disputed (*B J Psych* 1991, **159**, 584–85). See also bipolar (*1.10*).

Zotepine *

Delusional depressive patients may respond to zotepine (n=2, Konig and Wolfersdorf, *Tw Neurol Psych* 1994, **8**, 460–63).

▼ No efficacy

Benzodiazepines

Alprazolam (*J Aff Dis* 1990, **18**, 67–73) and diazepam (*B J Psych* 1989, **155**, 483–89) have been studied. Some depression rating scales include measures of anxiety and probably explain how an antidepressant effect can be shown. The BNF states that they should not be used to treat depression. Discontinuing drugs such as clonazepam prescribed for panic/anxiety control can often lead to improvement of depression (see *5.5*).

Caffeine

Some depressed people may have increased sensitivity to caffeine (*Am J Psych* 1988, **145**, 632–35).

1.15   DYSTHYMIA

See also depression (*1.14*)

Symptoms: *

Dysthymia (literally 'ill-humoured') is a low-grade chronic melancholic depression (often with anxiety) of insidious onset, chronic course (lasting at least two years with permanent or intermittent symptoms) and high risk of relapse. It has few of the physical symptoms of depression and is compatible with stable social functioning.

Almost all eventually develop super-imposed major depression (3yr follow-up, n=86, Klein *et al, Am J Psych* 2000, **157**, 931–39). The life-time prevalence rate may be around 3–6%, and higher in the elderly. It has been considered by some to be similar to depressive personality disorder or anxiety and by others as a way of medicalising (and hence ignoring) social problems or as a way of giving someone a medical diagnosis to allow insurance claims.

Role of drugs: *

It is clear that antidepressants are effective in dysthymia, with no proven significant differences between classes, and should form part of an overall treatment strategy including also, eg. IPT and marital therapy. A greater sensitivity to side-effects has been noted in dysthymics, with tricyclics most likely to cause these. MAOIs, SSRIs and moclobemide appear favoured. If one class does not work, switching to another may convey a 40–60% chance of response (Thase, *Curr Opin Psych* 1998, **11**, 77–83, 35 refs). Treatment for several months may be necessary for full response (de Lima and Moncrieff, Cochrane Review, reviewed by Thase, *EBMH* 1998, **1**, 111). A low (10–20%) placebo response is seen (Frances *et al, Int Clin Psychopharmacol* 1993, **7**, 197–200).

Reviews*: general (Thase, *Curr Opin Psych* 1998, **11**, 77–83, 35 refs), meta-analysis (de Lima *et al, Psychol Med* 1999, **29**, 1273–89), diagnosis and treatment (Rihmer, *Curr Opin Psych* 1999, **12**, 69–75, 48 refs), in the elderly (Bellino *et al, Drugs & Aging* 2000, **16**, 107–21).

● Unlicensed/Some efficacy

Fluoxetine

Fluoxetine at eight weeks may produce a significant improvement in dysthymic symptoms (n=35, p/c, Hellerstein *et al, Am J Psych* 1993, **150**, 1169–75). A further study showed fluoxetine to be more effective than placebo at 20mg/d, with 50% of the non-responders at 3 months improving with a dose increase to 40mg/d (n=140, RCT, Vanelle *et al, B J Psych* 1997, **170**, 345–50).

MAOIs

Phenelzine at 50–75mg/d and tranyl-cypromine have both been shown to be as effective as tricyclics, the latter over a two year period (mentioned in *B J Psych* 1995, **166**, 174–83). More studies are needed to confirm this.

Moclobemide

Moclobemide (mean 675mg/d) has been shown to be significantly more effective for dysthymia than imipramine (mean 220mg/d) and placebo, with fewer side-effects (n=315, RCT, Versiani *et al, Int Clin Psychopharmacol* 1997, **12**, 183–93), confirming previous studies (review by Petursson, *Acta Psych Scand* 1995, **91**[Suppl 386], 36–39).

Sertraline *

Two out-patient studies have shown sertraline (50–200mg/d) to be superior to placebo and as effective as imipramine (50–300mg/d), but better tolerated (12/52, RCT, n=416, Kocsis *et al, Am J Psych* 1997, **154**, 390; n=310, d/b, 12/52, Ravindran *et al, J Clin Psych* 2000, **61**, 821–27). There is some evidence that pre-treatment with a tricyclic may improve subsequent response to sertraline (Thase, *Curr Opin Psych* 1998, **11**, 77–83).

St John's wort

SJW seems effective in mild to moderate depression, including dysthymia (Laakmann *et al, Pharmacopsychiatry* 1998, **31**[Suppl], 54–59, Volz, *Pharmacopsychiatry* 1997, **30** [Suppl], 72–76).

Tricyclics

Amitriptyline and desipramine (Marin *et al, Am J Psych* 1994, **151**, 1079–80) have both been studied over 6–12 weeks and found at doses of 150–300mg/d to be 2–3 times more effective than placebo. 50–300mg/d imipramine has been shown to be as effective (but with more drop-outs, 18.4% *vs* 6%) as sertraline in long-standing dysthymia, and both were significantly better than placebo (n=416, 12/52, RCT, Kocsis *et al, Am J Psych* 1997, **154**, 390).

○ Unlicensed/Possible efficacy

Amisulpride *

A number of studies (review by Noble and Benfeld, *CNS Drugs* 1999, **12**, 471–83) have shown amisulpride to have some efficacy in dysthymia, eg. 50mg/d compared with amineptine (n=323, RCT, 3/12, Boyer *et al, Neuro-psychobiology* 1999, **39**, 25–32), and 50mg/d as effective as fluoxetine 20mg/d (n=268, retrospective, Smeraldi *et al, Eur Psychiatry* 1996, **11** [Suppl 3], 141S–43S). Amisulpride 50mg/d and imipramine 100mg/d are both more effective than placebo (n=156, RCT, 6/12, Lecrubier *et al, J Aff Dis* 1997, **43**, 95–103). Some dopaminergic side-effects are seen with amisulpride.

Chromium

Chromium (as the picolinate) provided a dramatic and complete resolution of dysthymia in a small trial (n=5, s/b, McLeod *et al, J Clin Psych* 1999, **60**, 237).

Fluvoxamine *

Fluvoxamine may be well tolerated and effective in dysthymic adolescents (n=21, open, Rabe-Jablonska, *J Child Adolesc Psychopharmacol* 2000, **10**, 9–18).

Lithium

This may be helpful in selected dysthymic patients (eg. Akiskal *et al, Arch Gen Psych* 1980, **37**, 777–83).

Mirtazapine *

Mirtazapine 15–45mg/d was effective in 73% of patients with dysthymia, 4 discontinuing because of sedation (n=15, open, 10/52, *Depress Anxiety* 1999, **10**, 68–72).

Valproate

There is a case of chronic depression and dysthymia responding to valproate (n=1, Kemp, *B J Psych* 1992, **160**, 121–23).

Venlafaxine *

An open study showed venlafaxine (up to 225mg/d) effective in 10 of the 14 patients who completed a 9-week trial (seven quickly to low dose, three only to high dose, n=17, Dunner *et al, J Clin Psych* 1997, **58**, 528–31). Although adverse effects were a problem in another trial, venlafaxine 100–250mg/d was effective (n=22, open, Hellerstein *et al, J Clin Psych* 1999, **60**, 845-49).

1.16   EATING DISORDERS

DSM-IV includes three eating disorders; anorexia nervosa (AN), bulimia nervosa (BN) and eating disorders, not otherwise specified (EDNOS), this latter including binge eating disorder. Remission is more likely in BN than AN.

Review*: drug treatment of adolescent eating disorders (Gillberg and Rastam, *Int J Psych Clin Pract* 1998, **2**, 79–82; Kruger and Kennedy, *J Psychiatry Neurosci* 2000, **25**, 497–508), general (Treasure, *Prescribers J* 1999, **39**, 227–33; Becker *et al, NEJM* 1999, **340**, 1092–98, 69 refs; Maddox and Long, *JAMA* 1999, **39**, 378–87; Kaye *et al, Ann Rev Med* 2000, **51**, 299–313), brain, bones and exercise (Bryant-Waugh and Lask, *Hosp Med* 1999, **60**, 472–73, editorial).

1.16.1   ANOREXIA NERVOSA

Symptoms:
The main diagnostic symptoms of anorexia nervosa are:
1. Amenorrhoea in females (absence of three consecutive menstrual cycles).
2. Refusal to maintain body weight over minimum normal for age and height.
3. Intense fear of becoming obese.
4. Disturbance in body perception, eg. feeling fat even when emaciated.

Anorexia usually starts in the late teens, with distorted body image and relentless dieting. Patients may avoid carbohydrates, induce vomiting, abuse laxatives, take excess exercise, binge eat and suffer depression and social withdrawal. It may occur in up to 2% of schoolgirls and up to 4 in 100,000 of the general population.

Role of drugs:
Drug therapy is generally most useful as a supportive measure to treat any concurrent conditions. In severely emaciated patients, enteral feeding or even TPN may be necessary.

Reviews*: overall management (Fairburn, *Adv Psych Treat* 1997, **3**, 2–8), in teenagers (Serpell and Treasure, *Prescriber* 1996, **7**[22], 19–25), SSRIs in anorexia (Ferguson *et al, Int J Eat Disord* 1999, **25**, 11–17) and general (Marcus and Levine, *Curr Opin Psych* 1998, **11**, 159–63).

● **Unlicensed/Some efficacy**

Nutritional feeding
TPN may be necessary in severely anorexic patients, where a life-threatening weight loss has occurred, particularly if accompanied by low potassium levels and where conventional therapies have failed. Weight gain can be significant in a relatively short period and TPN can help avert permanent damage or death. Great care is needed where patients are likely to interfere with the IV line with the possibility of infection in a compromised patient and of embolism. Supervised oral feeding with nutritional supplements can also be an effective acute treatment.

Treatment of any PMS
This may help any premenstrual exacerbations (see *1.26*).

Tricyclic antidepressants
The main role of the tricyclics may be in maintenance therapy. Doses of 150mg/d or more for 4–6 weeks may be needed.

○ **Unlicensed/Possible efficacy**

Antipsychotics *
Early trials showed a minor advantage over placebo for pimozide 4–6mg/d (d/b, c/o, Vandereycken and Pierloot, *Acta Psych Scand* 1982, **66**, 445–50) and sulpiride (*B J Psych* 1984, **144**, 288–92). OCD and anorexia have responded to olanzapine 5mg/d, with reduced fixed body perceptions, no weight loss and improved insight (n=1, Hansen, *B J Psych* 1999, **175**, 592), with further reports (n=3, Jensen and Mejlhede, *B J Psych* 2000, **177**, 87; n=2, La Vie *et al, Int J Eat Disord* 2000, **27**, 363–66). Risperidone has been used (Newman-Toker, *J Am Acad Child Adolesc Psych* 2000, **39**, 941–42).

Citalopram *
20mg/d has been used successfully (n=6, Calandra *et al, Eat Weight Disord* 1999, **4**, 207–10).

Cyproheptadine
Several reports of effectiveness at up to 32mg/d have appeared and a 4-week trial may be useful in some sufferers (n=72, RCT, Halmi *et al, Arch Gen Psych* 1986, **43**, 177–81).

Fluoxetine
Fluoxetine 60mg/d may not add significant benefit to in-patient treatment of anorexia (n=31, RCT, Attia *et al, Am J Psych* 1998, **155**, 548–51), but there is some evidence that it may be of use in preventing relapse in weight restored anorexics (Marcus and Levine, *Curr Opin Psych* 1998, **11**, 159–63).

Lithium
Only non-significant effects have been

shown, eg. increased weight (n=16, d/b, 16/52, Gross, *J Clin Psychopharmacol* 1981, **1**, 376–81), although sustained remission has occurred with long-term therapy in a number of cases (eg. Stein *et al, B J Psych* 1982, **140**, 526–28).

Sertraline

A case has been reported of complete response to sertraline at 50mg/d in a woman only partly responsive to fluoxetine (Roberts and Lydiard, *Am J Psych* 1993, **150**, 1753).

Zinc

Zinc has virtually no side-effects and a 4-week trial may help some people (eg. *Acta Psych Scand* 1990, **82**, 14–17) and 100mg/d produced an increase in BMI twice that of placebo (n=35, RCT, Birmingham *et al, Int J Eat Disord* 1994, **15**, 251–55).

1.16.2 BULIMIA NERVOSA

Symptoms:

The main diagnostic symptoms of bulimia nervosa are:

1. Recurrent binge eating.
2. An urge to overeat (including lack of control over eating during binges).
3. Regular self-induced vomiting/ laxative abuse/strict dieting/fasting etc.
4. Persistent over-concern with body shape and weight.

There must be a minimum of two binge episodes per week for at least 3 months. Weight and menses are normal.

Role of drugs*:

A recent meta-analysis concludes that CBT is the most effective single treatment for bulimia, and is superior to drug therapy, that there are advantages to the combination, but neither are effective in about 50% of cases (Whittal *et al, Behavior Therapy* 1999, **30**, 117–35, review by Waller, *EBMH* 1999, **2**, 89). Psychotherapy is also effective (5 RCT meta-analysis, Bacaltchuk *et al, J Clin Pharm & Ther* 1999, **24**, 23–31). However, antidepressants add modest but real benefits as adjunctive treatment (RCT, n=120, Walsh *et al, Am J Psych* 1997, **154**, 523–31), and not confined to people with a co-morbid depression. They are superior to placebo but do not work as antidepressants. Adequate doses are needed, eg. at least 150mg/d equivalent of a tricyclic for

adequate duration, eg. at least four weeks. Side-effects (especially anticholinergic) can be severe and result in non-compliance. Drugs should be part of an individualised programme with nutrition and psychotherapy/CBT, although the higher drop-out rates of the combination may produce lower acceptability (meta-analysis of 5 trials, Bacaltchuk *et al, Acta Psych Scand* 2000, **101**, 256–64).

Reviews*: general (McGilley *et al, Am Fam Physician* 1998, **57**, 2743–50; Freeman, *Neuropsychobiology* 1998, **37**, 72–79; Brewerton, *CNS Drugs* 1999, **11**, 351–61), systematic review (Bacaltchuk *et al, Aust NZ J Psych* 2000, **34**, 310–17), in teenagers (Serpell and Treasure, *Prescriber* 1996, **7**[22], 19–25).

BNF Listed
Fluoxetine *

60mg/d has a significant effect on binge eating and purging, eating attitudes, behaviour and food craving (Goldbloom & Olmsted, *Am J Psych* 1993, **150**, 770–74), being also safe and effective in longer-term treatment of bulimia (n=225, 16/52, Goldstein *et al, B J Psych* 1995, **166**, 660–66), a recent trial confirming this effect where psychological treatments have been inadequate (n=22, RCT, 8/52, Walsh *et al, Am J Psych* 2000, **157**, 1332–34). It does not work purely as an antidepressant as the improvement is independent of depression scores and uses higher doses, although any depression may also improve. Its long half-life may help with missed doses.

● Combinations
Naltrexone + fluoxetine

After a partial response to 60mg/d fluoxetine, addition of 100mg/d naltrexone produced a 'robust' reduction in binge frequency and amount (n=1, Neumeister *et al, Am J Psych* 1999, **156**, 797).

● Unlicensed/Some efficacy
MAOIs

MAOIs can be successful drugs if the dietary restrictions can be overcome.

PMS treatments

Pyridoxine and progesterones in particular may help to minimise the effects of premenstrual relapses.

SSRIs * (see also fluoxetine above)

One trial showed fluvoxamine to have a significant effect on reducing bulimic behaviour (n=72, d/b, p/c, Fichter, *J Clin Psychopharmacol* 1996, **16**, 9–18), and in binge-eating disorder (binge-eating without purging), with 50–300mg/d effective in most outcome measures in acute treatment (n=85, 9/52, RCT, Hudson *et al, Am J Psych* 1998, **155**, 1756–62). Sertraline was significantly superior to placebo in most measures in a short study (n=34, RCT, d/b, 6/52, McElroy *et al, Am J Psych* 2000, **157**, 1004-6). Citalopram 20mg/d has been used successfully (n=12, Calandra *et al, Eat Weight Disord* 1999, **4**, 207–10). Paroxetine has been reputed to have no beneficial effect in an unpublished study.

Tricyclics

Amitriptyline (*J Clin Psychopharmacol* 1984, **4**, 186–93), desipramine (*Am J Psych* 1990, **147**, 1509–13), doxepin and imipramine (*Arch Gen Psych* 1990, **47**, 149–57) have all been used but are of arguable potency. Poor relapse rates suggest serious limitations with long-term efficacy (*Am J Psych* 1991, **148**, 1206–12).

○ Unlicensed/Possible efficacy
Flutamide

The testosterone receptor antagonist flutamide (250–500mg/d) produced a rapid and marked improvement in bulimic behaviour in two women (Bergman and Eriksson, *Acta Psych Scand* 1996, **94**, 137–39).

Naltrexone

Reduced binge-purge symptomatology was seen in 18 of 19 bulimics treated with naltrexone (RCT, Marrazzi *et al, Int Clin Psychopharmacol* 1995, **10**, 163–72). See also naltrexone.

Ondansetron *

A small open study showed some effect (Hartman *et al, Arch Gen Psych* 1997, **54**, 969–70), and decreased binge-eating and vomiting has been shown with ondansetron 24mg/d, possibly due to pharmacological decrease in vagal neurotransmission (n=28, RCT, Faris *et al, Lancet* 2000, **355**, 792–97; editorial by Kiss, *Lancet* 2000, **355**, 769–70).

Reboxetine *

Successful use of reboxetine has been reported (n=7, open, El-Giamal *et al, Int Clin Psychopharmacol* 2000, **15**, 351–56).

Topiramate *

70% women with binge-eating disorder treated with topiramate showed a moderate or good response to topiramate, maintained for up to 30 months (case series, n=13, mean 18/12, Shapira *et al, J Clin Psych* 2000, **61**, 368–72).

Trazodone *

Trazodone has been shown to be well tolerated and superior to placebo (n=42, RCT, Pope *et al, J Clin Psychopharmacol* 1989, **9**, 254–59), although some patients worsened (n=3, *J Clin Psych* 1983, **44**, 275–76).

Valproate

There is a single reported case of a dramatic and dose-dependent response (*J Clin Pharmacol* 1985, **5**, 229–30).

Zinc

A 4-week trial showed zinc to be safe and potentially effective (*Arch Int Med* 1984, **100**, 317–18).

▼ No efficacy
Carbamazepine

No effect on bulimia was seen in one study (n=6, *Am J Psych* 1983, **140** 1225–26).

Clozapine

There is a single case of bulimia acutely worsening on clozapine 350mg/d (*Am J Psych* 1992, **149**, 1408).

Cyproheptadine

Although potentially useful in anorexia it appears to be detrimental in bulimia (*Arch Gen Psych* 1986, **43**, 177–81).

Lithium

Despite early enthusiasm, lithium is no more effective than placebo (n=91, Hsu *et al, J Nerv Mental Dis* 1991, **179**, 351–55).

Mianserin

No effect was seen at 60mg/d (n=50, 8/52, *B J Clin Pharmacol* 1983, **15**, 195S–202S).

1.17.1 EPILEPSY

See also status epilepticus (*1.17.2*)

The annual incidence of epilepsy is 50–70 cases per 100 000 (excluding febrile seizure), with a prevalence of 5–10 per 1000. The lifetime prevalence is 2–5% of the population. Of those people with epilepsy, up to 30–40% have seizures at unacceptably high rates or have additional problems (see Epilepsy Needs document, Brown *et al, Seizure* 1993, **2**, 91–103).

DISCONTINUING ANTICONVULSANTS*

All anticonvulsants have side-effects (eg. cognitive impairment, disturbed behaviour, alteration of bone and liver metabolism etc), especially when taken for long periods and even when optimum ranges are adhered to. They should be discontinued when no longer needed. About 70% of patients enter a prolonged remission. Relapse rates for children are about 20%, adults 45–50% (8-year follow-up — *Am J Mental Disorders* 1989, **93**, 593–99; comment *ibid* pp. 600–6). Little advice is given to adults on anticonvulsant discontinuation, with many stopping on their own initiative (Goodridge and Shorvon, *Epilepsia* 1983, 645–47). Withdrawal of anticonvulsants can also lead to emergence of seizures and psychiatric morbidity, particularly depression and anxiety (Ketter *et al, Neurology* **44**, 55–61).

A concentration of fits during or in the first few months after withdrawal suggest that at least some are provoked by drug withdrawal. Other withdrawal effects such as anxiety, agitation and insomnia are a problem but only occur with the barbiturates and benzodiazepines (Reviews in *Lancet* 1991, **337**, 1175–80; Kristmann *et al, Lancet* 1991, **338**, 53; Fenck & Reynolds, *Clin Pharm* 1990, **9**, 781–88). In one study of anticonfulsant withdrawal in 100 children, there was little improvement in cognitive function (Aldenkamp *et al, Neurology* 1993, **43**, 41–50).

Reviews*: withdrawing anticonvulsants (Schmidt and Gram, *Drugs* 1996, **52**, 870–74; Lhatoo and Sander, *Curr Pharm Des* 2000, **6**, 861–63; Buna, *Pharmacotherapy* 1998, **18**, 235–41), comparative study (n=1013, Chadwick, *Brain* 1999, **122**, 441–48), practical guide (Schmidt and Gram, *Drugs* 1996, **52**, 870–74).

One study of 149 children who were seizure-free for 2–4 years showed that seizure recurrence rates (40%) were not significantly different in those withdrawn from anticonvulsants quickly or slowly, six weeks or nine months respectively (Tennison *et al, NEJM* 1994, **330**, 1407–10).

A prognostic index for recurrence of seizures, either on continued treatment or discontinuation, has been advised by the MRC Antiepileptic Drug Withdrawal Study Group (Chadwick *et al, BMJ* 1993, **306**, 1374–78), based on a 4-year study of 1021 patients from six European countries, testing the potential for 26 possible risk factors. This is the only major study of withdrawal in patients in remission:

Starting score (all patients)	-175
Age 16 yrs or older	+45
Taking >1anticonvulsant	+50
Seizures after starting anticonvulsants	+35
History of 1° or 2° GTC seizures	+35
History of myoclonic seizures	+50
EEG in past year	
— not available	+15
— abnormal	+20
Period free from seizures (in years)	+200/t
Total scores=	=T
Then divide the total score by 100 and expontiate (e^x):	$z=e^{t/100}$
Thus the probability of recurrence of seizures is: Continued treatment:	
— by one year	$1-0.89^z$
— by two years	$1-0.79^z$
Slow withdrawal:	
— by one year	$1-0.69^z$
— by two years	$1-0.60^z$

It is suggested that this important and accessible paper be consulted in order to use this predictive model to its optimum. It should prove useful in counselling patients in the community who wish to withdraw from anticonvulsants. Further validation is being carried out. For guidelines for discontinuing antiepileptic drugs in seizure-free patients, see Rosenberg *et al* (*Neurology* 1996, **47**, 600–2).

Main risk factors on discontinuing anticonvulsants:

● Polypharmacy (4 or more anticonvulsants)

● Active epilepsy

● Age (50 years or older)

● 5 weeks or less between reductions

● Longer duration of treatment or illness (more than 30 months is a higher risk)

● Number of seizures before fits controlled (higher risk of relapse if more than 100 fits are experienced before control is achieved)

● Interval seizure less than one month at onset of illness

- Type of seizure: Complex partial seizures, tonic-clonic or combinations of seizures are more likely to relapse than simple partial seizures, except perhaps in children where atypical febrile seizures are a higher risk (*NEJM* 1985, **313**, 976–80)

- Number of drugs required before seizure control (and hence time taken to control fits): If fits are controlled by the drug of first choice, relapse rates are much less than where more drugs have to be tried or where polypharmacy is needed (*Lancet* 1991, **337**, 1175–80)

- Abnormal EEG: 'Class 4'/epileptiform are the highest risk

- Adult/late onset seizures (after 10 to 12 years of age)

- Underlying cerebral disorder (eg. mental retardation — *NEJM* 1981, **304**, 1125–29)

- Withdrawal in less than 6 months (*Epilepsia* 1984, **25**, 137–44)

- Age, especially in childhood, possibly related to maturation of the CNS (Murakami *et al, J Neurol Neurosurg and Psych* 1995, **59**, 477–81), and possibly including abnormal neonatal period

- Osteomalacia (case in *Postgrad Med J* 1992, **68**, 134–36)

References*: *NEJM* 1988, **318**, 942–46 + Editorial; *Drug & Ther Bull* 1989, **27**, 29–31; n=161, RCT, Peters *et al, Neurology* 1998, **50**, 724–30; n=226, Caviedes and Herranz, *Seizure* 1998, **7**, 107–14; n=409, RCT, Chadwick *et al, Epilepsia* 1996, **37**, 1043–50).

Favourable factors for discontinuing anticonvulsants:

- Primary generalised seizures

- Childhood onset (after the age of one)

- Short duration of epilepsy

- No cerebral disorder

- Normal IQ

- Normal EEG (or at least no gross abnormalities), persistently before and after discontinuation

- Few seizures documented, especially juvenile myoclonic epilepsy

- History of non-compliance/concordance without relapse (in which case withdrawal should be encouraged)

- Medication below therapeutic levels at time of discontinuation

- More than two years since last seizure, especially in children (*Lancet* 1991, **337**, 1175–80; *Drug & Ther Bull* 1989, **27**, 29–31; *Am J Mental Disorders* 1989, **93**, 593–99; comment *ibid* 600–6)

Role of drugs*:

Drug therapy is probably the single most important aspect in managing seizures. One study of 392 patients showed that treatment after a first fit reduced the recurrence rate at 24 months from 51% (untreated) to 26% (treated with first line anticonvulsant) (First Seizure Trial Group, *Neurology* 1993, **43**, 478–83). The most important risk factors for sudden unexpected death in epilepsy are polypharmacy, frequent changes in dose and seizure frequency (case-control study, Nilsson *et al, Lancet* 1999, **353**, 888–93). In a systematic review of the newer anticonvulsants, the NNTs for new anticonvulsants as add-on therapy for refractory epilepsy were topiramate (1000mg/d=2.9, 600mg/d=3.0), vigabatrin (300mg/d=3.3), tiagabine (32mg/d=6.5), lamotrigine (500mg/d=7.2) and gabapentin (1200mg/d=7.4) (Marson *et al, Epilepsia* 1997, **38**, 859–80, comment in *Bandolier* 1998, **5**, 4–5).

Plasma level monitoring for anticonvulsants is often over-used and should be restricted to:

1. Patients on phenytoin or polypharmacy where dosage adjustment is necessary due to poor control or dose-related toxicity.
2. People with learning disabilities, where assessing toxicity is difficult.
3. Patients with renal or hepatic disease.
4. Pregnant women.
5. Where compliance is suspect.

Reviews*: general (Wallace *et al, Hosp Med* 1998, **59**, 461–68; Feely, *BMJ* 1999, **318**, 106–9), managing severe epilepsy in the community (Brown, *Adv Psych Treat* 1998, **4**, 345–55; Sander, *Prescriber* 1998, **9**, 41–65), consensus statement on the medical management of epilepsy (Southern Clinical Neurological Society, *Neurology* 1998, **51**[Suppl 4], S39–S43), AED efficacy in adults according to seizure type (Mattson, *Neurology* 1998, **51**[Suppl 4], S15–S20, 28 refs), TDM of

AEDs (Eadie, *B J Clin Pharmacol* 1998, **46**, 185–93, 67 refs), practical TDM guidelines (Johannessen, *CNS Drugs* 1997, **7**, 349–65), modes of action (Rho and Sankar, *Epilepsia* 1999, **40**, 1471–83), Lennox-Gastaut Syndrome, (Schmidt and Bourgeois, *Drug Safety* 2000, **22**, 467–77, 51 refs), refractory seizures (Devinsky, *NEJM* 1999, **340**, 1565–70, 43 refs).

BNF Listed
First-line/monotherapy drugs
In a large comparison of phenobarbital, phenytoin, carbamazepine and valproate in childhood epilepsy, seizure outcome was good with all four drugs but phenobarbital had unacceptable side-effects and phenytoin had worse side-effects (9% withdrew) than valproate (4%) and carbamazepine (4%) (n=167, de Silva *et al, Lancet* 1996, **347**, 709–13).

Carbamazepine
Carbamazepine is a broad spectrum anticonvulsant, licensed in the UK for adjunctive or first-line therapy in partial or generalised epilepsy (excluding absence and myoclonus). It has been compared with valproate in complex partial and secondary GTC in a large adult study, where they were considered of similar efficacy but with carbamazepine better for complex partial seizures and with fewer long-term side-effects (Mattson *et al, NEJM* 1992, **327**, 765–71, comments in *NEJM* 1993, **328**, 207–9). Use of the sustained release tablet may reduce side-effects and improve control (*Arch Dis Child* 1990, **65**, 930–35). Although overall doses may need to be adjusted slightly upwards (*Br J Clin Pharmacol* 1991, **32**, 99–104), they can be used as a once-a-day dosage, with careful monitoring if seizures continue (study by Triscari *et al in B J Clin Pharmacol* 1993, **36**, 257, 263–65), although lower trough concentrations mean some patients may need twice daily dosing. For a review of population pharmacokinetics in adults, see Graves *et al* (*Pharmacotherapy* 1998, **18**, 273–81).

Lamotrigine *
Lamotrigine is indicated for adjunctive or monotherapy in partial or generalised epilepsy, Lennox-Gastaut, juvenile myoclonic epilepsy. It is well tolerated as monotherapy in adults with newly diagnosed epilepsy (review of published RCTs, Mullens, *Clinical Drug Investigation* 1998, **16**, 125–33) and at up to 500mg/d as monotherapy in adult patients with partial seizures (n=156, d/b, Gilliam *et al, Neurology* 1998, **51**, 1018–25). Lamotrigine is thought to stabilise pre-synaptic neuronal membranes by blockade of voltage-dependent sodium channels, with this secondarily inhibiting the release of excessive excitatory glutamate (Leach *et al, Epilepsia* 1986, **27**, 490–97) and aspartate. It may only be fully effective when rapid firing occurs, ie. before and during a seizure. This unique effect on the excitatory system may also reduce neuronal death (Leach *et al, Epilepsia* 1991, **32**, 4–8).

As monotherapy, a comparison with carbamazepine showed an equivalent effect in newly diagnosed epilepsy, but causing significantly less drowsiness (n=260, Brodie *et al, Lancet* 1995, **345**, 476–79). In a study of lamotrigine as add-on treatment in 30 children and adolescents with refractory generalised epilepsy, there was a clear statistically significant reduction of seizure frequency compared with placebo (n=30, RCT, Eriksson *et al, Epilepsia* 1998, **39**, 495–501). Lamotrigine has a good pharmacokinetic profile, eg. long half-life, low protein binding and few interactions.

Rash occurs in 2–5% of patients and may significantly limit treatment. To reduce the risk of skin reactions, an adult starting dose of 25mg/d for two weeks, then 50mg/d for two weeks, then increasing every 1–2 weeks is now recommended. These doses should be halved if the patient is also on valproate (where rash is also more likely to occur, Gilman, *Ann Pharmacother* 1995, **29**, 144–51) or allergic to trimethoprim, and doubled if combined with concurrent enzyme inducing drugs, eg. phenytoin, carbamazepine and phenobarbital.

SEIZURES—types, symptoms and treatment

	International Classification	Other names	Manifestation	Age of onset	Duration	Recovery
G E	Generalised Tonic-Clonic (G.T.C.)	Major motor	Sudden loss of consciousness, intense (tonic) muscle spasms, then intermittent seizures. Also flushing & incontinence	Any	1–5 minutes	Varies up to 1hr
N E	Absence (typical or atypical)	Petit mal	Sudden cessation of activity. Eyes rolling. Unresponsive. Immediate recovery, no awareness	3–15 years limit	Seconds	Immediate
R A	Myoclonic or Partial seizures with motor symptoms	Minor motor Infantile spasms Myoclonic jerks	Sudden jerk of limbs. May be followed by G.T.C. or atonic seizures	During 1st yr of life (3–9 mo)	Seconds to minutes	Varies
L I S E D	Atonic	Akinetic Astatic 'Drop attacks'	Sudden loss of consciousness	2+ yrs (3–7 most common)	Minutes	Varies
F O C A L	Simple Partial (Partial seizures with simple symptomatology)	Focal (localised) Simple motor Sensory	Spasmodic convulsions. Hallucinations of flashing lights. Numbness, paraesthesia dysphagia & visual phenomena. No loss of consciousness	Any	Minutes	Varies
P A R T I A L	Complex Partial (Partial seizures with complex symptomatology)	Temporal lobe Psychomotor	Unconscious behaviour (chewing, lip smacking, walking), acts of violence, hallucinations of taste, smell or hearing. Unreal feelings. Memory disturbance. Time disturbance. Fear, anxiety, distorted perception. Impaired consciousness	Adolescent and adult	Minutes to hours	Immediate. No awareness

Generalised epilepsy usually has genetic influence (eg. low threshold). Focal and partial epilepsy is probably due to a damaged brain area.
For further information on the International Classification of Epileptic Seizures (ICES), refer to *Epilepsia* 1981, **22**, 489–501.

Drug	Plasma levels		Half-life	Time to steady state	Peak plasma concs	Sample time	Sample frequency	Other checks	Comments
	'Optimum'	Toxic							
PHENYTOIN *TDM Essential	40–80 micromol/L (10–20mg/l) upper end for partial seizures, <20mmol unlikely to work	>80 micromol/L	20–40hrs (up to 140 at higher levels)	5 days minimum, 1–5 weeks possibly (variable, dose dependent)	3–12 hrs dependent on total daily dose	Aim for trough unless confirmation of toxicity required	Every 3–12 months for well stabilised patients	Folate, Calcium (both with phenytoin)	Non-linear kinetics, so missed doses, changes in absorption, tablet or capsule brand can all markedly affect plasma levels.
PHENOBARBITAL *TDM Useful	60–180 micromol/L ↑ (10–30mg/l) dependent upon response	>180 micromol/L chance of stupor	50–160 hrs, with age.	Adults: 10–25 days Children: 8–15 days	2–6 hrs	Long t½, so time not vital. Best to be consistent each time	Every 6/12 for well stabilised patients	Folate 6/12	Blood levels can also be useful as a measure of long-term compliance
CARBAMAZEPINE *TDM Fairly useful	20–50 micromol/L (4–12mg/l). 20–40 for G.T.C. + poly therapy, 30–50 for monotherapy	>50 micromol/L	5–38 hrs	1–4 weeks (enzyme induction). Changes stabilise in about a week	2.5–24 hrs (mean 6h) –less if taken with food	Aim for trough level unless side-effects suspected	Every six months for well stabilised patients	FBC in initial stages of treatment. Thyroid? Serum sodium	Plasma levels only of real use for anticonvulsant action. Are of limited use (eg toxicity) in affective disorders.
SODIUM VALPROATE/ VALPROIC ACID TDM Unproven	300–700 mmol/L (50–100mg/L) proposed. Care in elderly	>700mmol/L — but few side-effects or correlation proved	6–20 hrs, longer in liver disease + polytherapy	30–85 hrs	E/C tabs 2–4 hrs. Sol. tabs + syrup: 1–3 hrs.	Short t½ so need great care interpreting. Only serial levels are accurate	On request	LFT for 6/12 + Plasma amylase if in abdominal pain	Levels may be useful where control is poor or if toxicity suspected. Hepatotoxicity may be dose related

Unbound levels of phenytoin and valproate may be useful (*Neurology* 1992, **42**, 988–90).   ANTICONVULSANTS — Overuse of levels — *BMJ*,1987, **294**, 723

Therapeutic drug monitoring

Reviews*: pharmacokinetics in mono-therapy (Hussein and Posner, *Br J Clin Pharmacol* 1997, **43**, 457–66), safety (Messenheimer *et al, Drug Safety* 1998, **18**, 281–96, 28 refs), safety review of 68 trials, with particular emphasis on rash (Messenheimer *et al, Drug Safety* 1998, **18**, 281–96, 28 refs), overview (Leppil, *Neurology* 1998, **51**, 940–42, editorial; *Prescrire International* 1999, **8**, 80–82, 28 refs), use in children (Messenheimer *et al, Drug Safety* 2000, **22**, 303–12, 35 refs), saliva and serum monitoring (Tsiropoulos *et al, Ther Drug Monit* 2000, **22**, 517–21).

Phenytoin *

Phenytoin is a broad spectrum anti-convulsant licensed for adjunctive or first-line therapy in partial or generalised epilepsy (excluding absence and myoclonus) and status epilepticus, and is believed to stabilise seizure threshold. Phenytoin is not now routinely recommended for use in children as it can cause permanent learning difficulties. A wide range of side-effects and non-linear kinetics make it a difficult drug to use (review of optimising phenytoin by Valodia *et al, J Clin Pharm & Therap* 1999, **24**, 381). A study of 45 patients aimed at establishing dosing rules to minimise toxic effects with phenytoin produced the following:

1. Increase dose by 100mg/d if the steady state plasma level is less than 7mcg/ml.
2. Increase dose by 50mg/d if the steady state plasma level is 7 or more but less than 12mcg/ml.
3. Increase dose by 30mg/d when initial plasma levels are 12mcg/ml or more (Privitera, *Ann Pharmacother* 1993, **27**, 1169–73; advice on TDM of phenytoin by Aronson *et al, BMJ* 1992, **305**, 1215–18).

Valproate

An established drug licensed for adjunctive or first-line therapy in partial or generalised epilepsy (excluding absence and myoclonus), Lennox-Gastaut syndrome and juvenile myoclonic epilepsy. Monotherapy in partial seizures is less well-established. The sustained release preparations overcome the short plasma half-life. There is little correlation between blood levels and therapeutic effect (*BMJ* 1988, **296**, 1110–14) and so routine blood level monitoring is of limited use, although saturation protein binding may occur above 100mg/l, requiring great care. Serious toxicity is rare and careful supervision initially will guard against major problems, eg. liver toxicity. See carbamazepine for details of a comparative study.

Benzodiazepines

Benzodiazepines are excellent anti-convulsant drugs in the short-term but tolerance limits long-term use. They may be useful for 'rescue' or special events, eg. holidays, family events etc. (review by Henriksen, *Epilepsia* 1998, **39**[Suppl 1], S2–S6).

Clobazam

Clobazam is licensed as adjunctive therapy in partial or generalised epilepsy and as intermittent therapy. Tolerance can develop and so low doses (eg. 10–20mg/d) and intermittent administration may help minimise this. Sustained response is more likely in patients with a shorter duration of epilepsy, a known etiology and higher clobazam (but not n-desmethylclobazam) plasma levels (n=173, Singh *et al, Epilepsia* 1995, **36**, 798–803). It may be especially effective for stimulus-provoked attacks, catamenial epilepsy if given for one week in four and in intractable childhood epilepsy (n=63, Sheth *et al, J Child Neurol* 1995, **10**, 205–8).

Reviews: Shorvon, *Epilepsia* 1998, **39**[Suppl 1], S15–S23; Fisher and Blum, E*pilepsia* 1995, **36**[Suppl 2], S105–14; Schmidt, *Epilepsia* 1994, **35**[Suppl 5], S92–95.

Clonazepam

Clonazepam is licensed for adjunctive therapy in partial or generalised epilepsy (including absence and myoclonus), infantile spasms, status and Lennox-Gastaut syndrome. It has marked anticonvulsant properties but its usefulness is limited by tolerance (which may possibly be reversed with flumazenil 1.5mg IV — *Lancet* 1991, **337**, 133–37) and sedation. Review by Tassinari *et al, Epilepsia* 1998, **39**[Suppl 1], S7–S14.

Diazepam

Diazepam is occasionally useful orally

as an adjunct and in short-term therapy, although studies on it are limited. Use in status epilepticus is well established (see below). Review by Tassinari *et al, Epilepsia* 1998, **39**[Suppl 1], S7–S14.

Barbiturates
Methylphenobarbital
This barbiturate is to be discontinued in mid-2001.
Phenobarbital (phenobarbitone)
Phenobarbital and primidone are licensed as adjunctive or first-line therapy in partial or generalised epilepsy (excluding absence and myoclonus). Concerns about cognitive and psychomotor impairment and dependence have rightly limited its use.
Primidone
A barbiturate metabolised mainly to phenobarbital but also to phenylethyl-malonamide. Uses and actions are as for phenobarbital. Treatment failure due to toxicity is more common with primidone than other drugs. Increased adverse effects in a large study showed that its therapeutic action is not just that of phenobarbital (*BMJ* 1985, **313**, 145).

Add-on or adjunct therapy/others
Acetazolamide
Although a potent anticonvulsant, used for absence and other seizures, rapid tolerance and long-term side-effects render it of limited use (review by Reiss and Oles, *Ann Pharmacother* 1996, **30**, 512–19, 68 refs).
Ethosuximide
Ethosuximide is licensed as first-line or adjunctive therapy in generalised absence seizures but is poorly studied and due to its side-effects, eg. gastric upset, has largely now been replaced by valproate.
Gabapentin *
Gabapentin is an anticonvulsant licensed in the UK as adjunctive therapy in refractory partial and secondarily generalised epilepsy, with a reduction of 50% or more in partial seizures in 25–33% patients but few become seizure-free. There is a strong dose: response relationship, with much inter-patient variability (requiring individual optimisation), with 1200mg/d probably the minimum effective maintenance dose, although 600, 1200 and 2400mg/d have been shown to be equipotent in

refractory complex partial or secondarily generalized seizures (n=275, 6/12, RCT, Beydoun *et al, Neurology* 1997, **49**, 746–52). A four-year follow-up of gabapentin in drug-resistant epilepsy showed that 28% gained a significant improvement in seizures (n=25, Sivenius *et al, Arch Neurol* 1994, **51**, 1047–50). Gabapentin may be effective as add-on therapy in children with refractory partial seizures (n=247, RCT, 12/52, Appleton *et al, Epilepsia* 1999, **40**, 1147–54) and a beneficial effect on mood in partial epilepsy has been seen (n=40, Harden *et al, Epilepsia* 1999, **40**, 1129–34). The mode of action is not established (review by Kelly, *Neuropsychobiology* 1998, **38**, 139–44). It has a low order of toxicity, uncomplicated kinetics, no clinically important interactions and plasma levels are not necessary. A TDS dosage is recommended, with no more than 12hrs between doses. A Cochrane Review concluded that gabapentin has efficacy as an add-on in drug-resistant epilepsy, but trials are short-term, with long-term efficacy and monotherapy unproven (Marson *et al, CDSR* 2000, CD001415).

Reviews*: general (*Prescrire International* 2000, **9**, 40–42; Morris, *Epilepsia* 1999, **40**[Suppl 5], S63–70), as monotherapy (Beydoun, *Epilepsia* 1999, **40**[Suppl 6], S13–16).

Levetiracetam *
Levetiracetam is licensed for adjunctive therapy for partial seizures with or without secondary generalisations. Although structurally related to piracetam, it has a distinct pharmacological profile (Genton and Van Vleymen, *Epileptic Disord* 2000, **2**, 99–105) and the mode of action is unclear. It has good bioavailability, rapidly achieves steady-state concentrations, has linear kinetics, minimal protein binding, and minimal metabolism. It needs to be given twice a day. The main side effect of somnolence can be minimised by starting at a lower dose. It has been investigated at 1–3g/d for resistant partial seizures, where it has been effective and well tolerated (n=294, RCT, Cereghino *et al, Neurology* 2000, **55**, 236–42; n=286, d/b, p/c, Ben-Menachem and Falter,

Epilepsia 2000, **41**, 1276–83) and at 1–2g bd as add-on therapy in refractory epilepsy (n=119, RCT, 24/52, Betts *et al, Seizure* 2000, **9**, 80–87). 31% of patients had a greater than 50% reduction in seizures when used as add-on in another study in refractory partial seizures (n=324, RCT, 12/52, Shorvon *et al, Epilepsia* 2000, **41**, 1179–86). 4g/d may be the upper limit of efficacy in many patients (n=29, p/c, Grant and Shorvon, *Epilepsy Res* 2000, **42**, 89–95). A positive impact on epilepsy-related quality of life has been reported (Cramer *et al, Epilepsia* 2000, **41**, 868–74).

Reviews: pharmacokinetic profile (Patsalos, *Pharmacol Ther* 2000, **85**, 77–85), general (Dooley and Plosker, *Drugs* 2000, **60**, 871–93).

Oxcarbazepine *

Oxcarbazepine is an anticonvulsant that exerts its action primarily through its metabolite (the monohydroxy derivative, MHD). It is related to carbamazepine and its efficacy appears comparable, but oxcarbazepine may be better tolerated, and may prove particularly useful in patients unable to tolerate carbamazepine due to adverse effects or allergic reactions and in patients receiving concomitant medications with a high potential to interact with carbamazepine (*Formulary Monograph Service* 2000, 143–50, 34 refs). It is indicated for partial seizures with or without secondary GTC seizures (eg. n=79, RCT, Beydoun *et al, Neurology* 2000, **54**, 2245–51), as monotherapy or adjunctive therapy in adults and children, with an average maintenance dose of 2,400mg/day. Oxcarbazepine, 1200mg twice daily was effective and safe as monotherapy compared to placebo in hospitalised patients with refractory partial seizures (RCT, Schachter *et al, Neurology* 1999, **52**, 732–38). It has also been compared with valproate (d/b, Christe *et al, Epilepsy Res* 1997, **26**, 451–60), phenytoin (*Epilepsy Res* 1997, **27**, 195–204) and phenytoin in children and adolescents (Guerreiro *et al, Epilepsy Res* 1997, **27**, 205–13). It is less likely to induce enzymes than carbamazepine, and probably has minimal autoinduction.

About 25–30% of patients who have experienced hypersensitivity to carbamazepine may experience such reactions with oxcarbazepine. If signs and symptoms suggest such reactions, oxcarbazepine should be withdrawn immediately. Hyponatraemia can occur, and so regular sodium levels are advisable.

Reviews: general (Shorvon, *Seizure* 2000, **9**, 75–79; Castillo *et al, CDSR* 2000, **3**, CD002028; Tecoma, *Epilepsia* 1999, 40[Suppl 5], S37–S46), safety and efficacy (Beydoun, *Pharmacotherapy* 2000, **20**, 152S–58S).

Piracetam

Piracetam is a GABA derivative, licensed in the UK for cerebral myoclonus, especially of cortical origin (Brown *et al, Mov Disorder* 1993, **8**, 63–68 and n=20, RCT, Koskiniemi *et al, J Neurol Neurosurg Psychiatry* 1998, **64**, 344–48) and up to 70% may become seizure-free if they can swallow enough of it.

Tiagabine

Tiagabine is licensed in the UK as adjunctive therapy for partial seizures, with or without secondary generalisation. It is a potent GABA reuptake inhibitor in neuronal and glial cells, increasing GABA-mediated inhibition of the brain. Several studies have shown an effect in refractory partial seizures (14% achieving a 50% or greater increase in seizure-free days, n=154, d/b, p/c, Kalviainen *et al, Epilepsy Res* 1998, **30**, 31–40) and refractory complex partial seizures (up to 29% had a >50% reduction in seizures, n=297, RCT, Uthman *et al, Arch Neurol* 1998, **55**, 56–62). Data on monotherapy is limited. Tiagabine has linear kinetics, a short half-life (requiring bd to qds dosage), an inducable metabolism and a number of drug interactions (see *4.5.9*).

Reviews*: general (Leach and Brodie, *Lancet* 1998, **351**, 203–7; Stephen and Brodie, *Prescriber* 1999, **10**, 19–24; Luer and Rhoney, *Ann Pharmacother* 1998, **32**, 1173–80, 48 refs; *Drug & Ther Bull* 2000, **38**, 47–48, 17 refs), pharmacokinetics (Samara *et al, Epilepsia* 1998, **39**, 868–73), extensive (pharmacodynamics, therapeutic potential, Adkins and Noble, *Drugs* 1998, **55**, 437–60, 89 refs).

Topiramate *

Topiramate is licensed in the UK as adjunctive therapy for refractory partial seizures (eg. n=48, d/b, Sachdeo *et al, Epilepsia* 1997, **38**, 294–300) and secondary generalised seizures with or without secondary generalisation. In a pooled analysis of topiramate as add-on therapy, seizures were reduced by more than 50% in 43% of topiramate-treated and 12% of placebo-treated patients (n=743, 6 d/b, p/c trial, Reife *et al, Epilepsia* 2000, **41**[Suppl 1], S66–S71). The optimal dose appears around 400mg/d in many patients. No plasma levels are required, twice daily dosing is appropriate and the recommended starting dose is now 25mg/d for the first week, increased by 25–50mg/d every 1–2 weeks to 200–400mg/d. There is a multiple mode of action, including sodium channel blockade, GABA enhancement, glutamate inhibition and weak carbonic anhydrase inhibition, which may explain its effect in resistant epilepsy and severity of side-effects, eg. ataxia, dizziness and somnolence. These can be minimised by slower dose titration. Topiramate may have a role in refractory partial epilepsy (200–600mg/d, RCT, n=181, Faught *et al, Neurology* 1996, **46**, 1684–90), with 600mg/d as effective as 800mg/d as add-on therapy in refractory partial epilepsy (RCT, n=190, Privitera *et al, Neurology* 1996, **46**, 1678–83), in Lennox-Gastaut syndrome, (n=98, RCT, p/c, 11/52, Sachdeo *et al, Neurology* 1999, **52**, 1882–88; n=97, open extension to RCT, Glauser *et al, Epilepsia* 2000, **41**[Suppl1], S86–S90) in West syndrome (n=11, Glauser *et al, Epilepsia* 2000, **41**[Suppl 1], S91–S94), and in children (n=51, Mohamed, *Seizure* 2000, **9**, 137–41). A Cochrane Review concludes that topiramate has efficacy as add-on in partial epilepsy, but long-term and monotherapy were unproven (Jette *et al, CDSR* 2000, CD001417).

Reviews*: general (Kellett *et al, J Neurol, Neurosurg & Psych* 1999, **66**, 759–63; Garnett, *Epilepsia* 2000, **41**[Suppl 1], S61–S65; Glauser, *Epilepsia* 1999, **40**[Suppl 5], S71–80) and extensive (Sander, *Epilepsia* 1997, **38**[Suppl 1], S56–S58, Privitera, *Ann Pharmacother* 1997, **31**, 1164–73), pharmacokinetics and interactions (Johannessen, *Epilepsia* 1997, **38**[S1], S18–S23; Langtry *et al, Drugs* 1997, **54**, 752–73, 104 refs), pharmacology (Shank *et al, Epilepsia* 2000, **41**[Suppl 1], S3–9).

Vigabatrin *

Vigabatrin is a selective irreversible GABA-transaminase inhibitor licensed as adjunctive therapy in refractory partial and secondary generalised epilepsy, Lennox-Gastaut and infantile spasms and as monotherapy for West Syndrome (where it is first-line, Fejerman *et al, J Child Neurol* 2000, **15**, 161–65). An analysis of studies showed up to 50% (of epileptics) achieved a 50% or more reduction in seizures, mostly with complex partial seizures (Michelucci and Tassinari, *B J Clin Pharmacol* 1989, **27**, 119S–24S) and 10% may become seizure-free. No serum levels are necessary and once daily dosage is possible (n=50, RCT, d/b, 6/12, Zahner *et al, Epilepsia* 1999, **40**, 311–15). Visual changes occur in up to 50% patients (n=24, Gross-Tsur *et al, Ann Neurol* 2000, **48**, 60–64), including impaired contrast sensitivity (n=32, Nousiainen *et al, B J Ophthalmol* 2000, **84**, 622–25) and have limited the use of vigabatrin. The loss of visual field is not usually reversible (n=27, Hardus *et al, Br J Ophthalmol* 2000, **84**, 788–90) even when stopping the drug (n=13, Johnson *et al, Neurology* 2000, **55**, 40–45), although not invariably (n=1, Veggiotti, Lancet 1999, 354, 486). The CSM has expressed caution (*Pharm J* 1999, **263**, 848) and that it should not be initiated as monotherapy (*Cur Prob Pharmaco-vigilance* 1999, **25**, 13).

Reviews*: general (Gidal *et al, Ann Pharmacother* 1999, **33**, 1277–86, 115 refs; French, *Epilepsia* 1999, **40**[Suppl 5], S11–16), use in children (*BMJ* 2000, **320**, 1404).

+ Combinations

Valproate + lamotrigine *

The combination of valproate and lamotrigine may have some advantage over the drugs individually in refractory complex partial seizures, as well as being well tolerated if used with care (n=20, open, c/o, Pisani *et al, Epilepsia* 1999, **40**, 1141–46). See also lamotrigine.

● Unlicensed/Some efficacy

Clomethiazole (chlormethiazole)
Use in refractory cases, particularly children, can be successful (*Arch Dis Childhood* 1982, **57**, 242).

Nitrazepam
Nitrazepam has been used successfully for infantile spasms and myoclonic seizures. Although side-effects such as motor and cognitive impairment exist, it can still be useful in refractory cases (review by Shorvon, *Epilepsia* 1998, **39**[Suppl 1], S15–S23).

○ Unlicensed/Possible efficacy

Aromatherapy
Oils such as ylang ylang, camomile and lavender have been reported to be helpful in epilepsy (Anon, *Pharm J* 1993, **251**, 798).

Buspirone
Buspirone has been used in progressive myoclonus epilepsy (a syndrome of myoclonus, epilepsy, dementia and ataxia) but a small, uncontrolled study showed that it may exacerbate the myoclonus with no effect on the seizures (Pranzatelli *et al, J Neurol Neurosurg Psych* 1993, **56**, 114–15).

Calcium-channel blockers *
Nifedipine 60mg/d was successful in initial trials, producing a statistically significant reduction in seizures in 83% in one trial (n=18, *Am J Psych* 1991, **148**, 808–9) and preventing drop attacks (n=1, Mold, *J Fam Pract* 1995, **41**, 91–94), although of minimal effect in the only RCT (n=22, RCT, Larkin *et al, Epilepsia* 1992, **33**, 346–52). Nimodipine 1.5–2mg/kg/d, showed a greater than 50% reduction in fit frequency in 40% and two gained a full remission (n=20, *Develop Med & Child Neurol* 1990, **32**, 1114–16).

Carnitine *
Intractable epilepsy in a child who was found to have carnitine deficiency, was treated successfully with L-carnitine 100mg tds and valproate (n=1, Shuper *et al, Lancet* 1999, **353**, 1238).

Clomiphene
A number of successful uses have been reported, eg. at 25mg/d (n=1, *Arch Neurology* 1988, **45**, 209–10).

Flunarizine *
This has been used as an adjunct in refractory childhood fits (*Can J Neurol Sci* 1989, **16**, 191–93), although it is generally of limited use (n=14, open, Hoppu *et al, Pediatr Neurol* 1995, **13**, 143–47) and difficult to use (n=93, RCT, Pledger *et al, Neurology* 1994, **44**, 1830–36).

Fluoxetine
In a study in patients with complex partial seizures, addition of fluoxetine resulted in disappearance of seizures in six and a 30% reduction occurred in the other eleven (n=17, open, Favale *et al, Neurology* 1995, **45**, 1926–27).

Goserelin
Reduction in the number of attacks in catamenial epilepsy has been shown, although long-term treatment would have problems (*Lancet* 1992, **339**, 253).

Magnesium
Magnesium may have a true anticonvulsant effect, not just via neuromuscular paralysis (Walker *et al, Anaesthesia* 1995, **50**, 130–35 plus discussion in *Anaesthesia* 1995, **50**, 824–25).

Medroxyprogesterone
Some improvement in seizure frequency in women has been reported (*Epilepsia* 1985, **26**, S40–51; n=14, open, Mattson *et al, Neurology* 1984, **34**, 1255–58).

Midazolam
Acute childhood seizures have been managed with intranasal midazolam (n=20, *Lancet* 1998, **352**, 620).

Progesterone *
Progesterone produced reduced seizure frequency in 72% women with catamenial exacerbation of seizures (n=25, open, Herzog, *Neurology* 1995, **45**, 1660–62).

Propranolol
A synergistic effect with carbamazepine has been reported (n=1, *Am J Psych* 1990, **147**, 1687–88).

Pyridoxine
There is a case of a 3-month-old girl with resistant epilepsy who responded completely to pyridoxine 25mg/d, probably due to reduced GABA synthesis from an abnormal enzyme system (Gospe *et al, Lancet* 1994, **343**, 1133–34).

Vitamin E

300mg/d used as add-on therapy gave a 60% or more reduction in seizure frequency in 10 of 12 young epileptics in one trial (review in *DICP Ann Pharmacother* 1991, **25**, 362–63).

1.17.2 STATUS EPILEPTICUS

Status epilepticus is a state where multiple seizures occur without complete recovery between seizures, and there are a number of different types of status epilepticus. Mortality can be high, but a rapid and aggressive treatment reduces this, and any permanent neuronal damage.

Role of drugs :

To prevent permanent brain damage, first line therapy must be to support with oxygen and a glucose drip if possible. The American Epilepsy Foundation has produced a statement, review and guidelines for the treatment of status epilepticus (*JAMA* 1993, **270**, 854–59).

Status epilepticus refractory to first line drugs is frequently caused by acute neurological problems, eg. encephalitis, CVA or trauma. Hypoxia and ischaemia can add to brain disruption and respiratory depression and hypotension are side-effects of the drugs used. Transfer to an ITU may be preferred, where plasma expanders, ventilation and monitoring facilities are available. In a 5-year comparison of four treatments (diazepam 0.15mg/kg followed by phenytoin 18mg/kg, lorazepam 0.1mg/kg, phenobarbital 15mg/kg and phenytoin 18mg/kg) for generalized convulsive status epilepticus, treatment was successful for lorazepam on 64.9% of occasions, phenobarbital 58.2%, diazepam plus phenytoin 55.8% and phenytoin 43.6%. Lorazepam thus appears more effective than phenytoin, and easier to use than phenobarbital or diazepam plus phenytoin (n=384, RCT, Treiman *et al, NEJM* 1998, **339**, 792–98).

Reviews*: general (Lowenstein and Alldredge, *NEJM* 1998, **338**, 970–76, 57 refs; Fountain, *Epilepsia* 2000, **41**[Suppl 2], S23–30; Bleck, *Epilepsia* 1999, **40**[Suppl 1], S59–63), benzodiazepine routes (Rey *et al, Clin Pharmacokin* 1999, **36**, 409–24, 98 refs), risk factors and compliations (Fountain, *Epilepsia* 2000, **41**[Suppl 2], S23–30), new

concepts (Alldredge and Lowenstein, *Curr Opin Neurol* 1999, **12**, 183–90).

BNF Listed

Amylobarbital (sodium)

See the SPC for injection details, which are important for this potentially toxic drug.

Clomethiazole (chlormethiazole) *

The IV infusion has been discontinued in the UK.

Clonazepam

0.5–1.5mg by slow IV injection (possibly followed by an infusion) may be useful in refractory cases not responsive to diazepam. A prolonged effect may be seen. It is comparable with lorazepam and probably has the lowest respiratory depressant effect of the benzodiazepines (*Pharmacy World & Science* 1993, **15**, 17–28).

Diazepam

0.15–0.25mg/kg (ie. around 10–30mg) given as a slow IV injection over 5 minutes or rectal administration (eg. rectal tubes) is first choice treatment in the UK. Rates above 5mg/min IV are associated with respiratory depression. A diazepam infusion at 3mg/kg in 24 hours can be tried for maintenance (case in *Ann Pharmacother* 1993, **27**, 298–301). The speed of rectal absorption is second only to IV absorption (*Int J Pharmaceutics* 1980, **5**, 127).

Fosphenytoin *

Fosphenytoin is a water soluble parenteral pro-drug converted to phenytoin, and with complete IM absorption. It is licensed for status and as a substitute for oral phenytoin. It is better tolerated at injection sites, can be given up to three times more rapidly IV and can be given IM, where cardiac monitoring is not necessary. Conversion to phenytoin takes about 15 minutes and so fosphenytoin is less appropriate for the sole initial treatment of status epilepticus. Transient pruritis and paraesthesia are the main differential side-effects compared to phenytoin, although dilution and IV administration may minimise these. Although more expensive, fosphenytoin may be cost neutral due to reduced side-effects (Armstrong *et al, Pharmacotherapy* 1999, **19**, 844–53, 39 refs), although this has been disputed (editorial by Labiner, *Arch Int Med* 1999, **159**, 2631–32, 12 refs; review by DeToledo and Ramsay, *Drug Safety* 2000, **22**, 459–66, 58 refs). **Reviews***: general (Browne, *Clin Neuropharmacol* 1997, **20**, 1–12), IV use (Ramsay and Detoledo, *Neurology* 1996, **46**[S1], S17–S19; Marchetti *et al, Clin Therapeutics* 1996, **18**, 953–66).

Lorazepam

Lorazepam may be preferrable to diazepam, due to a longer duration of action (about 2 hours), shorter elimination half-life, no active metabolites and possibly less respiratory depression. Lorazepam appears more effective than phenytoin, and easier to use than phenobarbital or diazepam plus phenytoin (n=384, RCT, Treiman *et al, NEJM* 1998, **339**, 792–98).

Paraldehyde

Given by IM injection (up to 5ml per muscle site, glass syringe needed) or rectally (50/50 mixture with arachis oil, 2:1 in oil or cottonseed oil or mixed with 0.9% sodium chloride), paraldehyde can be rapidly effective, especially in infants and children where venous access is limited (*B J Psych* 1987, **150**, 654–55) but is painful at the site of injection. It is also active, albeit unpleasantly, by mouth and also by IV infusion (4–8% infusion in sodium chloride 0.9% — *Pharmacy World & Science* 1993, **15**, 17–28). **Reviews**: toxicology (von Burg and Stout, *J Appl Toxicol* 1991, **11**, 379–81) and kinetics (Ramsay, *Epilepsia* 1989, **30**[Suppl 2], S1–S3).

Phenytoin

Phenytoin (or fosphenytoin) is a useful second-line to the benzodiazepines, used as 10–20mg/kg intravenously over 15 minutes (not exceeding 50mg/minute) in 0.9% saline for recurrent or persistent seizures. It is effective from 20–30 minutes after injection but is not effective intramuscularly. It is not an easy drug to use due to the risk of hypotension and cardiac dysrhythmias.

● **Unlicensed/Some efficacy**

Midazolam *

Continuous IV infusion can be used for status (Koul *et al, Arch Dis Childhood* 1997, **76**, 445) with 1–3mg/hr rapidly successful in many patients (*Arch Emerg Med* 1987, **4**, 169–72). It has a rapid onset of action (30–90 seconds) but care is needed with this acute onset and the potentially fatal respiratory depression as midazolam half-life prolongs significantly after sustained infusion (n=2, Naritoku and Sinha, *Neurology* 2000, **54**, 1366–68). The IM (Towne and DeLorenzo, *J Emerg Med* 1999, **17**, 323–28), buccal liquid (n=42, RCT, Scott *et al, Lancet* 1999, **353**, 623–26, editorial, *ibid*, 608–9) and intranasal routes (n=47, RCT, *BMJ* 2000, **321**, 83) may be safe, effective, more socially acceptable and convenient alternatives to IV and rectal diazepam. **Reviews**: general (Shorvon, *Epilepsia* 1998, **39**[Suppl 1], S15–S23; Denzel *et al, Ann Pharmacother* 1996, **30**, 1481–83, 90 refs; Fountain and Adams, *Clin Neuropharmacol* 1999, **22**, 261–67; Molmes and Riviello, *Pediatr Neurol* 1999, **20**, 259–64).

Phenobarbital (phenobarbitone)

A parenteral loading dose of 10–20mg/kg (*Am J Hosp Pharm* 1993, **50**[Suppl 5], S5–S16) with a maintenance dose of 5–7mg/kg/day can be used, although some feel that this bolus dose of phenobarbital is too high and should not be given at a dose greater than 100mg/min (Zeisler and Beck, *Am J Hosp Pharm* 1994, **51**, 1578). It has a slow onset and causes cardiac and respiratory depression (reviews in *Pharmacy World & Science* 1993, **15**, 17–28; *Neurology* 1988, **38**, 202–7, 395–400 and 1035–40).

Thiopental (thiopentone)

Induction of anaesthesia with a 2.5% solution (4–8mg/kg) can be effective, continued with an infusion of 0.2% solution until seizure-free for 24 hours. Phenobarbital should be substituted once fitting stops, as thiopentone accumulates in fat and effects the myocardium.

Thiamine

The use of thiamine may be indicated and prevent serious complications when glucose IV is given as supportive therapy in status (*JAMA* 1994, **270**, 854–59; *JAMA* 1994, **271**, 980–81).

○ Unlicensed/Possible efficacy

Chloral

Doses of up to 30mg/kg at four hourly intervals given orally or rectally may be effective in resistant status although onset may be delayed (review in *Ann Emerg Med* 1990, **19**, 674–77).

Etomidate

This non-barbiturate induction agent has some anticonvulsant activity. Doses of 0.2–0.3mg/kg IV repeated after 20 minutes have been successful, as has infusion at 25mg/kg/min (*Intens Care Med* 1989, **15**, 255–59). Care would be needed as etomidate may cause involuntary muscle contractions and epileptiform seizures during prolonged IV infusion (*Lancet* 1983, **2**, 511–12).

Flumazenil *

IV doses may be effective as an anticonvulsant (*Lancet* 1991, **337**, 744, 133–37). In intractable epilepsy, flumazenil may be superior to diazepam, without sedation (n=12, d/b, c/o, Sharief *et al, Epilepsy Research* 1993, **15**, 53–60), although it may induce seizures (n=67, Schulze-Bonhage and Elger, *Epilepsia* 2000, **41**, 186–92). Review by Reisner-Keller and Pham in *Ann Pharmacother* 1995, **29**, 530–32.

Lidocaine (lignocaine)

A 1% solution given as a 2–3mg/kg bolus over 2 minutes can be rapidly effective (ie. within minutes) in cases refractory to other drugs (De Giorgio *et al, Epilepsia* 1992, **33**, 913–16). The effect lasts about 30 minutes but due to the relatively short duration, a second dose is needed in about 50% of cases (Pascual *et al, J Neurol Neurosurg Psychiatry* 1992, **55**, 49–51). If successful, IV infusion at 4mg/kg/hour may be considered. Enhanced seizure activity after high doses and cardiac arrhythmias are potential problems and so it should be used only with caution if any form of heart block or sinus bradycardia exists as it may induce ventricular arrhythmia or complete heart block.

Propofol *

Propofol has established anticonvulsant activities. There have been a number of reports of successful use by IV infusion, so far without serious problems (*Anaesthesia* 1988, **43**, 514, *Ibid* 1990,

45, 995–96, 1043–45; n=1, Begemann *et al, Epilepsia* 2000, **41**, 105–09). Propofol has been compared with barbiturates (n=16) in refractory status epilepticus and a protocol for use proposed (Stecker *et al, Epilepsia* 1998, **39**, 18–26).

Valproate *

Valproate has been used IV (n=3 and review, Morton and Quarles, *Pharmacotherapy* 2000, **20**, 88–92; n=3, Hovinga *et al, Ann Pharmacother* 1999, **33**, 579–84), including rectally and in patients with hypotension (n=13, Sinha and Naritoku, *Neurology* 2000, **55**, 722–24).

GILLES DE LA TOURETTE

See Tourette's Syndrome (*1.33*).

1.18 INSOMNIA

Insomnia, ie. difficulty in initiating or maintaining sleep, is a symptom of an illness, not an illness itself and should always be treated as such. It can be caused by a variety of external (eg. environment) and internal (eg. psychiatric illness, stress, physical illness, drugs, see *5.14* etc) stimuli, and can be transient, chronic, initial or early morning wakening. The causes, where possible, should be determined and treated, as well as emphasis on sleep hygiene.

Principles of sleep hygiene: *

1. Avoid excessive use of caffeine (particularly within 3-4 hours of going to bed), alcohol or nicotine. A hot milky drink at bedtime may promote sleep.

2. Do not stay in bed for prolonged periods if not asleep. Go to another dimly lit room – watching TV can have an alerting effect.

3. Avoid daytime naps or long periods of inactivity.

4. A warm bath or exercise a few hours before bedtime may promote sleep.

5. Avoid engaging in strenuous exercise or mental activity near bedtime.

6. Make sure that the bed and bedroom are comfortable and avoid extremes of noise, temperature and humidity.

7. Establish a regular bedtime routine, eg. going to bed at the same time and rising at the same time every morning, regardless of sleep duration.

8. Diet – carbohydrate (eg. pasta etc) helps sleep, but not eating a big meal within about 2 hours of going to bed. Sugar may inhibit sleep, as may some vitamin supplements.

Role of drugs:*

Assuming sleep hygiene is good, any hypnotics should always be used on a PRN basis, as tolerance may develop to the sedative effects within 2–3 weeks (especially with the benzodiazepines). Short-term use for short-term reasons is usually without problem and can be very useful and comforting for the patient. Longer-term use needs the risk:benefit analysis considered carefully. The principles of sleep hygiene should be discussed and any problems corrected before prescribing hypnotics. A meta-analysis of 22 RCTs of BDZs or zolpidem showed consistent superiority over placebo up to 5 weeks but the evidence beyond 5 weeks is unclear (Nowell *et al, JAMA* 1997, **278**, 2170–77, 86 refs). CBT, temazepam or both, have been shown to improve short-term outcomes for older people with persistent insomnia (Morin *et al, JAMA* 1999, **17**, 991–99, reviewed in *EBMH* 1999, **2**, 117). Guidelines for management of chronic insomnia are difficult to formulate.

Reviews*: comprehensive (Wilson and Nutt, *Adv Psych Treat* 1999, **5**, 11–18; Nishino and Mignot, *Clin Pharmacokinet* 1999, **37**, 305–30, 91 refs), general (Hallström, *Prescriber* 1999, **10**, 41–51; Cole, *Prescriber* 1999, **10**, 89–93; *Drugs & Ther Perspect* 2000, **15**, 5–9), sleep disorders in elderly (Jagus and Benbow, *Adv Psych Treat* 1999, **5**, 30–38; Ancoli-Israel, *Sleep* 2000, **23**[Suppl 1], S23–30), benzodiazepines and zolpidem (Nowell *et al, JAMA* 1997, **278**, 2170–77; reviewed by van Bemmel, *EBMH* 1998, **1**, 117), withdrawal (*Drugs & Ther Perspect* 1999, **14**, 12–14), non-drug methods of managing insomnia (Yang and Spielman, *Dis Manage & Health Outcomes* 1999, **5**, 209–24).

Predicting hypnotic dependence risk
(*BMJ* 1993, **306**, 706)

Factor	Score
Benzodiazepine hypnotic used	3
High mean dose *	2
Duration of treatment>3months	2
Dependent personality	2
Short elimination half-life drug	2
Tolerance or dose escalation	2
TOTAL	
*Dose higher than BNF mean	
No dependence, abrupt withdrawal	= 0
Some dependence risk, withdraw over two weeks recommended	= 1–4
Strong dependence risk, withdraw over 4–12 weeks	= 5–8
High risk of dependence, withdraw gradually plus support programme	= 8–13

BNF Listed

Benzodiazepines *

Benzodiazepines may be extremely useful in the short-term for insomnia, helping to facilitate essential high-quality sleep (rational defence of BDZ prescribing, Williams and McBride, *B J Psych* 1998, **173**, 361–62), and are certainly safer than older hypnotics, which may have worse dependence, abuse and overdose characteristics. A meta-analysis of 45 RCTs indicated benzodiazepines are effective in improving sleep latency and duration but ADRs (drowsiness, dizziness etc.) are common, although methodologically these studies are flawed (meta-analysis, n=2672, Holbrook *et al, CMAJ* 2000, **162**, 225–33, reviewed by Furukawa, *EBMH* 2000, **3**, 81). Users of benzodiazepines and zopiclone are also at greater risk of road-traffic accidents, especially if combined with alcohol (involved in accidents, n=19,386 over 3 years, Barbone *et al, Lancet* 1998, **352**, 1331–36).
Review: rational use (Ashton, *Drugs* 1994, **48**, 25–40).

Flunitrazepam

A longer-acting benzodiazepine, which may have an abuse potential (reviewed by Woods and Winger, *J Clin Psychopharmacol* 1997, **17**[3 Suppl 2], 1S–57S).

Flurazepam

A benzodiazepine with a short half-life but with longer-acting metabolites.

Loprazolam
An intermediate-acting benzodiazepine, with a half-life of 7–15 hours.

Lormetazepam
An intermediate acting benzodiazepine marketed in the UK as a hypnotic.

Nitrazepam
A longer-acting benzodiazepine similar to diazepam, which has active meta-bolites. Stable plasma levels can be attained in 5 days so avoid in the elderly.

Temazepam
A shorter-acting benzodiazepine, whose abuse potential has been well recognised.

Others

Antihistamines
Antihistamines may be effective. Promethazine has a relatively long half-life but low abuse potential. Diphenhydramine may have an abuse potential (de Nesnera, *J Clin Psych* 1996, **57**, 136–37).

Barbiturates
Barbiturates should only be used for severe and intractable insomnia where there are compelling reasons and only in patients already taking barbiturates (CSM warning in *Curr Problems* 1996, **22**, 7).

Chloral
Chloral has properties similar to the barbiturates and is relatively safe in the elderly (*Clin Pharmac* 1977, **21**, 355) as the half-life is not significantly lengthened. An abuse potential exists.

Clomethiazole (chlormethiazole)
A thiamine derivative with sedative-hypnotic and anticonvulsant properties. It has a rapid onset of action and short half-life, even in the elderly, although they may be more sensitive to it. Dependence and abuse has been reported but is not considered too important if the patient is not dependence prone (*Lancet* 1979, **ii**, 953–54). It is unsafe in overdose.

Triclofos
A chloral-related drug with similar actions to chloral but with less gastric irritation and a more palatable taste. Only available as a liquid in the UK.

Zaleplon *
Zaleplon is a pyrazolopyrimidine hypnotic, acting at the omega-1 benzodiazepine receptor. It can be taken at bedtime or after the person has failed to go to sleep, because peak plasma levels occur after 1 hour and it has a short half-life (1 hour). 5mg (elderly) and 10mg (adults) has been shown to be an effective hypnotic, with a significant reduction in sleep latency, comparable to zolpidem, but no rebound insomnia over four weeks nor withdrawal, unlike zolpidem (n=615, RCT, Elie *et al*, *J Clin Psych* 1999, **60**, 536–44). One study showed lack of residual effects even with 10mg zaleplon taken 2 hours before waking, while residual effects from zolpidem were detectable 5 hours after a dose (n=36, Danjou *et al*, *Br J Clin Pharmacol* 1999, **48**, 367–74). Lack of both long-term tolerance and rebound insomnia has been suggested (Dooley and Plosker, *Drugs* 2000, **60**, 413–45). Use in the elderly also appears safe and effective (RCT, 2/52, Hedner *et al*, *Int J Geriatr Psych* 2000, **15**, 704–12) as well as, anecdotally, for jet-lag.

Reviews*: general (Hurst and Noble, *CNS Drugs* 1999, **11**, 387–92; Anon, *Am J Health-Sys Pharm* 2000, **57**, 430–31; Wilson and Nutt, *Prescriber* 2000, **11**, 85–93; Anon, *Formulary Monograph Service* 1999, 75–80, ibid 395–402, 43 refs), extensive (Weitzel *et al*, *Clin Ther* 2000, **22**, 1254–67; Dooley and Plosker, *Drugs* 2000, **60**, 413–45), kinetics (Greenblatt *et al*, *Clin Pharmacol Ther* 1998, **64**, 553–61) and pharmacology (Rush *et al*, *Psychopharmacology [Berl]* 1999, **145**, 39–51; Heydorn, *Expert Opin Investig Drugs* 2000, **9**, 841–58).

Zolpidem *
Zolpidem is a imidazopyridine hypnotic which binds preferentially to the omega-1 benzodiazepine receptor. It decreases time to sleep and increases total sleep time and efficiency but does not affect sleep architecture. It has a rapid onset of action and a short (6–8hrs) duration. It has been shown in several studies to be equivalent to flunitrazepam but with few significant residual effects (eg. Bensimon *et al*, *B J Clin Pharmacol* 1990, **30**, 463–69). Indeed, lack of residual psychomotor effects in one study led to suggestions the drug be considered for use in navy fighter and other pilots (n=12, Sicard *et al*, *Aviat Space Environ Med* 1993, **64**, 371–75). Chronic abuse of zolpidem, at up to

600mg/d has been reported (n=1, Gericke and Ludolph, *JAMA* 1994, **272**, 1721–72; n=1, Aragona, *Clin Neuropharmacol* 2000, **23**, 281–83).

Reviews*: extensive (Holm and Goa, *Drugs* 2000, **59**, 865–89, 191 refs; Darcourt *et al, J Psychopharmacol* 1999, **13**, 81–93), comparison with placebo in heavy snorers (Quera-Salva *et al, B J Clin Pharmacol* 1994, **37**, 539–43), clinical pharmacokinetics (Salva and Costa, *Clin Pharmacokinetics* 1995, **29**, 142–53).

Zopiclone *

This non-benzodiazepine hypnotic has a low incidence of side-effects and hangover effect compared to temazepam. Zopiclone binds preferentially to two of the three benzodiazepine receptor subtypes. Treatment duration is recommended for up to 28 days. Zopiclone is equivalent, but not superior, to BDZs (meta-analysis, n=2672, Holbrook *et al, CMAJ* 2000, **162**, 225–33; reviewed by Furukawa, *EBMH* 2000, **3**, 81). Misuse and dependence has been reported (eg. Clee *et al, Addiction* 1996, **91**, 1389–90) and may be greater in those with dependent personalities (letters by Sikdar, Ayonrinde and Sampson, *BMJ* 1998, **317**, 146).

Reviews*: extensive (Noble *et al, Drugs* 1998, **55**, 277–302; Hajak, *Drug Saf* 1999, **21**, 457–69), kinetics (Fernandez *et al, Clin Pharmacokinet* 1995, **29**, 431–41), abuse potential/dependence (Lader, *J Neurol* 1997, **244**[4 Suppl 1], S18–S22).

● **Unlicensed/Some efficacy**

Other sedative drugs at night

Other sedative drugs the patient may already be taking, especially phenothiazines and antidepressants, may be prescribed as a single dose at night. In longer-term therapy most can be given this way. It is also important to avoid the use of 'stimulating' drugs at night, eg. anticholinergics, MAOIs etc. Trazodone and nefazodone are particularly useful if the insomnia is secondary to, eg. SSRIs.

Mirtazapine

Insomnia is reported by 90% depressed patients, but stimulation of 5-HT$_2$ receptors is thought to underlie insomnia

and the changes in sleep architecture seen with SSRIs/SNRIs. Mirtazapine and nefazodone block 5-HT$_2$ receptors and may improve sleep. In depressed patients, mirtazapine produces a significant shortening of sleep-onset latency, increases a total sleep time, and leads to a marked improvement in sleep efficiency (Thase, *J Clin Psych* 1999, **60** [Suppl 17], 28–31; discussion 46–48).

Nefazodone

See mirtazapine.

Phenothiazines

Promazine at 25–100mg can be fairly sedative with a low abuse potential, but a significant side-effect profile.

○ **Unlicensed/Possible efficacy**

Alcohol

Alcohol causes sedation, increases slow wave sleep, reduces and disrupts REM sleep, the diuretic effect is counterproductive and overdose can have serious consequences. Rebound arousal can occur with higher doses when blood concentrations reach zero, leading to awakening (Stradling, *BMJ* 1993, **306**, 573–75). Alcohol is thus not recommended for routine medical use. Having said that, it is used widely as self-medication and, unlike chloral, is available in a number of highly palatable formulations (eg. Adnams, Woodfordes), and in lager.

Antidepressants (sedative)

These are useful if the insomnia is a symptom of depression, but the depression must be treated with adequate antidepressant doses. Many are toxic in overdose and they may disrupt REM sleep.

Lavender oil

Ambient lavender oil odour may improve sleep duration in the elderly (understandably open study, n=4, Hardy *et al, Lancet* 1995, **346**, 701).

Nicotine

Low concentrations of nicotine can cause mild sedation and relaxation and so a cigarette could help sleep in an anxious person. Higher levels cause arousal and agitation (Stradling, *BMJ* 1993, **306**, 573–75).

Melatonin *

Not yet licensed in the UK, slow-release melatonin may be effective. It improved sleep *in* major depression, but had no effect *on* depression (n=24, open, Dolberg *et al, Am J Psych* 1998, **155**, 1119–21) and 2mg significantly improved sleep efficiency in chronic schizophrenics with poor sleep, but not in those with better sleep efficiency (RCT, n=19, Shamir *et al, J Clin Psych* 2000, **61**, 373–77). Review by Pepping (*Am J Health-Sys Pharm* 1999, **56**, 2520, 2523–24, 2527).

Paroxetine *

Paroxetine 20mg/d may be an effective treatment for primary insomnia (n=15, open, Nowell *et al, J Clin Psych* 1999, **60**, 89–95) although this might be a placebo response (Musa, *J Clin Psych* 1999, **60**, 795).

Tryptophan

Tryptophan at 1–2g may facilitate going off to sleep, reducing latency time and increasing total sleep time (*JAMA* 1989, **29**, 274–78).

▼ No efficacy
Caffeine

Caffeine competes with the inhibitory neurotransmitter adenosine, causing cortical arousal and decreased sleep. 150mg of caffeine before retiring has a marked effect on sleep latency, reduces sleep efficacy and REM periods. Its half-life of 5 hours means any ingested near bedtime will effect sleep latency (Stradling, *BMJ* 1993, **306**, 573–75). See caffeinism (*1.35*).

1.19 MANIA and HYPOMANIA

See also bipolar mood disorder (*1.10*), rapid-cycling disorder (*1.27*) and acute psychiatric emergency (*1.1*).

Symptoms:

Hypomania, the more common and milder form of mania, is defined as an abnormal elation of mood, alternating with irritability, great energy, inability to concentrate, flight of ideas (rapid changing of the subject with some connections), insomnia etc. Obsessive preoccupation with some idea, activity or desire may occur. The main presenting symptoms are a euphoric and labile mood (irritable, angry, grandiose), bright or untidy appearance, low sleep requirement, increased drive and energy, reduced insight, pressure of speech, flight of ideas, expansive thought, and an overactive and intrusive manner.

Role of drugs:*

Hypomania or mania represents a particular phase of a bipolar (or rarely a unipolar) illness. Both usually require specific long-term mood-stabiliser drug treatment for the bipolar component (ie. lithium, carbamazepine, valproate etc) and non-specific shorter-term treatments (eg. antipsychotics, benzodiazepines) for insomnia, agitation, hyperactivity, etc. to calm the patient and prevent exhaustion and harm. A night of sleep deprivation is likely to escalate any manic patient to a higher degree of mania and so hypnotic/sedative use should be considered appropriate (Wehr *et al, Arch Gen Psych* 1982, **39**, 559–65). Recovery from acute mania is poorer in people with a history of substance abuse (retrospective review, n=204, Goldberg *et al, J Clin Psych* 1999, **60**, 733–40).

Antipsychotics are potent antimanic agents, but generally should not be continued into the maintenance phase, although this frequently occurs. Lithium remains the best established mood-stabiliser, especially in hypomania. Evidence for an antimanic effect for valproate (particularly in mixed states) is better than carbamazepine, and the evidence for prophylactic effect for carbamazepine exceeds that of valproate. It may be that patients who have had more than about 10 previous manic episodes may respond less well to lithium than previously (n=154, Swann *et al, Am J Psych* 1999, **156**, 1264–66). This effect may not be true with valproate. See bipolar mood disorder (*1.10*) for maintenance strategies.

Treatment goals should be:
1. Discontinue any 'manicogenic' agents (see *5.7* for lists).
2. Stabilise any medical conditions.
3. Start non-specific calming medications, eg. BDZs, antipsychotics.
4. Start specific mood-stabilisers, eg. lithium, carbamazepine and valproate – preferably when the patient is able to consent to longer-term therapy.

Reviews*: treatment of acute mania and resistant mania (Tohen and Grundy, *J Clin Psych* 1999, **60**[Suppl 5], 31–36), concise

(Daly, *Lancet* 1997, **349**, 1157–60, 74 refs), comprehensive (Licht, *Acta Psych Scand* 1998, **97**, 387–97, 89 refs), loading strategies for lithium, valproate and CBZ (Keck *et al, Bipolar Disord* 2000, **2**, 42–46, 37 refs) and review of RCTs in acute mania (Keck *et al, J Aff Dis* 2000, **59**[Suppl 1], S31–37).

BNF Listed
Antipsychotics *
There is some evidence that hypomania has a hyper-dopaminergic component (eg. Pearlson *et al, Arch Gen Psych* 1995, **52**, 471–77) and so treatment with dopamine-blocking drugs may be rational (n=528, Chou *et al, Ann Pharmacother* 1996, **30**, 1396–98). Antipsychotics are certainly routinely and widely used, although the majority of even refractory bipolars can be stabilised without long-term neuroleptics (n=133, Brotman *et al, J Clin Psych* 2000, **61**, 68–72). A review of 15 RCTs of antipsychotics in acute mania showed that antipsychotics produce a more rapid antimanic effect than lithium (predictably) but lithium is superior at 3 weeks (Keck *et al, J Clin Psych* 1998, **59**[Suppl 6], 74–81). First episode manic patients tend to discontinue antipsychotics within a few months (70% within 6 months), independent of outcome (n=198, retrospective, Zarate and Tohen, *J Clin Psych* 2000, **61**, 33–38). Several studies have shown risperidone to be useful in bipolar disorder (e.g. n=14, open, out-patient, 64% improved, Ghaemi *et al, Can J Psych* 1997, **42**, 196–99; n=12, open, Ghaemi and Sachs, *Int Clin Psychopharmacol* 1997, **12**, 333–38). Risperidone may be effective in conjunction with mood stabilisers (eg. n=6, *Psychopharmacol Bull* 1996, **32**, 55–61), as may quetiapine (Dunayevich and Stratowski, *Am J Psych* 2000, **157**, 1341). See also unlicensed section.

Carbamazepine *
The 5 RCTs of carbamazepine in acute mania show a response rate equivalent to lithium and chlorpromazine (review by Keck *et al, J Clin Psych* 1998, **59**[Suppl 6], 74–81, 114 refs). It may be more effective in rapid cycling, early age of onset and predominant mania (Okuma, *Neuropsychobiology* 1993,

27, 138–45). Other trials have used combination therapy, eg. with lithium. Doses of up to 1600mg/d or more have been used in resistant patients (Ballenger, *J Clin Psych* 1988, **49**[Suppl 1], 13–19). No loading dose strategies have been published in bipolar (see Keck *et al, Bipolar Disord* 2000, **2**, 42–46). See also bipolar mood disorder (*1.10*).

Lithium *
Lithium may be effective in acute mania/ hypomania although onset of action may not be for 5–7 days or longer. A systematic overview of lithium concluded that it should remain first line in acute mania (n=658, 12 trials, Poolsup *et al, J Clin Pharm & Ther* 2000, **25**, 139–56). Serum levels of 0.9–1.4mmol/l may be necessary in the short-term for a therapeutic effect and should be reduced once mood is normalised (eg. Gelenberg *et al, NEJM* 1989, **320**, 535–8). Loading with lithium in mania has been tried with rapid success, many responding within 48 hours, but these preliminary findings have not been replicated (n=9, open, Moscovich *et al, Human Psychopharmacol* 1992, **7**, 343–45; see also Keck *et al, Bipolar Disord* 2000, **2**, 42–46). At least four previous depressive or 12 previous manic episodes are associated with reduced anti-manic response to lithium (Swann *et al, Acta Psych Scand* 2000, **101**, 444–51).
Review*: efficacy and side-effects in mania (Bowden, *J Clin Psych* 2000, **61**[Suppl 9], 35–40). See also bipolar mood disorder (*1.10*).

Valproate semisodium *
Valproate semisodium is licensed in UK for mania and hypomania. It may be more effective than lithium in mixed mania, rapid cycling and mania with co-morbid substance abuse, but less effective in severe mania or co-morbid BPD (review by Keck *et al, J Clin Psych* 1998, **59**[Suppl 6], 74–81, 114 refs). It is also a very effective adjunct to neuroleptics (see combinations). Plasma levels of between 45–125mcg/ml are much more likely to produce effective and well tolerated responses in acute mania than higher or lower levels (n=65, Bowden *et al, Am J Psych* 1996, **153**, 765–70). Compared to younger adults, valproate may have a different therapeutic window (65–90mcg/mL) in the elderly

(n=59, retrospective, Chen *et al, J Clin Psych* 1999, **60**, 181–86). More rapid control of mania is likely if loading doses are used to achieve plasma concentrations earlier. Divalproex loading doses of 20mg/kg/d have been shown to give a rapid response (often within 3 days) to manic and psychotic symptoms (McElroy *et al, J Clin Psych* 1996, **57**, 142–46). Oral loading doses of divalproex (30mg/kg/d on days 1 and 2, then 20mg/kg/d days 3–10) may produce more rapid therapeutic levels in acute mania, with no adverse effects (n=59, RCT, Hirschfeld *et al, J Clin Psych* 1999, **60**, 815–18). Valproate infusion (initially 125mg over 1 hour) may be rapidly effective (n=1, Herbert and Nelson, *Am J Psych* 2000, **157**, 1023–24).

Reviews*: loading dose strategies (Keck *et al, Bipolar Disord* 2000, **2**, 42–46).

+   Combinations

Lithium + carbamazepine

Carbamazepine can be used in resistant cases in combination with lithium (*Arch Gen Psych* 1989, **46**, 794–800, review of literature in *Comprehensive Psych* 1990, **31**, 261–65). See *4.4* for neurotoxicity warning.

Lithium + clonazepam

See zuclopenthixol + clonazepam.

Nifedipine + antipsychotics

Combination use in acute mania and schizoaffective disorders has been reported (Beaurepaire, *Am J Psych* 1992, **149**, 1614–15).

Valproate + lithium

Divalproex successfully augmented lithium in resistant rapid-cycling mania in 4 elderly patients (Schneider and Wilcox, *J Aff Dis* 1998, **47**, 201–5).

Valproate + antipsychotics *

Valproate is an effective adjunct in acute mania, producing a quicker response with lower neuroleptic doses (n=136, RCT, 3/52, Müller-Oerlinghausen *et al, J Clin Psychopharmacol* 2000, **20**, 195–203).

Zuclopenthixol + clonazepam

In a comparison of two drug combinations (zuclopenthixol plus clonazepam versus lithium plus clonazepam) in acute mania, approx-imately two thirds improved fully or partially on both combinations, with no statistical differences between the two (n=28, s/b, Gouliaev *et al, Acta Psych Scand* 1996, **93**, 119–24).

●   Unlicensed/Some efficacy

Benzodiazepines

Short-term medium or high doses of benzodiazepines can be used alone or as adjuvants to other therapies in acute phases of hypomania, eg. diazepam by itself, lorazepam (*Psychosomatics* 1986, **27**, 17–21) or clonazepam at 4–16mg/d (*Biol Psych* 1983, **18**, 451–66). For acute symptoms they have a rapid onset, are highly sedative and are well tolerated, with a low EPSE side-effect risk. Although benzodiazepines are mainly used as adjunctive therapy in the acute phase, it may be appropriate to continue them after recovery, eg. they are safer and can help reduce antipsychotic dosage. They may also be useful in atypical bipolar disorder (*Psychosomatics* 1988, **29**, 333).

Clomethiazole (chlormethiazole)

See benzodiazepines above for use of sedatives in controlling acute mania.

Clozapine *

Although problematic, clozapine may have some use. One study showed clozapine (mean 500mg/d) to be effective in 72% treatment-resistant manics or schizoaffectives (n=25, Calabrese *et al, Am J Psych* 1996, **153**, 759–64), another showed significant improvement relative to treatment as usual in bipolar (n=38, RCT, 1yr, Suppes *et al, Am J Psych* 1999, **156**, 1164–69) and up to 550mg/d was effective in treatment-refractory psychotic mania (n=22, open, 12/52, Green *et al, Am J Psych* 2000, **157**, 982–86).

Lamotrigine

Lamotrigine may have mood stabilising and mood elevating effects. Its primary action is on voltage-sensitive sodium channels, which stabilises neuronal membranes, inhibiting pathological release of glutamate. A case series with lamotrigine 50–250mg/d (mean of responders 141mg) in refractory bipolars showed a 50% response rate at 5 weeks (n=16, Sporn and Sachs, *J Clin Psychopharmacol* 1997, **17**, 185–89).

Olanzapine *

Olanzapine is approved in US for mania and hypomania, and awaits a UK licence. Several studies have shown some efficacy. In acute mania, response to olanzapine (49%) was better than placebo (24%) over three weeks (n=139, RCT, Tohen *et al, Am J Psych* 1999, **156**, 702–9), with other studies showing similar superiority to placebo (n=69, RCT, Tohen *et al, Schizoph Res* 1998, **29**, 204; n=14, open, 5–30mg/d, McElroy *et al, J Aff Dis* 1998, **49**, 119–22). Olanzapine was as effective as lithium in acute mania on most measures in a short trial (n=30, RCT, d/b, 4/52, Berk *et al, Int Clin Psychopharmacol* 1999, **14**, 339–43) and in manic or mixed bipolar disorder, 5–20mg/d was superior to placebo and generally well tolerated (n=115, 4/52, RCT, Tohen *et al, Arch Gen Psych* 2000, **57**, 841–49). A moderate-to-marked response may be more likely if the patient is younger, female and bipolar with a longer duration of trial (n=150, naturalistic, *J Clin Psych* 1998, **59**, 24–28).

Verapamil

120–450mg/d has shown promise as a mood stabiliser (*Biol Psych* 1989, **25**, 128–40), even in the elderly (*Int J Ger Psych* 1992, **7**, 913–15). A study showed that up to 320mg/d was as effective in acute mania as lithium (n=20, *Am J Psych* 1992, **149**, 121–2). However, a short random-assignment, parallel-group in-patient trial found no benefit for verapamil over placebo (n=32, RCT, 3/52, Janicak *et al, Am J Psych* 1998, **155**, 972–73), and so longer trials may be necessary.

O   Unlicensed/Possible efficacy
Dexamfetamine (dexamphetamine)

Small studies have shown a short-term effect (*Psychopharmacol Bull* 1988 **24**, 168; n=6, Garvey *et al, J Clin Psych* 1987, **49**, 412–13) and may reduce hypomanic activity in dementia (n=1, *Int J Geriatrics* 1991, **6**, 165–69).

Clonidine

This has been used successfully in antipsychotic-resistant mania but is possibly of low potency (*B J Psych* 1988, **152**, 293).

Doxepin

Response to 100mg/d has been reported (n=1, Kaye, *Am J Psych* 1992, **146**, 802–3).

Fish oils (omega-3 fatty acids) *

Fish oils may have some application (reviewed by Maidment, *Acta Psych Scand* 2000, **102**, 3–11, 40 refs).

Gabapentin

The only two double-blind placebo-controlled studies have failed to show any advantage over placebo in mania (eg. n=117, Pande, gabapentin study group, *Bipolar Disorders* 1999, 1[Suppl 1], 17). However, a number of case reports (eg. Stanton *et al, Am J Psych* 1997, **154**, 287) and open studies (n=9, 1600–4800mg/d, McElroy *et al, Ann Clin Psychiatry* 1997, **9**, 99–103; n=25, up to 1440mg/d, Cabras *et al, J Clin Psych* 1999, **60**, 245–48) have suggested a potential effect in mania in some people, a good advert for evidence-based approaches to treatment.

Levothyroxine (thyroxine)

0.3–0.5mg/d may be used for rapid or 48hr cycling mania (*Arch Gen Psych* 1982, **39**, 311–12).

Methylene Blue

Some effect has been suggested, as it may reduce pathotoxic vanadium ion concentrations (n=31, d/b, c/o, 2-yr, Naylor *et al, Biol Psych* 1986, **21**, 915–20; *Biol Psych* 1989, **26**, 850–52).

Oxcarbazepine *

See carbamazepine. Oxcarbazepine has been used successfully in acute mania at 1800–2100mg/d (open, n=6, Emrich *et al, Pharmacol Biochem Behav* 1983, **19**, 369–72) and at 2400mg/d compared with haloperidol 42mg/d, where it had a slower onset of action but fewer side effects (n=42, Emrich, *Int Clin Psychopharmacol* 1990, **5**[Suppl 1], 83–88). In a comparison with lithium in acute mania, oxcarbazepine was equally effective, but with a slower onset and less well tolerated (n=58, d/b, mentioned by Grant and Faulds, *Drugs* 1992, **43**, 873–88). Another comparison with lithium showed no clear oxcarbazepine responders, although the study deign was flawed (3yr, allegedly RCT, n=18, Wildegrube, *Int Clin Psychopharmacol* 1990, **5**[Suppl 1], 89–94).

Phenytoin *

Phenytoin augmentation of haloperidol in acute mania was more effective than haloperidol, and may indicate that blockade of voltage-activated sodium channels is a common therapeutic mechanism for anticonvulsants in acute mania (n=39, RCT, 5/52, Mishory *et al, Am J Psych* 2000, **157**, 463–65).

Spironolactone

A case report of combination with lithium has appeared (*BMJ* 1986, **292**, 661–62) and 100mg/d improved behaviour in a study (n=6, *J Nerv Ment Dis* 1978, **166**, 517–20).

Topiramate *

60% patients responded (>50% reduction in symptoms) to topiramate 100–300mg/d as adjunctive therapy in bipolar mania, with good tolerability and significant weight loss (n=18, open, 5/52, Chengappa *et al, Bipolar Disord* 1999, **1**, 42–53), with 50mg/d produced a rapid response in a treatment-resistant manic episode, confirmed by discontinuation and restarting (n=1, Normann *et al, Am J Psych* 1999, **156**, 2014).

▼ **No efficacy**

Tiagabine *

Tiagabine had no detectable antimanic activity as mono- or adjunctive therapy compared to standard treatments (14/7, n=8, open, Grunze *et al, J Clin Psych* 1999, **60**, 759–62).

1.20 MOVEMENT DISORDERS (Drug-induced)

Akathisia, pseudoparkinsonism, dyskinesias and dystonias have all been associated with antipsychotics and other drugs (see *5.8*). All can occur acutely or chronically.

Reviews*: extensive (Ebadi & Srinivasan, *Pharmacological Reviews* 1995, **47**, 575–604, 433 refs), role of atypicals in management (Fernandez and Friedman, *CNS Drugs* 1999, **11**, 467–83).

1.20.1 AKATHISIA *

Akathisia is described as uncontrolled physical restlessness with subjective (unpleasant inner feeling of restlessness, urge to move) and objective (constantly shifting posture, rocking, lifting feet as if marching on the spot and crossing and uncrossing the legs while sitting) components. Its prevalence may be high in schizophrenics treated with antipsychotics (Kahn *et al, Compr Psych* 1992, **33**, 233–36) eg. mild akathisia (41%), moderate-to-severe akathisia (21%) (Sachdev & Kruk, *Arch Gen Psych* 1994, **51**, 963–74), and chronic akathisia in up to 24% of in-patients (Halstead *et al, B J Psych* 1994, **164**, 177–83), a higher incidence than usually noticed. Antipsychotic-induced akathisia is classified according to the time of onset from start of antipsychotic treatment (acute, tardive, withdrawal or chronic akathisia). The cause is probably an imbalance of cortical and nigrostriatal dopaminergic innervation.

Role of drugs*:

Akathisia is usually related to the use of antipsychotic drugs, but if confused with agitation or psychosis, can result in an inappropriate increase in antipsychotic dose. Propranolol or other lipophilic beta-blockers seem to be the most consistent therapies for acute akathisia, with addition of benzodiazepines a sensible next choice. Amantadine, cyproheptadine, anticholinergics or clonidine can be tried.

Reviews*: editorial (Bakheit, *Postgrad Med J* 1997, **73**, 529–30), algorithm (Blaisdell, *Pharmacopsychiatry* 1994, **27**, 139–46), general (Miller and Fleischhacker, *Drug Safety* 2000, **22**, 73–81, 71 refs), effect on clinical outcome (n=34, Luthra *et al, Gen Hosp Psych* 2000, **22**, 276–80).

● **Unlicensed/Some efficacy**

Anticholinergics

These may be useful if the akathisia forms part of an extra-pyramidal side-effect profile but are generally considered less useful.

Benzodiazepines

Clonazepam 0.5–3mg/d (average 1.7mg/d) has been used for antipsychotic-induced akathisia and tardive akathisia (*Hum Psychopharmacol* 1991, **6**, 39–42). 81% patients in a study improved, with the effect prominent in two days (n=21, open, *Acta Psych Scand* 1989, **80**, 106–7).

Beta-blockers

30–80mg/d of propranolol can produce a dramatic and persistent improvement, particularly if the akathisia is not connected with Parkinsonian side-effects, but it may take up to three months to act in chronic cases (*Biol Psych* 1988, **24**, 823–27). Propranolol seems equipotent with the other lipophilic beta-blockers metoprolol (*Biol Psych* 1990, **27**, 673–75) and betaxolol (*Am J Psych* 1992, **149**, 647–50) and has been used for fluoxetine (*Biol Psych* 1991, **30**, 531–32) and olanzapine-induced akathisia (n=1, Kurzthaler *et al, Am J Psych* 1997, **154**, 1316). Nadolol (ineffective, n=20, d/b, *J Clin Psych* 1991, **29**, 1215–19), sotalol and atenolol are less effective.

○   **Unlicensed/Possible efficacy**

Amantadine

This can produce a relatively reliable effect, including if antidepressant-induced (*Nova Scotia Med J* 1991, **69**, 1012), but tolerance may develop in a week (n=4, Zubenko *et al, J Clin Psychopharmacol* 1984, **4**, 218–20).

Apomorphine

In a study of tardive akathisia, low dose apomorphine reduced objective (movement) effects but not subjective distress (Karstaedt and Pincus, *Neurology* 1993, **43**, 611–13).

Clonidine

Some effect has been noted but this may be sedation-related (*Am J Psych* 1987, **144**, 235–36).

Cyproheptadine

In a short trial of 16mg/d, antipsychotic-induced akathisia markedly improved in 15 and partly in 2, any psychosis or depression remained unchanged, and the improvement was reversed on withdrawal (n=17, 4/7, open, Weiss *et al, B J Psych* 1995, **167**, 483–86). Longer-term trials may thus be warranted.

Iron supplements

There is a disputed similarity with Ekbom's syndrome (*Lancet* 1987, **i**, 1234–36; *Biol Psych* 1991, **29**, 411–13) although no relationship between plasma iron and chronic akathisia has been found (Barnes *et al, B J Psych* 1992, **161**, 791–96).

Mianserin

Mianserin, a potent $5HT_{2A/2C}$ antagonist, at 15mg/d has been shown to produce a significant improvement in neuroleptic-induced akathisia and dysphoria (RCT, n=15, 5/7, Poyurovsky *et al, B J Psych* 1999, **174**, 238–42).

Moclobemide

Successful use has been reported (n=1, Ebert and Demling, *Pharmacopsychiatry* 1991, **24**, 229–31).

Tryptophan

Some improvement has been shown (n=6, open, *Biol Psych* 1990, **27**, 671–72).

1.20.2 PSEUDOPARKINSONISM or PARKINSONIAN SIDE-EFFECTS

Symptoms include akinesia, rigidity, bradykinesia and coarse tremor at rest (but not pill rolling). They can take a few weeks to occur and may remit spontaneously. EPSEs can occur even in untreated schizophrenics (Chatterjee *et al, Am J Psych* 1995, **152**, 1724–29).

BNF Listed

Anticholinergics (antimuscarinics) *

The case for anticholinergics:

1. Lack of use of anticholinergics in antipsychotic-treated schizophrenia is associated with *reduced* survival (n=88, 10-year prospective study, Waddington *et al, B J Psych* 1998, **173**, 325–29).

2. They may improve compliance with antipsychotics (McClelland, *B J Psych* 1974, **124**, 151–59).

3. PRN or low-dose regular use probably has a low impact.

4. Anticholinergics may partly help negative symptoms in acutely psychotic schizophrenics (eg. Mahaptra *et al, Biol Psych* 1993, **33**, 95) and so may only be detrimental to positive symptoms during *acute* phases (when excess dopaminergic activity is thought to occur) but not during stable phases (Tandon and Dequardo, *Am J Psych* 1995, **152**, 814–15, plus discussion by Goff).

The case against anticholinergics:

1. Most anticholinergics have been shown to adversely effect memory (especially visual) in schizophrenics and in the elderly (*B J Psych* 1984, **140**, 470–72), probably a result of their effect on the cholinergic system.

2. They may exacerbate tardive dyskinesia.
3. Abrupt withdrawal can produce rebound EPSEs (Carter, *B J Psych* 1983, **142**, 166–68), so a slow taper is necessary on withdrawal. Rapid withdrawal can lead to cholinergic rebound, myalgia, depression, anxiety, insomnia, headaches, g/i distress, vomiting, nightmares, rebound pesudoparkinsonism and malaise (n=110, Marken *et al, CNS Drugs* 1996, **5**, 190–99).
4. There is an abuse potential (eg. 6% in a cohort of n=214, Zemishlany *et al, Int Clin Psychopharmacol* 1996, **11**, 199–202), possibly due to an alleged euphorant effect, although this may be more of an attempt to self-medicate to treat EPSEs (Saran, *J Clin Psych* 1986, **47**, 130–32). True abusers may be identified as those who frequently 'lose' medication or request unnecessary dose increases. Use should be rational and if discontinued, should be over a 2-week period if high dose or long-term treatment.
5. Some studies have shown that anticholinergics significantly worsen positive symptoms in acutely psychotic schizophrenics (eg. Mahaptra *et al, Biol Psych* 1993, **33**, 95).

How to use:
1. Conventional wisdom is that when used for antipsychotic-induced side-effects, few patients need them regularly long-term, 'when required' being preferable, eg. often only for a couple of days after a depot to match peak blood levels. They are probably best prescribed only for overt symptoms and then discontinued gradually after three months, reinstated only if symptoms reappear. An attempt should be made to reduce the dose or discontinue any anticholinergic every three to six months, as up to 95% of patients may be able to continue without them (*B J Psych* 1989, **154**, 625–28). The standard recommendation of discontinuing after 3 months where EPSEs are under reasonable control is supported by a consensus statement from the WHO (WHO, *B J Psych* 1990, **156**, 412), although unless there is clear evidence of abuse, anticholinergics should not

be denied if the patient requests them, in moderate doses for EPSEs.
2. There is little, if any, clinically significant difference between the agents in this group.
Reviews: managing antipsychotic-induced parkinsonism (Mamo *et al, Drug Saf* 1999, **20**, 269–75, 49 refs; Holloman and Marder, *Am J Health-Sys Pharm* 1997, **54**, 2461–77), role of anticholinergic drugs (Barnes and McPhillips, *CNS Drugs* 1996, **6**, 315–30), anticholinergic abuse and misuse (Marken *et al, CNS Drugs* 1996, **5**, 190–99).
The drugs in this class are:

Benzhexol (trihexyphenidyl)
This is an anticholinergic agent with some smooth muscle effects. Abuse has been reported, with doses of up to 100mg/d taken (*Am J Psych* 1992, **149**, 574–75).

Benztropine
This is an anticholinergic agent with antihistaminic properties. It has a long half-life (up to 24 hours) and a prolonged action can be expected.

Biperiden
This drug is similar to benzhexol but with more potent antinicotinic effects.

Methixene
This drug is similar to atropine, with antimuscarinic, antihistaminic and direct antispasmodic properties. It is claimed to be a more potent anti-tremor agent than the others.

Orphenadrine
Orphenadrine is related to the antihistamine diphenhydramine and is similar in action to benzhexol. There is evidence that orphenadrine overdose is associated with greater death rates than with other anticholinergics, and also of overuse (Slørdal and Gjerden, *B J Psych* 1999, **174**, 275–76; Buckley and McManus, *B J Psych* 1998, **172**, 461–64). Best to avoid if possible.

Procyclidine
An anticholinergic similar to benzhexol. Abuse has been reported (*B J Psych* 1982, **141**, 81–4) but another study was unable to show a euphorant effect (*Acta Psych Scand* 1986, **74**, 519–23).

● **Unlicensed/Some efficacy**
Dose reduction of any antipsychotic.

○   Unlicensed/Possible efficacy

Amantadine

Amantadine is not usually recommended for drug-induced EPSEs (BNF) but has been found to be as effective as biperiden, with no worsening of any TD (d/b, c/o, Silver *et al, J Clin Psych* 1995, **56**, 167–70) although no comparison of cognitive function was made. Amantadine may be a better tolerated agent for EPSEs in elderly patients, with similar efficacy to the anticholinergic agents (review by Mamo *et al, Drug Saf* 1999, **20**, 269–75).

Calcium

Two cases of EPSEs treated with oral calcium have been reported (*B J Psych* 1988, **152**, 722–23).

Diphenhydramine

Oral or parenteral (25–50mg) diphenhydramine has been reported to produce rapid (within minutes) reversal of Parkinsonian side-effects of antipsychotics. Maintenance doses of 25–50mg tds have also been used widely.

Estrogen (oestrogen) *

High levels of estrogen have been reported to reduce hyperkinetic symptoms in women with psychosis (n=25, Thompson *et al, Acta Psych Scand* 2000, **101**, 130–34).

Quinine

This reduces muscle response to acetylcholine and may reduce symptoms (*Am J Psych* 1989, **146**, 801).

▼   No efficacy

Bromocriptine

This is not recommended for drug induced extrapyramidal side-effects (BNF).

Calcium-channel blockers

Verapamil, nifedipine and diltiazem showed no effect on EPSEs in one study (*B J Psych* 1989, **146**, 269).

1.20.3 TARDIVE DYSKINESIA

Symptoms:

Tardive dyskinesia (TD) is an involuntary hyperkinesia, which increases with anxiety, goes away during sleep and in some cases may be irreversible. Symptoms include choreas, tics, dystonias, orolingual dyskinesias etc but not tremor. It is generally seen as repetitive, involuntary and purposeless movements of, eg. the tongue, neck and jaw (the oro-facial dyskinesia or the buccolinguomasticatory [BLM] syndrome). TD can be consciously suppressed by the sufferer for limited periods but reappears when distracted and worsens during periods of stress. The incidence may be up to 30–40% in long-term patients (*B J Psych* 1986, **149**, 621–23) although figures of 10–20% seem more likely.

Causes:

There is growing evidence from treated and untreated schizophrenic populations that TD rates in both are roughly the same, implying that TD may be a late symptom of schizophrenia, and that antipsychotics might bring forward (rather than cause) such symptoms. There is a clear association between antipsychotic drug use and TD, but no established relationship with the length of treatment, dose nor actual drug used and the symptoms of TD also occur in non-antipsychotic treated people, especially the elderly. The main neurotransmitter theories are 'denervation super-sensitivity' caused by increased numbers of post-synaptic D_2 receptors occurring in response to chronic dopamine blockade, resulting in GABA transmission irregularities in the Substantia Nigra Pars Reticulate, or possibly a GABA defect. It may not be progressive and may improve with time (*Can J Psych* 1989, **34**, 700–3). Impaired neuroleptic metabolism may be important (n=18, Bates *et al, Acta Psych Scand* 1999, **99**, 294–99).

Risk factors:

These include length of exposure to antipsychotics in the elderly (Sweet *et al, Arch Gen Psych* 1995, **52**, 478–86), alcohol consumption (Duke *et al, B J Psych* 1995, **164**, 630–36), advancing age (*Am J Psych* 1992, **149**, 1206–11), being male (*Acta Psych Scand* 1990, **81**, 530–33, especially in elderly, n=706 chronic psychotics, van Os *et al, Acta Psych Scand* 1999, **99**, 288–93), having negative symptoms of schizophrenia (Liddle *et al, B J Psych* 1993, **163**, 776–80), previous head injury, presence of organic brain disease (eg. retardation, epilepsy) structural brain damage, earlier drug-induced Parkinsonism, akathisia or dystonias, lithium (Ghadirian *et al, J Clin Psych* 1996, **57**, 22–28), non-left-handedness (*Acta Psych Scand* 1990, **81**, 530–33), being diabetic (50% increase –

Woerner *et al, Am J Psych* 1993, **150**, 96–98), and concurrent affective or negative symptoms.

Treatment strategies*:

1. **Withdraw the antipsychotic** — if the drug was exacerbating the condition, the TD may improve. Psychosis may relapse, and this is an unproven and hazardous strategy (McGrath and Soares, *CDSR* 2000, CD000459). Ensuring that the original diagnosis is correct and valid is important. It may be possible to reintroduce the anti-psychotic again in the short-term or at reduced doses. Drug 'holidays' seem detrimental. Some predictors of improvement have been identified (*B J Psych* 1990, **157**, 585–92) but the risk of relapse (even in long-term patients without proper diagnosis) was noted to be high. Dose reduction may help.

2. **Withdraw or reduce any antichol-inergic drugs** if possible – these can provoke or exacerbate TD, although not a risk factor as such.

3. **Keep antipsychotic drug use down in the long-term to minimum effective doses**. A 10-year follow-up showed that reducing individual doses had little influence but overall the lower doses (<300mg/d chlorpromazine equivalents) tended to lead to improve-ment, so lower doses are appropriate (n=44, Yassa and Nair, *Acta Psych Scand* 1992, **86**, 262–66).

4. **Avoid increasing the dose or adding another drug** – this does **not** work in the long-term as it blocks any excess dopamine activity initially, but the condition will then worsen. This may, however, be useful in the short-term and can be useful for special occasions.

5. **Consider an alternative antipsy-chotic, eg. quetiapine** (eg. n=1, Vesely *et al, Int Clin Psycho-pharmacol* 2000, **15**, 57–60)**, olanzapine** (n=1714, RCT, Glazer, *J Clin Psych* 2000, **61**[Suppl 4], 21–26] **or risperidone** if an antipsychotic is needed. **Clozapine** also has a virtually clear record and some patients with severe TD make a clinically remarkable improvement on clozapine (see next page).

6. **GABA agonist treatment** (eg. valpro-ate, baclofen, progabide) may be effective (NNT=10, Soares *et al, CDSR*

2000, CD000203) or prophylactic against developing or re-developing TD.

7. **Consider other adjuncts** eg. benzodiazepine, buspirone, calcium antagonist or beta-blocker. ECT is also an option.

Reviews*: general (Duncan *et al, Psych Bull* 1997, **21**, 422–25; *Maudsley Prescribing Guidelines* 2001; Tarsy, *Curr Treat Options Neurol* 2000, **2**, 205–14; Sachdev, *Aust NZ J Psych* 2000, **34**, 355–69; Simpson, *J Clin Psych* 2000, **61**[Suppl 4], 39–44), 'miscellaneous' treatments (McGrath and Soares, *CDSR* 2000, CD000208).

BNF listed

Tetrabenazine *

Tetrabenazine is now licensed in the UK, with a starting dose of 12.5mg, titrated to 25–75mg/d (maximum 200mg/d). Patients with refractory TD receiving tetrabenazine (mean 58mg/d) had significantly improved AIMS scores over 20 weeks, as judged by 'blind videotape raters', a good trick if you can do it (n=20, Ondo *et al, Am J Psych* 1999, **156**, 1279–81). Informal follow-up of 400 patients with movement disorders, suggested a noticeable benefit from tetrabenazine in those (n=94) with TD (n=526, Jankovic and Beach, *Neurology* 1997, **48**, 358–62).

● **Unlicensed/Some efficacy**

Calcium-channel blockers

Nifedipine at 40–80mg/d (*Am J Psych* 1989, **146**, 1218–19) seems the most effective. Higher doses seem more effective and the elderly and people with more severe TD respond better (review by Cates *et al, Ann Pharmacother* 1993, **27**, 191–96, 14 refs). Verapamil (Obad and Ovsiew, *B J Psych* 1993, **162**, 554–56) and diltiazem may also be useful.

Valproate

There is evidence for the efficacy of valproate in TD (*Curr Opin Psych* 1989, **2**, 12–16), although it is not always suc-cessful (Fisk and York, *B J Psych* 1987, **150**, 542–46).

○ **Unlicensed/Possible efficacy**

Amantadine *

Amantadine was superior to placebo in one study (d/b, c/o, 18/52, Angus *et al, J Clin Psychopharmacol* 1997, **17**, 88–91).

Benzodiazepines *

A Cochrane Review concluded that benzodiazepines had no proven advantage over placebo (McGrath and Soares, *CDSR* 2000, CD000205), although there have been reports of clonazepam decreasing dystonic symptoms (n=19, RCT, Thacker *et al, Am J Psych* 1990, **147**, 445–51).

Beta-blockers

Propranolol has been used with equivocal results (*Biol Psych* 1983, **18**, 391–94).

Botulinum toxin

A successful use in severe TD with dystonia has been reported (*B J Psych* 1992, **161**, 867–68).

Bromocriptine

There has been limited success with low doses, eg. 0.75–7.5mg/d (*Arch Gen Psych* 1989, **46**, 908–13; *Integr Psych* 1989, **6**, 171–79).

Buspirone *

High-dose buspirone (up to 180mg/d) may be useful (n=8, open, 12.52, Moss *et al, J Clin Psychopharmacol* 1993, **13**, 204–9) and even in severe TD at up to 240mg/d (n=1, Neppe, *Lancet* 1989, **2**, 1458).

Clozapine *

In approximately 43% of cases of TD, especially with dystonic features, improvement (ie. >50% reduction in symptoms) has been seen when the current antipsychotic was replaced with clozapine (*B J Psych* 1991, **158**, 503–10; see also n=7, open, Bassitt *et al, Eur Arch Psych Clin Neurosci* 1998, **248**, 209–11).

Cyproheptadine

In a study of patients with TD taking haloperidol, significant improvement in symptoms occurred when cyproheptadine 8–24mg/d was added, the authors suggesting this warrants a double-blind trial (n=10, open, Lee *et al, J Serotonin Res* 1994, **1**, 91–95).

Gabapentin *

Some suggestion of efficacy has been made (n=16, Hardoy *et al, J Aff Dis* 1999, **54**, 315–17).

Insulin *

Low-dose insulin has been suggested as superior to placebo (see McGrath and Soares, *CDSR* 2000, CD000208).

Olanzapine

There are several cases of a marked reduction in pre-existing symptoms of TD when treated with olanzapine (n=4, Littrell, *Arch Gen Psych* 1998, **55**, 279–80; n=2; Soutullo *et al, J Clin Psychopharmacol* 1999, **19**, 100–1).

Ondansetron *

Ondansetron (a 5-HT3 antagonist) 12mg/d produced a significant reduction in neuroleptic-induced TD and in psychotic symptoms (n=12, 12/52, open, Sirota *et al, Am J Psych* 2000, **157**, 287–89).

Piracetam

There is a case report of piracetam improving chlorpromazine-related TD (Chaturvedi, *J Clin Psych* 1987, **48**, 255).

Pyridoxine

There are several case reports of pyridoxine 200mg/d producing a rapid and sustained reduction in TD symptoms (eg. n=1, Lerner and Liberman, *J Clin Psych* 1998, **59**, 623–24).

Risperidone

There are a number of case reports of remission of TD (eg. Santone *et al, Clin Drug Invest* 1997, **14**, 502–6; Rangwani *et al, Ann Clin Psych* 1996, **8**, 27–29).

▼ No efficacy

Anticholinergics *

Discontinuing may result in improvement in TD (*B J Psych* 1984, **145**, 304–10) although the evidence for any effect is poor (Soares and McGrath, *CDSR* 2000, CD000204), and it may be that they just exacerbate the movement disorder.

Citalopram

One study showed citalopram had no effect on the symptoms of TD (n=13, Korsgaard *et al, Clin Neuropharmacol* 1986, **9**, 52–57).

Lithium

One study showed lithium to have no consistent effect on the symptoms of TD (n=11, d/b, c/o, Mackay *et al, Psychol Med* 1980, **10**, 583–87), supported since by other studies (Yassa *et al, Can J Psych* 1984, **29**, 36–37). Lithium may even exacerbate TD (see *5.8.4*).

Vitamin E *

Two RCTs have failed to find any significant effect from Vitamin E (up to 1600iu/d) in long-term tardive dyskinesia (n=40, RCT, 20/52, Dorevitch *et al, Biol Psych* 1997, **41**, 114; n=158, RCT, up to 2 years, Adler *et al, Arch Gen Psych* 1999, **56**, 836–41). There is lack of evidence to support the theory that low vitamin E levels are a contributory factor to TD (n=128, McCreadie *et al, B J Psych* 1995, **167**, 610–17), although some trials have shown an effect (eg. n=35, 12/52, RCT, Lohr and Caligiuri, *J Clin Psych* 1996, **57**, 167–73) and vitamin E may be effective in a subgroup of patients with TD (18 trial review, Boomershine *et al, Ann Pharmacother* 1999, **33**, 1195–1202). A Cochrane Review concludes that Vitamin E may have some effect, but that the evidence is inadequate (Soares and McGrath, *CDSR* 2000, CD000209)

1.20.4 DYSTONIA (tardive or acute) (subtype of TD)

Dystonia is a syndrome of sustained or slow involuntary muscular contractions, resulting in twisting of the neck, limbs, trunk or face. Acute dystonia from antipsycotics is more likely to occur in younger, more severely ill patients, especially antipsychotic-naive schizophrenics with predominantly negative symptoms (Aguilar *et al, Am J Psych* 1994, **151**, 1819–21) and so care should be taken with antipsychotic use in this group. Dystonias related to dopamine-blocking drug use may occur several years after these are started.

Reviews*: general (*Am J Psych* 1993, **150**, 1035–41; Adityanjee *et al, Biol Psych* 1999, **45**, 715–30), extensive review and algorithm (Raja, *Drug Safety* 1998, **19**, 57–72, 176 refs).

● **Unlicensed/Some efficacy**
Anticholinergics
These can be effective in acute dystonia but are less useful in chronic dystonia, although some symptoms may partially respond (*Am J Psych* 1991, **148**, 1055–59). Biperiden has been shown to prevent dystonias from occurring in first-onset psychotic patients treated with haloperidol (Agular *et al, Am J Psych* 1994, **151**, 1819–21).

+ **Combinations**
Clozapine + clonazepam
There is a case of multiple drug-resistant disabling tardive dystonia, after five years of antipsychotics, responding partly to clozapine and virtually completely when clonazepam was then added (n=1, Shapleske *et al, B J Psych* 1996, **168**, 516–18).

○ **Unlicensed/Possible efficacy**
Baclofen
Baclofen has been used for idiopathic adult-onset and secondary dystonia, but no prospective trials have been carried out (Greene, *Clin Neuropharmacol* 1992, **15**, 276–88; mentioned in Narayan, *Drugs* 1991, **41**, 889–926).

Benzodiazepines
See combinations.

Botulinum toxin
This may relieve the pain and symptoms of strabismus and possibly dystonias. It is a powerful neurotoxin which destroys nerve terminals at the end plates (*Neurology* 1990, **40**, 1332–36) and may help tardive dystonia (n=34, open, Tarsy *et al, Clin Neuropharmacol* 1997, **20**, 90–93).

Bromocriptine *
A modest and variable effect has been seen (n=15, d/b, c/o, Newman *et al, Clin Neuropharmacol* 1985, **8**, 328–33) and a therapeutic window effect has been suggested (*Arch Gen Psych* 1989, **46**, 908–13).

Clozapine
Severe and persistent tardive dystonia showed marked improvement during clozapine therapy, up to 300mg/d (n=1, *J Nerv Ment Dis* 1993, **181**, 137–38). It is possible that many patients with tardive dystonia improve on clozapine. See also combinations.

Diphenhydramine
Oral or parenteral (50mg) diphenhydramine has been reported to produce rapid reversal of dystonic reactions to antipsychotics, such as oculogyric crisis (Leigh *et al, Ann Neurol* 1987, **22**, 13–17).

Levodopa
Beneficial effects from combined levodopa and a central anticholinergic have been reported in a patient with severe drug-induced tardive dystonia (Looper and Chouinard, *Can J*

Psychiatry 1998, **43**, 646–47, letter).

Ondansetron *

Olanzapine 15mg/d over 7 months reduced symptoms of tardive dystonia in one patient (Jaffe and Simpson, *Am J Psych* 1999, **156**, 2016).

Tetrabenazine

Use has been reported (Kong *et al, Mov Disorder* 1986, **1**, 193–208).

▼ **No efficacy**

Carbamazepine

This has been shown to be ineffective *(Psychopharmacol Bull* 1985, **21**, 345–46).

1.21 NARCOLEPSY

Symptoms:

Narcolepsy is a rare and often mis-diagnosed disabling neurological disorder of excessive daytime sleepiness, sleep paralysis, hypnagogic hallucinations, cataplexy (sudden loss of muscle tone provoked by strong emotions, eg. laughter) and abnormalities in REM sleep, with a strong genetic linkage, and normally starting in the 20s or 30s. The incidence ranges from 1 in 1,000 to 10,000 in Europe. About 70% of sufferers also experience cataplexy during the day. The hallucinations have led it to be confused with schizophrenia (*J Nerv Mental Dis* 1991, **179**, 12–18) and sleepiness to a diagnosis of depression.

Role of drugs:

The use of stimulants is considered first-line treatment, with some antidepressants useful in some resistant cases.

Reviews*: drug and non-drug treatment options (Hublin, *CNS Drugs* 1996, **5**, 426–36, 80 refs), general (Green and Stillman, *Arch Fam Med* 1998, **7**, 472–78; Gerhardstein *et al, Respir Care Clin N Am* 1999, **5**, 427–46; Stores, *Arch Gen Child* 1999, **81**, 519–24; Bassetti, *Curr Treat Options Neurol* 1999, **1**, 291–98).

BNF Listed

Dexamfetamine (dexamphetamine)

5–50mg/d can be highly effective although doses of 40–60mg/d have been shown to be more effective than lower doses (Mitler *et al, Sleep* 1993, **16**, 306–17). If tolerance develops, drug holidays may be necessary. Although dexamfetamine is not immune from problems of chronic

stimulant ingestion, many can take it for decades without apparent adverse consequences. Dexamfetamine acts by enhancing release of noradrenaline, dopamine and serotonin, but the stimulant effect appears to be mainly via dopamine.

Modafinil *

Modafinil is a wake-promoting agent chemically and pharmacologically unrelated to methylphenidate, amfetamine or pemoline. Its precise mechanism of action is unknown. Modafinil is indicated for the improvement of wakefulness in patients with excessive daytime sleepiness associated with narcolepsy. It significantly increases daytime sleep latency but does not suppress cataplexy. Modafinil offers advantages because of its lack of rebound phenomena after treatment withdrawal and its low abuse potential. Modafinil 600mg/d appears the maximum tolerated dose (n=32, RCT, Wong *et al, J Clin Pharmacol* 1999, **39**, 30–40; see also RCT, n=75, Broughton *et al, Neurology* 1997, **49**, 444–51), with 200–400mg/d optimum (RCT, n=283, 9/52, Modafinil study group, *Ann Neurol* 1998, **43**, 88–97) and with no tolerance in a 40-week follow-on, nor withdrawal (RCT, 9/52, n=271, Modafinil study group, *Neurology* 2000, **54**, 1166–75). Studies directly comparing it to amfetamines and methylphenidate, currently the preferred therapies for narcolepsy, are not yet available.

Reviews*: pharmacology and efficacy (McClellan and Spencer, *CNS Drugs* 1998, **9**, 311–24), general (Anon, *Formulary Monograph Service* 1999, 93–102, 22 refs; *Drugs & Ther Perspect* 1996, **8**, 7–10; *Prescrire International* 1999, **8**, 5–7).

● **Unlicensed/Some efficacy**

Methylphenidate *

2.5–5mg bd (up to 60mg/d) can be used (see also dexamfetamine above). In a controlled study of methylphenidate, pemoline and protriptyline, methyl-phenidate improved performance and waking, pemoline only performance and protriptyline neither, although all three were better than placebo (*Sleep* 1986, **9**, 371–72). Tolerance can be a problem, with drug holidays helpful. Generally considered as good as dexamfetamine (n=40, open, Zwicker *et al, J Sleep Res* 1995, **4**, 252–55) but with a better side-effects profile (reviewed by Challman and Lipsky, *Mayo Clin Proc* 2000, **75**, 711–21).

SSRIs

These are generally considered less effective than tricyclics but some positive results have been reported, eg. fluvoxamine (Schachter and Parkes, *J Neurol Neurosurg Psychiatry* 1980, **43**, 171–74) and fluoxetine (Langdon *et al, Sleep* 1986, **9**, 371–72).

Tricyclics

Clomipramine and imipramine can be used for cataplexy and sleep paralysis, particularly in stimulant-resistant or intolerant patients. Clomipramine at 10–25mg/d is highly effective and may have the most specific effect on cataplexy (Guilleminault *et al, Acta Neurol Scand* 1976, **54**, 71–87). Side-effects from tricyclics can be considerable and rebound cataplexy can occur with abrupt withdrawal ('Status Cataplecticus').

○ Unlicensed/Possible efficacy
Benzodiazepines

Clonazepam (1–4mg/d) has been used successfully, but sedation has been a problem (Thompson *et al, Ann Neurol* 1982, **12**, 62–63).

Clonidine

One paper indicated clonidine 150–300mcg/d may have positive effects (Salin-Pascual *et al, J Clin Psych* 1985, **46**, 528–31).

Codeine *

Codeine has a limited efficacy on subjective measures (n=8, RCT, Fry *et al, Sleep* 1986, **9**, 269–74) but it has been dramatically effective (n=1, Benbadis, *Pharmacotherapy* 1996, **16**, 463–65) and up to 240mg/d was as effective as pentazocine (n=1, 8yrs, *Lancet* 1981, **i**, 92).

Levodopa

Levodopa may improve vigilance and performance but with no effect on the capacity to fall asleep rapidly (n=6, Boivin and Montplaisir, *Neurology* 1991, **41**, 1267–69).

MAOIs *

MAOIs may be useful in refractory cases, albeit difficult to use (eg. tranylcypromine, n=1, Gernaat *et al, Pharmacopsychiatry* 1995, **28**, 98–100).

Pentazocine

See codeine, above.

Propranolol

Whilst initial response may be good in some patients, it may begin to wear off after six months or so (n=48, 18/12, Meier-Ewart *et al, Sleep* 1985, **8**, 95–104; see also n=4, Kales *et al, Ann Int Med* 1979, **91**, 741).

Selegiline *

Two trial have shown a potent and dose-related effect, at doses of at least 20mg/d (n=30, RCT, Mayer *et al, Clin Neuropharmacol* 1995, **18**, 306–19; n=17, d/b, c/o, Hublin *et al, Neurology* 1994, **44**, 2095–101), and may be useful in patients who get disturbing side-effects with stimulants.

1.22 NEUROLEPTIC MALIGNANT SYNDROME (NMS)

Symptoms:

This is a rare and potentially fatal idiosyncratic dose-independent adverse drug reaction resulting in a sudden loss in control of body temperature during drug therapy. The main diagnostic symptoms are hyperthermia or fever and severe muscle rigidity, with two or more of: diaphoresis, dysphagia, tremor, incontinence, altered consciousness, tachycardia, altered blood pressure, leucocytosis and raised creatinine phosphokinase concentration (*B J Psych* 1991, **158**, 706–7). Body temperature rises rapidly and can be fatal in a short time (eg. 24–72hrs) due to renal and respiratory failure. Clinical features progress over 24–72 hours and subside over 5–10 days (oral drugs) or 10–21 days (depots). The incidence is unknown but it may possibly occur in up to 0.15% of all patients given antipsychotics although this may be reducing due to increased awareness, early intervention and reduction in risk factors (*Am J Psych* 1991, **148**, 880–82). Death rates have been reported to be 14% for oral antipsychotics and 38% for depots. The cause is thought to be a sudden over-blockade of dopaminergic function, resulting in a 'crash', and leading to disruption to the thermoregulatory centre. Anaesthetists see a similar syndrome as malignant hyperthermia. It has been confused (or linked) with lethal catatonia (*1.12*) and serotonin syndrome (Carbone, *Emerg Med Clin North Am* 2000, **18**, 317–25).

Risk factors include*:

History – previous NMS, known cerebral compromise, previous ECT (Sachdev *et al, Am J Psych* 1997, **154**, 1156–58).

Mental state – agitation (Sachdev *et al, Am J Psych* 1997, **154**, 1156–58), overactive and/or in need of restraint or seclusion (Sachdev *et al, Am J Psych* 1997, **154**, 1156–58), catatonia, affective disorder (*Am J Psych* 1989, **146**, 914–18).

Physical state* – dehydration (Sachdev *et al, Am J Psych* 1997, **154**, 1156–58), postpartum (n=4, *Ann Clin Psych* 1999, **11**, 13–15), Parkinson's disease (n=98, Ueda *et al, Neurology* 1999, **52**, 777–82), young, male.

Drugs – (see *5.9*) high potency antipsychotics, IM therapy (eg. depot fluphenazine, *Am J Psych* 1990, **147**, 1149–55, or haloperidol *Am J Psych* 1989, **146**, 717–25), high doses over short periods (Sachdev *et al, Am J Psych* 1997, **154**, 1156–58), recent changes, rapid neuroleptisation, concurrent MAOIs.

Symptoms may be modified (eg. absence of fever) in the presence of carbamazepine (*B J Psych* 1990, **157**, 437–38).

Neuroleptic re-challenge:

Re-challenge with antipsychotics may show a high NMS recurrence rate. In one review of 41 re-challenges, 7 were re-challenged with the same drug, 4 were successful and of 27 re-challenges with another drug, 16 were fully successful (*Drug Intell Clin Pharm* 1988, **22**, 475–80). Another study showed that 87% were able to tolerate antipsychotics again if a two-week recovery period was allowed (*J Clin Psych* 1989, **50**, 295–98, 472), and monitored carefully. Re-challenge with clozapine has been successful (*B J Psych* 1992, **161**, 855–56) but care is needed with the widespread advice to use clozapine in patients with previous NMS as the safety in NMS is as yet unproven (Buckley and Meltzer, *B J Psych* 1993, **162**, 566). Depots are contra-indicated.

Guidelines for the re-introduction of antipsychotics following NMS (Williams and MacPherson, *Irish J Psych Med* 1997, **14**, 147–48):

1. Review diagnosis of NMS to ensure the key features were present.
2. Review psychiatric diagnosis and need for further antipsychotics.
3. Consider alternative strategies, eg. benzodiazepines for anxiety/agitation, carbamazepine for behaviour, ECT.
4. Leave as long a gap as possible (eg. 5–14 days), considering risk of untreated psychosis.
5. Chose a drug from a different group, particularly any previously used without problem, or a low potency drug. Use a low starting dose and small increments. Contraindicate depots.
6. Perform alternate day CPK assays, interpreted in the context of the global clinical picture.
7. Perform daily temperature, pulse and muscle tone measures, weekly wbc's and ensure adequate hydration and nutrition.
8. Obtain an informal or formal second opinion, as informed consent may not be possible. Inform family and carers of the decisions and risks (and document).
9. Educate patients and carers of the symptoms of early NMS and of the appropriate action to take, ie. seek urgent medical advice. Ensure the primary care team is also aware of these symptoms and required actions.

Role of drugs*:

NMS is potentially life-threatening and treatment should be immediate and intensive. The main treatment strategies are:

1. Withdrawal of antipsychotics, lithium and antidepressants immediately.
2. Correct dehydration and hyperpyrexia, eg. using ice packs, rehydration and sedate with benzodiazepines if necessary.
3. Measure WCC, U&E, LFT and CK.
4. Drug treatment of acute symptoms is usually essential (review of responses to treatment in *Arch Int Med* 1989, **149**, 1927–31). Dantrolene or bromocriptine are probably most useful. ECT is used (review, Trollor and Sachdev, *Aust NZ J Psych* 1999, **33**, 650–59).

Reviews*: general (Bristow and Kohen, *B J Hosp Med* 1996, **55**, 517–20; Kohen and Bristow, *Adv Psych Treat* 1996, **2**, 151–57; Velamoor, *Drug Safety* 1998, **19**, 73–82; McDonough *et al, Ir Med J* 2000, **93**, 152–54), case control study (Sachdev *et al, Am J Psych* 1997, **154**, 1156–58), novel antipsychotics and NMS (n=32, Hasan and Buckley, *Am J Psych* 1998, **155**, 1113–16).

● **Unlicensed/Some efficacy**

Amantadine

Amantadine is often recommended as second or third choice and has been reported to be successful in a number of cases at 100mg bd (mentioned in *B J Psych* 1987, **150**, 752–59; Blumlein, *Psychiatr Prax* 1997, **24**, 257–58).

Bromocriptine

Bromocriptine is usually used at doses of 7.5–60mg/d and has been shown to reduce the duration and mortality of NMS (Sakkas *et al, Psychopharmacol Bull* 1991, **27**, 381–84). It has, however, been suggested that it might prolong the course of symptoms when compared to supportive therapies (Rosebush *et al, B J Psych* 1991, **148**, 709–12).

Dantrolene *

IV dantrolene (a skeletal muscle relaxant licensed for malignant hyperthermia) has been used successfully (eg. n=21, Tsutsumi *et al, Psych Clin Neurosci* 1998, **52**, 433–38) and is probably the treatment of choice. It has been shown to reduce the duration and mortality of NMS (Nisijima and Ishiguro, *Biol Psych* 1993, **33**, 45–48). It reduces body temperature in 2–24 hours but muscular rigidity may take 4–16 days (*Arch Int Med* 1989, **149**, 1927–31). As with bromocriptine it has been suggested that it might prolong the course of symptoms compared to supportive therapy (Rosebush *et al, B J Psych* 1991, **148**, 709–12).

Lorazepam

IV lorazepam has been used if dantrolene and bromocriptine have failed (see also diazepam).

○ **Unlicensed/Possible efficacy**

Anaesthetics

Anaesthetics have been used for emergency treatment in a person recovering from NMS (Parke and Wheatley, *Anaesthesia* 1992, **47**, 908–9).

Anticoagulants

Since death can be from pulmonary embolism, complete anticoagulation has been suggested as adjunctive therapy (*Am J Psych* 1995, **152**, 1103).

Diazepam

There may be a benzodiazepine responsive sub-type of NMS, with predominantly catatonic symptoms, rapidly responsive to bolus diazepam, and where continuous IV administration is effective (Miyaoka *et al, Am J Psych* 1997, **153**, 882). Its longer half-life has been reported to complicate recovery (*B J Psych* 1992, **160**, 135–36).

Levodopa

Intravenous levodopa has been used as an effective alternative to dantrolene for NMS (Nisijima *et al, Biol Psych* 1997, **41**, 913–14, letter), as has the carbidopa/ levodopa combination (Shoop and Cernek, *Ann Pharmacother* 1997, **31**, 119, letter).

Nifedipine

25mg s/l has been used (*Clin Neuropharmacol* 1988, **11**, 552–55, Talley and Taylor, *Psychosomatics* 1994, **35**, 168–70).

1.23 OBSESSIVE-COMPULSIVE DISORDER (OCD)

Symptoms:

OCD is characterised by recurrent and intrusive thoughts of compulsive, stereotyped, repetitive behaviour or thoughts, eg. recurrent checking, hand-washing etc. Functioning is impaired by obsessive thoughts and rituals. Resisting these thoughts results in heightened anxiety. OCD probably has a lifetime prevalence of 2.5–3%.

Role of drugs*:

There is much evidence for the cause of OCD being related to a dysfunctional serotonin system, and serotonin reuptake blocking drugs have been shown to be effective eg. an SSRI (sertraline) was more effective and tolerable than a noradrenergic agent (desipramine) in concurrent OCD and major depression (n=166, d/b, Hoehn-Saric *et al, Arch Gen Psych* 2000, **57**, 76–82).

Two extensive meta-analyses (covering 1975 to 1994) have been published (Piccinelli *et al, B J Psych* 1995, **166**, 424–43; Greist *et al, Arch Gen Psych* 1995, **52**, 53–60) and both draw the same conclusions:

1. Only antidepressants affecting the serotonin system are effective, in the short-term, eg. clomipramine can be

shown to be clearly superior to placebo and has a surprisingly low drop-out rate (12% overall).

2. The SSRIs as a class are similarly effective to clomipramine and both are superior to non-serotonergic drugs. Although there are some published differences in clomipramine and individual SSRIs, comparative trials show similar efficacy.

3. Concomitant depression does not seem necessary for improvement in obsessive-compulsive symptoms.

4. Relapse is common on discontinuation.

5. Dosage usually needs to be high, eg. 250–300mg clomipramine, or 60–80mg fluoxetine. Response is slow and may not occur for several weeks.

Although drugs may only reduce symptomatology by 30–60%, many patients consider this a significant benefit. SSRIs may also have lower side-effects and lower drop-out rates in OCD (reviewed by Piggott and Seay, *J Clin Psych* 1999, **60**, 101–6, 50 refs). SSRIs (inc. clomipramine) are likely to be less effective when hoarding obsessions and compulsions are present (n=354, Mataix-Cols *et al, Am J Psych* 1999, **156**, 1409–16).

Psychotherapy, behaviour therapy and cognitive therapy are also useful. A meta-analysis of these treatments showed little difference, except that behavioural therapy plus SSRIs was more effective than SSRIs alone on self-ratings (van Balkom *et al, Clin Psychol Rev* 1994, **14**, 359–81). Neurosurgery is also developing as a treatment for OCD.

Reviews*: options and flowchart (*Drugs & Therapy Perspectives* 1998, **11**, 5–8, 13 refs), drug treatment options (Hollander *et al, Psychiatr Clin North Am* 2000, **23**, 643–56; Greist and Jefferson, *B J Psych* 1998, **173**[Suppl 35], 64–70), algorithms for pharmacotherapy (Zohar *et al, Int J Psych Clin Pract* 1997, **1**, S17–23; *B J Psych* 1998, **173**[Suppl 35], 1–70).

BNF Listed
Clomipramine
Of the 11 double-blind crossover studies published, 10 show clomipramine clearly superior to placebo. A meta-analysis showed clomipramine to be clearly superior to antidepressants with no selective serotonin activity (Piccinelli *et al, B J Psych* 1995, **166**, 424–43), with clomipramine (but not N-desmethylclomipramine, more a NA reuptake inhibitor) levels correlating significantly with positive treatment outcome (Mavissakalian *et al, J Clin Psychopharmacol* 1990, **10**, 261–68, evidence for the lack of noradrenergic component; Barr *et al, Am J Psych* 1997, **154**, 1293–95). Intravenous clomipramine may be effective in patients intolerant or non-responsive to oral clomipramine (n=54, RCT, Fallon *et al, Arch Gen Psych* 1998, **55**, 918–24; n=15, RCT, Koran *et al, Am J Psych* 1997, **154**, 396–401). See also introduction.

Fluoxetine
Fluoxetine has shown a significant clinical effect at 20mg/d, developing over 13 weeks, and continuing to be effective for at least 9 months with few side-effects (reviewed by Wood *et al, Int Clin Psychopharmacol* 1993, **8**, 301–6). The response is not related to plasma levels (Koran *et al, Am J Psych* 1996, **153**, 1450–54), although higher doses (eg. 60–80mg/d) may be needed.

Fluvoxamine *
Fluvoxamine has been shown to be partially or very effective in several trials (*Am J Psych* 1990, **147**, 1209–15), and as good as clomipramine but better tolerated (n=133, RCT, 1/52, Mundo *et al, Int Clin Psychopharmacol* 2000, **15**, 69–76), showing a clinical effect in about 4–6 weeks, although it may not be of any additional benefit in patients non-responsive to fluoxetine or clomipramine, except where side-effects had been limiting (open, Mattes, *Am J Psych* 1994, **151**, 1524). A therapeutic window may occur as increasing the dose above 200mg/d reversed the improvement seen (n=1, *Lancet* 1992, **339**, 689).

Paroxetine *
Paroxetine is licensed in the UK for the symptoms of OCD at doses of 40–60mg, being more effective than placebo, equipotent to clomipramine, but better tolerated in adults (n=406, 6/12, RCT, Zohar *et al, B J Psych* 1996, **169**, 468–74) and in children with OCD (n=20, open 12/52, Rosenberg *et al, J Am Acad Child Adolesc Psych* 1999, **38**, 1180–85).

Sertraline *

Sertraline has been shown to be effective in several studies (eg. RCT, n=167, 12/52, p/c, Kronig *et al, J Clin Psychopharmacol* 1999, **19**, 172–76), with a possible dose-response relationship, eg. 50mg/d and 200mg/d were more potent than 100mg/d, but adverse effects were dose-related (n=324, p/c, Greist, *Arch Gen Psych* 1995, **52**, 289–95). High dose sertraline (300mg/d) may be effective in treatment-resistant OCD (n=1, Byerly *et al, Am J Psych* 1996, **153**, 1232–33). Reviewed by Perry and Benfield (*CNS Drugs* 1997, **7**, 480–500).

+ Combinations *

Carbamazepine + clomipramine *

Carbamazepine may be useful as SSRI augmentation in refractory OCD (n=1, Iwata *et al, J Clin Psych* 2000, **161**, 528–29).

Citalopram + clomipramine *

Citalopram plus clomipramine was markedly more effective than clomipramine in treatment-resistant OCD (n=16, 3/12, open, Pallanti *et al, Eur Psychiatry* 1999, **14**, 101–6).

Clomipramine + risperidone

Risperidone-augmentation of clomipramine-resistant OCD was effective in 50% (open, Raviza *et al, Psychopharmacol Bull* 1996, 32, 677–82).

Inositol + SSRIs*

One trial showed inositol at 18g/d to significantly reduce Y-BOCS rating scale scores (n=13, d/b, c/o, 6/52, Fux *et al, Am J Psych* 1996, **153**, 1219–21). 30% patients responded to inositol augmentation of SSRIs (n=10, open, Seedat and Stein, *Int Clin Psychopharmacol* 1999, **14**, 353–56).

Lithium + SSRIs

The only controlled study of lithium augmentation of fluvoxamine was unable to show a clinically significant effect (n=30, d/b, p/c, McDougle *et al, J Clin Psychopharmacol* 1991, **11**, 175–84).

Pindolol + SSRIs *

In one study, pindolol 7.5mg/d significantly improved respose to paroxetine in multiple SSRI-resistant OCD (n=14, d/b, p/c, 6/52, Dannon *et al, Eur Neuropsychopharmacol* 2000, **10**, 165–69).

SSRIs + antipsychotics *

Risperidone can augment SSRIs in resistant cases (eg. n=70, RCT, McDougle *et al, Arch Gen Psych* 2000, **57**, 794–801), with doses of 3mg/d more effective than lower doses (Baker, *J Clin Psych* 1998, **59**, 131–33). Antipsychotics may improve outcomes in fluvoxamine-resistant OCD (eg. *B J Psych* 1990, **157**, 762–65), including risperidone (n=3, McDougle *et al, J Clin Psych* 1995, **56**, 526–28) and olanzapine 5mg/d (43% responders, n=23, open, Bogetto *et al, Psychiatry Res* 2000, **96**, 91–98).

SSRIs + buspirone

A trial of **fluvoxamine** and buspirone was not successful (McDougle, *Am J Psych* 1993, **150**, 647–49, 819–21), but there are case reports with other SSRIs eg. **sertraline** (n=2, Menkes, *B J Psych* 1995, **167**, 823–24; n=1, Veivia *et al, J Pharm Technology* 1995, **11**, 50–52) and **fluoxetine** (*Am J Psych* 1991, **148**, 1605).

Tricyclics (combined)

Addition of desipramine to clomipramine in SSRI-resistant OCD patients did not enhance its action (Barr *et al, Am J Psych* 1997, **154**, 1293–95), but addition of nortriptyline 50mg/d to clomipramine 150mg/d produced a more rapid onset of action than clomipramine alone (n=30, RCT, Noorbala *et al, J Clin Pharm Ther* 1998, **23**, 155–59).

● Unlicensed/Some efficacy

Citalopram *

Citalopram has been shown to be as effective as fluvoxamine and paroxetine (n=30, s/b, Mundo *et al, J Clin Psychopharmacology* 1997, **17**, 267–71; review by Pato, *Int Clin Psychopharmacol* 1999, **14**[Suppl 2], S19–26). Very high dose citalopram (160mg/d) may be effective in severe, resistant OCD (n=1, Bejerot and Bodlund, *Acta Psych Scand* 1998, **98**, 423–24).

Tricyclics (except clomipramine)

Many tricyclics have been studied and some have been shown to be superior to placebo but generally they are not as potent as clomipramine or the SSRIs, eg. imipramine (Volavka *et al, Psych Res* 1985, **14**, 85–93) and amitriptyline.

Nortriptyline (Thoren *et al, Arch Gen Psych* 1980, **37**, 1281–85) has been shown to be ineffective.

○ **Unlicensed/Possible efficacy**

Antipsychotics *

Although widely used, there are no controlled studies (*B J Psych* 1988, **153**, 650–70). A multiple drug-resistant case of concomitant OCD and Tourette's syndrome responded rapidly to risperidone 6mg/d (Glakas, *Am J Psych* 1995, **152**, 1097–98), which may be dose-dependent, with doses of 3mg/d more effective than lower doses (Baker, *J Clin Psych* 1998, **59**, 131–33). Olanzapine augmentation (up to 10mg/d) was successful in one and partly in three fluoxetine-refractory OCD patients (n=10, open, 8/52, Koran *et al, J Clin Psych* 2000, **61**, 514–17; n=2, Marazziti and Pallanti, *Am J Psych* 1999, **156**, 1834–35). See also combinations.

Buspirone

Up to 60mg/d was as effective as clomipramine in one study (Pato *et al, Am J Psych* 1991, **148**, 127–29; extensive review in *Ann Pharmacother* 1992, **26**, 1248–51). See also combinations.

Clonazepam

One study showed clonazepam (up to 10mg/d) to be equipotent with clomipramine (up to 250mg/d) and superior to diphenhydramine up to 250mg/d (d/b, c/o, 6/52, Hewlett *et al, J Clin Psychopharmacol* 1992, **12**, 420–30).

Diphenhydramine

One study showed diphenhydramine (up to 250mg/d) to be inferior to clonazepam and clomipramine (d/b, c/o, 6/52, Hewlett *et al, J Clin Psychopharmacol* 1992, **12**, 420–30).

Gabapentin

There is some evidence that gabapentin up to 3600mg/d is useful in patients only partially responsive to fluoxetine 30–100mg/d (n=5, open, 6/52, Cora-Locatelli *et al, J Clin Psych* 1998, **59**, 480–81).

Phenelzine

75mg/d was shown to be equipotent with clomipramine 225mg/d in a trial (n=30, d/b, Vallejo *et al, B J Psych* 1992, **161**, 665–70) but in a randomised comparison (n=60, Jenike *et al, Am J Psych* 1997, **154**, 1261–64), phenelzine 60mg/d was shown to be inferior to fluoxetine (80mg/d) except in patients with asymmetry or other atypical obsession, and no preferential response in patients with high anxiety levels was detected.

Tramadol

There is a case of rapid reduction in OCD symptoms with 100mg/d tramadol in the short-term, allowing fluoxetine to be introduced as the long-term treatment (Goldsmith *et al, Am J Psych* 1999, **156**, 660–61).

Venlafaxine

One trial showed a slight positive effect for venlafaxine 225mg/d in OCD (n=16, d/b, p/c, 8/52, Yaryura-Tobias and Neziroglu, *Arch Gen Psych* 1996, **53**, 653–55). There are case reports of response in treatment-resistance (n=1, Zajecka *et al, J Clin Psychopharmacol* 1990, **10**, 152–53) and rapidly and dramatically to 150–300mg/d (n=3, Ananth *et al, Am J Psych* 1995, **152**, 1832; Grossman and Hollander, *Am J Psych* 1996, **153**, 576–77).

▼ **No efficacy**

Clozapine

An open study of clozapine was unable to show any effect for clozapine in refractory OCD (n=10, McDougle *et al, Am J Psych* 1995, **152**, 1812–14). There are a number of reported cases of OCD being unmasked or induced by clozapine (Baker *et al, J Clin Psych* 1992, **53**, 439–42).

Flutamide

The anti-androgen flutamide was almost completely ineffective in one trial (n=8, Altemus *et al, J Clin Psych* 1999, **60**, 442–45).

Oxytocin

Initial reports that oxytocin may help OCD (*Psychiatry Psychobiol* 1989, **4**, 11–16) were not repeated in a study of intranasal administration in three patients (*Am J Psych* 1992, **149**, 713–14).

Tricyclics

See possible efficacy section.

Trazodone

A study showed trazodone up to 300mg/d to be equipotent with placebo (d/b, c/o, 10/52, Pigott *et al, J Clin Psychopharmacol* 1992, **12**, 156–62).

1.24 PANIC DISORDER

See also anxiety (*1.6*)

Symptoms:

Panic attacks present as sudden attacks of anxiety, where physical symptoms predominate and with a fear of serious consequences, eg. heart attack. These attacks need to include four of the following: palpitations, abdominal distress/nausea, numbness/tingling, inability to breathe or shortness of breath, choking, sweating, chest pains, dizziness, depersonalisation, flushes/chills, fear of dying and trembling/ shaking (extensive review by Johnson *et al, Drugs* 1995, **49**, 328–44, 150 refs).

Role of drugs: *

In general, short-term benefits may be gained with drug therapy, but relapse rates at 6–12 months can be as high as 75%, and so continued treatment and support is necessary in most patients (*B J Psych* 1989, **155**[Suppl 6], 46–52). Of all the serotonergic agents, only the SSRIs are effective in panic disorder and are better tolerated than the TCAs long-term (review of serotonin and panic by Bell and Nutt, *B J Psych* 1998, **172**, 465–71; meta-analysis of 27 RCTs of SSRIs vs. imipramine and/or alprazolam, Boyer, *Int Clin Psychopharmacol* 1995, **10**, 45–49). Placebo responders tend to show an early and temporary remission but quality of life does not necessarily improve (Rapaport *et al, Am J Psych* 2000, **157**, 1014–16). An alternative treatment eg. CBT should be strongly considered if there is no significant improvement within 6–8 weeks (APA, *Am J Psych* 1998, **155** [Suppl:1–3]). Although paroxetine and clomipramine may be superior to CBT and placebo (SB funded, 12/52, n=131, d/b, Bakker *et al, J Clin Psych* 1999, **60**, 831–38), combined therapy is generally better than for either therapy alone in the maintenance phase (n=326, RCT, 12/12, Barlow *et al, JAMA* 2000, **283**, 2529–36; Glass, *JAMA* 2000, **283**, 2573–74).

Reviews: long-term issues (Rosenbaum *et al, J Clin Psych* 1996, **57**[Suppl 10], 44–48), practice guidelines (APA, *Am J Psych* 1998, **155** May Suppl), algorithm for pharmacotherapy (Lepine *et al, Int J Psych Clin Pract* 1997, **1**, S13–15) and the risk-benefit with pharmacotherapy (Bennett *et al, Drug Safety* 1998, **18**, 419–30, 92 refs).

BNF Listed

Benzodiazepines

Benzodiazepines are rapidly effective and so are useful in patients needing immediate relief, although claims for the effectiveness of the benzodiazepines have been strongly challenged (*Arch Gen Psych* 1989, **46**, 668–70). Many benzodiazepines have been studied eg. **alprazolam** at 2–6mg/d (review in *B J Psych* 1992, **161**, 465–71; Kilic *et al, Psychother Psychosom* 1997, **66**, 175–78), which may be no better than placebo for anxiety, better for hostility but produce more aggression in response to provocation (n=23, d/b, p/c, Bond *et al, J Aff Dis* 1995, **35**, 117–23). **Clonazepam** is longer-acting, with 1–2mg/d the best balance between benefit and tolerability (n=413, Rosenbaum *et al, J Clin Psychopharmacol* 1997, **17**, 390–400). Diazepam may also be effective (8/52, n=241, Noyes *et al, J Clin Psych* 1996, **57**, 349–55). The main problems are discontinuation, where relapse may be more common with shorter-acting benzodiazepines, eg. alprazolam (*Am J Psych* 1991, **148**, 517–23) and transfer to an SSRI in due course is advised. People with panic disorder may have abnormal benzodiazepine receptors (*Biol Psych* 1989, **26**, 744–48).

Reviews: general (Davidson, *J Clin Psych* 1997, **58**[Suppl 2], 26–28).

Citalopram *

The starting dose for citalopram in panic disorder is 10mg/d for one week, increasing to 20–30mg/d as the optimum dose (n=475, Wade *et al, B J Psych* 1997, **170**, 549–53), to a maximum of 60mg/d. Citalopram may also control phobic symptoms in panic, especially at 20–30mg/d (n=475, RCT, 8/52, Leinonen *et al, J Psychiatry Neurosci* 2000, **25**, 25–32). After an 8-week trial (n=475), an optional continuation phase (n=279) showed 20–60mg/d citalopram to be effective and well tolerated over one year (d/b, Lepola *et al, J Clin Psych* 1998, **59**, 528–34). It appears quicker acting than paroxetine, but is the same at one year (review, *Prescrire International* 1999, **8**, 18–19).

Paroxetine

Paroxetine is licensed for panic disorder and for the prevention of relapse. A 10mg/d starting dose is recommended. Large studies have shown a significant effect, eg. as effective clomipramine, with a more rapid onset of action and less side-effects (eg. 12/52, d/b, p/c, n=367, Lecrubier *et al, Acta Psych Scand* 1997, **95**, 145–52), with continued improvement, maintained efficacy and low drop-outs (36/52 follow-on, Lecrubier *et al, Acta Psych Scand* 1997, **95**, 153–60) and with an optimum effective dose of 40mg/d (n=278, d/b, p/c, Ballenger *et al, Am J Psych* 1998, **155**, 36–42). In a multi-centre RCT, paroxetine plus CBT was significantly more effective than placebo plus cognitive therapy in reducing the number of panic attacks in the study group, as well as being well tolerated (n=120, Oehrberg *et al, B J Psych* 1995, **167**, 374–79). Reviewed by Foster and Goa (*CNS Drugs* 1997, **8**, 163–88, 158 refs).

Tricyclics *

Tricyclics were generally accepted as first line treatment. Initial jitteriness is a common problem with many tricyclics although this may be subtly different with clomipramine (Ramos *et al, J Psychopharmacol* 1993, **7**, 265–69). It is usually necessary to start at a low dose (10–25mg/d) and warn patients that they may feel more jittery and anxious initially (*J Aff Dis* 1989, **17**, 261–70). **Clomipramine** has been shown to be effective at less than 100mg/d (eg. *Arch Gen Psych* 1988, **45**, 453–59; n=180, d/b, Caillard *et al, Acta Psych Scand* 1999, **99**, 51–58) and with a biphasic response, symptoms worsening over 12 weeks before improving. It is as effective as paroxetine in panic disorder, but with a slower onset of action and more side-effects (n=367, d/b, p/c, 12/52, Lecrubier *et al, Acta Psych Scand* 1997, **95**, 145–52), and with efficacy maintained over 36 weeks (Lecrubier *et al, Acta Psych Scand* 1997, **95**, 153–60). **Imipramine** is effective (*vs* placebo) in all studies using doses above 150mg/d (*B J Psych* 1989, **155**[Suppl 6], 46–52). There may be a therapeutic window, with response tapering off at about 110ng/ml and with no improvement after 140ng/ml (n=63, Mavissakalian and Perel, *Am J Psych* 1995, **152**, 673–82) and so plasma level monitoring may be useful. There is a proven and potent prophylactic protective effect over six months (n=56, RCT, Mavissakalian and Perel, *Arch Gen Psych* 1999, **56**, 821–27). Relapse only occurs with a minority of patients who are in stable remission prior to treatment discontinuation (n=110, d/b, Mavissakalian and Perel, *Arch Gen Psych* 1999, **56**, 821–27).

● Unlicensed/Some efficacy

MAOIs

Phenelzine at 45–90mg/d may be at least as effective as imipramine in patients with panic attacks as part of 'endogenous depression' (*J Clin Psych* 1987, **48**, 55–59) and in atypical depression with panic attacks (*Arch Gen Psych* 1988, **45**, 129–37). Generally considered third line for tricyclic-resistant cases (*B J Psych* 1989, **155**[Suppl 6], 46–52).

SSRIs (except paroxetine and citalopram above, which are licensed)

Fluoxetine is effective when initial doses are kept very low (2.5–5mg/d) then increased as higher doses produce side-effects as well as anxiety and over-stimulation, possibly due to serotonergic supersensitivity. Fluoxetine 20mg/d was clearly superior to placebo over a range of symptoms in panic disorder (RCT, n=243, Michelson *et al, Am J Psych* 1998, **155**, 1570–77), and over 24 weeks compared to placebo (Michelson *et al, B J Psych* 1999, **174**, 2113–18). Once weekly fluoxetine dosing (10–60mg/week) has proved successful as maintenance over two years (Emmanuel *et al, J Clin Psych* 1999, **60**, 299–301). **Sertraline** has been shown to be superior to placebo in reducing panic attacks, with no advantage of a dose above 50mg/d (multisite d/b, p/c, n=178, Londborg *et al, B J Psych* 1998, **173**, 54–60), and well tolerated (n=168, 10/52, RCT, Pohl *et al, Am J Psych* 1998, **155**, 1189–95; n=176; 10/52, RCT, Pollack *et al, Arch Gen Psych* 1998, **55**, 1010–16). **Fluvoxamine** compared favourably with placebo and cognitive therapy (n=55, Black *et al, Arch Gen Psych* 1993, **50**, 44–50) and is equipotent with clomipramine *Arch Gen Psych*

1990, **47**, 926–32) and cognitive therapy (*Arch Gen Psych* 1993, **50**, 44–50). It may have a biphasic response, with symptoms worsening over 12 weeks before improving. For panic with agoraphobia, fluvoxamine augmentation of exposure therapy can help improve the response (study by de Beurs *et al, Am J Psych* 1995, **152**, 683–91; review by Ninan, *J Clin Psych* 1997, **58**[Suppl 5], 24–31).

○ Unlicensed/Possible efficacy

Carbamazepine

400mg/d has been reported to be successful (*Am J Psych* 1989, **146**, 558–59; review by Keck *et al, J Clin Psychopharmacol* 1992, **12**[Suppl] 36S–41S).

Clonidine

Short-term studies with clonidine have not shown a consistent effect but may be useful as a last-line in treatment-resistant cases (reviewed by Puzantian and Hart, *Ann Pharmacother* 1993, **27**, 1351–53).

Inositol

In one study, inositol 12g/d improved panic symptoms, whereas lorazepam did not (n=25, d/b, p/c, c/o, Benjamin *et al, Am J Psych* 1995, **152**, 1084–86).

Moclobemide

The efficacy of moclobemide mono-therapy in panic disorder with agoraphobia was unable to be shown in one study, although the long-term effects of CBT were enhanced with concomitant moclobemide (n=55, RCT, Loerch *et al, B J Psych* 1999, **174**, 205–12).

Mirtazapine

60% patients showed a sustained response to mirtazapine at 16 weeks (n=10, open, Carpenter *et al, Ann Clin Psychiatry* 1999, **11**, 81–86) and it may be effective in treatment-intolerant individuals (n=2, Berigan and Harazin, *Primary Psych* 1999, **6**, 36).

Nefazodone

There is a case report of successful use 400mg/d (Berigan *et al, J Clin Psychiatry* 1998, **59**, 256–57) and an open study (Demartinis *et al, J Clin Psych* 1996, **57**, 245–48).

Ondansetron

Ondansetron has been tried (Schneier *et al, Anxiety* 1996, **2**, 199–202).

Oxcarbazepine *

Increasing an oxcarbazepine dose from 600mg/d to 900mg/d has successfully treated panic disorder (n=1, Windhaber *et al, J Clin Psych* 1997, **58**, 404–5).

Propranolol

Propranolol has been compared to diazepam (Noyes *et al, Arch Gen Psych* 1984, **41**, 287–92) and alprazolam (n=29, RCT, 6/52, Ravatis *et al, Jo Clin Psychopharmacol* 1991, **11**, 344–50), where it appears less effective in agoraphobia with panic attacks but may have some use in the treatment of somatic symptoms.

Trazodone

Trazodone was effective in some studies (eg. *Am J Psych* 1987, **144**, 785–87) but ineffective due to side-effects in another (n=74, d/b, 8/52, Charney *et al, J Clin Psych* 1986, **47**, 580–86), possibly because its principal metabolite mCPP has been shown to be panicogenic (*Psych Res* 1988, **25**, 101–4).

Valproate

Valproate 1500mg/d may be useful for resistant panic disorder (eg. cases by Marazziti and Giovanni, *Am J Psych* 1996, **153**, 842–43; Roberts *et al, Am J Psych* 1994, **151**, 1521; review by Keck *et al, J Clin Psychopharmacol* 1992, **12**[Suppl] 36S–41S). Divalproex sodium (300–600mg/d) improved affective symptoms, particularly panic, in all 10 study completers, in patients with panic disorder and mood instability who have not responded to conventional therapy (n=13, open, 8/52, Baetz and Bowen, *Can J Psychiatry* 1998, **43**, 73–77).

Venlafaxine

One trial suggested low-dose (mean 47mg/d) venlafaxine may be highly effective in panic attacks (n=13, 10/52, open, Papp *et al, Psychopharmacol Bull* 1998, **34**, 207–9).

▼ No efficacy

Buspirone

Buspirone was not superior to placebo in one study (d/b, c/o, *J Clin Psych* 1988, **49**[8, Suppl], 30–36), in an open study (*Am J Psych* 1988, **145**, 1285–86) and in combination with CBT (Bouvard *et al, Psychother Psychosom* 1997, **66**, 27–32).

Caffeine

Caffeine is anxiogenic and panic

patients seem to be more sensitive to its effects (*Am J Psych* 1988, **145**, 632–35).

Maprotiline

This has been shown to be ineffective at doses of up to 150mg/d (*Int Clin Psychopharmacol* 1988, **3**, 59–74).

1.25 POST-TRAUMATIC STRESS DISORDER

Symptoms:

PTSD is an anxiety disorder resulting from an extreme stressful event, eg. serious threat to life or involvement of a loved one in a catastrophic event. The person then re-experiences the event recurrently by dreams, feelings etc. PTSD may be quite common yet often unrecognised and may lead to significant morbidity and mortality. The lifetime prevalence in the community may be 1–9%. A number of sub-types of PTSD have now been recognised (*Curr Opin Psych* 1995, **8**, 98–101). It has been shown that severe trauma can produce long-lasting neurobiological changes (mentioned in McIvor and Turner, *B J Hosp Med* 1995, **53**, 501–6) and drugs which affect these changes may thus have a beneficial effect. Interestingly, only drugs with a significant effect on the serotonin system seem to work.

Role of drugs:

Drug treatment is still relatively poorly studied but from current data it seems that positive symptoms (eg. nightmares etc) respond better whereas 'negative' symptoms of avoidance (eg. social withdrawal etc) are less responsive to drugs. There is an almost total lack of response to placebo in chronic PTSD. Most drugs shown to be active are also antidepressants, although depression and PTSD are quite distinct entities (eg. Dinan *et al, Biol Psych* 1990, **28**, 665–72). Higher doses for longer periods (at least 5 weeks) seem necessary.

Reviews*: general (McIvor, *Progress Neurol Psych* 1998, **2**, 18–21; Turner, *Lancet* 1999, **354**, 1404–5, 7 refs; Cyr and Farrar, *Ann Pharmacother* 2000, **34**, 366–76, 99 refs), pharmacotherapy (Pearlstein, *J Clin Psych* 2000, **61**[Suppl 7), 40–43).

BNF Listed

Paroxetine

Paroxetine is now licensed in the UK for PTSD, with a standard 20mg dose, increasing gradually to 50mg/d if needed. Paroxetine has been used successfully for post-traumatic grief (n=15, open, Zygmont *et al, J Clin Psych* 1998, **59**, 241–45) and non-combat-related, chronic PTSD (n=17, open, 12/52, Marshall *et al, J Clin Psychopharmacol* 1998, **18**, 10–18).

● **Unlicensed/Some efficacy**

Fluoxetine *

Fluoxetine (up to 60mg/d) was shown to be superior to placebo over 12 weeks in civilians with PTSD (41% response), with a low placebo response rate of 4% (n=53, RCT, Connor *et al, B J Psych* 1999, **175**, 17–22), confirming previous studies (particularly regarding avoidant symptoms, PTSD *Research Quarterly*, Summer 1990, 7, *J Traumatic Stress* 1991, **4**, 419–23; n=64, RCT, 5/52, van der Kolk *et al, J Clin Psych* 1994, **55**, 517–22). Care may be needed initially with use in patients with co-morbid panic attacks, as fluoxetine may increase panic/anxiety (short review of fluoxetine in PTSD by Marshall *et al, Am J Psych* 1995, **152**, 1238–39), so start low and go slow.

Sertraline *

Sertraline has recently been licensed in the US for PTSD, but may only be effective in women. The main trial in PTSD showed sertraline (mean dose 150mg/d) was superior to placebo in measures of global and functional outcomes and symptom severity (n=187, RCT, 12/52, Brady *et al, JAMA* 2000, **283**, 1837–44).

Tricyclics

Amitriptyline (Davidson *et al, Arch Gen Psych* 1990, **4**, 259–69) and imipramine (Frank *et al, Am J Psych* 1988, **145**, 1289–91) have been shown to produce a modest and clinically meaningful effect. The main feature is that doses of 300mg/d for at least 8 weeks are needed.

○ **Unlicensed/Possible efficacy**

Antipsychotics *

Antipsychotics are generally considered to be poorly effective (*Psychopharmacol* 1981, **74**, 263–68), although risperidone has been used (Leyba and Wampler, *Psychiatr Serv* 1998, **49**, 245–46) and at 1mg/d has been highly effective for hyperarousal, irritable aggression and dyscontrol in PTSD (n=1, Monnelly and Ciraulo, *J Clin Psychopharmacol* 1999, **19**, 377–78).

Benzodiazepines

The potential anti-arousal effect could be useful and beneficial effects have been seen with alprazolam (mentioned in *B J Psych* 1992, **160**, 309–14) and clonazepam at 4–5mg/d (*Dissociation* 1988, **1**, 3–12). Care is needed with possible abuse, induction of depression and the potential for the release of impulsive or antisocial behaviour.

Beta-blockers

Propranolol at 120–160mg/d may improve some symptoms (mentioned in *B J Psych* 1992, **160**, 309–14).

Bupropion *

In one study, bupropion decreased depressive symptoms and most patients reported global improvement, although PTSD symptoms remained mostly unchanged (n=17, open, Canive *et al, J Clin Psychopharmacol* 1998, **18**, 379–83).

Carbamazepine

Some effect on hyperarousal, hostility and intrusive symptoms has been reported (*Psychsomatics* 1986, **27**, 845–49).

Clonidine

0.1–0.4mg/d may effect some self-mutilatory behaviour (*J Aff Dis* 1987, **13**, 203–13) and may enhance some actions of imipramine (*J Nerv Ment Dis* 1989, **177**, 546–50).

Clozapine

Clozapine has been used successfully in a man with co-morbid psychosis and PTSD (Hamner, *Am J Psych* 1996, **153**, 841).

Fluvoxamine

An open trial in Vietnam veterans showed an effect at 4–6 weeks, maintained at 10 weeks (Marmar *et al, J Clin Psych* 1996, **57**[Suppl 8], 66–70).

Lithium

Two uncontrolled studies have suggested some effects (*Military Med* 1985, **150**, 378–81).

MAOIs

Phenelzine exerted a notable effect on intrusive and avoidance symptoms when used in an 8-week trial (see tricyclics) and appeared more effective than imipramine (*Psych Res* 1988, **24**, 149–55).

Mirtazapine

In a pilot study of mirtazapine 45mg/d for PTSD, 50% showed a 50% or more improvement (n=6, open, 8/52, Connor *et al, Int Clin Psychopharmacol* 1999, **14**, 29–31).

Nefazodone *

A number of open trials have suggested some efficacy, eg. 100–600mg/d (n=36, open, 8/52, Davis *et al, J Clin Psychopharmacol* 2000, **20**, 159–64). It was well-tolerated and produced a 25–33% reduction in key symptoms in treatment-refractory Vietnam veterans who had failed at least three previous drugs (open, n=19, Zisook *et al, J Clin Psych* 2000, **61**, 203–8) and where three primary PTSD symptom clusters, sleep and anger improved (n=10, 12/52, open, Hertzberg *et al, J Clin Psych* 1998, **59**, 460–64).

Prazosin *

Trauma nightmares in PTSD may be responsive to prazosin 2–5mg/d (open, n=4, Raskind *et al, J Clin Psych* 2000, **61**, 129–33).

Valproate *

Intrusion, hyperarousal and depressive symptoms may respond to valproate, (n=16, 8/52, Clark *et al, J Trauma Stress* 1999, **12**, 395–401) and use in combat-related PTSD has been reported (Fesler, *J Clin Psych* 1991, **52**, 361–64).

PSYCHIATRIC EMERGENCY, ACUTE

See acute psychiatric emergency (*1.1*).

1. 26 PSYCHOSIS and SCHIZO-PHRENIA

See also catatonia (*1.12*)

Symptoms:

Schizophrenia can be considered a 'perceptive disorder' and Schneider's 'First rank symptoms' are often quoted as the main diagnostic features. They include hearing thoughts spoken aloud, 'third person' hallucinations, hallucinations in the form of a commentary, somatic hallucinations, thought withdrawal or insertion, thought broadcasting, delusional perceptions and feelings or actions experienced as being made or influenced by external agents.

Schizophrenics most frequently have a lack of insight, auditory hallucinations, ideas of reference, suspiciousness, flatness of affect, voices speaking to them, delusional mood, delusions of persecution and thoughts spoken aloud.

Possible causes of schizophrenia *

The dopamine hypothesis, ie. excess dopamine activity remains the most widely quoted theory, but is clearly not the whole story and there are many other theories. These include hypofunction of glutamate neuronal systems (antipsychotics may work partly by increasing glutamate activity, Tsai *et al, Arch Gen Psych* 1995, **52**, 829–36), particularly at the NMDA sub-type of glutamate receptor, (as stimulation of it by ketamine produces a thought-disorder similar to schizophrenia, Adler *et al, Am J Psych* 1999, **156**, 1646–49), combined dopamine hyperfunction and glutamate hypofunction (Olney and Farber, *Arch Gen Psych* 1995, **52**, 998–1007, plus 1015–18, 1019–24) and 5-HT$_2$ hyperfunction. The balance between D$_2$ and 5-HT$_2$ may be important. Abnormal connections between nerves involving amino acid neurotransmitters may be a consequence of developmentally reduced synaptic connectivity (during perinatal and adolescent periods) rather than loss of neuronal or glial cells (McGlashan and Hoffman, *Arch Gen Psych* 2000, **57**, 637–48).

Antipsychotics are thought to exert a significant part of their clinical effect via blockade of mesolimbic D$_2$ receptors (the 'short' D$_2$ receptors). Although receptor blockade takes hours and the clinical effect takes weeks, it has been noted that homovanillic acid (the principal metabolite of dopamine) levels take several weeks (not hours or days) to decrease.

Role of drugs in schizophrenia:

Antipsychotics are the mainstay in the treatment of schizophrenic illnesses. Two separate treatment phases can be considered:

1. Acute phase*:

Many antipsychotics have an immediate calming effect, which is useful in relieving patient distress in the acute situation. They also eliminate or reduce the intensity of psychotic experiences, the onset usually being delayed by one or two weeks from the start of full-dose treatment.

There is little proven advantage of using higher doses of drugs, eg. above about 12–15mg/d of high-potency antipsychotics (eg. haloperidol) or 400–1000mg chlorpromazine equivalents. Naturalistic studies have suggested that patients most at risk of excessive antipsychotic dosing include those on depots, Afro-Americans, with a history of hospitalisations and being more thought disordered (e.g. n=293, Walkup *et al, J Clin Psych* 2000, **61**, 344–48). Most response is likely to occur within 3–4 weeks and if little occurs by 6–8 weeks, raising doses is unlikely to help. Early treatment is associated with better long-term outcome (Loebel *et al, Am J Psych* 1992, **149**, 1183–88).

'Treatment-resistance' in the acute phase may include true resistance and those with sub-optimal treatment (eg. non-compliance etc, short review by Johnson and Sandler, *BMJ* 1996, **312**, 325–26).

2. Relapse prevention:

Antipsychotics suppress symptoms with tolerable side-effects in about a third of people with schizophrenia but poor compliance compromises long-term treatment effectiveness. Side-effects, particularly the underrated akathisia and weight gain, and the unpleasant feeling of dysphoria (*B J Psych* 1996, **168**, 655–56) tend to reduce compliance. Compliance therapy has been show to improve attitude, concordance and insight on an intensive one-to-one basis (Kemp *et al, BMJ* 1996, **312**, 345–49), although some service users consider this brain-washing. Concordance implies an agreement between the prescriber and patient as to the degree of drug taking acceptable to both. In patients, this will balance the positive effects of the drug (eg. symptom suppression) and the negative effects (eg. side-effects). Schizophrenia is very sensitive to psychosocial factors often requiring comprehensive, continuous and individualised therapy.

Relapse of schizophrenia occurs in somewhere around 80% of untreated schizophrenics and so maintenance therapy, which reduces relapse rates significantly, is usually indicated. Sadly, it is not yet possible to identify the 20% who do not relapse and thus do not need long-term drug therapy (review by Johnstone and

The Royal College of Psychiatrists 1994: Consensus statement on 'The Use of High-Dose Antipsychotic Medication'
(Thompson, *B J Psych* 1994, **164**, 448–58)

The upper end of BNF antipsychotic dose ranges is often not clearly established and usually defined by limits of safety and the SPC. The BNF states that doses above these limits should only be used 'with caution and under specialist supervision'. 'Chlorpromazine equivalents' have been used to compare drugs or calculate total doses of multiple drugs but maximum doses vary between drugs and dosage equivalents are of only limited use (see *2.2.1*). BNF maximum doses can also be used

The evidence and scientific rationale for the effectiveness of high doses is limited.

Main dangers of high dose antipsychotics:
1. Sudden cardiac-related death — eg.QT prolongation etc.
2. CNS toxicity, eg. CNS and respiratory depression, hypoxia, seizures etc.

Main uses of antipsychotics above BNF limits:
1. **Psychiatric Emergency**: See Acute Psychiatric Emergency (Chapter *1.1*).
2. **Acute Treatment:** ie. After the emergency, but before the antipsychotic takes full effect. Doses should be reduced as soon as possible, once the patient has responded. ECT can be a suitable alternative.
3. **Long-term treatment:** eg. in treatment-resistant schizophrenia where residual symptoms impair living or rehabilitation:
   i) **As polypharmacy:** the BNF describes the prescribing of multiple antipsychotics as 'not recommended' as it 'may constitute a hazard' and side-effects are not minimised.
   ii) **Poor resources:** Inadequate resources/environment often result in the need for more medication at higher doses.

Factors to be considered before prescribing high-dose antipsychotics:
a. the diagnosis is fully correct
b. plasma levels are therapeutic and drug compliance occurring/assured
c. treatment duration has been fully adequate
d. reduced doses for a trial period have been tried
e. adverse social and psychological factors minimised
f. alternative drug therapies tried, eg. 'atypicals', lithium, antidepressants, carbamazepine, etc

If exceeding BNF antipsychotic doses, the following should be routine:
a. multidisciplinary team and patient (or advocate) discussion, obtaining valid consent if possible, making a thorough record of the decision and reasoning, including target signs and symptoms, and outcome evaluation.
b. consideration of any contra-indications, eg. cardiac, age, renal, hepatic, weight, smoker etc., and any interactions, eg. with tricyclics, terfenadine etc.
c. ECG pre-treatment to exclude 'QT' prolongation, repeated every 1–3 months.
d. doses increased only slowly.
e. regular checks carried out on pulse, bp, temperature and hydration
f. Prescription reviewed regularly and reduced after 3 months if no improvement.

See also Jusic and Lader, *B J Psych* 1994, **165**, 787–91. Polypharmacy is still widespread in the UK (Chaplin and McGuigan, *Psych Bull* 1996, **20**, 452–54) which may in part be a result of the 'Consensus Statement' as prescribers may now use several drugs at lower dose instead of one at higher dose and now partly as a result of non-evidence-based augmentation with atypicals.

Geddes, *Acta Psych Scand* 1994, **89** [Suppl 382], 6–10). If treatment is stopped, relapse may be delayed for 2–6 months, with the patient often feeling better (due to reduced side-effects) before the relapse. Although intermittent anti-psychotic treatment has been advocated, restarting when prodromal symptoms appear, studies have not shown it to be an effective treatment strategy (review by Gaebel, *Acta Psych Scand* 1994, **89**[Suppl 382], 33–38). Anticholinergics use in schizophrenia is actually associated with improved survival (n=88, 10-year prospective study, Waddington *et al, B J Psych* 1998, **173**, 325–29).

3. Withdrawal/discontinuation:
See 2.2.1.6.

First episode schizophrenia *
Recent data show that individuals with a first episode of schizophrenia appear particularly responsive to pharmaco-therapy, as well as quite sensitive to side-effects (review, McGorry *et al, Curr Opin Psych* 2000, **13**, 37–43). A delay in treating schizophrenia may narrow the therapeutic window of opportunity (Stephenson, *JAMA* 2000, **283**, 2091–92). Early treatment of schizophrenia is better because:

1. The time between the onset of positive symptoms and proper diagnosis is often delayed beyond one year, although probably predictable (n=20, Yung *et al, B J Psych* Suppl 1998, **172**, 14–20).
2. Delays in diagnosis delay treatment, leading to longer untreated psychosis (n=43, Larsen *et al, Schizophr Bull* 1996, **22**, 241–56). This is important, as 10% schizophrenics commit suicide within 10 years of diagnosis (Linzen *et al, Int Clin Psychopharmacol* 1998, **13** [Suppl 3], S31–34).
3. Earlier intervention seems to produce better outcomes than delayed treatment (delayed and incomplete remission, poorer compliance, eg. Opjordsmoen, *Psychopathology* 1991, **24**, 287–92), and longer untreated schizophrenia leads to poorer treatment response and outcomes.
4. Earlier treatment seems to allow the use of low-dose antipsychotics. Low-dose olanzapine has been shown to be preferable to haloperidol in first-episode schizophrenia (superior

efficacy, reduced side-effects, n=83, 6/52, d/b study, Sanger *et al, Am J Psych* 1999, **156**, 79–87).

Reviews*: general (Canales *et al, CNS Drugs* 1999, **12**, 179–88), Consensus panel statements (*Am J Psychiatry* 1997, **154**[Suppl], 1–56), GP guide (Livingstone, *Prescriber* 1999, **10**, 103–19; Launer and MacKean, *Prog Neurol Psych* 2000, **4**, 24–27), drug-resistant schizophrenia review of options (Jalenques, *CNS Drugs* 1996, **5**, 8–23), clinical features, diagnosis and management (Turner, *BMJ* 1997, **315**, 108–11), long-term management (Mortimer, *Adv Psych Treat* 1997, **3**, 339–46), drug treatment of newly diagnosed schizo-phrenic (Travis and Kerwin, *Adv Psych Treat* 1997, **3**, 331–38; Remington *et al, B J Psych* 1998, **172**[Suppl 33], 66–70), adolescent schizophrenia (Hollis, *Adv Psych Treat* 2000, **6**, 83–92), schizo-phrenia and atypicals in the elderly (Sweet and Pollock, *Drugs & Aging* 1998, **12**, 115–27; Wynn Owen and Castle, *Drugs & Aging*, 1999, **15**, 81–89) and new *vs* old drugs (Stanniland and Taylor, *Drug Safety* 2000, **22**, 195–214, 86 refs).

BNF Listed

Phenothiazines
Chlorpromazine
The prototype phenothiazine, chlor-promazine has a wide range of effects on many transmitter systems. It is used for a wide range of psychotic conditions but use in the elderly is problematical. IV use is not recommended unless the injection is diluted and the patient is in a supine position. A Cochrane Review showed chlorpromazine to reduce relapse and improve global improvement *cf* placebo, but with the (obvious) risk of side- effects (summary, plus comment by Barnes, *EBMH* 1998, **1**, 83).

Fluphenazine
An oral preparation is available but is usually used as a depot (see depots).

Levomepromazine (methotrimeprazine)
This phenothiazine is related to promethazine, has a strong anti-histaminic effect and is better known for its use as a pre-operative sedative and analgesic. It has significant sedative effects but causes little respiratory depression (study *vs* haloperidol and

risperidone, Blin *et al, J Clin Psychopharmacol* 1996, **16**, 38–44).

Pericyazine

A piperidine phenothiazine similar to thioridazine, with marked sedative and hypotensive side-effects.

Perphenazine

A piperazine phenothiazine with a relatively short half-life (8–12 hours).

Prochlorperazine

A piperazine phenothiazine better known for its use as an antiemetic and in Ménières disease.

Promazine

Promazine retains a minor role as a non-dependence-prone hypnotic, although the potential for side-effects should not be ignored.

Thioridazine *

Due to recent concerns about the long-known issue of QT prolongation, the UK MCA and US FDA now only approve of thioridazine for resistant schizophrenia, and consider it inappropriate for patients with a history of cardiac arrhythmias and require a baseline ECG and serum potassium, plus monitoring throughout treatment. A dose-related increase in risk of lengthened QT-interval has been reported, detectable at doses as low as 10mg/d (n=596, Reilly *et al, Lancet* 2000, **355**, 1048–52).

Trifluoperazine

A piperazine phenothiazine widely used as an antipsychotic and sometimes claimed to have 'activating' effects at low doses.

Butyrophenones
Benperidol

Marketed originally as specific for anti-social forms of sexual behaviour, uncontrolled studies and reports claiming beneficial effects (*Drug & Ther Bull* 1974, **12**, 12). See benperidol under sexual deviancy disorders (*1.31*).

Droperidol *

Droperidol was discontinued world-wide in 2001 due to concerns over a dose-related increase in risk of lengthened QT-interval (n=596, Reilly *et al, Lancet* 2000, **355**, 1048–52).

Haloperidol *

Haloperidol is the prototype butyro-phenone, widely used throughout the world for the treatment of acute and chronic psychosis, both orally and as an injection (aqueous and depot). Although frequently used in the acute situation at relatively high dose, there is no additional antipsychotic advantage from doses higher than 12mg/d in psychosis (eg. *Arch Gen Psych* 1991, **48**, 166–70; *Arch Gen Psych* 1992, **49**, 354–61), and in acute mania (Rifkin *et al, B J Psych* 1994, **165**, 113–16). Indeed, 4mg/d may be as effective as 10mg/d and 40mg/d in newly-admitted in-patients, mostly schizophrenics (Stone *et al, Am J Psych* 1995, **152**, 1210–12). Studies even show that haloperidol doses of 2mg/d for two weeks produces 53–74% D_2 receptor occupancy, with substantial clinical improvement and minimal side-effects (n=7, Kapur *et al, Am J Psych* 1996, **153**, 948–50; n=2, Hirsschowitz *et al, Am J Psych* 1997, **154**, 715–16) and a mean dose of haloperidol 2.1mg/d was effective in first-episode schizophrenia (McEvoy *et al, Arch Gen Psych* 1991, **48**, 739-45). There thus appears no clinically significant benefit from doses above 12–20mg/d, with dose-related increases in side-effects and possible deterioration (review of dosage of haloperidol by Hilton *et al, Psych Bull* 1996, **20**, 359–62). Any dose above 20mg/d should be the exception rather than the rule. This is illustrated by a 63% dose reduction in chronic treatment-resistant schizophrenics on high dose haloperidol resulting in improvement of symptoms and side-effects, further improved by intensive behaviour therapy (Liberman *et al, Am J Psych* 1994, **151**, 756–59).

The therapeutic window appears to lie between about 5.6–16.9mcg/L and plasma level monitoring may be indicated in some people (n=552, Ulrich *et al, Clin Pharmacokinet* 1998, **34**, 227–63). The elimination half-life in brain tissue is about 6.8 days, with significant amounts still detectable after 2 weeks. Thus, residual side-effects may continue for many weeks or months after stopping the drug, due to persistence of active CNS levels (Kornhuber *et al, Am J Psych* 1999, **156**, 885–90). See also haloperidol decanoate. There have been some concerns over a dose-related increase in risk of lengthened QT-interval (n=596, Reilly *et al, Lancet* 2000, **355**, 1048–52), especially if given by the IV, rather than IM route.

Reviews*: Pharmacokinetics (Kudo and Ishizaki, *Clin Pharmacokinetics* 1999, **37**, 435–56, 231 refs).

Thioxanthenes
Flupentixol
See under depots. An oral preparation is also available.

Zuclopenthixol
Longer-term therapy is well tolerated and established (eg. *B J Clin Res* 1991, **2**, 140–56), as an oral preparation and as a shorter- and longer-acting depot. In hostile and aggressive elderly, zuclopenthixol and thioridazine have been shown to be equally effective (*Int J Ger Psych* 1992, **7**, 369–75). A slow onset and long half-life makes use in acute psychiatric emergencies less useful (*Acta Psych Scand* 1981, **64** [Suppl 294], 1–77), where zuclopenthixol acetate ('Acuphase') is preferable.

Diphenylbutylpiperidines
Fluspirilene
See depots.

Pimozide *
Pimozide is a pure dopamine antagonist effective against a wide range of positive symptoms (Sultana and McMonagle, *CDSR* 2000, CD001949), but with potential cardiotoxic effects (see *3.2*). With a long half-life (about 55 hours), once weekly oral therapy has been tried (*B J Psych* 1982, **140**, 280) but was not particularly successful, although twice weekly therapy is unreported.

Benzamides, substituted
Amisulpride *
Amisulpride is related to sulpiride, with specific D_2 and D_3 receptor blocking and little effect on other receptors. It has been shown to be effective against negative symptoms, where 50–100mg/d seems optimum (eg. 6/12, RCT, p/c, n=141, Loo *et al, B J Psych* 1997, **170**, 18–22; 6/12, RCT, n=85, Boyer *et al, B J Psych* 1995, **166**, 68–72; n=232, d/b, p/c, Danion *et al, Am J Psych* 1999, **156**, 610–16) and against fluphenazine

(Saletu *et al, Neuropsychobiology* 1994, **29**, 125–35) and haloperidol (eg. n=488, RCT, 12/12, Colonna *et al, Int Clin Psychopharmacol* 2000, **15**, 13–22; n=21, RCT, d/b, c/o, 5/7, Ramaekers *et al, J Clin Psychopharmacol* 1999, **19**, 209–21). A short trial in schizophrenics showed that 400–800mg/d was effective for positive symptoms, with less EPSEs than haloperidol 16mg/d and apparently not dose-related between 400–1200mg/d compared to amisulpride 100mg/d (RCT, n=319, 4/52, Peuch *et al, Acta Psych Scand* 1998, **98**, 65–72). In a one-year, low-dose neuroleptic study of in-patients with chronic schizophrenia characterised by persistent negative symptoms, amisulpride was well tolerated, had some effect on positive but little on negative effects, when compared with haloperidol (n=60, RCT, Speller *et al, B J Psych* 1997, **171**, 564–68). EPSEs and raised prolactin are generally considered to be dose-dependent. Oral bio-availability is poor. Animal studies suggest some limbic specificity.

Reviews: Coukell *et al, CNS Drugs* 1996, **6**, 237–56; Saleem, *Prescriber* 1998, 49–53.

Sulpiride
Sulpiride is a specific dopamine (D_2, plus some D_3 and D_4) receptor blocker, well-established in the UK. The incidence of EPSEs is much reduced, making it a useful drug (extensive review by Caley and Weber, *Ann Pharmacother* 1995, **29**, 152–60, 55 refs).

'Atypicals'
'Atypical' is a widely-used term used to describe a wide range of antipsychotics with specific characteristics, eg. minimal EPSEs, lack of sedation etc. It may be better to either consider antipsychotics on a spectrum, from typical (eg. chlorpromazine) at one end to atypical (eg. clozapine) at the other, or to base it upon a particular definition of atypical.

Reviews of atypicals: pharmacology, pharmacokinetics and efficacy (Marko-witz *et al, Ann Pharmacother* 1999, **33**, 73–85, 87 refs) and adverse effects, interactions and costs (Brown *et al, Ann Pharmacother* 1999, **33**, 210–17), general (Worrel, *Am J Health-Sys Pharm* 2000, **57**,

238–58, 155 refs; Pandarakalam, *Hosp Med* 2000, **61**, 10–14; Marder *et al, Curr Opin Psych* 2000, **13**, 11–14; *J Clin Psych* 2000, **61**, 223–32), pharmacoeconomics (Amin, *Hosp Med* 1999, **60**, 410–13).

Clozapine * (see also separate tables)
Clozapine is the prototype atypical antipsychotic, indicated for treatment-resistant schizophrenia, including the elderly (Barak *et al, Comp Psych* 1999, **40**, 320–25). Although considered more effective in all aspects of schizophrenia by many, some remain unconvinced of this (discussion by Carpenter *et al* and Meltzer, *Am J Psych* 1995, **152**, 821–25).

Clozapine is probably effective in up to 30–50% of treatment-resistant schizophrenics (Kane *et al, Arch Gen Psych* 1988, **45**, 789–96) and this may rise to 60% if adequate doses are given for up to 12 months (Meltzer *et al, Eur Arch Psychiatry Neurol Sci* 1989, **238**, 332–39). A one-year study of treatment refractory or antipsychotic-intolerant schizophrenics showed that 50% of the former and 76% of the latter groups responded to clozapine over 52 weeks, the peak response occurring at 12–24 weeks (n=84, Lieberman *et al, Am J Psych* 1994, **151**, 1744–52). Improvement in BPRS at the end of the first week of clozapine is more likely to predict later response than those showing little or no improvement at one week (Stern *et al, Am J Psych* 1994, **151**, 1817–18). There is probably little clinical gain in prolonging exposure to clozapine beyond 8 weeks at any particular dose if no response is seen (n=50, open, Conley *et al, Am J Psych* 1997, **154**, 1243–47). Clozapine has been shown to be superior to risperidone in positive symptoms, EPSEs and prolactin, but not on negative symptoms (n=29, 6/52, b/d, parallel, Breier *et al, Am J Psych* 1999, **156**, 294–98).

Delaying treatment with clozapine until after an extended period of poorly effective treatment with other antipsychotics may reduce its eventual effectiveness (Kerwin and Lofts, *BMJ* 1993, **307**, 199–200).

Valproate is usually used as prophylaxis of clozapine-induced seizures, but gabapentin may be an alternative (n=1, Usiskin *et al, Am J Psych* 2000, **157**, 482–83). Hyper-salivation (possibly due to an altered swallow reflex) can be managed with hyoscine tablets, or atropine eye drops orally (*J Psych & Neurosci* 1999, **24**, 250).

Blood levels: These may be useful in optimising therapy if poor response occurs. Plasma clozapine levels of 200–450ng/ml have been shown to be superior to levels of 150ng/ml and below (n=56, VanderZwaag *et al, Am J Psych* 1996, **153**, 1579–84). Although there is some evidence that levels of over 350ng/ml may be needed for a good response (Kronig *et al, Am J Psych* 1995, **152**, 179–82), such levels should only be reached with extreme care (review by Duncan and Taylor, *Psych Bull* 1995, **19**, 753–55) and blood levels may not necessarily be related to therapeutic efficacy (n=41, Kurz *et al, B J Psych* 1998, **173**, 341–44). Reviewed by Olesen (*Clinical Pharmacokinetics* 1998, **34**, 497–502, 20 refs.). Low plasma levels may occur in CYP1A2 rapid metabolisers.

Mode of action: Clozapine's mode of action is open to some debate, eg. it has a low occupancy of D_2 receptors (30–60%) and thus may act via D_1, 5-HT$_2$, ACh, 5-HT$_6$ and 5-HT$_7$ receptors (Roth *et al, J Pharmacol Exp Ther* 1994, **268**, 1403–10; Jones *et al, Am J Psych* 1998, **155**, 838–40) and inhibition of pre-synaptic alpha-2 autoreceptors (Litman *et al, J Clin Psychopharmacol* 1993, **13**, 264–67). Some D_2 limbic specificity has been detected.

CLOZAPINE UK PRESCRIBING AND MONITORING SUMMARY

Clozapine is indicated in the UK for treatment-resistant schizophrenia, ie. patients 'non-responsive' or 'intolerant' of conventional antipsychotics (*Table 1*). It can be dispensed on a weekly, fortnightly or four-weekly basis (*Table 2*), but only following a satisfactory blood result (*Table 3*). The Clozaril Patient Monitoring Service (CPMS) controls these tests in the UK.

Table 1. Summary of UK clozapine prescribing restriction

'Non-responsive'	Lack of satisfactory clinical improvement despite the use of at least two marketed antipsychotics prescribed at adequate dose for an adequate duration.
'Intolerance'	The impossibility of achieving clinical benefit with conventional antipsychotics because of severe or untreatable neurological or other adverse reactions eg. extrapyramidal or tardive dyskinesia.
Patient requirements	Hospital based originally. Normal white cell and differential blood counts. Enrolled with CPMS.
Prescriber and dispensing requirements	Consultant must be registered with CPMS. Hospital or nominated community pharmacy must be registered with CPMS.

Table 2. Summary of UK clozapine minimum blood test requirements

Blood tests	Required frequency	Validity
Pre-treatment	Single full blood screen	Two weeks, if satisfactory (green)
First 18 weeks of treatment First sample at 3 days	Weekly (usually Monday or Tuesday with result on Wednesday or Thursday).	11 days from date of sampling, if satisfactory (green)
Weeks 19–52	Every 2 weeks, if blood results have been satisfactory	21 days from date of sampling, if satisfactory (green)
Week 53 onwards	Every 4 weeks, if 'stable haematological profile'	42 days from date of sampling, if satisfactory (green)
Discontinuation (temporary or permanent)	Weekly (up to 18 weeks) or fortnightly (19 weeks onward) for four occasions	If test result has not been or does not go red, clozapine may be restarted See table 4

Table 3. Summary of UK Clozaril Patient Monitoring Service Test Result

Result	Meaning	Action
Green	Satisfactory	Routine tests
Amber	wbc or neutrophil counts below accepted levels.	Repeat test twice a week until either red or green
Red	wbc below 3000/mm^3 and/or absolute neutrophils below 1500/mm^3.	Immediate cessation of therapy. Four weeks follow-up blood levels. No further prescribing allowed unless an error has occurred or consultant takes full responsibility.

Table 4. Temporary breaks in clozapine therapy (*Clozaril Newsletter* 1995, Issue 12)

1. Dose

Dose on discontinuing	Break	Dose on restart
Any	<48 hours	Restart on previous dose
Any	>48 hours	Restart at 25mg and build up gradually to previous dose to minimise dose-related side-effects

2. Sampling frequency

Previous monitoring frequency	Break	Monitoring on restart
Weekly	<1 week	Weekly, no need to restart 18 week period
Weekly	>1 week	Weekly. MUST restart 18 week period
Fortnightly	<4 weeks	Fortnightly
Fortnightly	>4 weeks	Weekly for 18 weeks, then fortnightly
4 weekly	<4 weeks	Four weekly
4 weekly	>4 weeks	Weekly for 18 weeks, then 4 weekly

Blood dyscrasias*: Clozapine can cause a usually reversible neutropenia in 3% of patients which may lead to agranulocytosis in 0.8% of patients over one year, with a non-dose-related higher risk in older people and those with lower base-line wbc counts (Alvir *et al, NEJM* 1993, **329**, 162–67). Onset occurs usually around 8–10 weeks (range 0.5–24+ weeks) and treatment is thus restricted as per *Table 2*. A recent meta-analysis concluded the incidence of dyscrasias in long-term therapy may be as high as 7% (n=2530, Wahlbeck *et al, Am J Psych* 1999, **156**, 990–99). A CPMS database study indicated that agranulocytosis rises 2.4-fold in Asians compared to Caucasians, and there is an age-related increase in risk of 53% per decade, but no dose-relationship (n=12,760, Munro *et al, B J Psych* 1999, **175**, 576–80). Clozapine (and olanzapine) are both able to induce transient granulocytopenia without the usual rise in granulocyte colony stimulating factor (G-CSF) levels. The use of G-CSF in neutropenia is both effective and logical (eg. n=1, Schuld *et al, Acta Psych Scand* 2000, **102**, 153–55; Sperner-Unterweger *et al, B J Psych* 1998, **173**, 82–84).

Cost-effectiveness: Despite the high acquisition costs of clozapine in the UK, it can still be a very cost-effective treatment for resistant schizophrenia. Savings result almost exclusively from reduced costs of hospitalisation (Meltzer *et al, Am J Psych* 1993, **150**, 1630–38; review in *Lancet* 1993, **306**, 1427–28; UK study of efficacy and safety in *B J Psych* 1993, **163**, 150–54) but are partly off-set by increased demands on active rehabilitation resources in outpatient care (n=21, Jonsson and Walinder, *Acta Psych Scand* 1995, **92**, 199–201). Clozapine may reduce suicide rates in schizophrenics, eg. a study showed reduction in both suicides and suicidal ideation (n=88, Meltzer and Okayli, *Am J Psych* 1995, **152**, 183–90), making a contribution to the risk:benefit analysis of clozapine. The UK CPMS database has shown a suicide rate of only 0.05% pa, a tenth of the expected rate (Kerwin, *Lancet* 1995, **345**, 1063–4), eg. to late 1997, 11,140 patients in the UK had been exposed to clozapine. The total deaths have been 153, including 2 haematological deaths (both early 1990s) and 20 suicides (ie. 1 in 500). The suicide rate for schizophrenia can be as high as 1 in 20, so this figure is around 530 less suicides than would have been expected.

Reviews*: management of clozapine side-effects (Young *et al, Schizophr Bull* 1998, **24**, 381–90), GP role (Launer, *Prescriber* 2000, **11**, 35-38), predicting response (Hu *et al, CNS Drugs* 1999, **11**, 317–26).

Olanzapine *

Olanzapine is licensed for the treatment of schizophrenia and for relapse prevention. It blocks a wide variety of receptors, eg. $5\text{-}HT_{2A/C}$, $5\text{-}HT_3$, $5\text{-}HT_6$, D_{1-5}, M_{1-5}, alpha-one and H1, with some mesolimbic dopamine selectivity. The $5\text{-}HT_{2A}:D_2$ ratio is high, as with clozapine. The starting and main therapeutic dose is reportedly 10mg/d (range 5–20mg/d), although doses of up to 60mg/d have been used (eg. n=1, Reich, *Am J Psych* 1999, **156**, 661). Many studies have shown a clinical effect, eg. where olanzapine (mean dose 15mg/d) was more effective than haloperidol (10–20mg/d) on negative symptoms (n=335, 12/12, RCT, Tollefson and Sanger, *Am J Psych* 1997, **154**, 466–74), superior to haloperidol for all symptoms of schizophrenia, with fewer side-effects, including EPSEs and prolactin levels (n=1996, d/b, 6/52, Tollefson *et al, Am J Psych* 1997, **154**, 457–65) and superior to risperidone for primary negative symptoms and with less side-effects (Lilly study, n=339, d/b, 28/52, Tran *et al, J Clin Psychopharmacol* 1997, **17**, 407–18, reviewed by Cunningham Owens, *EBMH* 1998, **1**, 55). It may also be effective for secondary negative symptoms, but not necessarily in having a direct beneficial effect on primary negative symptoms (n=39, 12/52, open, Kopelowicz *et al, Am J Psych* 2000, **157**, 987–93). Neuropsychological changes in early phase schizophrenia during 12 months of treatment with olanzapine (5–20mg/d), risperidone (4–10mg/d), or haloperidol (5–20mg/d) showed olanzapine may have some superior cognitive effects (n=65, Purdon *et al, Arch Gen Psych* 2000, **57**, 249–58). Olanzapine was also shown to be superior to haloperidol in schizoaffective disorder, with less drop-outs and fewer EPSEs, but more weight gain (n=300, 12/12, Tran *et al, B J Psych* 1999, **174**, 15–22). The main side-effects are somnolence and weight gain, but with low EPSEs and may have a lower incidence of treatment-emergent tardive dyskinesia than haloperidol (re-analysis of data from three studies, Tollefson *et al, Am J Psych* 1997, **154**, 1248–54, n=1714; Beasley *et al, B J Psych* 1999, **174**, 23–30). A transient rise in prolactin levels can occur. Although olanzapine is more expensive than traditional drugs, it may over one year be cheaper, considering efficacy, in-patient and out-patient costs (n=817, RCT, Hamilton *et al, Pharmacoeconomics* 1999, **15**, 469–80). Most of the cost-pressures in the community due to olanzapine are the the result of off-license use.

Reviews: general (Kando *et al, Ann Pharmacother* 1997, **31**, 1325–34), pharmacology and kinetics (Falsett, *Hosp Pharm* 1999, **34**, 423–35, 91 refs; Callaghan *et al, Clin Pharmacokinetics* 1999, **37**, 177–93; Stephenson and Pilowsky, *B J Psych* 1999, **174**[Suppl 38], 52–58), pharmacoeconomics (Sacristan *et al, Clin Drug Invest* 1998, **15**, 29–35; Foster and Goa, *Pharmaco-Economics* 1999, **15**, 611–40, 122 refs).

Quetiapine *

Quetiapine is structurally related to clozapine but without the need for blood nor ECG monitoring. Many double-blind randomised trials indicate that the drug is as effective in schizophrenia as reference drugs (eg. n=101, Peuskens and Link, *Acta Psych Scand* 1997, **96**, 265–73; n=448, RCT, 6/52, Copolov *et al, Psychol Med* 2000, **30**, 95–105), and has a very low incidence of EPSE, prolactin elevation and related side-effects (eg. Arvantis and Miller, *Biol Psych* 1997, **42**, 233–46; Small *et al, Arch Gen Psych* 1997, **54**, 549–57). Doses of 300–450mg/d (range 150–750mg/d) are quoted as the most effective. Doses need to be increased gradually over several days initially, and a starter pack is available in the UK. Headache, somnolence and dizziness are common adverse events. Quetiapine shows transiently high D2 occupancy which drops rapidly over 12–14 hours, which may explain the low EPSE and prolactin elevation (n=12, Kapur *et al, Arch Gen Psych* 2000, **57**, 553–59). The Cochrane review concludes that although quetiapine is more effective than placebo, no difference could be detected against traditional antipsychotics, drop-outs due to adverse effects were lower with quetiapine, but still high (Srisurapanont *et al, CDSR* 2000, **3**, CD000967). **Reviews***: general (McDonald, *Prescriber* 1998, 65–66; Green, *Curr Med Res Opin* 1999, **15**, 145–51), safety (Dev and Raniwalla, *Drug Saf* 2000, **23**, 295–307).

Risperidone *

Risperidone is licensed for acute and chronic psychosis. It has D_2 and 5-HT$_2$ blocking actions and has been shown to be effective against both positive and negative symptoms with few side-effects, eg. low EPSEs (meta-analysis showing risperidone to have greater efficacy and fewer EPSEs than haloperidol, de Oliveira *et al, J Clin Pharm & Therapeut* 1996, **21**, 349–58).

Dose: The optimum dose is around 4–8mg/d (eg. analysis of d/b studies, Lemmens *et al, Acta Psych Scand* 1999, **99**, 160–70) with little or no advantage in exceeding this dose. 60% acutely exacerbated schizophrenics can tolerate and respond well to risperidone 6mg/d and, in the remaining 40%, most then tolerate and respond to lower doses (3–4mg/d), with equivalent plasma levels to the higher dose, illustrating the effect of slower metabolism (n=31, 6/52, open, Lane *et al, J Clin Psych* 2000, **61**, 209–14). PET-measured D_2 and 5-HT$_{2A}$ receptor occupancy indicates that 4mg/d is the suitable initial dose (Nyberg *et al, Am J Psych* 1999, **156**, 869–75). Although titration to 6mg/d over 3 days is recommended, a slower titration has been recommended (over weeks rather than days, stabilising on 2–4mg/d initially before proceeding to higher doses), particularly in drug-naïve first-episode schizophrenics as this markedly reduces the final doses needed, EPSE and the risk of non-compliance (n=17, Kontaxakis *et al, Am J Psych* 2000, **157**, 1178–79), and may lead to better outcomes (retrospective review; n=1056, Love *et al, J Clin Psych* 1999, **60**, 771–75; n=96, McGorry, *J Clin Psych* 1999, **60**, 794).

Efficacy: Risperidone has shown efficacy across a wide range of symptoms of schizophrenia, eg. against positive and negative symptoms, disorganised thoughts, hostility and affective symptoms (Marder *et al, J Clin Psych* 1997, **58**, 538–46; Moller *et al, Eur Arch Psychiatry Clin Neurosci* 1997, **247**, 1–5) and superior at 4 weeks and better tolerated than haloperidol (b/d, n=67, 8/52, Wirshing *et al, Am J Psych* 1999, **156**, 1374–79). A multicentre study indicated that risperidone was as effective as haloperidol (but much better tolerated) in reducing a wide range of first psychotic episode symptoms (n=183, RCT, Emsley *et al, Schizophr Bull* 1999, **25**, 721–29; review by McIntosh, *EBMH* 2000, **3**, 77). Risperidone may be more effective than olanzapine, with comparable side-effects (open, n=42, 6/12, Ho *et al, J Clin Psych* 1999, **60**, 658–63), with lower relapse rates over 2 years (naturalistic retrospective study, n=142, Chengappa et al, *J Clin Psych* 1999, **60**, 373–78). Long-term open studies have shown a trend to continuous improvement and in relapse prevention (open, Moller *et al, Int Clin Psychopharmacol* 1998, **13**, 99–106), but current data is mostly short-term (eg. 4–8 weeks), and some used short treatment periods and wash-outs (critical review by Cardoni, *Ann Pharmacother* 1995, **29**, 610–18). There appears to be a significantly lower incidence of tardive dyskinesia with risperidone compared with haloperidol in older patients (n=122, 9/12, rater-blind, Jeste *et al, J Am Geriatr Soc* 1999, **47**, 716–19).

Efficacy in refractory schizophrenics was not encouraging in one study (n=33, open, Tanner *et al, Am J Psych* 1995, **152**, 1233) but a comparison with clozapine in treatment-resistant/intolerant schizophrenia claimed similar efficacy (n=86, d/b, Bondolfi *et al, Am J Psych* 1998, **155**, 499–504, although

this study has been fiercely criticised by Meltzer and others, *Am J Psych* 1999, **156**, 1126–28; see also open study, n=13, Cavallaro *et al, Human Psychopharmacol* 1995, **10**, 231–34). Other studies show risperidone to be only slightly less effective than clozapine in neuroleptic-refractory patients, but with fewer side-effects (n=35, open, 12/52, Lindenmayer *et al, J Clin Psych* 1998, **59**, 521–27) and equivalent to clozapine on negative symptoms, but not on positive symptoms (n=29, 6/52, b/d, parallel, Breier *et al, Am J Psych* 1999, **156**, 294–98). In another study, 25% refractory schizophrenics responded to risperidone (mean 7mg/d) and 58% responded to clozapine (mean 520mg/d), suggesting that risperidone may be worth a try before clozapine (n=24, Sharif *et al, J Clin Psych* 2000, **61**, 498–504). Risperidone is better tolerated and more effective than haloperidol in patients with treatment-refractory schizophrenia (d/b, n=67, Wirshing *et al, Am J Psych* 1999, **156**, 1374–79).

Cognitive function: There is growing evidence for the role of poor cognitive function (especially working memory) in poor outcome of schizophrenia, and risperidone has been shown to produce an improvement in cognitive function (n=25, Rossi *et al, Acta Psych Scand* 1997, **95**, 40–43; n=13, Stip and Lussier, *Can J Psych* 1996, **41**[Suppl 2], 35S–40S), including against haloperidol (n=59, Green *et al, Am J Psych* 1997, **154**, 799–804).

Reviews*: general (Jones, *J Serotonin Res* 1997, **4**, 17–28, Mattes, *Schizophrenia Bull* 1997, **23**, 155–61, TDM (therapeutic range of 25–150microg/L, n=50, Odou *et al, Clin Drug Investigat* 2000, **19**, 283–92).

Sertindole

Lundbeck has voluntarily suspended the availability of sertindole pending a full evaluation of its risks and benefits in collaboration with the Medicines Control Agency and other European regulatory authorities. The company is currently completing certain studies which will further define the safety profile of sertindole.

Zotepine *

Zotepine is a tricyclic dibenzothiepine antipsychotic, licensed in some European countries for schizophrenia. Both zotepine and its active metabolite norzotepine have a high affinity for a range of dopamine and serotonin receptor sub-types, and some NARI activity. To minimise hypotension, the dose should be titrated from 25mg tds every 4 days to a maximum of 300mg/d (as a tds dose). The risk of seizures is dose-related and rises above 300mg/d (open study, n=129, Hori *et al, Jpn J Psychiatry Neurol* 1992, **46**, 161–67). It has been compared with haloperidol (n=124, Petit *et al, Psychopharmacol Bull* 1996, **32**, 81–87), low dose chlorpromazine (n=159, Cooper *et al, Eur Neuropsychopharmacol* 1996, **6**[Suppl 3], 148) and higher dose chlorpromazine 300–600mg/d (less EPSE and greater improvement in BPRS, n=158, RCT, 8/52, Cooper *et al, Acta Psych Scand* 2000, **101**, 218–25). Relapse prevention has been shown (n=121, 6/12, d/b, p/c, Cooper *et al, Psychopharmacol* [*Berl*] 2000, **150**, 237–43). The Cochrane meta-analysis of 10 studies indicated that zotepine was as effective as typical and atypical antipsychotics and superior to placebo, but with the need for more studies (n=1006, Fenton *et al, CDSR*, reviewed by Remington, *EBMH* 2000, **3**, 78). Improvement in cognitive function has been reported to be superior to clozapine (n=26, RCT, Meyer-Lindenberg, *Pharmacopsychiatry* 1997, **30**, 35–42, although why some patients were excluded from the analysis is unclear). An ECG is recommended pre-treatment in people with CHD, at risk of hypokalaemia or taking other drugs known to prolong QTc. A white cell count (WCC) is recommended if low white cells are suspected.

Review: Prakash and Lamb (*CNS Drugs* 1998, **9**, 153–75, 115 refs).

Others

Loxapine *

Loxapine is a dibenzoxazepine, possibly of similar efficacy to chlorpromazine (*Am J Psych* 1986, **143**, 116–17). There is some PET evidence that loxapine is an equipotent blocker of 5-HT$_2$ and D$_2$ receptors, and hence might be claimed to be 'atypical' (Kapur *et al, Am J Psych* 1997, **154**, 1525–29), but a Cochrane Review concluded that whilst loxapine was an antipsychotic, it was under-researched and had no clear advantages over other typical drugs.

Oxypertine

This is a dopamine depleter which, unlike other similar drugs (eg. reserpine and tetrabenazine), is not reported to have depression as a major side-effect (mentioned in *Acta Psych Scand* 1986, **74**, 446–50) as it only depletes dopamine and not noradrenaline.

Depot injections *

Depot administration of antipsychotics is widely used in Europe. The major advantage is of assured compliance, with associated and proven reduction in relapses, rehospitalisation and severity of relapse, plus reduction in bio-availability problems (some people metabolise antipsychotics extensively via the first-pass effect). By being sure of doses received, depots **should** be able to facilitate better downward titration of doses to reduce the incidence of side-effects. The major disadvantages include the impossibility of altering a dose if side-effects develop (eg. dystonia, NMS), patients seeing depot administration as 'being controlled', having no control over their treatment or, worse still, as being a punishment. Many patients and families/carers are insufficiently educated about the pros and cons of depot administration. Used properly they can lead to reduced relapses, low side-effects and stable therapeutic effects. It should not be enough just to prevent relapse with a depot.

The Cochrane reviews of depots note the lack of decent trials and low patient numbers. For fluspirilene, the 7 studies, have low numbers, no advantage over oral and no outcome data (Quraishi and David, *CDSR* 2000, CD001718). Haloperidol decanoate has 2 studies *vs* placebo which show lower drop-outs on depot, but no difference against oral haloperidol (n=22), and the 8 trials *vs* other depots showed no discernable difference (Quraishi and David, *CDSR* 2000, CD001361). Pipothiazine has 14 studies, with no advantage over oral (n=166) and no differences against other depots (9 studies, n=455, Quraishi and David, *CDSR* 2000, CD001720). The data for fluphenazine decanoate is very limited, the 6 studies showing no difference between depot and oral (Adams and Eisenbruch, *CDSR* 2000, CD000307). Flupentixol decanoate has no trials against placebo, no difference against oral (but possibly less EPSE), high dose is no better than low dose, and no advantage over other depots (Quraishi and David, *CDSR* 2000, CD001470). Although there are no placebo trials for zuclopenthixol decanoate, the 4 trials showed reduced relapse against other depots (possibly more side effects) but the data suggests 'real differences' over other depots (Coutinho *et al*, *CDSR* 2000, CD001164).

The incidence of problems and complications (eg. bleeding or haematoma, leakage, inflammatory nodules etc) associated with long-term depot injections have probably been under-reported (retrospective study by Hay, *BMJ* 1995, **311**, 421). The need for a meticulous (Z-tracking) injection technique (Belanger-Annable, *Canadian Nurse* 1985, **81**, 1–3) and using the most appropriate preparation and dose for that individual are essential for long-term success (Muldoon, *BMJ* 1995, **311**, 1368).

Reviews*: overview (Gerlach, *Acta Psych Scand* 1994, **89**[Suppl 382], 28–32; Taylor, *Psych Bull* 1999, **23**, 551–53; Kennedy and Mikhail, *Lancet* 2000, **356**, 594), extensive review of depots place in therapy (Davis *et al*, *Drugs* 1994, **47**, 741–73, 170 refs), optimising the use of depots (Dencker and Axelsson, *CNS Drugs* 1996, **6**, 367–81).

Pharmacokinetics

The graph with each depot show plasma levels against time for each depot. All are single first-dose profiles. Chronic treatment will show considerably less fluctuation but, surprisingly, there is still evidence of large variations in the plasma levels of haloperidol decanoate and flupenthixol decanoate, although there was no relationship between side-effect ratings and fluctuations in plasma levels (n=30, 3-year study, Tuninger and Levander, *Br J Psych* 1996, **169**, 618–21).

Flupentixol decanoate ('Depixol', 'Depixol Conc.', 'Depixol Low Volume')

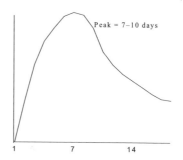

Peak = 7–10 days

*Flupentixol decanoate ('Depixol') is the most widely prescribed depot in the UK. It is a dopamine specific thioxanthene antipsychotic with potentially activating effects at low dose, and has been dubbed a 'partial atypical' (Kuhn *et al, Fortschr Neurol Psychiatr* 2000, **68**[Suppl 1], S3841):
- Duration of action = 3–4 weeks
- Peak = 7–10 days
- Rate limiting half-life = 8 days (single dose), 17 days (multiple doses)
- Time to steady state = 10–12 weeks.

Fluphenazine decanoate

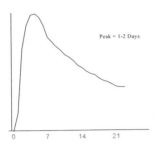

Peak = 1-2 Days

Fluphenazine is a phenothiazine that can be given up to four-weekly as a depot. Responders have been shown to have greatest improvement at fluphenazine levels above 1.0ng/ml and doses above 0.2–0.25mg/kg/d (Levinson *et al, Am J Psych* 1995, **152**, 765–71; Miller *et al, J Clin Pharm Ther* 1995, **20**, 55–62). 25mg fluphenazine every 6 weeks and every 2 weeks produces similar side-effects, symptom relief and relapse rates, but with reduced drug exposure with the longer dosage interval (n=50, RCT, 54/52, Carpenter *et al, Am J Psych* 1999, **156**, 412–18).

- Duration of action = 1–3 weeks
- Peak = 6–48 hours
- Rate limiting half-life = 6–10 days (single doses), 14–100 days (multiple doses)
- Time to steady state = 6–12 weeks (*B J Psych* 1991, **158**, 658–65).

Fluspirilene ('Redeptin')

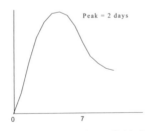

Peak = 2 days

Fluspirilene is now only available in the UK as an import from Belgium, as a waterbased micro-crystalline injection.

- Duration of action = 1.5 weeks
- Peak within 2 days
- Rate limiting half-life = 7–9 days
- Time to steady state = 5–6 weeks.

Haloperidol decanoate ('Haldol Decanoate')

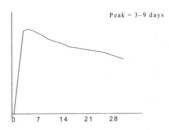

Peak = 3–9 days

Haloperidol decanoate is a longer-acting depot and a 4-week interval between injections is possible. It is probably best reserved for chronic relapsing schizophrenics responsive to haloperidol (full review in *Drug Intell Clin Pharm* 1988, **22**, 290–95).

- Duration of action = 4 weeks
- Peak = 3–9 days
- Rate limiting half-life = 18–21 days (single + chronic)
- Time to steady state = 10–12 weeks at monthly dosing (*Pharmacopsychiat* 1985, **58**, 240–45).

Pipothiazine palmitate ('Piportil Depot')

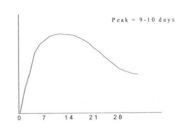

Peak = 9-10 days

Pipothiazine is a piperidine phenothiazine marketed in the UK as the palmitate:

- Duration of action = 4 weeks
- Peak = 9–10 days
- Rate limiting half-life = 14–21 days (chronic)
- Time to steady state = 8–12 weeks.

Zuclopenthixol acetate ('Clopixol-Acuphase')

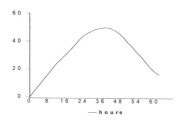

— hours

Zuclopenthixol acetate is available as 'Clopixol-Acuphase' in the UK. 50–150mg as a single dose provided a rapid and effective reduction in psychotic symptoms in 25 patients (*Curr Med Res Opin* 1990, **12**, 58–65) over about 78 hours. It is a drug of choice in acute psychiatric emergency in many areas. A Canadian economic evaluation study indicated a potential cost saving over haloperidol injection in some circumstances eg. reduced nursing time and reduced repeat injections (Laurier *et al, Clin Ther* 1997, **19**, 316–29). Use in psychotic anxiety may also be possible (open study, n=46, Romain *et al, Encephale* 1996, **22**, 280–86). See also acute psychiatric emergencies (*1.1*).

- Duration of action = 2–3 days
- Peak = 24–40hrs *(Psychopharmacology*, 1986, **90**, 412–16)
- Rate limiting half-life = 32hrs +/- 7 hrs
- Time to steady state = 6 days.

Zuclopenthixol decanoate ('Clopixol', 'Clopixol Conc')

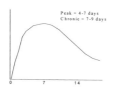

Peak = 4-7 days
Chronic = 7-9 days

This is an established antipsychotic which has also been used in high dose in aggression, particularly in learning disabilities and forensic patients but is not indicated for this.

- Duration of action = 2–4 weeks
- Peak = 4–9 days
- Rate limiting half-life = 17–21 days (multiple doses)
- Time to steady state = 10–12 weeks.

+ Combinations *

Despite widespread use, there is in fact only one RCT of combination antipsychotics in schizophrenia (review, *Drugs & Ther Perspect* 2000, **16**, 9–12, 14 refs).

Clozapine + lamotrigine *

A small open study suggested that adjunctive lamotrigine (125–250mg/d) could produce a significant improvement in schizophrenics only partly responding to clozapine (n=6, open, 24/52, Dursun and McIntosh, *Arch Gen Psych* 1999, **56**, 950).

Clozapine + olanzapine *

One patient responded to clozapine 100mg/d and olanzapine 10mg/d when individually neither was satisfactory (n=1, Rhoads, *J Clin Psych* 2000, **61**, 678–80).

Clozapine + ondansetron

There is a case report where ondansetron (4mg bd) enhanced the action of clozapine in a treatment-refractory schizophrenic (Briskin and Curtis, *Am J Psych* 1997, **154**, 1171). See also entry for ondansetron under unlicensed/possible efficacy.

Clozapine + risperidone *

Resistant schizophrenics may respond quickly and noticeably to a combination of clozapine and risperidone (n=2, Morera *et al, Acta Psych Scand* 1999, **99**, 305–7; n=3, Raskin *et al, Acta Psych Scand* 2000, **101**, 334–36).

Clozapine + sulpiride

In the only RCT of combined antipsychotics, in previously unresponsive schizophrenics, clozapine and sulpiride produced a substantially greater improvement than clozapine alone (n=24, Shiloh *et al, B J Psych* 1997, **171**, 569–73), although the two study groups had some initial differences. The rationale was additional D2 blockade, enhancing that of clozapine.

Clozapine + quetiapine *

After 6-months on clozapine (200–

800mg/d), randomly selected patients had 25% dose converted to quetiapine (1mg clozapine:2mg quetiapine). The average weight loss was 0.22–10.5kg after one-month, and maintained, with '100% user satisfaction' reported, and improvement in those (n=13) who had developed diabetes (open, 10/12, n=65, Reinstein *et al, Clin Drug Invest* 1999, **18**, 99–104).

Loxapine + cyproheptadine

In patients treated with loxapine 15mg/d plus cyproheptadine 8mg twice a day, a 33% to 43% improvement in BPRS scores in the first two weeks was shown (n=3, open, Kapur and Zipursky, *Arch Gen Psych* 1998, **55**, 666–67). The letter was entitled, 'Do loxapine plus cyproheptadine make an atypical antipsychotic?', the question mark revealing the author's lack of confidence.

Risperidone + olanzapine *

This combination has been used, with some success (n=5, open, Lemer *et al, Clin Neuropharmacol* 2000, **23**, 284–86).

Valproate + antipsychotics

There is some data that valproate may be able to reduce the doses of antipsychotics needed in schizoaffective disorder, or even replace them (eg. Reutens and Castle, *B J Psych* 1997, **170**, 484–85).

● Unlicensed/Some efficacy

Benzodiazepines

Benzodiazepines have no antipsychotic effect but may reduce anxiety, tension and insomnia and high doses may have symptomatic effects. They may also be used to allow lower doses of antipsychotics to be used, as high doses of antipsychotics are often used for their additional sedative properties. Diazepam, lorazepam (*Lancet* 1986, **i**, 510) and clonazepam (*Biol Psych* 1983, **18**, 451–66) have been used as adjuvants, eg. against hallucinations (review in *Acta Psych Scand* 1991, **84**, 453–59) although they are probably most useful in psychotic agitation. For acute psychiatric symptoms they have a rapid onset, are highly sedative, well-tolerated and a low EPSE risk. Relatively high doses may occasionally be needed and, although the effects develop rapidly, they may

diminish after several weeks in some patients (review in *Am J Psych* 1991, **148**, 714–26). Diazepam has been shown to be equivalent to fluphenazine and superior to placebo in treating prodromal signs of exacerbation of schizophrenia, either in antipsychotic refusers or as an adjunct to low-dose antipsychotics (n=53, d/b, Carpenter *et al, Am J Psych* 1999, **156**, 299–303). See also Acute Psychiatric Emergency (*1.1*).

Carbamazepine

Carbamazepine is often used in addition to antipsychotics to improve behaviour in overactive or aggressive schizophrenics. The effect on 'core' symptoms is likely to be secondary or small (*Psycholog Med* 1989, **19**, 591–604) and only in schizophrenics, not schizoaffectives (*Acta Psych Scand* 1989, **80**, 250–59). It is ineffective as maintenance (*Arch Gen Psych* 1991, **48**, 69–72) although some patients do improve (*Am J Psych* 1988, **145**, 748–50).

Clonidine

This NA agonist has been tried successfully in combination with antipsychotics as augmentation but possibly has only a low potency (*B J Psych* 1988, **152**, 293).

○ Unlicensed/Possible efficacy

Amoxapine

This tricyclic at 100mg/d may possibly be equivalent to 15mg/d of haloperidol (*Am J Psych* 1983, **140**, 1232–35). It can cause EPSEs.

Azathioprine

There is a case of a long-standing paranoid schizophrenia improving markedly when concurrent SLE was treated with 50–150mg/d azathioprine (n=1, Levine, *Lancet* 1994, **344**, 59–60).

Beta-blockers

High dose propranolol has been tried for rage outbursts or schizophrenia, with minimal efficacy *(Lancet* 1980, **ii**, 627–28), as has nadolol at up to 120mg/d for verbal or physical aggression in chronic schizophrenia (*Clin Pharm* 1989, **8**, 132–35).

Bromocriptine

There has been some speculation that increasing some dopaminergic function may improve negative symptoms of schizophrenia. Bromocriptine (Levi-

Minzi *et al, Compr Psych* 1991, **32**, 210–16), and dexamfetamine (mentioned by Breier in *Curr Opin Psych* 1995, **8**, 41–44) have been shown to decrease these negative symptoms, at least in some sub-groups of patients.

Calcium-channel blockers

Nifedipine has been used, combined with antipsychotics (*Am J Psych* 1992, **149**, 1615). A short review of the possible use of verapamil can be found in *Drug Intell Clin Pharm* 1990, **24**, 838–40.

Cycloserine

D-cycloserine is a partial agonist of a glutamate receptor sub-type and, in one study, 50mg/d significantly reduced negative symptoms and improved cognitive function (n=9, Goff *et al, Am J Psych* 1995, **152**, 1213–15), supporting the view that glutamate function may be important in schizophrenia. However, in another trial of clozapine-treated patients, successive placebo and increasing cycloserine doses failed to show an improvement in negative symptoms (n=10, Goff *et al, Am J Psych* 1996, **153**, 1628–30). Dietary supplementation with high-dose glycine is a possible adjuvant treatment option.

Cyproheptadine

The addition of cyproheptadine 24mg/d to haloperidol 30mg/d significantly reduced negative symptoms (n=30, RCT, Akhondzadeh *et al, J Clin Pharm & Ther* 1999, **24**, 49), supporting an earlier study against negative symptoms, where 32mg/d showed a good response in 40%, with two relapsing on withdrawal (n=10, open, *Biol Psych* 1989, **25**, 502–4).

Dexamfetamine (dexamphetamine)

A single trial showed some potential effect on negative symptoms of schizophrenia (van Kammen and Bornow, *Int Clin Psychopharmacol* 1988, **3**, 111–21). See also bromocriptine.

Dipyridamole *

Combined dipyridamole (75mg/d) and haloperidol (16–20mg/d) was superior to haloperidol alone in schizophrenia, possibly suggested as being via an effect on the interaction between the adenosine and dopamine systems (n=30, RCT, Akhondzadeh *et al, J Clin*

Pharm Ther 2000, **25**, 131–38).

Estradiol (oestradiol) *

In 10 women with postpartum psychosis, estradiol reversed symptoms in 100% over two weeks, a remarkable outcome that deserves further study, say the authors (open, n=10, 6/52, Ahokas *et al, J Clin Psych* 2000, **61**, 166–69). There is also a report of daily percutaneous estradiol gel alone abolishing all psychotic symptoms in a woman whose schizo-affective psychosis appeared premenstrually (n=1, Korhonen *et al, Acta Psych Scand* 1995, **92**, 237–38).

Famotidine *

There is a single case of famotidine 40mg/d markedly improving negative symptoms in a male schizophrenic (letter in *Lancet* 1990, **335**, 1312; review by Martinez, *Ann Pharmacother* 1999, **33**, 742–47, 14 refs).

Folate

15mg/d in addition to psychotropic drugs significantly improved clinical response and recovery from acute psychiatric disorders (*Lancet* 1990, **336**, 392–95; *B J Psych* 1992, **160**, 714–15).

Glycine *

In a trial of this excitatory amino acid as adjunct therapy, 2 responders were found at 15g/d in chronic treatment-resistant schizophrenics (n=6, *J Clin Psychopharmacol* 1990, **10**, 71–72). A trial of glycine in treatment-resistant schizophrenics showed a significant reduction in negative symptoms and cognitive symptoms (n=11, RCT, Heresco-Levy *et al, B J Psych* 1996, **169**, 610–17). Best results were in patients with low pre-treatment plasma glycine levels. However, glycine 60g/d had no statistically significant effects when used as augmentation of clozapine in schizophrenia (n=30, d/b, p/c, Evins *et al, Am J Psych* 2000, **157**, 826–28).

Levodopa

This has been suggested as a possible treatment for the negative symptoms of schizophrenia (*Am J Psych* 1988, **145**, 1180) although theoretically this could be detrimental.

Lithium

Lithium-responsive psychosis does occur and may be familial and perhaps genetically distinct from the bulk of schizophrenias (*J Aff Dis* 1990, **20**, 63–69). Responders have little obvious difference to non-responders but may have only a few negative symptoms and an absence of a family history of schizophrenia (n=66, Schexnayder *et al, Am J Psych* 1995, **152**, 1511–13). Generally, use of lithium does not result in symptomatic improvement (*Acta Psych Scand* 1991, **84**, 150–54) but may help where affective symptoms are prominent (n=21, d/b, p/c, c/o, Terao *et al, Acta Psych Scand* 1995, **92**, 220–24) and enhance the action of some antipsychotics (Jefferson, *J Clin Psych* 1990, **51**[Suppl], 4–8).

Melatonin *

Melatonin 2mg significantly improved sleep efficiency in chronic schizophrenics with poor sleep, but not in those with better sleep efficiency (RCT, n=19, Shamir *et al, J Clin Psych* 2000, **61**, 373–77).

Naltrexone/naloxone

Opiate antagonists have been tried in schizophrenia. Naltrexone appears ineffective but some trials have shown naloxone to have a positive effect on auditory hallucinations in some patients (review by Welch and Thompson, *J Clin Pharm Ther* 1994, **19**, 279–83).

Ondansetron

Ondansetron may block raised dopamine function without sedating. There is an isolated case report of a good response at 4mg/d in a drug-resistant patient (*Lancet* 1991, **i**, 1173). In a study of psychosis in advanced Parkinson's Disease, 94% responded to ondansetron, with reduced hallucinations, paranoid delusions and confusion (n=16, open, 8/52, Zoldan *et al, Neurology* 1995, **45**, 1304–8). See also combinations.

Prednisone

There is one case of a relapsing psychosis resolving with prednisone (Cohen *et al, Lancet* 1996, **347**, 1228).

SSRIs

There has been some interest in the SSRIs as adjuvant therapy. **Citalopram** has been trialled successfully for the depressive/anxiety symptoms of PANSS (Taiminen *et al, Int Clin Psychopharmacol* 1997, **12**, 31–35) and has been

shown to improve subjective well-being (n=90, d/b, p/c, Salokangas *et al, Acta Psych Scand* 1996, **94**, 175–80). **Fluoxetine** 20mg/d significantly improved positive and negative symptoms in conjunction with antipsychotics in two open studies of treatment-resistant schizophrenics (*Am J Psych* 1990, **147**, 492–94; *Am J Psych* 1991, **148**, 274–75), but may increase the incidence of EPSEs (*J Clin Psychopharmacol* 1990, **10**, 48–50) and in a trial of adjunctive fluoxetine or placebo in 33 clozapine-treated patients, no significant differences were shown (n=33, open, 8/52, Buchanan *et al, Am J Psych* 1996, **153**, 1625–7). **Fluvoxamine** should not be used with clozapine unless with extreme care (see *4.2.2*).

Tetrabenazine

This has been used for the treatment of psychoses and psychoneuroses but the high incidence of side-effects makes this a relatively unsuitable drug.

▼ **No efficacy**

Buspirone

Buspirone has various receptor activities, eg. 5-HT$_{1A}$ partial antagonism and dopamine antagonism. No improvement was seen in 10 schizophrenics given up to 2400mg/d over 4 weeks (*Curr Therap Research* 1975, **18**, 701–5), and exacerbation of psychosis with buspirone has been reported (n=1, Pantelis and Barnes, *J Psychopharmacol* 1993, **7**, 295–300). There is, however, a single case of antipsychotic-resistant psychotic symptoms responding to buspirone 10mg/d (Medrano and Padierna, *Am J Psych* 1996, **153**, 293).

Caffeine

Excess caffeine consumption can present as psychosis, increased arousal (eg. *Biol Psych* 1990, **28**, 35–40) and has a psychotogenic effect (*B J Psych* 1991, **159**, 565–67). However, moderate use of caffeine has probably little effect on anxiety, depression and psychosis (eg. Mayo *et al, B J Psych* 1993, **162**, 543–45).

Methylphenidate

Bolus IV methylphenidate has been used to induce an exacerbation of symptoms, in an attempt to predict those people most likely to relapse when antipsychotics are discontinued (mentioned in Klein and Wender, *Arch Gen Psych* 1995, **52**, 429–33).

Tricyclics

Tricyclics seem ineffective in treating depressive symptoms during acute psychotic episodes (*Arch Gen Psych* 1989, **46**, 922–28 and may even be counterproductive (mentioned in *Drug Dev Res* 1988, **12**, 259–66).

1.27 RAPID-CYCLING BIPOLAR DISORDER

See also bipolar mood disorder (*1.10*), mania/hypomania (*1.19*) and depression (*1.14*)

Rapid-cycling bipolar disorder is a sub-class of bipolar mood disorder, where four or more mood episodes occur in one year. Although it is a relatively uncommon (eg. 5–15% of all bipolars seen at mood disorder clinics) and often transient condition, the clinical significance of the sub-group is that it accounts for up to 80% of lithium non-responders, that antidepressant therapy of depressive phases can induce or worsen cycling in some patients (eg. Wehr and Goodwin, *Am J Psych* 1987, **176**, 633–36) and that rapid-cycling is a risk factor for suicide. Some studies suggest rapid-cycling may be associated with an underlying thyroid abnormality (Joffe *et al, Psych Res* 1988, 25, 117–21; Bauer *et al, Arch Gen Psych* 1990, **47**, 427–32).

Role of drugs:
There will probably always be a lack of quality data on drug use in rapid-cycling as research is complicated by the unpredictable and spontaneously remitting nature of the condition. The best plan is to immediately stop any anti-depressants or other contributory drugs. Carbamazepine, valproate and lithium (although up to 80% may be lithium non-responders) are the first line monotherapy options. If ineffective, they may then be used in combination. Levothyroxine, nimodipine and clozapine may be effective in some patients not responsive to first line drugs and may be worth a therapeutic trial.
Reviews: definitions (Maj *et al, Am J Psych* 1999, **156**, 1421–24), general (Sharma and Persad, *Lithium* 1994, **5**, 117–25; Taylor and Duncan, *Psych Bull* 1996, **20**, 601–3).

BNF listed
Carbamazepine

Several studies (eg. Joyce, *Int Clin Psychopharmacol* 1988, **3**, 123–29) have shown a long-term response rate ranging from 20% to 70% and so more work is needed. The original carbamazepine study (*Kishimoto et al, B J Psych* 1983, **143**, 327–31) showed a particular effect in rapid-cycling. Doubt has, however, been raised about the long-term efficacy of carbamazepine as many people seem to lose the therapeutic response over several years (Post *et al, J Clin Psychopharmacol* 1990, **10**, 318–27).

Lithium

Although initial studies showed that around 82% of rapid-cyclers were lithium non-responsive (as opposed to 41% of non-rapid cyclers), lithium un-doubtedly has some effect, probably by reducing the intensity of relapses rather than the actual number (Misra and Burns, *Acta Psych Scand* 1977, **55**, 32–40). So-called 'Ultra-rapid cyclers' (cycle length of around 48 hours) may do very well on lithium (Paschalis *et al, B J Psych* 1980, **137**, 332–36). It has been noted that lithium response is better if the sequence of relapse is mania, depression and then remission rather than depression, then mania and remission (Grof *et al, Prog Neuropsycho-pharmacol Biol Psych* 1987, **11**, 199–203). Poor compliance, particularly if intermittent (eg. frequent abrupt stopping), may complicate treatment by inducing relapse.

+ Combinations
Carbamazepine + valproate

Synergy in rapid-cycling has been reported (case and review by Ketter *et al, J Clin Psychopharmacol* 1992, **12**, 276–81).

Lithium + carbamazepine

The combination can be useful in rapid-cyclers non-responsive to the individual drugs (eg. retrospective study by Di Costanzo and Schifano, *Acta Psych Scand* 1991, **83**, 456–59). See inter-actions for cautions on the use of this combination (*4.5.1*).

Lithium + levothyroxine/thyroxine

One case has been reported of low dose levothyroxine added to lithium in a rapid-cycler producing complete euthymia within seven days (Bernstein, *J Clin Psychopharmacol* 1992, **12**, 443–44).

Lithium + valproate

Open studies have included this combination in rapid-cyclers, and reported an additive or potentiating effect, sometimes within a matter of days (mentioned by Sharma and Persad, *Lithium* 1994, **5**, 117–25).

Thyroid + tricyclic

Sub-therapeutic doses of T_3 tri-iodothyronine 25–50mcg/d (*Am J Psych* 1990, **147**, 255) or T_4 levothyroxine up to 0.1mg/d have been used as augmentation to tricyclics and phenelzine (although care is needed with any use of antidepressants in rapid-cycling). This may be effective particularly in rapid-cycling disorder (*Arch Gen Psych* 1990, **47**, 435–40) rather than equally in all depressions. See also levothyroxine/liothyronine.

● Unlicensed/Some efficacy

Levothyroxine/thyroxine/liothyronine *

Levothyroxine has potential efficiacy at 0.3–0.5mg/d (or liothyronine 140–400mcg/d) for rapid or 48-hour cycling mania. 91% patients in one study showed clear-cut improvement of rapid-cycling on levothyroxine, supranormal free levothyroxine levels being necessary for clinical response, with minimal side-effects (n=11, open, Bauer and Whybrow, *Arch Gen Psych* 1990, **47**, 435–40) and significant response was seen in a 2-year study (n=6, open, Afflelou *et al*, *Encephale* 1997, **23**, 209–17).

Valproate

No controlled studies have been carried out with valproate but several open studies have found a significant effect, with up to 83% showing a good response, particularly against manic episodes and perhaps less so with depressive episodes (reviewed by Sharma and Persad, *Lithium* 1994, **5**, 117–25), logical bearing in mind a probable GABA-enhancing mode of

action. There are suggestions that the response does not wear off with time, unlike carbamazepine.

Reviews: easily digestible review of its use in rapid-cycling disorder (Calabrese *et al*, *Can J Psych* 1993, **39**[Suppl 2], 57–61), predictors of response (Calabrese *et al*, *J Clin Psychopharmacol* 1993, **13**, 280–83).

○ Unlicensed/Possible efficacy

Calcium-channel blockers

There has been one trial and case reports of the use of nimodipine in rapid-cycling with a very marked response in some patients (n=8, Pazzaglia *et al*, *Psychiatr Res* 1993, **49**, 257–72; Goodnick, *J Clin Psych* 1995, **56**, 330). Nimodipine is highly lipophilic, allowing adequate CNS concentrations and minimal peripheral effects. A dose of 90–180mg/d may be optimal. As verapamil is poorly lipophilic and has a low central effect, nimodipine has been preferred. See bipolar disorder (*1.10*).

Clonazepam

Anecdotal cases exist of clonazepam being useful as an adjunct to lithium in lithium-refractory bipolars (Aronson *et al*, *Am J Psych* 1989, **146**, 77–80).

Clozapine

A number of case reports indicate clozapine may be effective in treatment-resistant rapid cycling (n=2, Calabrese *et al*, *J Clin Psychopharmacol* 1991, **11**, 396–97; n=3, Suppes *et al*, *Biol Psych* 1994, **36**, 338–40).

Lamotrigine

One case report (200mg/d over 20 weeks, Calabrese *et al*, *Am J Psych* 1996, **153**, 1236) and an open trial (n=6, Jusumakar and Yatham, *Am J Psych* 1997, **154**, 1171–12) have shown lamotrigine to have a potential effect in rapid-cycling.

Mexiletine *

Mexiletine (200–1200mg/d) may have some role in the adjunctive management of treatment-resistant rapid-cyclers (n=20, open, 6/52, Schaffer *et al*, *J Aff Dis* 2000, **57**, 249–53).

Primidone

One anecdotal case exists of primidone acting prophylactically in a rapid-cycling lithium non-responder (Brown *et al*, *Lancet* 1993, **342**, 925).

▼ No efficacy
Antidepressants

Up to 50% of cases of rapid-cycling may be antidepressant-induced and so discontinuation of such drugs has been suggested as first line treatment (Wehr *et al, Am J Psych* 1988, **145**, 179–84) although this has been challenged by Coryell *et al (Arch Gen Psych* 1992, **49**, 126–31). If necessary, antidepressants should be used in rapid-cyclers only in severe depression, in low dose and only in the acute stage.

1.28 SEASONAL AFFECTIVE DISORDER (SAD) *

See also depression (*1.14*), mania/hypomania (*1.19*) and bipolar mood disorder (*1.10*).

Seasonal affective disorder is a recurrent affective disorder (predominantly major depression, but can include mania or hypomania). It has a characteristic seasonal pattern relationship, usually autumn or winter, for at least two or three years, with full remission at a characteristic time of the year and out-numbering any non-seasonal episodes that may occur. The incidence may be around 0.9–9.7% and peaks in winter (20 studies, Magnusson, *Acta Psych Scand* 2000, **101**, 176–84). Atypical depressive features include hypersomnia, increased appetite and weight and carbohydrate cravings. Theories for the cause include excess melatonin secretion, delayed or reduced amplitude circadian rhythms and serotonergic dysfunction (short review by Benca in *Curr Opin Psych* 1995, **8**, 64–67). Although the latter is supported by the antidepressant effect of bright light being reversed by rapid tryptophan depletion (Lam *et al, Arch Gen Psych* 1996, **53**, 41–44), rapid tryptophan depletion in depressives with SAD (n=11) did not exacerbate symptoms in another study, suggesting dysfunctional serotonin activity is not necessarily involved with the primary pathogenesis of winter depression (Neumeister *et al, Am J Psych* 1997, **154**, 1153–55).

Role of drugs*: Phototherapy is established, first choice for seasonal affective disorder (review and algorithm, *Drugs & Therapy Perspectives* 1998, **12**,

6–9, 14 refs), although it is not without risk, with side-effects including jumpiness (9%), headache (8%), and nausea (16%), despite a beneficial effect on improving bothersome symptoms (n=83, open, Terman and Terman, *J Clin Psych* 1999, **60**, 799–808). It's effects may be dose-related (meta-analysis, Lee and Chan, *Acta Psych Scand* 1999, **99**, 315–23). Preliminary data from controlled trials indicates that drug treatment may also be effective, with the SSRIs fluoxetine and sertraline, and the MAO-A inhibitor moclobemide suggested as effective.

Reviews : general (Rodin and Thompson, *Adv Psych Treat* 1997, **3**, 352– 59, 27 refs; Jepson *et al, JAMA* 1999, **39**, 822-29; Zulman and Oren, *Curr Opin Psych* 1999, **12**, 81–86, 51 refs), guide to diagnosis and management (Partonen and Lonnqvist, *CNS Drugs* 1998, **9**, 203–12).

○ Unlicensed/Possible efficacy
Beta-blockers

In a trial of up to 60mg/d propranolol administered pre-sunrise (5.30–6am), 73% of those with winter depression responded, and those transferred to placebo showed varying degrees of relapse. The effect may be via short-term, short-acting beta-blocker-induced truncation of nocturnal melatonin secretion early morning but not in the evening (Schlager, *Am J Psych* 1994, **151**, 1383–85). Atenolol appeared less effective in another trial (Rosenthal *et al, Am J Psych* 1988, **145**, 52–56), but a small group of patients showed a sustained and substantial response.

Fluoxetine

Fluoxetine may produce clinically useful improvements in SAD symptoms at 20mg/d (open, Childs *et al, B J Psych* 1995, **166**, 196–98). An out-patient study of 20mg/d showed improvement in both groups and although the fluoxetine group improved more (59% to 34%), this was not quite statistically significant (n=68, p/c, 5/52, Lam *et al, Am J Psych* 1995, **152**, 1765–70).

Melatonin

A small study showed that low dose melatonin taken in the early afternoon reduced depression, possibly by a 'phase shift' mechanism (n=5, Lewy *et al, Psychiatry Res* 1998, **77**, 57–61).

Mirtazapine

One study has shown a rapid and well-tolerated effect in SAD (4/52, open, n=8, Hesselmann *et al, Hum Psychopharmacol Clin Exp* 1999, **14**, 59–62).

Moclobemide

Moclobemide 400mg/d for SAD was superior to placebo in a trial (n=34, Lingjaerde *et al, Acta Psych Scand* 1993, **88**, 372–80).

St. John's wort

One study showed some effect (s/b, see Kasper, *Pharmacopsychiatry* 1997, **30**[Suppl 2], 89–93).

Tranylcypromine

86% responded completely to tranylcypromine (mean dose 30mg/d) in winter depression (n=14, open, Dilsaver and Jaeckle, *J Clin Psych* 1990, **51**, 326–29).

▼ No efficacy

Ginkgo biloba

One study was unable to show an effect from 'Bio-Biloba' in preventing winter depression (n=27, RCT, 10/52, Lingaerde et al, *Acta Psych Scand* 1999, **100**, 62–66).

1.29 SELF-INJURIOUS BEHAVIOUR (SIB)

SIB is a self-destructive behaviour resulting in significant tissue damage, but without lethal intent. It can occur in learning disabilities (eg. Lesch-Nyhan syndrome), as well as in OCD, sado-masochism, schizophrenia, borderline personality disorder etc. There seems to be a variety of causes, eg. relief of dysphoria, poor impulse control, dissociation etc.

Role of drugs:

Opiate antagonists may be useful where a reward mechanism seems to exist. There is some evidence of a serotonergic involvement. Antipsychotics seem to work mainly via a non-specific sedating mechanism. **Review**: psychopharmacology of severe SIB associated with learning disabilities (Clarke, *B J Psych* 1998, **172**, 389–94).

+ Combinations

Clozapine + clomipramine

This combination was successful in treating compulsive self-mutilation in a drug-resistant mild learning disability patient (n=1, Holzer *et al, Am J Psych* 1996, **153**, 133).

● Unlicensed/Some efficacy

Antipsychotics

Chlorpromazine and haloperidol are frequently prescribed but evidence for their efficacy is suggestive rather than conclusive (*J Am Acad Child & Adoles Psych* 1987, **26**, 296–302). Low dose fluphenazine may effect SIB rates in Lesch-Nyhan syndrome (*Lancet* 1985, **i**, 338–39). Antipsychotics with a relatively high D_1 blockade may have greater potency.

Buspirone

In a trial of developmentally disabled individuals with self-injury and anxiety, 64% responded to doses of 20–45mg/d with a maximal response seen more than three weeks later (n=14, open, Ratey *et al, J Clin Psych* 1989, **50**, 382).

Lithium

Studies suggest that lithium is effective in both aggression and self-injury. In one study, response was seen in 2–8 weeks with a lithium serum concentration of 0.7–1.0mEq/L (d/b, Caraft *et al, B J Psych* 1987, **150**, 685).

Naltrexone/naloxone

There is conflicting data about the efficacy of naltrexone in SIB. Two trials have shown a lack of efficacy. Mentally retarded and autistic adults failed to show an effect of naltrexone on reducing SIB, and indeed many patients worsened (n=33, d/b, p/c, c/o, Willemsen-Swinkels *et al, Arch Gen Psych* 1995, **52**, 766–73) and although 50–100mg/d showed some improvement in hand-to-head and head-to-object SIB, the 14-day duration and variation in behaviour made statistical evaluation invalid (n=8, d/b, Thompson *et al, Am J Mental Retard* 1994, **99**, 85–102). Other studies have, however, shown some efficacy. 25–100mg/d orally had been shown to reduce SIB (n=4, *Am J Mental Retardation* 1990, **95**, 93–102). However, some studies showed that SIB may get worse over the first few weeks of naltrexone but *then* improves and so short studies may miss the effect. It may be that lower doses (eg. 10–50mg/d) may be more effective and it undoubtedly helps some patients. There is some evidence of raised opioid peptide activity in autism, fragile-X syndrome and other mental handicaps, which would explain the effect. (Discussion of the hypotheses in *Am J Mental Retard* 1991, **95**, 692–96).

Propranolol

Case reports and open trials suggest that propranolol may decrease self-injurious behaviour. Response may be seen with average doses of 120mg/d which may be immediate or gradual over several weeks. Dose limited side-effects include bradycardia and hypotension (Ruedrich *et al, Am J Ment Retard* 1990, **95**, 110).

○   **Unlicensed/Possible efficacy**

Clomipramine

Clomipramine 25–125mg/d reduced SIB target symptoms rapidly in many subjects (n=11, open, Garber *et al, J Am Acad Child Adolesc Psych* 1992, **31**, 1157–60).

Dextromethorphan

30mg/d successfully controlled SIB and aggression in a man with learning disabilities (*B J Psych* 1992, **161**, 118–20).

Fluoxetine

Some benefit (reductions in SIB from 20–85%) has been shown in mentally retarded young adults (Ricketts *et al, J Am Acad Child Adolesc Psych* 1993, **32**, 865–69).

1.30 SEROTONIN SYNDROME

Serotonin syndrome (SS) is a condition caused by drug-induced serotonin hyperstimulation. It probably goes largely unreported as it is usually mild. It can be managed by drug withdrawal, although it can be severe, with death reported. It is difficult to diagnose (Sampson and Warner, *Br J Gen Pract* 1999, **49**, 867–68, editorial).

Sternbach's Diagnostic Criteria:

1. At least three of the following: agitation/restlessness, sweating, diarrhoea, fever, hyperreflexia, lack of co-ordination, mental state changes (confusion, hypomania), myoclonus, shivering, tremor.
2. Other causes, eg. infection, metabolic, substance abuse or withdrawal ruled out.
3. No concurrent antipsychotic dose changes prior to symptom onset.

Other symptoms can include nausea, vomiting, tachycardia and myoclonus. Hypertension, convulsions and multiple organ failure have been reported. Onset is usually within a few hours of drug/dose changes and usually resolves in 24 hours. Recurrent mild symptoms may occur for weeks before a full-blown syndrome appears. Severe cases have on occasion been confused with neuroleptic malignant syndrome (*1.22*).

Causes:

SS has been reported with SSRIs, MAOIs (including moclobemide and selegiline), tricyclic and related drugs, dextromethorphan and levodopa, usually in combination but can be with single drugs or in overdose (see *5.13* for sample list).

Role of drugs:

First-line treatment should be to discontinue identifiable serotonergic drugs (including over-the-counter sympathomimetics), then provide symptomatic support, eg. cooling blankets etc. Mild cases can usually be managed with drug discontinuation and benzodiazepines. More severe cases require major supportive measures. No prospective studies are available yet to compare the reported drug treatments for serotonin syndrome.

Reviews: Brown *et al, Ann Pharmacother* 1996, **30**, 527–33; Mills, *Crit Care Clin* 1997, **13**, 763–83; LoCurto, *Emerg Med Clin North Am* 1997, **15**, 665–75.

●   **Unlicensed/Some efficacy**

Benzodiazepines

Lorazepam (1–2mg by slow IV injection every 30 minutes until excessive sedation occurs) has been recommended as being effective and superior to clonazepam for serotonin toxicity. Clonazepam has a lower affinity for peripheral benzodiazepine receptors than lorazepam and diazepam which may explain its lower efficacy (eg. Nierenberg and Semprebon, *Clin Pharmacol Ther* 1993, **53**, 84–88).

Chlorpromazine

IM chlorpromazine has been used for its sedative effect (letters from Gillman and Norman, *Med J Aust* 1996, **165**, 345–46 and Graham, *Med J Aust* 1997, **166**, 166–67).

Cyproheptadine

Cyproheptadine (a non-specific 5-HT blocker) at 4–8mg orally, repeated every 2–4 hours up to 0.5mg/kg/d maximum (beware of urinary retention) has been claimed to be the best antiserotonergic drug strategy, with case reports of rapid success (Lappin and Auchincloss, *NEJM* 1994, **331**, 1021–22).

○ **Unlicensed/Possible efficacy**

Mirtazapine

Mirtazapine has been proposed as a possible treatment as it blocks 5-HT$_2$ and 5-HT$_3$ receptors (Hoes, *Pharmacopsychiatry* 1996, **29**, 81).

Nitroglycerin

A single case of rapidly successful use of nitroglycerin (2mg/kg/min) in a severe case of SS has been reported (Brown and Skop, *Ann Pharmacother* 1996, **30**, 191).

Propranolol

Propranolol (1–3mg every 5 minutes, up to 0.1mg/kg) may be useful as it also blocks 5-HT$_{1A}$ and 5-HT$_2$ receptors (Guze and Baxter, *J Clin Psychopharmacol* 1986, **6**, 119–20).

1.31 SEXUAL DEVIANCY DISORDERS

Sexual deviancy disorders are recognised psychiatric syndromes, and include exhibitionism, fetishism, sexual masochism or sadism, paedophilia and voyeurism. Rape is not included as it is considered a sexual expression of aggression rather than an aggressive expression of sexuality. The main characteristic is of intense, recurrent sexual arousal and fantasies, particularly connected with inanimate objects, children, non-consenting adults or the self.

Role of drugs:

Drug therapy may sometimes be a useful adjunct to other therapies, due to the chronic nature of the disease and its high and unpredictable relapse rates, but must be carried out with care and is controversial. Deviant sexual behaviour is rare in women and so drug therapy is usually aimed at reducing sexual drive in men.

BNF listed

Benperidol

Benperidol is a standard and expensive butyrophenone which, although licensed for control of deviant antisocial sexual behaviour, has no proven use other than as an antipsychotic. The only double-blind study published showed a slight reduction in sexual thoughts but not in behaviour (*Drug Ther Bull* 1974, **12**, 2).

Cyproterone (acetate)

Cyproterone is available in many countries to treat severe hypersexuality and sexual deviation in men. It has both antiandrogenic and antigonadotropic actions and probably acts by disrupting the receptors' response to androgens (Cooper, *Can J Psych* 1986, **31**, 73–79) and can reduce sexual interest, drive and arousal, as well as deviant fantasies and behaviour (eg. Cooper, *Comp Psych* 1981, **22**, 458–65). Few proper trials exist to support the use of cyproterone and there are no adequate double-blind crossover trials in learning disability. Onset of action may be delayed for 2–3 weeks and is reversible within 3–6 weeks of stopping. An adequate trial of 4 months is thus usually recommended. A depot injection is available on a named patient basis and a syrup can be made. Cyproterone 100mg/d rapidly cured a woman of severe sexual obsessions, maintained over two years and after discontinuation (Eriksson, *B J Psych* 1998, **173**, 351) and so may have other applications.

● **Unlicensed/Some efficacy**

Medroxyprogesterone (acetate)

Medroxyprogesterone has antiandrogenic activity which prevents testosterone release from the testicles (Cooper, *Can J Psych* 1986, **31**, 73–79), resulting in suppression of sexual arousal and libido. A direct effect on neurotransmitters has also been suggested (Berlin and Meinecke, *Am J Psych* 1981, **138**, 601–7). Dose, action and adverse effects are as for cyproterone, except that feminisation has not been reported. Again, few proper trials have been carried out. Due to a possible central tranquillising effect, care is needed on ethical grounds (Berlin, *Bull Am Acad Psych Law* 1989, **17**, 233–39).

○ Unlicensed/Possible efficacy

Flutamide
See LHRH antagonists.

Imipramine
Some improvements in paraphilic and nonparaphilic sexual addictions and depressive symptoms were noted in 9 of 10 patients treated with imipramine, fluoxetine or lithium (Kafka, *J Clin Psych* 1991, **52**, 60–65).

LHRH antagonists
Luteinising hormone-releasing hormone (gonadorelin, LHRH) antagonists can produce complete chemical castration and thus have a potent effect on sexual deviancy (Rousseau *et al, Can J Psych* 1990, **35**, 338–41). Nafarelin has been used for this purpose. Flutamide, a pure antiandrogen similar to cyproterone, has been used in conjunction with nafarelin and in one case resulted in rapid discontinuation in exhibitionism (n=1, Rousseau *et al, Can J Psych* 1990, **35**, 338–41).

Lithium
See imipramine.

Methylphenidate *
Methylphenidate may be cautiously but effectively used to augment the effect of SSRIs in paraphilias and related disorders (n=26, Kafka and Hennen, *J Clin Psych* 2000, **61**, 664–70).

SSRIs *
SSRIs may have a significant effect in reducing the daily frequency and duration of paraphilia and related disorders (n=26, Kafka and Hennen, *J Clin Psych* 2000, **61**, 664–70). A similarity between sexual deviancy and obsessive-compulsive disorders has been postulated and there are case reports of the successful use of fluoxetine to decrease the intensity and intrusiveness of sexual fantasies, resulting in more conventional sexual behaviour and impulse control (eg. Perilstein *et al, J Clin Psych* 1991, **52**, 169–70; Kafka, *B J Psych* 1991, **158**, 844–47; n=10, fluoxetine, imipramine or lithium, Kafka, *J Clin Psych* 1991, **52**, 60–65). Fluoxetine-induced anorgasmia may be a contributory factor to this effect. Controlled clinical trials are needed to confirm a definite effect.

1.32 SOCIAL PHOBIA (social anxiety disorder)
See also anxiety disorder (*1.6*).

Social phobia is the second most common phobia, where the sufferers fear public ridicule, scrutiny and negative evaluation, with fear of making a public mistake, embarrassment or criticism. Situations include public speaking, social gatherings, writing under supervision or eating and drinking in public. Anticipatory anxiety leads to impaired performance. Two sub-divisions include general and specific social phobia.

Role of drugs*: Drugs and behavioural approaches are commonly used. SSRIs are clearly superior to placebo and are emerging as the gold standard drug therapy, with another SSRI or moclobemide second line and MAOIs and benzodiazepines third. Combined drugs and psychological treatments do not generally provide better results than psychological therapies alone.

Reviews*: general (Logan and Freeman, *Prescriber* 1997, 79–84; Van Ameringen *et al, CNS Drugs* 1999, **11**, 307–15; *Drugs & Therapy Perspectives* 2000, **16**, 8–9; Lipsitz and Schneier, *Pharmaco-Economics* 2000, **18**, 23–32; Sareen and Stein, *Drugs* 2000, **59**, 497–509, 66 refs).

BNF listed

Paroxetine
Paroxetine is licensed for generalised social phobia, with several studies showing it superior to placebo, eg. at 20–50mg/d reducing symptoms and avoidance compared to placebo (RCT, n=187, 12/52, Stein *et al, JAMA* 1998, **280**, 708–13), although with a high drop-out rate, some caution over confidence in the study has been expressed (Dahl, *EBMH* 1999, **2**, 53). Paroxetine 20–50mg/d significantly improved symptoms in another study, with the effect measurable from week 4 onwards (RCT, n=290, 12/52, Baldwin *et al, B J Psych* 1999, **175**, 120–26; review by Wilson, *EBMH* 2000, **3**, 41), another similar design study showing similar results (RCT, n=92, Allgulander, *Acta Psych Scand* 1999, **100**, 193–98). Review by Prakash and Foster, *CNS Drugs* 1999, **12**, 151–69.

○ Unlicensed/Possible efficacy

Beta-blockers

There is no evidence for efficacy, except perhaps in people where management of tremor is essential, eg. musicians.

Bupropion *

Bupropion may be a potential treatment for social phobia (n=10, 12/52, open, Emmanuel *et al, Depress Anxiety* 2000, **12**, 111–13).

Gabapentin *

Gabapentin (900–3600mg/d) was well tolerated and significantly reduced symptoms of social phobia in one trial (n=69, RCT, d/b, p/c, 14/52, Pande *et al, J Clin Psychopharmacol* 1999, **19**, 341–48).

Moclobemide

Moclobemide has been compared favourably with phenelzine (Versani *et al, B J Psych* 1992, **161**, 353–60), building up to 600mg/d over two weeks and maintaining for twelve weeks to produce a therapeutic effect (Nutt and Bell, *Adv Psych Treat* 1997, **3**, 79–85). Another trial showed some efficacy but the advantage over placebo was relatively small and often not significant (n=77, p/c, Schneier *et al, Br J Psych* 1998, **172**, 70–77).

MAOIs/phenelzine

In a complex trial, phenelzine was slightly superior to CBGT (Group CBT), and both were superior to placebo in social phobia (n=133, 12/52, Heimberg *et al, Arch Gen Psych* 1998, **55**, 1113–14; reviewed by Thyer, *EBMH* 1999, **2**, 80).

Nefazodone

16 of 21 patients completing a trial of nefazodone (variable dose) improved, and it may thus have a role (n=23, 12/52, open, Van Ameringen *et al, J Clin Psych* 1999, **60**, 96–100). More studies are warranted.

SSRIs *

One trial showed some effect from **sertraline** (n=12, d/b, c/o, Katzelnick *et al, Am J Psych* 1995, **152**, 1368–71). **Citalopram** 40mg/d may be effective (n=22, open, Bouwer and Stein, *J Aff Dis* 1998, **49**, 79–82) and **fluvoxamine** may have some role, 200mg/d (average dose) being shown to be superior to placebo (n=92, RCT, Stein *et al, Am J Psych* 1999, **156**, 756–60) and in treating clozapine-induced social phobia (n=12, 12/52, open, Pallanti *et al, J Clin Psych* 1999, **60**, 819–23).

1.33 TOURETTE'S SYNDROME (Gilles de la Tourette)

See also OCD (*1.23*) and self-injurious behaviour (1.29).

Symptoms:

The main diagnostic symptoms of this hereditary multiple tic disorder include multiple tics, vocal tics (grunts, snarls etc. including obscenities), stereotyped movements (jumping and dancing), over-activity, learning difficulties and emotional problems. It occurs in 1–5 per 10,000 of the population and is more common in males. It has an onset at 5–6 years, beginning with respiratory or vocal tics with grunting or barking noises. Psychiatric co-morbidity is common, eg. OCD, anxiety, depression, ADHD etc.

Role of drugs:

If the disease is affecting the person's ability to function, drug therapy may be useful. Low starting doses, gradual increases and adequate trials are necessary. Dysregulation of presynaptic dopamine function has been proposed (Malison *et al, Am J Psych* 1995, **152**, 1359–61), and drugs such as haloperidol (a D_2 blocker) are often effective. Some possible relationship with OCD has been postulated, as has a high incidence of SIB (*Psychol Med* 1989, **19**, 611–25).

Reviews: Case study and review (Hyde and Weinberger, *JAMA* 1995, **273**, 498–501), general review (Robertson and Stern, *B J Hosp Med* 1997, **58**, 253–55).

BNF Listed

Haloperidol

0.5–40mg/d is the licensed drug of choice. Side-effects may be limiting and its efficacy has been questioned (n=22, p/c, d/b, Sallee *et al, Am J Psych* 1997, **154**, 1057–62). Comparisons with pimozide (see separate entry) have tended to favour pimozide. See also nicotine chewing gum.

● Unlicensed/Some efficacy

Clonidine

0.1–0.6mg/d may be as effective as haloperidol in some patients. In one trial, clonidine was more effective than placebo (n=47, d/b, *Arch Gen Psych* 1991, **48**, 324–28), but in another of clonidine (up to 0.2mg/d) and desipramine (up to 100mg/d) in children with both ADHD and Tourette's syndrome, desipramine was superior to clonidine in reducing ADHD and tic symptoms (d/b, p/c, c/o, Singer *et al, Pediatrics* 1995, **95**, 74–81).

Lorazepam

1.5–10mg/d may be useful as adjuvant therapy.

Pimozide *

Two trials have shown pimozide 1–20mg/d to be superior to haloperidol, eg. in children with Tourette's and ADHD (Sallee *et al, Acta Psych Scand* 1994, **90**, 4–9) and with less side-effects than haloperidol and a superior therapeutic effect, where haloperidol was not significantly better than placebo (n=22, p/c, d/b, Sallee *et al, Am J Psych* 1997, **154**, 1057–62). Long-term therapy has been shown to be more effective than treating acute exacerbations with short-term acute therapy (n=10, Tourette Syndrome Study Group, *Neurology* 1999, **52**, 874–77).

Sulpiride

200–400mg/d has been used, and has been considered by some as a treatment of choice.

+ Combinations

Naltrexone + codeine

Sequential use of naltrexone (100–300mg/d) and codeine phosphate (15–120mg/d) has proved effective (n=2, McConville *et al, Lancet* 1994, **343**, 601). See also naltrexone/opiate antagonists.

O Unlicensed/Possible efficacy

Cannabinoids

In a survey of people with Tourette's who had tried marijuana, 82% reported a reduction or complete remission in motor and vocal tics, urges and OCD symptoms (n=17, Muller-Vahl *et al, Acta Psych Scand* 1998, **98**, 502–6). A report of effective use of Delta-9-THC has been published (n=1, Muller-Vahl *et al, Am J Psych* 1999, **156**, 495), with RCT's now planned.

Buspirone

Drug-resistant Tourette's has been treated successfully with buspirone 30mg/d (n=1, Dursun *et al, Lancet* 1995, **345**, 1366–67).

Calcium-channel blockers

Tourette's has been treated with verapamil and nifedipine, but diltiazem produced no response (n=2, Walsh *et al, Am J Psych* 1986, **143**, 1467–68).

Clomiphene citrate

50mg/d was effective in one case (*Postgrad Med J* 1987, **63**, 510).

Fluoxetine

81% patients with OCD in Tourette's syndrome had improved symptoms on fluoxetine (n=32, open, *Neurology* 1991, **41**, 872–74). A potential effect for fluoxetine has been suggested in children with obsessive-compulsive symptoms in Tourette's syndrome (n=11, Kyrlan *et al, Clin Neuropharmacol* 1993, **16**, 167–72).

Fluvoxamine

This may help any OCD-related symptoms which may be present.

Methadone

Up to 110mg/d has been used successfully in one treatment-resistant case (*Am J Psych* 1992, **149**, 139–40).

Methylphenidate

Methylphenidate can aggravate tics or be associated with their appearance (Klein and Wender, *Arch Gen Psych* 1995, **52**, 429–33) but one study has shown that although some tics are significantly worse, generally these are not to the extent of contraindicating a trial, eg. in ADHD with Tourette's (Gadow *et al, Arch Gen Psych* 1995, **52**, 444–55).

Naltrexone/opiate antagonists

One study of a selective opioid antagonist suggested that Tourette's syndrome does not arise from a primary abnormality of opioid receptor dysfunction (n=6, Weeks *et al, Lancet* 1994, **343**, 1107–8).

Nicotine chewing gum

This preparation enhanced the symptomatic effects of haloperidol when used in combination (n=2, *Lancet* 1988, **i**, 592) and in a small study (n=10, open *Am J Psych* 1991, **148**, 793–94). Transdermal nicotine patches have been used to potentiate haloperidol in Tourette's syndrome in six patients (Silver and Sanberg, *Lancet* 1993, **342**, 182) and a further open study (n=16, aged 9–15 years) has shown that a single transdermal nicotine patch (7mg/24 hours) shows a significant effect over 1–2 weeks, with considerable individual variation (Silver *et al, J Am Acad Child Adolesc Psychiatry* 1996, **35**, 1631–36).

Nifedipine

Nifedipine has been used (Berg, *Acta Psych Scand* 1985, **72**, 400–1; Goldstein, *J Clin Psych* 1984, **45**, 360).

Olanzapine *

There are case reports of response (eg. n=1, Bhadrinath, *B J Psych* 1998, **173**, 366) and olanzapine may be as effective but better tolerated than pimozide (n=4, d/b, c/o, 52/52, Onofrj *et al, J Neurol* 2000, **247**, 443–46).

Paroxetine

Paroxetine may have a role in treatment of episodic rage in Tourette's (n=45, 8/52, open, 75% had reduced or absent rage episodes, Bruun and Budman, *J Clin Psych* 1998, **59**, 581–84).

Pergolide *

Pergolide (up to 300mcg/d) was shown to be safe and effective in chilldren with Tourette's disorder, chronic motor tic disorder, or chronic vocal tic disorder (n=245, RCT, 6/52, Gilbert *et al, Neurology* 2000, **54**, 1310–16).

Pentazocine

This has been suggested (*Clin Pharm* 1985, **4**, 494). See also methadone.

Risperidone

There are cases of response in multiple drug-resistant Tourette's syndrome and OCD responding rapidly to risperidone 6mg/d (Giakas, *Am J Psych* 1995, **152**, 1097–98; Shulman *et al, Neurology* 1995, **45**, 1419) and one trial (n=38, Bruun and Budman, *J Clin Psych* 1996, **57**, 29–31).

Selegiline

Selegiline (L-deprenyl) was just significantly superior to placebo in children with Tourette's syndrome and attention deficit hyperactivity disorder (n=24, d/b, p/c, c/o, Feigin *et al, Neurology* 1996, **46**, 965–68). Selegiline may improve both ADHD and tics in children with TS and warrants further study.

1.34 TRICHOTILLOMANIA

See also OCD (*1.23*)

Symptoms:

Trichotillomania is the recurrent failure to resist impulses to pull out one's own hair (scalp, eyebrows, and eyelashes as well as pubic, chest etc), resulting in noticeable hair loss. It is associated with obsessive-compulsive behaviour, and can also occur in the presence of learning disability, anxiety, depression, schizophrenia and borderline personality disorder.

Role of drugs*:

A range of psychological and behaviour therapies are used and may be most effective when combined with drug therapies (Swedo and Leonard, *Psych Clin North Am* 1992, **15**, 777–90). Drug therapy is still unproven and drug trials need to be of at least 8–10 weeks duration to prove or disprove an effect in an individual case. There is evidence that longer-term treatment with SSRIs may be of benefit (Swedo *et al, NEJM* 1993, **329**, 141–42). A retrospective review of treatment outcomes, showed significant benefit from behavioural and pharmacological treatments (n=63, Keuthen *et al, Am J Psych* 1998, **155**, 560–61). One trial showed that CBT was more effective than clomipramine, and both were superior to placebo (n=23, RCT, 9/52, Ninan *et al, J Clin Psych* 2000, **161**, 47–50).

Reviews: treatment options (Christenson and O'Sullivan, *CNS Drugs* 1996, **6**, 23–34), diagnosis (Hanna, *Child Psychiatry Hum Dev* 1997, **27**, 255–68), general (Christenson and Crow, *J Clin Psych* 1996, **57** [Suppl 8], 42–44).

+ **Combinations**

Olanzapine + fluoxetine

A case has been reported of improvement in trichotillomania when olanzapine 10mg/d was added to fluoxetine 40mg/d (Potenza *et al, Am J Psych* 1998, **155**, 1329–30).

● **Unlicensed/Some efficacy**

Clomipramine

Several studies (eg. Swedo *et al, NEJM* 1989, **321**, 497–501) have shown clomipramine in doses of around 180mg/d to be effective in some patients with trichotillomania and thus appears the drug of choice. Some patients non-responsive to fluoxetine have then responded to clomipramine (eg. Naylor and Grossman, *J Am Acad Child Adolesc Psych* 1991, **30**, 155–56).

○ **Unlicensed/Possible efficacy**
Citalopram

Citalopram may be safe in trichotillomania, with modest but significant improvements (n=14, open, 12/52, Stein *et al, Eur Arch Psychiatry Clin Neurosci* 1997, **247**, 234–36).

Fluoxetine

Although a positive effect has been suggested by several reports, (eg. Winchel *et al, J Clin Psych* 1992, **53**, 304–8; d/b, c/o, Christenson, *Am J Psych* 1991, **148**, 1566–71), a subsequent study failed to show an effect on hair-pulling at up to 80mg/d on any of the measures used (n=23, d/b, c/o, 31/52, Streichenwein and Thornby, *Am J Psych* 1995, **152**, 1192–96). The effect therefore appears minimal, the doses required are high (up to 80mg/d) and if response occurs, relapse is not uncommon. There are case reports of response (eg. Hamdan-Allen, *J Autism Dev Disorder* 1991, **21**, 79–82; Alexander, *J Clin Psych* 1991, **52**, 88–89). It is generally considered second line to clomipramine.

Fluvoxamine

Some potential use has been reported in reducing overall distress but not hair pulling (n=21, open, 12/52, Stanley *et al, J Clin Psychopharmacol* 1997, **17**, 278–83).

Lithium

80% patients tried on lithium for chronic hair pulling showed reduced hair pulling and some hair re-growth, possibly via an effect on aggressive behaviour (n=10, Christenson *et al, J Clin Psych* 1991, **52**, 116–20).

Nortriptyline

There is a case report where minor improvement occurred (Alexander, *J Clin Psych* 1991, **52**, 88–89).

Paroxetine

40mg/d was effective in one resistant case (Reid, *Am J Psych* 1994, **151**, 290).

Pimozide

Pimozide has been used as augmentation of SSRI therapy (eg. *J Clin Psych* 1992, **53**, 123–26).

Trazodone

Responsive cases have been reported (eg. Sunkureddi and Markovitz, *Am J Psych* 1993, **150**, 523–24).

Unlicensed/non-UK drugs

Two UK sources of special, foreign and unlicensed drugs are *PharmaSeek*, Suite 48, 78, Marylebone High St, London W1M 4AP, and *IDIS*, 6/7 Canbury Business Park, Elm Crescent, Kingston upon Thames, Surrey KT2 6BR.

1.35–6 OTHER DRUG RELATED TOPICS

1.35 CAFFEINISM

Caffeine consumption at 250–500mg/d is regarded as moderate use. Caffeinism is estimated to start at a consumption of between 600mg and 750mg/d, with above 1000mg/d well into the toxic range. 12mcg/mL is the US Olympic Committee upper limit for caffeine levels (*Am J Hosp Pharm* 1990, **47**, 303). One study showed that caffeine-dependence displays features of a typical psychoactive substance dependence, ie. withdrawal, continued use despite caffeine-induced problems, tolerance and persistent desire or unsuccessful attempts to cut down or control use. It may be useful to remember this when dealing with such a dependence (n=16, Strain *et al, JAMA* 1994, **272**, 1043–48). Withdrawal abruptly even from moderate doses may lead to depression, anxiety (in 10%) and increased use of OTC analgesics (Silverman *et al, NEJM* 1992, **327**, 1109–14).

Intake can be calculated thus:

Source	caffeine content	
	per 100ml	per container
Brewed coffee	55–85mg	140–210mg/mug
Instant coffee	35–45mg	85–110mg/mug
Decaffeinated coffee	2mg	5mg/mug
Cocoa	3mg	7mg/mug
Brewed tea	25–55mg	55–140mg/mug
Coca Cola	11mg	36mg/can
Pepsi Cola	7mg	22mg/can
Milk chocolate		22mg/100g
Hedex Seltzer		60mg/sachet
Aqua Ban		100mg/tablet
a mug is taken as being 250ml		

Symptoms of caffeinism (acute or chronic):

Side-effects of low to moderate doses: Diuresis, increased gastric secretion, fine tremor, increased skeletal muscle stamina, mild anxiety, palpitations, nervousness

Side-effects of high doses: chronic insomnia, persistent anxiety, restlessness, tension, irritability, agitation, tremulousness (*Arch Gen Psych* 1991, **48,** 611–17), panic, poor concentration, confusion, disorientation, paranoia, delirium, tremor, muscle twitching and tension, convulsions, vertigo, dizziness, tinnitus, auditory and visual hallucinations, facial flushing, hyperthermia, hypertension, nausea, vomiting, abdominal discomfort, headaches, tachypnoea and disturbed sleep.

Caffeine withdrawal is a DSM-IV diagnosis and thus should be taken seriously. Sudden withdrawal can produce headaches (52%), rebound drowsiness, fatigue/lethargy and depression (*J Psychopharmacol* 1991, **5**, 129–34; *NEJM* 1992, **327**, 1109–14), with many other effects reported.

Adverse consequences*: There is some contradictory evidence about the effect of caffeine on people with mental health problems. Clearly, high doses can cause significant effects. Acute high doses (10mg/kg) significantly increase arousal and have a psychotogenic effect in schizophrenics (n=13, d/b, Lucas *et al, Biol Psych* 1990, **28**, 35–40). Schizophrenics often have higher caffeine intakes and average intake should be routinely monitored (Rihs *et al, Eur Arch Psychiatry Clin Neurosci* 1996, **246,** 83–92) as it can exacerbate schizophrenia (n=2, Mikkelsen, *J Clin Psych* 1978, **39**, 732–36). Ward studies have shown that, '*chronic caffeine use created clinically significant levels of anxiety and tension that could be reduced by decreasing caffeine consumption*'. Caffeinism can present as anxiety neurosis, precipitate or exacerbate psychosis and make these more resistant (*B J Psych* 1991, **159**, 565) to drug treatment, especially antipsychotics. The clinical signs of affective diseases can be modified. 150mg of caffeine at bedtime has been shown to have a marked effect on sleep latency, total sleep time and reduced sleep efficacy and REM periods. Consumption may be influenced by some genetic factors (twin study, Kendler and Prescott, *Am J Psych* 1999, **156**, 223–28).

Alternatively, there are reports of lack of correlation between caffeine consumption and anxiety and depression, with no changes when a ward moved to decaffeinated products (n=26, d/b, c/o, Mayo *et al, B J Psych* 1993, **162**, 543–45) and little difference in behaviours between caffeinated and decaffeinated periods (Koczapski *et al, Schizophr Bull* 1989, **15**, 339–44). Withdrawal of caffeine from a group of severely retarded and highly disturbed patients produced no improvement in sleep patterns, but reintroduction was accompanied by a highly significant increase in ward disturbances (Searle, *J Intellect Disabil Res* 1994, **38**, 383–91), which may explain the contradictions in evidence.

Methods of caffeine reduction:

1. Recognition of problems of excess (>750mg/d) caffeine and likely benefits of reduction.
2. Identification of all current caffeine sources and pattern of consumption.
3. Gradual reduction, eg. making weaker drinks, taken less often, increasing use of caffeine-free equivalent drinks, particularly at 'usual' drinking times of the day.
4. Use of analgesia (caffeine-free, of course) for withdrawal headaches.
5. Setting a target for consumption, which will not need to be complete abstinence, eg. caffeine drinks only at set times in the day, eg. on rising etc.

Causes:

Patients may drink large quantities of tea and coffee to relieve thirst/dry mouth caused by tricyclic and phenothiazine side-effects. In-patient settings, especially in the evening, often build in caffeine consumption.

Reviews*: general (Glass, *JAMA* 1994, **272**, 1065–66; Pickworth, *Lancet* 1995, **345**, 1066; *Am J Psych* 1992, **149**, 33–40), in psychiatric patients (Kruger, *Psychol Rep* 1996, **78**, 915–23; Hyde, *Schizophr Bull* 1990, **16**, 371–75).

1.36 ELECTRO-CONVULSIVE THERAPY

ECT was first used in its current form in 1938 (*BMJ* 1988, **297**, 1354–55) and is an established treatment for major depression, especially if marked with melancholia, psychomotor retardation, psychosis or delusions. It is also used in mania (especially manic delirium), more rarely catatonia (*Convulsive Therapy* 1990, **6**, 1–4) and drug-resistant Parkinsonism (*Acta Neurol Scand* 1987, **76**, 191–99). ECT is probably superior to, or at least as effective as, drugs and tends to be quicker-acting in severely depressed patients, although there remains some dispute about this.

ECT facilitates monoaminergic transmission by increasing receptor sensitivity and increasing the turnover and release of noradrenaline (Ottoson *et al, Biol Psych* 1985, **20**, 933–46).

Contraindications: Raised intracranial pressure (due to the brief increase in cerebral blood flow).

High-risk patients: These include those with severe cardiovascular disease, arrhythmias, pacemakers, obstructive pulmonary disease, asthma, pregnancy, osteoporosis, cerebral tumours (*Curr Opin Psych* 1990, **3**, 58–61), hydrocephalus and multiple sclerosis. If the patient has hypertension, sublingual nifedipine 20 minutes prior to ECT attenuates the hypertensive response (*Anaesth Intensive Care* 1989, **17**, 31–33).

Adverse effects: Confusion, headache and memory disturbance, usually mild and transitory.

Premedication: Atropine or glycopyrrolate are used as antimuscarinics occasionally, mainly in patients with cardiovascular risks (*Convulsive Therapy* 1989, **5**, 48–55).

Muscle relaxants: Suxamethonium is used to prevent fractures that can occur during the procedure secondary to the tonic-clonic muscular contractions (*Anaesthesia* 1988, **43**, 474–76).

Induction agents*: Propofol is now widely used since methohexital was withdrawn. It is well tolerated and short-acting with quick recovery, but shortens seizure length by up to 25% (*Anaesthesia* 1989, **44**, 168–69). It may effect seizure threshold and may be associated with bradycardia and hypotension. Some small studies indicate that seizure duration does not affect overall efficacy (*J Drug Dev* 1991, **4**[Suppl 3], 117–18; *Aust NZ J Psych* 1991, **25**, 255–61; n=20, d/b, Fear *et al, B J Psych* 1994, **165**, 506–9), although ECT courses may be prolonged. **Etomidate** is short-acting, has a rapid recovery, less hypotension than propofol and may lengthen seizure duration compared to methohexital and propofol (Ilivicky *et al, Am J Psych* 1995, **152**, 957–58). It may perhaps cause convulsions pre-ECT (n=1, Nicoll and Callender, *B J Psych* 2000, **177**, 373), is painful at the injection site, has a high incidence of extraneous muscle movements, and rarely causes adrenocortical dysfunction with repeated doses (a major concern which limits use with longer courses). Sodium **thiopentone** has little documented effect on seizure threshold or duration but the longer duration of action can delay recovery (a particular problem in the elderly). Review by Freeman, *Psych Bull* 1999, **23**, 740–41.

Seizure induction: Bilateral ECT has been shown to be markedly superior to unilateral ECT in 12 of the 23 studies carried out, the rest showing an equal or slightly poorer effect.

Maintenance: ECT has been used at 2-, 3- and then 4-weekly intervals for six months to prevent relapse (*Convulsive Therapy* 1987, **3**, 260–68; review by Rabheru and Persad, *Can J Psych* 1997, **42**, 476–84).

Mode of action: See *Curr Opin Psych* 1990, **3**, 58–61 for review, drugs and ECT.

Reviews: current practice, concomitant medications and clinical indications (Khan *et al, Psychiatr Clin North Am* 1993, **16**, 497–513), general (Prudic and Sackeim *Curr Opin Psych* 1996, **9**, 35–39; Budden, *Pharm J* 1997, **258**, 669), systematic review of 115 studies (Wijeratne *et al, Med J Aus* 1999, **171**, 250–54).

Drug considerations
Antipsychotics
Antipsychotics lower the seizure threshold and would be expected to lead to seizures at lower ECT doses.

Benzodiazepines

Benzodiazepines may lessen the improvement with unilateral ECT (*B J Psych* 1992, **161**, 129–30, 717–18; n=124, Jha and Stein, *Acta Psych Scand* 1996, **94**, 101–4), and reduce the effectiveness, even several months after treatment is stopped (n=1, *B J Psych* 1992, **160**, 545–46). The reduced effect of ECT is probably by raising seizure threshold, having an effect on seizure duration, number of sub-maximal seizures or increasing the number of treatments needed.

Bupropion *

Use with ECT has been reported (n=2, Kellner *et al, J Clin Psychopharmacol* 1994, **14**, 215–16).

Caffeine

240mg IV of caffeine has been used to augment seizure duration (reported by the ideally named Coffey *et al, Am J Psych* 1990, **147**, 579–85) or 300–1000mg orally (n=30, Ancill and Carlyle, *Am J Psych* 1992, **149**, 137), as has 125mg IV during treatment (Jaffe and Dubin, *Am J Psych* 1992, **149**, 1610). A small study showed a complex effect which deserves a full study to determine the optimum dose, timing etc. (Francis *et al, Am J Psych* 1994, **151**, 1524–26).

Carbamazepine

Logic would dictate that since carbamazepine is an anticonvulsant it would have an effect on reducing seizures (as benzodiazepines above). A small retrospective study showed that in 7 patients taking either valproate or carbamazepine, seizure durations were slightly shorter but that this appeared to have no dramatic effect on the efficacy nor side-effects of ECT (n=7, Zarate *et al, Ann Clin Psych* 1997, **9**, 19–25).

Clozapine *

Novartis recommend suspending clozapine for 24 hours pre-ECT to reduce the risk of unwanted seizures. A meta-analysis of reported cases (n=36, Kupchik *et al, Clin Neuropharmacol* 2000, **23**, 14–16) indicates that 67% benefit but adverse events occur in 17%, including prolonged seizures (n=1, Bloch *et al, B J Psych* 1996, **169**, 253–54), and supraventricular

tachycardia (Beale *et al, Convul Ther* 1994, **10**, 228–31).

Flumazenil

Effective ECT was possible in a benzodiazepine-dependent depressed woman when the anticonvulsant effect of clonazepam was reversed by flumazenil 0.1mg (Berigan *et al, Am J Psych* 1995, **152**, 957).

Ketamine

Enhanced ECT seizure duration has been reported (mentioned in review by Weiner *et al, Psych Clin North Am* 1991, **14**, 857–67).

Lithium

The use of lithium with ECT has been reported to cause severe memory loss, neurological abnormalities and a reduced antidepressant effect (*Am J Psych* 1988, **145**, 1178) although a retrospective study of 31 patients on lithium given ECT showed no increase in side-effects nor other problems (Jha *et al, B J Psych* 1996, **168**, 241–43). It has been suggested that ECT facilitates lithium toxicity (see also *Psychopharmacol Bull* 1991, **27**, 595), possibly by releasing lithium from cells, producing a pure toxicity. Elderly patients may be more susceptible to this combination. Some sources recommend discontinuing lithium 48 hours before ECT to prevent this neurotoxicity (see Lithium Encyclopaedia for Clinical Practice 1987, 274–83) and not re-started for several days after the last treatment (Ferrier *et al, Adv Psych Treat* 1995, **1**, 102–10). A review of the pros and cons of the use of lithium in ECT (Lippmann and El-Mallakh, *Lithium* 1994, **5**, 205–9) concluded that there must be clear indications for concurrent use of both treatments. However, discontinuing lithium would risk discontinuation effects and be potentially dangerous (see lithium in *1.10*).

MAOIs

MAOIs are normally contraindicated with surgery as they can interact with opiates but there may be no great problem with the ECT itself (*Convulsive Therapy* 1985, **1**, 190–94).

Mirtazapine *

An open study indicated that there were no problems with mirtazapine, either started before or during the course of ECT (n=19, Söderström, poster, XI World Congress Psychiatry, August 1999, Germany). There are cases of successful and uneventful use (n=2, Farah, *Convul Ther* 1997, **13**, 116–17).

Moclobemide

The manufacturers recommend, as a precaution, suspending moclobemide for 24hrs pre-ECT, although there is no data on its use with ECT.

Naloxone

Naloxone has no detectable effect (Rasmussen *et al, Convuls Ther* 1997, **13**, 44–46).

Nefazodone

No studies have been done to assess the combination.

SSRIs

A small study showed a significantly longer seizure duration in patients taking SSRIs compared to other antidepressants (n=13, Potokar, Wilson and Nutt, *Int J Psych Clin Pract* 1997, **1**, 277–80), although there have been some case reports of prolonged seizures (*Convulsive Therapy* 1991, **7**, 145–47). An earlier review did not support the theory that fluoxetine causes prolonged seizures (n=12, *Convulsive Therapy* 1989, **5**, 344–48). There are rare reports of prolonged seizures with ECT and paroxetine and in a rater-blinded comparison, seizure length was twice as long in those taking paroxetine (n=14, Curran, *Acta Psych Scand* 1995, **92**, 239–40). There are several reports of prolonged seizures with fluvoxamine and ECT and Duphar recommend a 4-day interval between stopping fluvoxamine and giving ECT. There is only limited experience with ECT and sertraline or citalopram.

Theophylline

Theophylline is related to caffeine and at 100–400mg IV has been reported to facilitate ECT seizures in previously resistant patients (n=8, Swartz and Lewis, *Psychosomatics* 1991, **32**, 47–50; n=7, Leentjens *et al, Convuls Ther* 1996, **12**, 232–37). There are two reports of status epilepticus and increase in seizure duration with concomitant ECT (Devanand *et al, J Clin Psychopharmacol* 1988, **8**, 153; Peters *et al, Mayo Clin Proc* 1984, **59**, 568–70).

Trazodone

A prolonged seizure duration has been reported (*Am J Psych* 1993, **150**, 525).

Tricyclics

Combined tricyclic and ECT therapy is often used and would seem to present no routine problems. The use of anaesthetics could enhance the risk of cardiac arrhythmias and hypotension.

Valproate

A small retrospective study showed that in patients taking either valproate or carbamazepine, seizure durations were slightly shorter but that this appeared to have no dramatic effect on the efficacy nor side-effects of ECT (n=7, Zarate *et al, Ann Clin Psych* 1997, **9**, 19–25).

Zopiclone

Reduced seizure length has been reported with 7.5–15mg of zopiclone the previous night (n=2, *J Psychopharmacol* 1991, **5**, 268–69) and so it is best avoided.

CHAPTER TWO

SELECTING DRUGS, DOSES and PREPARATIONS
Table 2.1.1: HYPNOTICS — RELATIVE EFFECTS *

Gp	Drug	Usual night dose mg/d	Adult max. dose mg/d	Elderly max dose mg/d	Elim half-life (hours) adult	elderly	G/I upset	Hang-over	Depen-dence potent-ial
Shorter acting Benzodiazepines									
1a	Loprazolam	1	2	1	7–15	20	○	●	●
1a	Lormetazepam	1	1.5+	<Ad	10	14	○	●	●
1a	Temazepam	10-20	40	20	5–11	14+	○	●	●●
Longer acting Benzodiazepines									
1b	Flunitrazepam	1	2	1	35	35	○	●●	●
1b	Flurazepam	15	30	15+	47–95	?	○	●●●	●●
1b	Nitrazepam	5	10	5	18–36	40+	○	●●●	●
Chloral and derivatives									
2	Chloral betane	707	5tabs	<Ad?	7–10	Same	●●●	●	●
2	Triclofos	1g	2g	1g	?	?	●	?	?
Other hypnotics									
3	Clomethiazole	N/A#	2caps#	Same	4–5	Same	○	●	●●
4	Promethazine	25	50	–	?	?	○	○	○
5	Zaleplon	10	10	5	2	3	○	○	○
6	Zopiclone	7.5	7.5	<Ad	3.5–6	8	●	●	●
7	Zolpidem	10	(10)	10	2(2–5)	longer	○	○	○

Groups:

1a	=	Shorter acting or minimally-accumulating benzodiazepines
1b	=	Longer acting or accumulating benzodiazepines
2	=	Chloral and derivative
3	=	Clomethiazole (chlormethiazole)
4	=	Antihistamine
5	=	Pyrazolopyrimidine
6	=	Imidazopyridine
7	=	Cyclopyrrone

Side-effects:

●●● = Marked effect   ○ = Little or nothing reported
●● = Moderate effect   ? = No information available
● = Mild effect

Other abbreviations:

Nightly dose	=	Usual dose for an adult as stated in the BNF
Adult max. dose	=	Maximum adult hypnotic dose as stated in the UK SPC
Eld. max dose	=	Maximum elderly hypnotic dose as stated in the UK SPC
#	=	1 capsule is therapeutically equivalent to 5ml syrup (1cap = 192mg clomethiazole base, and 5ml syrup = 157 mg clomethiazole base). Indicated for severe insomnia in the elderly only.

Table 2.1.2: ANXIOLYTICS — RELATIVE EFFECTS *

Gp	Drug	Average dose mg/day	Adult max. dose mg/d	Eld. max. dose mg/d	Half-life (hrs) adult (+range)	Half-life (hrs) elderly	Drowsi-ness	Depend-ence potent-ial
Shorter acting Benzodiazepines								
1a	Alprazolam	1	3	0.75	14(6–20)	L	●●	●●
1a	Bromazepam	9	18–60	<Ad	16(9–20)	?	●●	●●
1a	Lorazepam	4	4	<Ad	12(8–25)	Same	●●●	●●●
1a	Oxazepam	30	120	80	8(5–15)	Same	●●●	●●
Longer acting Benzodiazepines								
1b	Chlordiazepoxide	30	100	<50	12(6–30)	L	●●●	●●
1b	Clobazam	30	60	20	18(9–77)	L	●	●●
1b	Clorazepate	15	15?	<Ad	PD	L	●●●	●●
1b	Diazepam	6	30	15	32(21–50)	L	●●●	●●
Beta-blockers								
2	Oxprenolol	80	80	80	4# (3–6)	Same	●	○
2	Propranolol	80	120	–	2# (1–2)	Same	●	○
Other Anxiolytics								
3	Buspirone	30	45	45	7(2–11)	Same	○	○

Groups:

1a	=	Shorter acting or minimally-accumulating benzodiazepines
1b	=	Longer acting benzodiazepines. These also have active metabolites which enhance their length of action
2	=	Beta-blockers
3	=	Azapirone (Azaspirodecanedione)

Side-effects:

●●●	= Marked effect	○	= Little or nothing reported
●●	= Moderate effect	?	= No information available
●	= Mild effect		

Other abbreviations:

Adult max dose	=	Maximum adult anxiolytic dose as stated in UK SPC. Most only recommend treatment for up to four weeks at this dose
Eld. max. dose	=	Maximum elderly anxiolytic dose as stated in UK SPC. Most state that half the adult dose should be adequate.
PD	=	Pro-drug metabolised to desmethyldiazepam (t½ 48–200 hrs).
#	=	Pharmacological action longer than t½ suggests.

The data on the previous and three following pages is based on a large number of papers. Note was taken of presentation of data, equivalence of doses used etc. When non-comparable papers are excluded, there is a surprisingly high level of consistency on reported relative side-effects. Individuals responses may, of course, vary widely.

Table 2.1.3: ANTIDEPRESSANTS — RELATIVE SIDE-EFFECTS *

Gp	Drug	Adult max. dose mg/d	Eld. max. dose mg/d	Anti-cholin-ergic	Card-iac	Nausea ‡	Seda-tion	Over-dose §	Pro-con-vulsant
Tricyclics									
1a	Amitriptyline	200	75	●●●	●●●	●●	●●●	●●●	●●
1a	Amoxapine	300	150	●●●	●	●	●	●●●	●●●
1a	Clomipramine	250	75	●●●	●●	●●	●●	●	●●
1a	Dothiepin (dosulepin)	150	75	●●	●●	○	●●●	●●●	●●
1a	Doxepin	300	<Ad	●	●●	●	●●	●●	●●
1a	Imipramine	300	50	●●	●●	●●	●	●●●	●●
1a	Lofepramine	210	<Ad	●●	●	●	●	○	○
1b	Maprotiline	150	75	●●	●●	●●	●	●●●	●●●
1a	Nortriptyline	150	50	●●	●	●●	●	●●	●●●
1a	Trimipramine	300	<Ad	●●●	●●	●	●●	●●	●
Selective serotonin reuptake inhibitors									
2a	Citalopram	60	40	○	○	●●	○	○	○
2b	Fluoxetine	(20)	(80)	○	○	●●	○	○	○
2c	Fluvoxamine	300	300	●	○	●●●	●	○	○
2d	Paroxetine	50	40	○	○	●●	○	○	○
2e	Sertraline	200	200	○	○	●●	○	○	○
Mono-amine oxidase inhibitors									
3a	Isocarboxazid	60	<Ad	●●	●●	●●	○	●●	○
3a	Phenelzine	90	(90)	●	●	●●	○	●●	○
3b	Tranylcypromine	CA30	(30)	●	●	●●	●	●●●	○
Others									
4	Mianserin	90+	<Ad	●	○	○	●●●	○	○
5	Mirtazapine ▼	45	45	○	○	○	●●	○	○
6	Moclobemide	600	600	●	○	●	○	○	?
7	Flupentixol	3	2	●●	○	○	●	●	?
8	Nefazodone	600	400	●	○	●●	●	?	?
9	Reboxetine ▼	12	NR	●	●	●	○	○	○
8	Trazodone	600	≅300	●	●	●●●	●●	●	○
10	Tryptophan	6g	6g	○	○	●	●●	●	○
11	Venlafaxine	375	375	○	●●	●●	●	?	●

Groups:

1a	= Tricyclic	4	= Tetracyclic
1b	= Tricyclic with a middle ring bridge	5	= 'NaSSA'
2a	= Bicyclic isobenzofuran	6	= 'RIMA'
2b	= Benzenepropanamine	7	= Thioxanthene
2c	= Aminoethyl oximer of aralkyl ketone	8	= Triazolopyridine
2d	= Phenylpiperidine	9	= 'NARI'
2e	= Naphthylamine derivative	10	= Amino acid
3a	= Hydrazine MAOI	11	= 'SNRI'
3b	= Non-hydrazine MAOI		

Side-effects:

●●●	= Marked effect	○	= Little or minimal effect
●●	= Moderate effect	?	= No information or little reported
●	= Mild effect		

Other abbreviations:

‡ = Typical serotonergic side-effect

Adult max. dose = Maximum adult antidepressant dose in UK SPC

Eld. max. dose = Maximum elderly antidepressant dose as stated in UK SPC. Most state that half adult dose may be sufficient

§ Overdose = Based on UK Fatal Toxicity Index (Henry *et al*, *BMJ* 1995, **310**, 221–24, Henry *et al*, *Eur J Med* 1992, **1**, 343–48). For a review of epidemiology and relative toxicity of antidepressant drugs in overdose see Henry (*Drug Safety* 1997, **16(6)**, 374–90, 92 refs).

Table 2.1.4: ANTIDEPRESSANTS — PHARMOKINETICS etc

Drug	Major active metabolites	Half-life (hrs)	Transmiter/receptor profile			Peak plasma conc (hrs)
			5-HT	NA/NE	DA	
Tricyclics						
Amitriptyline		8–24	+++	++++	+	6
	Nortriptyline	18–96	+	++++	+	(4–5)
Amoxapine		8	+	+++	+	1–2
	7+8-hydroxy			Weak		–
Clomipramine		17–28	+++	+	O	2.5
	Desmethyl-	>36	+	+++		4–24
Dothiepin		14–40	+	+	+	3
(dosulepin)	Desmethyl-	22–60				–
Doxepin		8–24	+	+		4
	Desmethyl-	30–72				
Imipramine		4–18	+++	+	+	2
	Desipramine	12–24	+	++++	O	(4–5)
Lofepramine		1.6-5	+	++++	O	1–2
	Desipramine	12–24	+	++++	O	4–5
Maprotiline		12–108	+	+++	O	8–24
	Desmethyl-					
Nortriptyline		18–96	+	+++		(4–5)
Trimipramine	(Desmethyl-)	7–23	+	+	+	3
Selective Serotonin Reuptake Inhibitors						
Citalopram		33	++++	O	O	2–4
Fluoxetine		24–140	++++	O	+	6–8
	Norfluoxetine	168–216	+	O	O	–
Fluvoxamine	None	13–22	+++	O	O	2–8
Paroxetine	None	24	++++	O	O	6
Sertraline		25–26	+++	O	O	4–10
	Desmethyl-	66–109	+	O	O	8–12
Mono-amine oxidase inhibitors						
Isocarboxazid			↑	↑	↑	
Phenelzine		1.5	↑	↑	↑	
Tranylcypromine		2.5	↑	↑	↑	2.5
Others						
Mianserin	Desmethyl-8-hydroxy-	12–29	O	O	+	1–3
Mirtazapine	None	20-40	+++	+++	O	1-3
Moclobemide	None	1–2	↑	↑	↑	1
Flupentixol		35				3–8
Nefazodone	Several	2–4	++#			30min(1–3h)
Reboxetine	NK	13	O	+++	O	2
Trazodone		3–7	++#	O	O	½–2
	mCPP		♠			
Venlafaxine		1–2	+++	+++	+	5(2–7)
	-desmethyl	1–11				10(8–13)

Abbreviations used:
++++	= Marked potency/selective reuptake inhibition	+	= Minimal
+++	= Moderate potency	O	= Nil or virtually nil
++	= Minor potency		= Not known

Other abbreviations:
mCPP = m-Chlorphenyl-piperazine

Desmethyl = Metabolite is desmethyl-parent drug

♠ = Potent postsynaptic 5-HT agonist

\# = Also potent central 5-HT antagonist

NA/NE = Noradrenaline or norepinephrine

5-HT = 5-hydroxytryptamine or Serotonin

↑ = Cytoplasmic levels increase

DA = Dopamine

Table 2.1.5: ANTIPSYCHOTICS — RELATIVE SIDE-EFFECTS *

Gp	Drug	Adult oral max. dose mg/d	Eld oral max dose mg/d	Relative side-effects at average dose					
				Anti-cholin-ergic	Card-iac	EPSE	Hypo-tension	Seda-tion	Minor O/D
Phenothiazines									
1a	Chlorpromazine	1g	<Ad	●●●	●●	●●	●●●	●●●	●●●
1a	Levomepromazine (methotrimeprazine)	1000	NR	●●●	●●	●●?	●●●	●●●	?
1a	Promazine	800	<Ad	●●	●●	●	●●	●●	●●
1b	Thioridazine	600	<Ad	●●	●●●	●	●●	●●	●
1b	Pericyazine	(300)	<Ad	●	●●	●	●●	●●●	●●
1c	Fluphenazine	CA20	CA10	●●	●●	●●●	●	●●	●●
1c	Perphenazine	24	<Ad	●	●●	●●●	●	●	●●
1c	Trifluoperazine	–	<Ad	○	●●	●●●	●	●	●●
Butyrophenones									
2	Benperidol	1.5	<Ad	?	?	?	●	●●	?
2	Droperidol	120	<Ad	●●	●●●	●●●	●●	●●	●
2	Haloperidol	30	30	●	●●	●●●	●	●	●
Others									
3	Flupentixol	18	<Ad	●●	○	●●	○	●	●
3	Zuclopenthixol	150	<Ad	●●	●	●●●	●	●●	●●
4	Pimozide	20	<Ad	●	●●●	●●	●●	●	●
5	Amisulpride ▼	1200	1200	○	○	●	○	○	○
5	Sulpiride	2400	2400	○	○	●	○	●	●
6	Loxapine	250	–	●●	●●	●●●	●	●●	●●●
7	Clozapine	900	(900)	●●●	●●●	○	●	●●●	?
8	Olanzapine ▼	20	20	●	○	○	○	●●	○
9	Quetiapine	750	<Ad	●	●	○	●	●	?
10	Risperidone	(16)	4	○	○	●	●	●?	?
11	Zotepine ▼	300	150	●●	●●	●	●●	●	?
Depot Injection ◆									
1b	Pipothiazine	200–4	<Ad	●●	●●	●●	●	●	?
1c	Fluphenazine	100–2	<Ad	●●	●●	●●●	●	●●	●
2	Haloperidol	300–4	<Ad	●	●●	●●●	●	●●	?
3	Flupentixol	400–1	<Ad	●●●	○	●●	○	●	●
3	Zuclopenthixol	600–1	<Ad	●●	●	●●●	●	●●	?
4	Fluspirilene	20–1	<Ad	●	●	●●	●●	●	?

Groups:
1a = Phenothiazine – aliphatic side chain
1b = Phenothiazine – piperidine side chain
1c = Phenothiazine – piperazine side chain (also includes prochlorperazine)
2 = Butyrophenones   5 = Benzamide/orthopramide
3 = Thioxanthene   6 = Dibenzoazepine
4 = Diphenylbutylpiperidines   7 = Dibenzodiazepine

Side-effects:
●●● = Marked effect   ○ = Little or nothing reported
●● = Moderate effect   ? = No information available
● = Mild effect

Other abbreviations:
Adult max. dose = Maximum adult oral antipsychotic dose as stated in UK SPC. May be smaller for other indications.
Eld. max. dose = Maximum oral antipsychotic dose in the elderly as stated in UK SPC. Most state that a starting dose of half to a quarter of the adult dose should be adequate, with small dose increments.
◆ = 2–200 means 200mg every 2 weeks. 400–1 means 400mg every week etc.

List of other Abbreviations used in Tables 2.1.1 to 2.1.5

L = Half-life is longer in elderly.
<AD = Maximum dose is less than the adult dose
Anticholinergic = Anticholinergic or
antimuscarinic side-effects

Pro-convulsant = Pro-convulsive effect
CA = Care above
EPSE = Extra-pyramidal side-effects
NR = Not recommended

2.2 SWITCHING OR DISCONTINUING PSYCHOTROPICS

Switching psychotropics can be achieved using a variety of methods, varying in rate, overlap, gap and complexity. These are summarised in the graphs and comments shown. Those remarks specifically relating to antipsychotics are marked with #.

Switch 1 – drug-free interval

(discontinue first drug, leave drug-free interval, introduce second drug):
Advantages:
1. Minimises combined ADRs.
2. Low relapse risk, if the patient is relatively stable and the gap is not prolonged.
3. Minimal interaction potential.
4. Side-effects from the second drug are less likely to be confused with discontinuation effects from first drug
5. Anticholinergic drug doses can be titrated as needed #.
6. Recommended for switches to clozapine to reduce additive myelo-suppressive potential #.
7. Low medication error potential.

Disadvantages:
1. Takes time, which delays the desired relief of symptoms or side-effects and may extend inpatient stays #.
2. Fear of relapse during gap and changeover (probably rare).
3. Early relapse might be interpreted as lack of efficacy of the second drug.

Switch 2a and 2b: No interval

(stop first drug, start second immediately)
Advantages:
1. Straightforward.
2. Low medication error potential.
3. Appropriate for in-patient settings with better supervision.
4. Appropriate where an acute, severe reaction to a drug has occurred, eg. statutory abrupt withdrawal of clozapine due to a blood dyscrasia #.
5. Sometimes acceptable for high-risk switches to clozapine to reduce additive myelosuppressive potential # .

Disadvantages:
1. May raise unrealistic expectations from patient and family of a rapid improvement on the second drug.
2. Less suitable for clozapine #.
3. Combined ADRs may occur, albeit short-lived.
4. Potential for drug interactions if the first drug has a long half-life.
5. Rapid discontinuation of the first drug may produce higher relapse rates.
6. Discontinuation effects from the first drug might be interpreted as side-effects of the second.

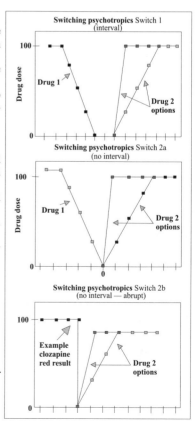

Switch 3a, 3b, 3c, 3d: Partial overlap

(Add new drug, either at standard dose or quickly titrated upwards, while slowly tapering the first drug)

Advantages:

1. Appropriate when side-effect relief is needed but a high relapse risk.
2. No sudden changes occur, which might destabilise the patient.

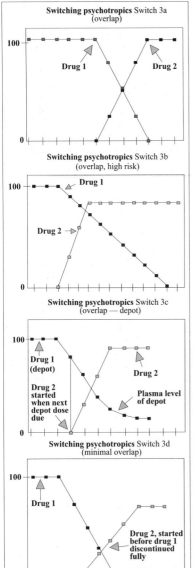

Switching psychotropics Switch 3a
(overlap)

Drug 1   Drug 2

Switching psychotropics Switch 3b
(overlap, high risk)

Drug 1

Drug 2

Switching psychotropics Switch 3c
(overlap — depot)

Drug 1 (depot)

Drug 2 started when next depot dose due

Drug 2

Plasma level of depot

Switching psychotropics Switch 3d
(minimal overlap)

Drug 1

Drug 2, started before drug 1 discontinued fully

3. 3c may be appropriate for depot to oral switches, where plasma levels of depot will decline slowly and withdrawal reactions have not been reported #.
4. Useful for high potency antipsychotics to an atypical, and from a low potency drug where cholinergic rebound may occur. Either way, anticholinergic cover can be retained for several weeks #.

Disadvantages:

1. If taper is too quick, two drugs may be given at sub-therapeutic doses.
2. Combined ADRs may occur.
3. Potential for drug interactions, especially with antidepressants.
4. Potential for medication errors if not planned fully in advance – involve carers and patient if patient is at home.
5. High potential for polypharmacy if switch never completed, eg. if discharged and message not passed on, or the patient improves and there is a reluctance to discontinue the first drug and possibly destabilise the patient #.

Switch 4: Full overlap

(add new drug to therapeutic dose and then slowly taper previous drug)

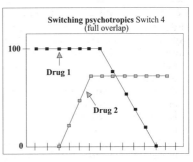

Switching psychotropics Switch 4
(full overlap)

Drug 1

Drug 2

Advantages:

1. Safest if relapse prevention of greatest concern.
2. Most appropriate if the patient has recently (eg. <3 months) recovered from acute relapse with the first drug.
3. Low risk of discontinuation effects of the first drug.
4. If depot to oral antipsychotic, this may be lowest risk opportunity to assess compliance with oral drugs #.
5. Slow taper is possible and is better for drugs with high anticholinergic activity.

Disadvantages:

1. Combined ADRs may occur (but not necessarily with antipsychotics, Gardner *et al, Can J Psych* 1997, **42**, 430–31).

2. Potential for drug interactions.

3. Potential for medication errors if not planned and completed fully.

4. High potential for polypharmacy if switch never completed, eg. if discharged and message not passed on, or patient improves and there is a reluctance to discontinue the first drug and possibly destabilise the patient #.

2.2.1 SWITCHING OR DISCONTINUING ANTIPSYCHOTICS

Reviews: switching from typical to atypical antipsychotics (Taylor, *CNS Drugs* 1997, **8**, 285–92), switching to risperidone (Borison *et al, Clin Therapeutics* 1996, **18**, 592–607), general (Weiden *et al, J Clin Psych* 1997, **58**[Suppl 10], 63–72, 60 refs; Amery and Marder, *Int J Psych Clin Pract* 1998, **2**, S43–S49), discontinuing antipsychotics (review, Tranter and Healy, *J Psychopharmacol* 1998, **12**, 401–6).

2.2.1.1 General advice on switching

Indications for switching antipsychotics include (Weiden *et al, J Clin Psych* 1997, **58**[Suppl 10], 63–72):

1. Persistent positive (distressing and disruptive) symptoms.

2. Persistent negative (restrictive and burdening) symptoms.

3. Relapse despite compliance.

4. Persistent distressing adverse effects such as EPSEs, akathisia, hyperprolactinaemia, poor self-image and sexual dysfunction.

5. Oral to depot or other formulation change.

There are as yet no published controlled trials on switching antipsychotics.

Risks of discontinuing (or switching) antipsychotics (review and guidance, Keks *et al, CNS Drugs* 1995, **4**, 351–56):

1. Cholinergic rebound (eg. nausea, vomiting, restlessness, anxiety, insomnia, fatigue, malaise, myalgia, diaphoresis, rhinitis, paraesthesia, GI distress, headaches, nightmares). It may occur after discontinuation or if a second drug has less anticholinergic effects or anticholinergic drugs are withdrawn too soon (Luchins *et al, Am J Psych* 1980, **137**, 1395–98). It can be severe but tends to be relatively brief and predictable.

2. Withdrawal dyskinesias, eg. extrapyramidal symptoms, rebound akathisia (which may be confused with anxiety or psychosis, Dufresne and Wagner, *J Clin Psych* 1988, **49**, 435–38), rebound dystonia and worsening tardive dyskinesia (Glazer *et al, Biol Psych* 1989, **26**, 224–33). Withdrawal EPSEs may, in part, be related to cholinergic rebound. These have been reported in mentally healthy people taking metoclopramide as an antiemetic (see Tranter and Healy, *J Psychopharmacol* 1998, **12**, 401–6) and can be minimised by slow tapering (n=81, d/b, p/c, Battegay, *Comp Psych* 1966, **7**, 501–9).

3. Other discontinuation symptoms, eg. NMS (Spivak *et al, Acta Psych Scand* 1990, **81**, 168–69).

4. Relapse or destabilisation – this may present an unacceptable risk to the patient. Relapse rates of up to 50% at 6 months after abrupt discontinuation has been reported (n=1210, Viguera *et al, Arch Gen Psych* 1997, **54**, 49–55), gradual discontinuation reducing this risk (reviewed by Tranter and Healy, *J Psychopharmacol* 1998, **12**, 401–6). True relapses tend to occur from 1–6 months after even abrupt withdrawal of oral drugs (eg. Prien *et al, B J Psych* 1968, **115**, 679–86) and 3–6 months with depots (Wistedt, *Acta Psych Scand* 1981, **64**, 65–84), probably due to persistence of drug at receptor level (Cohen *et al, Arch Gen Psych* 1988, **45**, 879–80). There may be a particular problem with clozapine, where relapse or rebound psychosis can be more severe (eg. Baldessarini *et al, Arch Gen Psych* 1995, **52**, 1071–72, see also *2.2.1.4*).

5. Anxiety or stress from the switch causing symptom flare-up.

6. Medication errors.

7. The replacement drug being less effective than the former, or having different but still unacceptable side-effects, resulting in premature abandonment and an inadequate trial of the new drug.

General principals for switching antipsychotics:

1. Ensure a treatment target is set and measured (take care that the key aims of a switch are not easier and less risky to achieve by, eg. dose or timing adjustment of the first drug).
2. Avoid switches coinciding with major life stress events.
3. Avoid switching after a change in treatment team. Allow full assimilation into the new treatment team first.
4. Avoid switching within 3–6 months of recovery from a drug which was successfully used to treat a major relapse.
5. In patients previously non-compliant with oral drugs now stable for under a year on a depot (Weiden *et al, J Clin Psych* 1997, **58**[Suppl 10], 63–72).
6. If possible, slowly taper the first antipsychotic, probably over at least eight weeks, as this reduces the risk of relapse (Wyatt, *Arch Gen Psych* 1995, **52**, 205–8) and emergent extrapyramidal and psychotic symptoms.
7. Slowly taper any anticholinergic, which may also be allowed to continue for a time after the drug has been discontinued. Reintroduce if necessary for any emergent symptoms.
8. Monitor mental and physical state regularly (particularly during the first month).

Advice to patients before switching to atypicals:

1. Warn about possible ADRs, eg. weight gain, short-term sedation, time course and implications of reduced prolactin inhibition.
2. Need for adequate trial and need to complete switch, plus time scale.
3. How to define success.
4. How to measure success and the chances thereof.
5. The new drug isn't perfect.

2.2.1.2 Antipsychotic dose equivalents

The antipsychotic dose(s) of each drug within each heading of this section are approximately equivalent to others under the same heading (eg. perphenazine 24mg/d is equivalent to chlorpromazine 300mg/d and to flupentixol 60mg 2/52), based on the references indicated.

There is a genuine lack of agreement about antipsychotic equivalents. This is mainly because the three methods of assessing antipsychotic equivalence (clinical studies, non-clinical/receptor binding studies and manufacturers' information) can produce up to a five-fold difference in the equivalents then recommended (full discussion by Rey *et al, Int Clin Psychopharmacol* 1989, **4**, 95–104), particularly true in the case of high-potency antipsychotics. Ranges quoted here are thus unweighted for individual variation and are valid, but imprecise. For example, antipsychotics (excluding some atypical drugs) displace ligands from dopamine receptors (particularly D2 receptors) at a rate that highly correlates with their antipsychotic potency (eg. Peroutka & Snyder, *Am J Psych* 1980, **137**, 1518–22) and so roughly equivalent antipsychotic doses can be calculated. However, some dose relationships, eg. haloperidol, are unlikely to be linear and sedation and anxiety may not be directly related to dopamine blockade (reviewed by Hilton *et al, Psych Bull* 1996, **20**, 359–62). High-potency drugs, eg. haloperidol, fluphenazine etc have the highest quoted variance, over 1000% in some cases. This may lead to prescribing in higher doses than necessary (Dewan and Koss, *Acta Psych Scand* 1995, **91**, 229–32). Additionally, higher doses of antipsychotics tend to be used to control disruptive behaviour rather than just to control psychotic symptoms (Peralta *et al, Acta Psych Scand* 1994, **90**, 354–57). Using the percentage of the maximum BNF dose has been proposed as an alternative, but is also imprecise, as maximum doses may not be equivalent, eg. is flupentixol decanoate 400mg a week really equivalent to 50mg a week of fluphenazine decanoate?

Antipsychotic equivalence is specifically quoted here and the doses are as accurate as data allows but to avoid any confusion you **must** consider the following:

i. Antipsychotic equivalence should not be confused with **sedation**, which in some cases, eg. haloperidol (with a relatively low sedative effect) causes confusion over equivalence. Indeed, there may be no extra antipsychotic effect from haloperidol above 12–20mg/d (see *1.27*).

ii. With some drugs there may not be a

linear relationship between dose and antipsychotic effect.

iii. Dose frequency with depots may be important (*Curr Ther Res* 1982, **31**, 982) as the first pass effect may reduce the effective doses of oral preparations.

iv. If using a 'broad-spectrum' drug (eg. the so-called 'dirty' drugs, such as chlorpromazine) and converting to a D2 receptor selective drug (eg. flupenthixol, sulpiride etc), the use of conversion tables may not thus be appropriate and may result in enhanced side-effects or over-dosage.

v. Differing half-lives may complicate the calculations and final dose recommendation.

vi. Haloperidol and fluphenazine seems a particular problem.

vii. These equivalent doses are not necessarily equivalent in terms of maximum doses in the BNF/SPC.

viii. For 'atypicals', therapeutic doses are better defined and so no equivalent doses are appropriate.

You should always check your answer against the SPC limits to ensure an inappropriately high dose (eg. beyond BNF/SPC limits) is not inadvertently considered (review, Atkins *et al, Psych Bull* 1997, **21**, 224–26).

Antipsychotic equivalent doses

	Oral	mg/d (+range)
1	Chlorpromazine	100mg ($\cong$25–50mg IM[7] or 250mg rectally)
	Fluphenazine	2mg (1.25–5mg)
	Levomepromazine	NK
	Pericyazine	24mg
	Perphenazine	8mg (7–15mg)
	Prochlorperazine	15mg (14–25mg)
	Promazine	100mg (50–200mg)
	Thioridazine	100mg (75–104mg)
	Trifluoperazine	5mg (2–8mg)
2	Benperidol	2mg
	Droperidol	4mg (Short t½) or 3mg IM/IV
	Haloperidol[9]	3mg (1–5mg) or 1.5mg IM/IV* for doses up to 20mg/d
3	Flupentixol	2mg
	Zuclopenthixol	25mg (25–60mg) up to 150mg/d
4	Pimozide	2mg (1–3) (Long t½)
5	Remoxipride	75mg
	Amisulpride	100mg (40–150mg)
	Sulpiride	200mg (200–333mg)
6	Loxapine	10mg (6–25mg)
7	Clozapine	100mg (30–150mg)
	Olanzapine	NK
	Quetiapine	NK
	Zotepine	NK
8	Risperidone[4]	1.5mg (0.5-3mg)

	Depot	mg/week
1	Fluphenazine[3]	5–10mg (1–12.5mg)
1	Pipothiazine	10mg (5–12.5mg)
2	Haloperidol[5]	15mg (5–25mg)
3	Flupentixol	10mg (8–20mg)
3	Zuclopenthixol	100mg (40–100mg)
4	Fluspirilene	2mg (NE)

Bioavailability from oral haloperidol is about 50% of IM, with IV approximately equivalent to IM.

Key:
NE = Not fully established.
90mg (75–100) = Recommended average dose +ranges quoted in the literature. The wider the range, the greater the uncertainty about the exact equivalent.

Further reading

1. Peroutka and Synder, *Am J Psych* 1980, **137**, 1518–22

2. *Acta Psych Scand* 1980, **65**, 356–63

3. *Am J Psych* 1990, **147**, 258–60 + Refs

4. Remington *et al, Am J Psych* 1998, **155**, 1301–2

5. Hemstrom *et al, Drug Intell Clin Pharm* 1988, **22**, 290–95

6. *Am J Psych* 1989, **146**, 1233

7. Dewan and Koss, *Acta Psych Scand* 1995, **91**, 229–32 (excellent review)

8. Schwartz and Brotman, *Drugs* 1992, **44**, 981–92

9. Hilton *et al, Psych Bull* 1996, **20**, 359–62

The Actual Dose of a new drug required =

$$\frac{\text{Current total daily (oral) or weekly (depot) drug dose}}{\text{Equivalent dose stated for that drug in that form}} \times \text{equivalent dose of the new drug as stated in that table}$$

2.2.1.3 Switching antipsychotic doses and/or preparations
Depot switches
Oral antipsychotic to depot
Anecdotal evidence shows that the change can usually be made uneventfully (eg. review in *Clin Pharmacokinet* 1985, **10**, 315–33) although no studies have been published on the process. Converting to the same drug as a depot should present no problems if doses are chosen carefully (eg. 3c, see also *2.2.1.4*)

Altering the frequency of a depot
Such a change should present no great problems, provided antipsychotic levels do not drop too low.

Changing from one depot to another depot
No significant problems are usually experienced (Soni *et al, Acta Psych Scand* 1992, **85**, 354–59) and a direct exchange from one depot to another can often be made uneventfully (eg. 3c).

Combined oral antipsychotic plus depot to depot alone
This can be an unusually difficult procedure and relapses may occur more frequently with this change when compared to other changes. Relapses can occur particularly in the first 3–4 months, when antipsychotic levels can be inadvertently sub-therapeutic (*Acta Psych Scand* 1992, **85**, 354–59). Any change should be done verging on the side of caution, eg. increasing the depot dose, then reducing the oral dose later.

2.2.1.4 Specific antipsychotic drug switches (where specific information is available)
Switching from clozapine
Converting clozapine to other antipsychotics seems particularly problematic (Shiovitz *et al, Schizophr Bull* 1996, **22**, 591–95). Relapse after clozapine discontinuation seems to be of a higher incidence, may be more rapid (Shore, *Schizophr Bull* 1995, **21**, 333–37) and withdrawal symptoms may be more severe (Still *et al, Psychiatr Serv* 1996, **47**, 1382–84) than with other drugs. For gradual discontinuation of clozapine, it is best to simultaneously introduce and escalate the doses of another antipsychotic.

Switching to clozapine
Due to the potential for an increased risk of agranulocytosis, ideally, a previous drug should be completely withdrawn before clozapine is started, including depots (eg. switch 1), but this is not always practical. Clozapine is a very sedative and hypotensive drug, so care is needed with additive effects, so start with gradual dose titration. Pharmacokinetic interactions are unlikely (see *4.2.2*).

Switching to risperidone
Risperidone can cause hypotension, so gradual dose titration over at least 3 days to 6mg/d is recommended. Slower increases may help some people. Additive hypotension with low potency drugs may occur during a switch. A sudden switch (along with gradual withdrawal of anticholinergics) may be successful in about 60% patients, but a more gradual switch would be preferrable (n=36, Kirov *et al, Acta Psych Scand* 1997, **95**, 439–43). A review of switching to risperidone recommended reducing the existing antipsychotic dose, then overlapping risperidone and the existing therapy, rather than making an abrupt switch (Borison *et al, Clin Ther* 1996, **18**, 592–607). Risperidone may be a suitable replacement if introduced before slow clozapine withdrawal, ie. switch 4 (Zimbroff, *Am J Psych* 1995, **152**, 1102).

Switching to olanzapine:
Additive EPSEs, hypotension and drug interactions are unlikely to occur and so switch 3a is usually suitable with care. In one open study of a clozapine to olanzapine switch by patients wishing to avoid blood monitoring, 8 of 19 successfully completed the switch (using switch 4) and the others required restabilised on clozapine (Henderson *et al, J Clin Psych* 1998, **59**, 585–88).

Switching from oral to depot fluphenazine
If transferring from oral fluphenazine, multiply the total daily oral dose by 1.2 and administer as fluphenazine decanoate IM every one to two weeks. Accumulation occurs and so the dosing interval may be increased to every three weeks or so after four to six weeks of therapy (Ereshefsky *et al, J Clin Psych* 1984, **45**, 50). Concomitant oral therapy

should be limited to the initial period or during times of decompensation.

Switching from oral to depot haloperidol

If transferring from stabilised oral haloperidol to depot, multiply the total daily oral dose by 15–20, to a maximum of 300mg, preferably much lower. Accumulation occurs and so the decanoate dose should be decreased by 25% a month until the minimum effective dose is achieved. The average maintenance dose appears to be about 200mg every four weeks. Elderly patients or those stabilised on less than 10mg/d oral haloperidol should receive haloperidol decanoate in an IM dose that is 10–15 times the oral dose every four weeks. Concomitant oral therapy should be limited to the initial period or during times of decompensation.

2.2.1.5 Post-switching issues

(Based on an extensive review by Weiden *et al, J Clin Psych* 1998, **59**[Suppl 19], 36–49)

A. Assessing response:

1. For all drugs, aim for a minimum of 3 months at full therapeutic dosage.
2. Be cautious of any significant gains (eg. reduced side-effects) within 6/52 of the last drug stopping, as drug concentrations at receptor level may outlast plasma levels (see haloperidol, *1.27*).
3. Even if gains occur, make sure full therapeutic dose is achieved, as discontinuation of the previous drug will lead to a gradual loss of its side-effects (including cognitive impairment), which may be interpreted as improvement.
4. If gains occur, it has been suggested to delay discontinuing any anticholinergic and/or antiakathisia drugs until during the second month.
5. Raised prolactin levels may take over 3/12 to resolve, so women need to be warned about this, and to ensure they have adequate contraceptive cover.
6. If positive changes occur, the patient should be cautioned not to risk relapse by 'over doing it'.

B. Managing a sub-optimum response to a switch

1. No improvement by 6/52 – exclude non-compliance with the switch, substance misuse and inadequate dosage. Try to work towards 12/52 at full dose.
2. Some response by 6/52 – don't get too excited, continue to 12/52.
3. Partial response between 6/52 and 12/52 – consider an increase in dose, and try to go for an 6/12 trial.
4. Initial response followed by worsening of positive symptoms – check worsening is not actually improvement (eg. previous positive symptoms hidden by the patient now surfacing), try to restabilise and aim for 12/52 at full dose.

C. Long-term issues

1. With improvements in insight, increased psychosocial support and monitoring will be needed to reduce the risk of post-psychotic depression and self-harm.

Long-term polypharmacy with antipsychotics

(extensive review, Weiden *et al, J Clin Psych* 1998, **59**[Suppl 19], 36–49)

The advantages of long-term monotherapy are that one is better able to judge the effectiveness of any given drug accurately and medication regimens is simple and not confused by polypharmacy.

Appropriate justifications for polypharmacy might include:

1. Clozapine intolerance, as augmentation of a low clozapine dose.
2. Clozapine partial response, as augmentation.
3. When discontinuing a depot poses an unacceptable risk eg. forensic patients.
4. Patients refusing to stop an old drug or refusing to try clozapine.

Inappropriate reasons for polypharmacy, however, include:

1. As a substitute for failing to plan and communicate a switch, which is then never fully completed.
2. Where clinical improvement occurs before a switch is completed, and the clinician 'quits while ahead' rather than risking completing the change.

2.2.1.6 Discontinuing antipsychotics

Withdrawal symptoms (eg. tardive psychosis, dyskinesias etc) have been reported upon abrupt discontinuation (eg. *J Clin Psych* 1991, **52**, 346–48) eg.

cholinergic rebound-headache, restlessness, diarrhoea, nausea and vomiting (Lieberman, *Psychosomatics* 1981, **22**, 253–54). In 1006 schizophrenics withdrawing from antipsychotics abruptly, the risk of relapse reached 25% in 10 weeks and 50% within 30 weeks, with little additional relapse risk up to 3.7 years. With gradual withdrawal, risk of relapse was lower (Viguera *et al, Arch Gen Psych* 1997, **54**, 49–55). For a comprehensive and fascinating review of neuroleptic discontinuation syndrome, see Tranter and Healy (*J Psychopharmacol* 1998, **12**, 401–6).

2.2.2 SWITCHING BENZODIAZEPINES

Switching benzodiazepines may be advantageous for a variety of reasons, eg. to a drug with a different half-life prediscontinuation. Whilst there is broad agreement in the literature about equivalent doses, clonazepam has a wide variety of reported equivalalences and particular care is needed with this drug. Inter-patient variability and differing half-lives means the figures can never be exact and should be interpreted using your own pharmaceutical knowledge.

BENZODIAZEPINES [1,2,3,4]

See note in introduction re: half lives	
Diazepam	5mg (oral, im or iv)
Alprazolam	0.5mg
Bromazepam	3mg
Chlordiazepoxide	15mg (10–25mg)
Clobazam	10mg
Clonazepam	0.5mg (0.25-4) [4]
Clorazepate	7.5mg (7.5-10)
Flunitrazepam	0.5mg
Flurazepam	7.5–15mg
Loprazolam	0.5–1mg
Lorazepam	[4]0.5–1mg at ≤ 4mg/d 2mg at ≥ 5mg/d
Lormetazepam	0.5–1mg
Nitrazepam	5mg (2.5–20mg)
Oxazepam	15mg (15–40mg)
Temazepam	10mg

References

1. *B J Pharm Pract* 1989, **11**, 106–10.
2. *B J Psych* 1991, **158**, 511–16.
3. *Clinical Handbook of Psychotropic Drugs*, 4th edn, Bezchlibnyk-Butler *et al*, Hogrefe and Huber, Toronto.
4. Cowen, *Adv Psych Treat* 1997, **3**, 67.

2.2.3 SWITCHING ANTICHOLINERGICS

See *1.20.1* about the overall indications for the use of anticholinergics. Equivalent doses are:

Benztropine	1mg
Biperiden	2mg
Orphenadrine	50mg
Procyclidine	2mg
Benzhexol (trihexyphenidyl)	2mg

(Saklad, personal communication)

2.2.4 SWITCHING DRUGS OF ABUSE OR DEPENDENCE

Switching drugs of abuse/dependence, usually to methadone, is a common treatment strategy. The following table may be of some use, although caution is obviously necessary regarding, eg. the potency of individual samples of street drugs etc. Many dose equivalents are also derived from analgesic equivalents, which may not necessarily be the same as those necessary to prevent withdrawal symptoms.

NARCOTICS

Drug	Qty	Methadone
Actified Compound	100ml	6mg
Buprenorphine	0.3mg	2.5mg
Codeine linctus	100ml	10mg
Codeine Phosphate	15mg	1mg
Diamorphine BP	10mg	10mg
Diamorphine inj[4]	5mg	10mg
Diconal	1 tab	5mg
Dihydrocodeine	30mg	2.5mg
Dr Collis Browns	100ml	10mg
Gees Linctus	100ml	10mg
Morphine inj	10mg	10mg
Morphine oral[4]	15mg	10mg
MST tablets [2]	10mg	3.25mg
Palfium	5mg	5–10mg
Pentazocine	25mg	2mg
Pethidine tabs/inj	50mg	5mg
Street Heroin	¼g*	20mg*
Street Morphine*	¼*	15mg*

*This is obviously highly variable depending upon its purity

2.2.5 SWITCHING OR STOPPING ANTIDEPRESSANTS

Switching from one antidepressant to another, either for reasons of side-effects or lack of efficacy, can be problematical and present unexpected problems for the unwary. It is often necessary to leave gaps of drug-free days, eg. the 14-day gap after stopping an MAOI before starting another antidepressant is well known. However, other problems may occur and the prescriber must be aware of these to avoid unnecessary adverse events. For a summary of sequential strategies for switching antidepressants, see Thase and Rush, *J Clin Psych* 1997, **58**[Suppl 13], 23–29.

Factors which must be considered before choosing a switch regimen:

i. Speed at which the switch is needed, eg. with less urgency a more cautious regimen can be used. Since many drugs are used in combination, faster switches can obviously be made, but additional monitoring is recommended.

ii. Current dose of the first drug.

iii. Individual drugs and their effects, neurotransmitter effects, kinetics etc.

iv. Individuals susceptibility to (additive) side-effects.

Potential problems:

i. Cholinergic rebound, eg. headache, restlessness, diarrhoea, nausea and vomiting (Lieberman, *Psychosomatics* 1981, **22**, 253–54) from withdrawal of drugs affecting ACh, eg. tricyclics.

ii. Antidepressant withdrawal or discontinuation symptoms (see *13*).

iii. Serotonin Syndrome for drugs affecting serotonin (see *1.31*).

iv. Interaction between the two drugs, eg. altered drug levels from altered metabolism (see *4.3*).

v. Discontinuation effects from the first drug being interpreted as side-effects of the second.

Lithium has been suggested to help cover the gap between antidepressants, eg. starting as one is tapered off and finishing after the second has reached therapeutic doses (Gitlin and Altshuler, *Arch Gen Psych* 1997, **54**, 21–23).

How to use the table overleaf:

i. Look down the vertical column headed 'from' and find the drug or drug group the patient is currently taking.

ii. Follow that line along until you come to the column of the drug or drug group to which you wish to change.

iii. The details there give the current known information. For further details look up the reference number quoted.

Example: Changing from tranylcypromine to a tricyclic requires a 14-day drug-free gap (reference 9) but changing from a tricyclic to tranylcypromine only requires a 7-day drug-free gap (reference 9).

1. A two-week gap is recommended, especially if the MAOI is changed **to** tranylcypromine. The SPC for tranylcypromine recommends leaving at least a seven-day gap after stopping other antidepressants, then starting tranylcypromine at half the usual dosage for one week. Careful observation is essential. An open study of switching MAOIs with less than a 14-day gap showed that only one of the eight suffered adverse events, indicative of either tranylcypromine withdrawal or a mild serotonin syndrome. A shorter gap may be feasible with full dietary control, good compliance and close monitoring (n=8, Szuba *et al, J Clin Psych* 1997, **58**, 307–10). However, since deaths have been reported with such a switch (eg. Bazire, *Drug Intell Clin Pharm* 1986, **20**, 954–56), caution is recommended.

2. Fluoxetine, paroxetine and fluvoxamine (but probably not citalopram and sertraline at standard doses) can double or triple tricyclic levels (particularly of amitriptyline, imipramine, desipramine, nortriptyline and clomipramine), by CYP2D6 inhibition and so care is needed. Prescribing both drugs together over a change-over period is not advised unless the drugs are chosen carefully and specific care is taken. Ideally, 'drop-and-stop' before starting the next drug is recommended.

Factors to be considered:

i. **Speed** at which the switch is needed, eg. faster switches can obviously be made, but additional monitoring, eg. tricyclic levels and cardiac status is recommended.

ii. **SSRI dose** – CYP2D6 inhibition appears to be dose-related for some drugs, eg. paroxetine.

iii. **Tricyclic** – stronger serotonin re-uptake inhibitors are more likely to produce serotonin syndrome (eg. clomipramine), and tertiary tricyclics (eg. imipramine, amitriptyline, clomipramine) are metabolised by CYP3A3/4 and CYP1A2, inhibited by fluvoxamine.

iv. **P450 status** of the patient.

To / From	MAOIs		Tricyclics	SSRIs				
	Hydra-zines	Tranyl-cypromine		Citalopram	Fluvox-amine	Fluoxetine	Sertraline	Parox-etine
MAOIS — Hydra-zines	14/7[1]	14/7[1]	7-14/7[9]	14/7[7]	14/7[7]	14/7[7]	14/7[7]	14/7[7]
MAOIS — Tranyl-cypro-mine	14/7[1]	■	14/7[9]	14/7[7]	14/7[7]	14/7[7]	14/7[7]	14/7[7]
Tricyclics	7/7[9]	7/7[9]	NSPR[4]	Care[2]	Great Care[2]	Great Care[2]	Care[2]	Great Care[2]
Citalopram	7/7[7]	7/7[7]	Care[2]	■	SSP[5]	SSP[5]	SSP[5]	SSP[5]
Fluvoxamine	4/7[7]	7-14/7[7]	Great care[2]	SSP[5]	■	SSP[5]	SSR[5]	SSR[5]
Fluoxetine	5/52[7]	5/52[7]	Great care for 28/7[2]	SSP[5]	SSP[5]	■	SSP[5]	SSP[5]
Sertraline	7/7[7]	7-14/7[7]	Care[2]	SSP[5]	SSP[5]	SSP[5]	■	SSP[5]
Paroxetine	14/7[7]	14/7[7]	Great care[2]	SSP[5]	SSP[5]	SSP[5]	SSP[5]	■
Trazodone Nefazodone	7/7[6,7]	7/7[6,7]	OP[13]	Care[3,6]	Care[3,6]	Care[3,6]	Care[3,6]	Care[3,6]
Tryptophan	14/7[10] or care	7-14/7[10] or care	NSPR	Care[11]	Care[11]	Care[11]	Care[11]	Care[11]
Moclobemide	NSPR[7]	NSPR[7]	OP[15]	NSPR[8]	NSPR[8]	2/52[8]	NSPR[8]	NSPR[8]
Venlafaxine	7/7[16]	7/7[16]	NSPR[16]	Care[16]	Care[16]	Care[16]	Care[16]	Care[16]
Mirtazapine	7/7[7]	7/7[7]	NSPR[12]	NSPR[12]	NSPR[12]	NSPR[12]	NSPR[12]	NSPR[12]
Mianserin	14/7[1]	14/7[1]	NSPR	NSPR	NSPR	NSPR	NSPR	NSPR
Reboxetine	1/52[17]	1/52[17]	NSPR[17]	NSPR[17]	NSPR[17]	NSPR[17]	NSPR[17]	NSPR[17]
Just plain stopping:[17]	Over 4/52[17]	Over 4/52[73]	Over 4/52[17]	Over 4/52[17]	Over 4/52[17]	Reduce to 20 mg/d, then stop	Over 4/52[17]	Over 4/52[17] or longer

NSPR = No significant problems reported, careful cross-taper
OP = Occasional problems
SSP = Serotonin Syndrome possible (see ref 5)
NB: Patients with bipolar mood disorders should be monitored closely for manic episodes following discontinuation or change of any antidepressant medication (*J Clin Psych* 1985, **5**, 342–3)

To / From	Trazodone[16] Nefazodone	Tryptophan	Moclo-bemide	Venla-faxine[16]	Mirtazapine	Mianserin	Reboxetine
MAOIS Hydra-zines	14/7[6,7]	14/7[10] or care	1/7[7] with care	14/7[16]	2/52[7]	14/7[1]	2/52[17]
MAOIS Tranyl-cypro-mine	14/7[6,7]	1/7[10]	7/7[1,7] with care	14/7[16]	2/52[7]	14/7[1]	2/52[17]
Tricyclics	NSPR	NSPR[10]	NSPR[15]	Variable [16]	NSPR[12]	NSPR	NSPR[17]
Citalopram	Care[3,6]	Care[11]	7/7[14]	Care[16]	NSPR[12]	NSPR	NSPR[17]
Fluvoxamine	Care[6]	Care[11]	4-5/7[14]	Care[16]	NSPR[12]	NSPR	NSPR[17]
Fluoxetine	Care[6]	Care[11]	4-45/7[14]	Care[16]	NSPR[12]	NSPR	NSPR[17]
Sertraline	Care[6]	Care[11]	4-13/7[14]	Care[16]	NSPR[12]	NSPR	NSPR[17]
Paroxetine	Care[6]	Care[11]	4-5/7[14]	Care[16]	NSPR[12]	NSPR	NSPR[17]
Trazodone Nefazodone		NSPR	NSPR	Care[16]	NSPR[12]	NSPR	NSPR[17]
Tryptophan	NSPR		NSPR	NSPR	NSPR[12]	NSPR	NSPR[17]
Moclobemide	NSPR[6,8]	NSPR		NSPR	NSPR[12]	NSPR	NSPR[17]
Venlafaxine	Care[16]	NSPR[16]	NSPR[16]		NSPR[16]	NSPR[16]	NSPR[17]
Mirtazapine	NSPR[12]	NSPR[12]	NSPR[12]	NSPR[12]		NSPR[12]	NSPR[17]
Mianserin	NSPR	NSPR	NSPR	NSPR	NSPR[12]		NSPR[17]
Reboxetine	NSPR[17]	NSPR[17]	NSPR[17]	NSPR[17]	NSPR[17]	NSPR[17]	
Just plain stopping:	Over 4/52[17]	Over 4/52[17]	Over 4/52[17]	Over 4/52[17] or longer	Over 4/52[17]	Over 4/52[17]	Over 4/52[17]

NSPR = No significant problems reported, careful cross-taper
OP = Occasional problems
SSP = Serotonin Syndrome possible (see ref 5)
NB: Patients with bipolar mood disorders should be monitored closely for manic episodes following discontinuation or change of any antidepressant medication (*J Clin Psych* 1985, **5**, 342–43)

v. **Individual** susceptibility to tricyclic and SSRI side-effects.

Main potential problems (see also introduction for details):

i. Cholinergic rebound.

ii. Tricyclic/SSRI discontinuation symptoms (see ref 13).

iii. Serotonin Syndrome (see *1.31*).

iv. Increased tricyclic levels from decreased metabolism via SSRI CYP450 inhibition (see *4.3.1*).

Suggested switch regimens:

Tricyclic → fluoxetine, paroxetine or fluvoxamine: Taper tricyclic dose to around 50mg/d, start SSRI at usual starting dose and discontinue tricyclic over next 5–7 days, with careful observation.

Main potential problems (see above for details): Serotonin syndrome, raised tricyclic levels by P450 inhibition, cholinergic rebound or tricyclic withdrawal.

Tricyclic → citalopram or sertraline: As above, but less potential for interaction so problems less likely. A serotonin syndrome has been reported with sertraline and amitriptyline (Alderman *et al, Ann Pharmacother* 1996, **30**, 1499–500).

Fluoxetine → tricyclic: Stop fluoxetine, wait several days for peak levels to fall, then add tricyclic cautiously at low dose and build up slowly. Care is needed for up to four weeks as the interaction potential may be prolonged (see SSRI interactions *4.3.2*). An abrupt switch from fluoxetine 20mg/d to amitriptyline 50–100mg/d resulted in 14% dropping out due to adverse reactions, the rest tolerating the switch (Rutten *et al*, MI).

Main potential problems (see above for details): Serotonin syndrome (especially with drugs such as clomipramine) and higher tricyclic levels via CYP2D6 inhibition.

Paroxetine → tricyclic: Taper paroxetine dose to about 10mg/d, and introduce tricyclic at low dose. After several days, discontinue paroxetine and increase tricyclic dose to therapeutic levels.

Main potential problems (see above for details): Paroxetine withdrawal (see *17*), serotonin syndrome (especially with drugs such as clomipramine) and higher tricyclic levels via CYP2D6 inhibition.

Fluvoxamine → tricyclic: As paroxetine. Main potential problems (see above for details): Fluvoxamine withdrawal (rare, see *17*), serotonin syndrome (especially with drugs such as clomipramine) and higher tricyclic levels via CYP1A2 and 3A3/4 inhibition (especially with tertiary tricyclics).

Citalopram or sertraline → tricyclic: If necessary, reduce to minimum doses of citalopram (20mg/d) or sertraline (50mg/d). Stop SSRI and introduce tricyclic, titrating dose upwards as tolerated. With standard doses of SSRIs, few problems should be seen. A serotonin syndrome has been reported with sertraline and amitriptyline (Alderman *et al, Ann Pharmacother* 1996, **30**, 1499–500).

Main potential problems (see above for details): SSRI withdrawal (rare, see *17*), serotonin syndrome (especially with eg. clomipramine) and higher tricyclic levels via CYP2D6 inhibition (low risk).

3. **Trazodone** and **fluoxetine** have been used together but enhanced sedation (eg. *J Clin Psych* 1992, **53**, 83) and serotonin syndrome (George and Godleski, *Biol Psych* 1996, **39**, 384–85) have been reported. Fluoxetine can slightly raise trazodone levels (see *4.3.2.2*). A serotonin syndrome with low dose trazodone added to **paroxetine** would indicate the need for similar care (n=1, Reeves and Bullen, *Psychosomatics* 1995, **36**, 159–60). There is no information on changing from trazodone to the other SSRIs at present but a gradual switch, with close observation of the patient would seem sensible for all SSRIs. See also *5*.

4. No significant problems reported. A gradual switch from one **tricyclic** to another is recommended as per normal practice.

5. Any combination of **SSRIs** can precipitate a serotonin syndrome (see *1.30*). Thus, careful observation initially and a gentle change-over is recommended. A washout period would further minimise the possibility of problems. An example of potential problems has been shown in a report of a 'therapeutic substitution', where outpatients were abruptly swapped from **fluoxetine to sertraline** (20mg:50mg respectively dose substitution). 63%

swapped successfully but 37% failed, including 18% with intolerable adverse effects, (nervousness, jitters, nausea and headache), suggestive of a serotonin-like syndrome (n=54, Stock and Kofoed, *Am J Hosp Pharm* 1994, **51**, 2279–81). One study showed that abrupt switching from **fluoxetine to paroxetine** produced an increased level of side-effects such as insomnia, nausea, dry mouth, nervousness and tremor in the immediate switch group when compared to a two-week washout, which was well tolerated (n=240, d/b, Kreider *et al, J Clin Psych* 1995, **56**, 142–45). However, paroxetine had no effect on the kinetics of fluoxetine and norfluoxetine in a study (n=9, Dominguez *et al, J Clin Psychopharmacology* 1996, **16**, 320–23).

6. If **MAOIs** are stopped shortly before **nefazodone** is started, then initial care and a gradual dose introduction is appropriate. No other recommendations are available at the time of writing, but the **SSRI to nefazodone** switch may have problems. SSRIs typically have an antagonistic effect at 5-HT$_{2C}$ receptors, which is lost when discontinued, and mCPP (a major metabolite of nefazodone) has 5-HT$_{2C}$ agonist activity. When switching from an SSRI to nefazodone, this change in 5-HT$_{2C}$ status may produce some central effects, with dysphoria, anxiety and anxiety reported. It is best to taper the SSRI and introduce nefazodone gradually.

7. **MAOIs to/from SSRIs:** The time to wait between stopping an SSRI and starting an MAOI depends upon the respective SSRI. The SPC for tranylcypromine recommends leaving at least a seven-day gap after stopping other antidepressants, then starting tranylcypromine at half the usual dosage for one week. The BNF recommends a two-week gap from the SSRIs before an MAOI is started but this appears only to be strictly correct for paroxetine.

Fluvoxamine → MAOI: fluvoxamine has a short half-life and so isocarboxazid/phenelzine may be started 4–5 days after stopping fluvoxamine (4–5 x half-life) or 7 days for tranylcypromine.

Paroxetine → MAOI: two-week gap (MI).

Fluoxetine → MAOI: a serotonin syndrome has been reported when tranyl-cypromine was started six weeks after fluoxetine was stopped, due to persistence of norfluoxetine (but not fluoxetine) in the blood (letter in *Am J Psych* 1993, **150**, 837). Since several reported interactions exist, it might be better to allow 6 weeks after stopping fluoxetine before starting an MAOI (*Drug & Ther Bull* 1990, **28**, 334, BNF). The isocarboxazid SPC recommends a gap longer than 2 weeks.

Sertraline → MAOI: a one-week gap should elapse before starting an MAOI. A serotonergic syndrome has been reported with sertraline and tranyl-cypromine (see SSRI interactions 4.3.2). The manufacturer suggests that a two-week gap between sertraline and MAOI therapies would be prudent.

Trazodone → MAOI: the SPC recommends a one-week gap. In one study, combined treatment did not show hypertensive reactions but an increase in side-effect severity, eg. sedation, postural hypotension etc occurred (n=13, *J Clin Psychopharmacol* 1989, **9**, 42).

Moclobemide → MAOI: moclobemide has a half-life of 14 hours and so stopping moclobemide one day and starting another antidepressant the next day is adequate.

Mirtazapine → MAOI: a one-week wash-out period is recommended, by the UK manufacturers.

MAOI → SSRIs: a two-week gap (*Drug & Ther Bull* 1990, **28**, 33–34, BNF) has been suggested but longer may be safer as a severe serotonin syndrome has been reported with a two-week gap between stopping tranylcypromine and starting fluoxetine (Ruiz, *Ann Emerg Med* 1994, **24**, 983–85), even although tranylcypromine has a relatively short action (ie. reversible MAO inhibition).

MAOI → trazodone: the SPC recommends a two-week gap after stopping trazodone before MAOIs (see also trazodone to MAOI above).

MAOI → moclobemide: a gap is not needed between stopping an MAOI and starting moclobemide, provided MAOI dietary restrictions are maintained for 10–14 days.

MAOI → mirtazapine: a two-week wash-out period is recommended.

8. Due to a lack of clinical information, the manufacturers of **fluoxetine** recommend that normal MAOI procedures be observed for **moclobemide**, and so a two-week gap after stopping moclobemide is stated. This would appear over-cautious and Roche recommend that when changing to an SSRI only an 8–12 hour gap is needed.

9. **Tricyclics and MAOIs:** These have been used together uneventfully (see *1.14*) but have also interacted (see *4.3.4*):

MAOIs → tricyclic: a 10–14-day gap is often recommended (isocarboxazid '1–2 weeks') particularly if imipramine, desipramine, clomipramine or tranylcypromine are involved. Using initial low doses of the tricyclic is essential.

Tricyclic → MAOI: A one-week gap is recommended (BNF) and is advisable particularly if imipramine, clomipramine or tranylcypromine are involved. Using initial low doses of the MAOI is essential.

10. Behavioural and neurological toxicity has been reported with concomitant high dose **tryptophan** and **MAOIs** and so initial observation and care would seem advisable. See also *1*.

11. **Tryptophan** and **fluoxetine:** Cases of central toxicity, agitation and nausea have occurred with the combination and are suggested as likely to occur with other SSRIs. It would thus be prudent to observe the patient carefully and consider the possibility of a serotonergic syndrome developing.

12*.**Mirtazapine** has multiple routes of metabolism (2D6, 3A4 and 1A2) so switching problems will be unlikely in terms of P450 inhibition. The only recommendation is for MAOIs (see *7*). Fluoxetine 20–40mg/d has been switched abruptly to mirtazapine 15mg/d, without problems (n=40, Preskorn *et al, Biol Psych* 1997, **41**, 96S).

13. Two isolated cases exist of hypomania after abrupt change from **trazodone** to **imipramine** (*J Clin Psych* 1985, **5**, 342–43).

14. **SSRIs and moclobemide:** The SPC recommends a gap of 4–5 half-lives after stopping an SSRI before starting moclobemide, as serotonin syndromes have been reported (see *4.3.3.3*). However, in a study where up to 600mg/d moclobemide was added to established fluoxetine therapy, there was no change in the number, intensity, or type of adverse events. Fluoxetine markedly inhibited the metabolism of moclobemide but did not lead to excessive accumulation, and there was no evidence of the development of a 'serotonin syndrome' (Dingemanse *et al, Clin Pharmacol Ther* 1998, **63**, 403–13).

Citalopram → moclobemide: a 7-day gap is recommended.

Fluoxetine → moclobemide: with fluoxetine's long half-life, the gap should be as much as six weeks if five times the half-life of norfluoxetine is calculated. A gap of three weeks together with careful monitoring would seem a reasonably practical figure. See also above, where no clinically significant problem was apparent and a shorter gap may be appropriate.

Fluvoxamine → moclobemide: a 3-day gap is recommended (but see above).

Paroxetine → moclobemide: a 5-day gap is recommended (but see above), although paroxetine's half-life can be longer in the elderly.

Sertraline → moclobemide: with the long half-life of desmethylsertraline, the gap should be up to 13 days but 5 and 7 days is recommended by Roche and Pfizer respectively (but see above).

15. **Tricyclics and moclobemide:**

Tricyclic → moclobemide: a gap is recommended if the tricyclic concerned is a 5-HT reuptake inhibitor. Roche only mention clomipramine needing a 7-day gap (study by Laux *et al, Psychopharmacology Berlin* 1988, **96** [Suppl], 230) although theoretically amitriptyline (5-day gap) and imipramine (4-day gap) might be included as well. However, healthy volunteers taking either clomipramine 100mg/d or amitriptyline 75mg/d for at least a week, were swapped abruptly to moclobemide (150mg first day, 300mg/d thereafter) or placebo. There was no increase in incidence or severity of side-effects nor any significant pharmacokinetic interaction between the drugs (n=24, Dingemanse *et al, J Clin Psychopharmacol* 1995, **15**, 418).

Moclobemide → tricyclic: in an open study, patients on moclobemide were abruptly switched to maprotiline, doxepin or amitriptyline without incident, but switching to clomipramine caused some problems (Luax *et al, Psychopharmacology* 1988, **Suppl 96**, 230).

16. **Venlafaxine:**

MAOI → venlafaxine: Wyeth recommend a 14-day gap between stopping an MAOI and starting venlafaxine. This is appropriate as there are a number of reports of interactions, eg. extreme agitation, diaphoresis, rapid respiration and raised CPK after a 37.5mg dose of venlafaxine seven days after phenelzine 45mg/d was stopped (Phillips and Ringo, *Am J Psych* 1995, **152**, 1400–1) and serotonin syndrome (eg. n=4, Diamond *et al, Neurology* 1998, **51**, 274–76). In the first reported case, the reaction did not occur a further seven days later and strongly suggests that a 14-day gap is indeed required.

Venlafaxine → MAOI: Wyeth recommend a 7-day gap (see above).

Tricyclic → venlafaxine: 5 times the first drugs half-life should be allowed as a wash-out time before starting venlafaxine (MI). For some tricyclics this would require leaving a 2–3-week gap, an unnecessarily extended period. The company, however, have no evidence of any problems.

Venlafaxine → other drugs: no information.

Other drugs → venlafaxine: no information.

17*. **Withdrawal or discontinuation:**
Adverse discontinuation events have been reported for many antidepressants. Such symptoms are not, however, indicative of dependence, which usually requires **three** of the following:
- Tolerance
- Withdrawal symptoms
- Use greater than needed
- Inability to reduce doses
- Excessive time taken procuring drug
- Primacy of drug taking over other activities
- Continued use despite understanding of adverse effects.

Discontinuation symptoms have a number of characteristics, eg. they usually start within 1–2 days of stopping and resolve within 24hrs of restarting the drug, and are more common with longer courses or higher doses. They can occur with missed doses. The UK *Drug and Therapeutics Bulletin* (*Drug & Ther Bull* 1999, **37**, 49–52) recommends:
- After less than 8 weeks treatment, withdraw over 1–2 weeks
- After 6–8 months treatment, taper over a 6–8 week period
- After long-term maintenance treatment, reduce the dose by 25% every 4–6 weeks.

Management:
1. Reduce the dose stepwise every week or so, stabilising between reductions, eg. paroxetine 20mg/d, 10mg/d, 10mg alternate days (but not less frequently). Use of the syrup, gradually diluted, may also be effective
2. Transfer to a long half-life drug, eg. fluoxetine (care with switching), then reduce (clomipramine case, Benazzi, *Am J Psych* 1999, **156**, 661–62; venlafaxine case, Giakas and David, *Psychiatr Ann* 1997, **27**, 85–92)
3. Treat the emerging syndrome symptomatically, eg. nausea, headache and diarrhoea have been managed with ondansetron (n=1, Raby, *J Clin Psych* 1998, **59**, 621–22) and ginger root (Schechter, *J Clin Psych* 1998, **59**, 431–32).

Reviews: recognition, prevention and management of antidepressant withdrawal syndromes (Lejoyeux *et al, CNS Drugs* 1996, **5**, 278–92), general (Haddad, *J Clin Psych* 1998, **59**, 541–48; editorial, Edwards, *Prescriber* 1998, **11**, 107–9), WHO reporting system (Stahl *et al, Eur J Clin Pharmacol* 1997, **53**, 163–69).

Main withdrawal symptoms:
Tricyclics: cholinergic rebound, eg. headache, restlessness, diarrhoea, nausea and vomiting (Lieberman, *Psychosomatics* 1981, **22**, 253–54), flu, lethargy, abdominal cramps, sleep disturbance, movement disorders.

MAOIs: psychosis, hallucinations, disorientation, catatonia (n=2, Liskin *et al, J Clin Psychopharmacol* 1985, **5**, 46–47), irritability, hypomania (Rothchild, *J Clin Psychopharmacol* 1985, **5**,

340–41), nausea, sweating, palpitations, nightmares, delirium (Liebowitz *et al, Am J Psych* 1978, **135**, 1565–66).

SSRIs: dizziness, vertigo/lightheadedness, nausea, fatigue, headache, sensory disturbance, 'electric shocks' in the head, insomnia, abdominal cramps, chills, flu-like symptoms, increased dreaming, anxiety/agitation and volatility, not caused by anything else, eg. physical illness, other drugs etc. (occur if you 'FINISH' treatment, ie. Flu-like symptoms, Insomnia, Imbalance, Sensory disturbance, Hyperarousal; Berber, *J Clin Psych* 1998, **59**, 255).

Reviews of SSRI withdrawal (Zajecka *et al, J Clin Psych* 1997, **58**, 291–97; *J Clin Psych* 1997, **58**[Suppl 7], 5–40).

Specific drugs:

SSRIs

Comparative data: There have been a number of comparative studies. Interruption for 5–8 days of maintenance therapy produced few discontinuation symptoms with fluoxetine (long half-life), some with sertraline and most with paroxetine (n=242, RCT, d/b, 4/52, Rosenbaum *et al, Biol Psych* 1998, **44**, 77–87, study funded by Lilly). In another study, suddenly discontinuing fluoxetine showed slightly more dizziness and somnolence at weeks 2–4, but no difference at week 6 compared to continuous treatment (RCT, n=395, 12/52, Zajecka *et al, J Clin Psychopharmacol* 1998, **18**, 193–97; review, Kendrick, *EBMH* 1999, **2**, 31). A third study of 5-day interruption showed increased symptoms after a second missed dose with paroxetine, with impaired functional performance at five days, sertraline with less pronounced changes, and fluoxetine with no significant symptoms (n=107, RCT, Michelson *et al, B J Psych* 2000, **174**, 363–68).

Paroxetine: has been associated with more discontinuation reports than other SSRIs (Young *et al, B J Psych* 1997, **170**, 288). Cases reports include fever, severe fatigue, headache, nausea, vomiting and agitation (eg. Debattista and Schatzberg, *Am J Psych* 1995, **152**, 1235–36) and electrical shock-like sensations (Frost and Lal, *Am J Psych* 1995, **152**, 180). This phenomenon may

be more frequent because paroxetine inhibits its own CYP2D6 metabolism and, as concentrations fall, less inhibition occurs and levels fall quicker, leading to a more rapid drop (discussed by Preskorn, *Int Clin Psychopharmacol* 1994, **9**[Suppl 3], 139). Discontinuation symptoms tend to resolve in a few days or on reintroduction of paroxetine. The CSM recommends tapering if withdrawal symptoms occur, ie. stop if problems occur then restart and taper over 12 weeks, with either half-tablet doses or alternate day (but not less frequently) therapy. However, even a four-week gradual dose reduction may not prevent significant symptoms of vertigo, light-headedness and gait instability, so care is needed (n=5, Pacheco *et al, B J Psych* 1996, **169**, 384).

Fluoxetine: has a long half-life and discontinuation problems are rare eg. isolated cases of extreme dizziness 3–14 days after fluoxetine stopped (Einbinder, *Am J Psych* 1995, **152**, 1235), of severe, dull, aching pain in the left arm after abrupt withdrawal, which remitted after reintroduction (Lauterbach, *Neurology* 1994, **44,** 983–84) and of reversible delirium (Kasantikul, *J Med Assoc Thailand* 1995, **78**, 53–54).

Sertraline: discontinuation reactions are relatively uncommon, eg. fatigue, cramps, insomnia etc, which resolved on restarting and where tapering over about 14 weeks was successful (Louie *et al, Am J Psych* 1994, **151**, 450–51), electrical shock-like sensations (Frost and Lal, *Am J Psych* 1995, **152**, 180) and postural hypotension (Amsden and Georgian, *Pharmacotherapy* 1996, **16**, 684–86).

Citalopram*: even rapid discontinuation appears only to produce mild and transient effects (n=225, Markowitz *et al, Int Clin Psychopharmacol* 2000, **15**, 329–33).

Fluvoxamine: a slow withdrawal may be preferred (Szabadi, *B J Psych* 1992, **160**, 283–84).

Nefazodone: 'electrical sensations down the legs', dizziness and nausea have been reported for 2–3 days after abrupt cessation of nefazodone (final dose 200mg bd, 9/7 course, n=1,

Kotlyar *et al, Am J Psych* 1999, **156**, 1117).

Tryptophan: many patients had their tryptophan stopped abruptly after it was withdrawn from the market without apparent serious withdrawal problems, other than recurrence of depression.

Venlafaxine: if used for more than six weeks, withdrawal over at least a week is recommended by the manufacturers. A 1999 UK SPC change includes withdrawal reactions from abrupt cessation, dose reduction or tapering of venlafaxine, and includes fatigue, headache, nausea, vomiting, dizziness, dry mouth, diarrhoea, insomnia, nervousness, confusion, paraesthesia, sweating and vertigo. Other symptoms include, abdominal distension and congested sinuses (n=1, resolving within 12 hours of restarting, Farah and Lauer, *Am J Psych* 1996, **153**, 576), gastrointestinal upset (which responded to re-introduction and then slow reduction over 1–4 weeks, n=3, Louie *et al, Am J Psych* 1996, **153**, 1652) and classic SSRI-type discontinuation symptoms (eg. confusion, headache, agitation, abdominal distension and sweating) occurring 16 and 20 hours after stopping (n=2, Agelink *et al, Am J Psych* 1997, **154**, 1473–74; review of similarity to SSRI symptoms, n=13, Boyd, *Med J Aus* 1998, **169**, 91–92). An outpatient study showed that 7 of the 9 patients discontinuing sustained-release venlafaxine reported the emergence of adverse reactions, compared to 2 of the 9 stopping placebo (n=9, d/b, p/c, Fava *et al, Am J Psych* 1997, **154**, 1760–62).

Mirtazapine*: a withdrawal hypomania is all that has been reported to date (n=1, MacCall and Callender, *B J Psych* 1999, **175**, 390).

Reboxetine: no withdrawal or discontinuation syndrome has been observed in studies with reboxetine, with few additional effects on abrupt withdrawal (SPC). There is no data on switching antidepressants, other than a requirement for a gap with MAOIs.

Table 2.3 — SELECTING DRUGS, DOSES & PREPARATIONS: LIQUIDS & INJECTIONS

Drug	Commercial liquid	Extemporaneous liquid[1]	Injection[2]	Other
Antidepressants[1,2]				
Amitriptyline	10mg/5ml[3] 25mg/5ml[3] syrup 50mg/5ml[3] syrup	Possible[27]	10mg/ml IM/IV s/c possible[28]	Suppositories[22]
Amoxapine	-	Possible[34]	N/K	N/K
Citalopram	-	1mg/drop??	Reported[53]	N/K
Clomipramine	25mg/5ml syrup	-	25mg/2ml IM/IV	N/K
Dothiepin (dosulepin)	25mg/5ml SF syrup[3] 75mg/5ml SF syrup[3] Any strength[7]	-	N/K	Suppositories[7]
Doxepin	-	Mentioned in USP[25]	N/K	Suppositories[43]
Fluoxetine	20mg/5ml liquid	-	N/K	Sub-lingual[50]
Flupentixol	-	Import possible[39]	Depot	N/K
Fluvoxamine	-	No hard data[40]	N/K	N/K
Imipramine	25mg/5ml syrup	-	N/K	N/K
Isocarboxazid	-	1/52 expiry possible	N/K	N/K
Lofepramine	70mg/5ml susp[3]		N/K	N/K
Maprotiline	-	?	N/K	N/K
Mianserin	-	Yes[19]	N/K	N/K
Mirtazapine	-	NK	IV[48]	-
Moclobemide	-	Yes[44]	N/K	N/K
Nefazodone	-	NK	N/K	N/K
Nortriptyline	-	Yes[20]	N/K	N/K
Paroxetine	10mg/5ml	-	N/A	N/A
Phenelzine	-	Not possible[18]	N/K	N/K
Reboxetine	-	NK	N/K	N/K
Sertraline	-	Just possible[29]	N/K	N/K
Tranylcypromine	-	3/12 expiry possible	N/K	N/K
Trazodone	50mg/5ml syrup	-	N/A[21]	N/K
Tryptophan	-	-	N/K	N/K
Venlafaxine	-	-	N/K	N/K
Benzodiazepines and anxiolytics				
Alprazolam	-	Tabs can be crushed	N/K	N/K
Bromazepam	-	N/K	N/K	N/K
Buspirone	-	N/K	N/K	N/K
Chlordiazepoxide	-	Yes[47]	N/K	N/K
Clorazepate	-	-	N/K	N/K?
Diazepam	2mg & 5mg/5ml susp[9] 1mg & 2.5mg/5ml SF syrup[3] Variable[9]	-	5mg/ml IV/IM[8]	Rectal tubules[45] Suppositories
Hydroxyzine	-	N/K	N/K	N/K
Loprazolam	-	N/K	N/K	N/K
Lorazepam	-	N/K	4mg/ml IV/IM[4]	Rectal, sub-lingual tabs[4]
Meprobamate	-	Mentioned in USP	N/K	N/K
Midazolam	-	Yes[42]	2mg/ml 5mg/ml	Intranasal[17] Buccal[17]
Nitrazepam	2.5mg/5ml susp 5mg/5ml susp[3]	-	N/K	N/K
Oxazepam	-	N/K	N/K	N/K
Propranolol	Various[3]	-	1mg/ml	N/K
Temazepam	10mg/5ml syrup	-	N/K	N/K
Antipsychotics				
Benperidol	-	N/K	N/K	N/K
Chlorpromazine	25mg/5ml syrup 50mg/5ml SF syrup[3] 100mg/5ml syrup[3] 100mg/5ml susp	-	25mg/ml IM 100mg/ml[5]	Suppositories

Table 2.3 — SELECTING DRUGS, DOSES & PREPARATIONS: LIQUIDS & INJECTIONS

Drug	Commercial liquid	Extemporaneous liquid[1]	Injection[2]	Other
Clozapine	-	Possible[6]	N/K	N/K
Flupentixol	-	Import possible[39]	Depot	N/K
Fluphenazine	-	2/52 expiry possible	Depot	N/K
Fluspirilene	-	N/K	Depot	N/K
Haloperidol	1mg & 2mg/ml 1, 1.5 & 2mg/5ml SF syrup3 10mg/ml concentrate	-	5mg/ml IM/IV 10mg/ml IM/IV Depot	N/K
Levomepromazine	-	Yes[32]	25mg/ml IV/IM/SC	N/K
Loxapine	-	Known in USA[35]	Known in USA[35]	N/K
Olanzapine	-	Velotabs, plus Extemp possible[51]	Awaited [54]	-
Pericyazine	10mg/5ml syrup	-	N/K	N/K
Perphenazine	2mg/5ml SF syrup[3] 4mg/5ml SF syrup[3]	-	Known[30]	N/K
Pimozide	-	N/K	N/K	N/K
Prochlorperazine	5mg/5ml syrup	-	12.5mg/ml IV	Suppositories
Promazine	12.5mg/5ml SF syrup[3] 50mg/5ml susp 50mg/5ml SF syrup[3]	-	50mg/ml IM	N/K
Quetiapine	-	NK	NK	NK
Risperidone	Img/ml	-	Depot planned	N/K
Sulpiride	200mg/5ml SF syrup[3]	-	N/K	N/K
Thioridazine	10mg/5ml syrup[3] 25mg/5ml syrup 50mg/5ml SF syrup[3] 100mg/5ml SF syrup[3] 100mg/5ml susp	-	N/K	N/K
Trifluoperazine	1mg/5ml syrup 5mg/5ml SF syrup[3] 10mg/ml concentrate	-	1mg/ml IM	N/K
Zuclopenthixol	-	2/52 expiry extemp[13] plus imports[13]	Depot + Acuphase	N/K

Anticonvulsants

Drug	Commercial liquid	Extemporaneous liquid[1]	Injection[2]	Other
Carbamazepine	100mg/5ml liquid	-	N/K	Rectal[15]
Clomethiazole	192mg/5ml syrup	-		?
Clonazepam	2.5mg/5ml [3]	-	1mg/ml see BNF	N/K
Clobazam	-	Any strength[24]	N/K	N/K
Diazepam	See benzodiazepines			
Ethosuximide	250mg/5ml syrup	Capsules [46]	N/K	N/K
Gabapentin	-	Not advised[26]	N/K	N/K
Lamotrigine	-	Dispersable tablets[38]	N/K	Rectal possible[38]
Levetiracetam	-	-	-	-
Oxcarbazepine	-	-	-	-
Paraldehyde	Pure	Various	Pure[16]	Enema[10]
Phenobarbital	15mg/5ml	-	200mg/ml IM/IV	?
Phenytoin	30mg/5ml susp 90mg/5ml SF susp[3]	-	50mg/ml IM/IV	Rectal possible [49]
Primidone	250mg/5ml susp	-	N/K	N/K
Tiagabine				
Topiramate		Sprinkle capsules[52]		
Valproate	200mg/5ml syrup 200mg/5ml SF liquid	Others known[33]	400mg IV	Suppositories[12]
Vigabatrin	-	Sachets[41]	N/K	N/K

Hypnotics

Drug	Commercial liquid	Extemporaneous liquid[1]	Injection[2]	Other
Benzodiazepines	See benzodiazepines			
Chloral	'Welldorm' 500mg/5ml syrup[3]	-	N/K	Rectal possible
Clomethiazole	See anticonvulsants			
Promethazine	5mg/5ml syrup	-	N/K	N/K
Triclofos	500mg/5ml syrup	-	N/K	N/K
Zaleplon	-	N/K	N/K	N/K
Zolpidem	-	N/K	N/K	N/K
Zopiclone	-	N/K	N/K	N/K

Drug	Commercial liquid	Extemporaneous liquid[1]	Injection[2]	Other
Table 2.3 — SELECTING DRUGS, DOSES & PREPARATIONS: LIQUIDS & INJECTIONS				
Anticholinergics				
Benzhexol	2mg/5ml SF soln[3] 5mg/5ml syrup	Yes[31]	N/K	N/K
Benztropine	-	N/K	1mg/ml IM/IV	N/K
Biperidin	-	N/K	N/K	N/K
Orphenadrine	25mg/5ml syrup 50mg/5ml SF syrup[3]		N/K	N/K
Procyclidine	2.5mg & 5mg/5ml syrup	Injection used [36]	5mg/ml IV/IM?	N/K
Miscellaneous				
Cyproterone	-	3/12 expiry	Named pt basis	N/K
Disulfiram	-	Disp. tablets[11]	Implants tried[23]	N/K
Lithium	5.4 mmol/5ml 10.8 mmol/5ml	-	N/K	Vaginal [14]
Tetrabenazine	50mg/5ml SF syrup[3]	Yes[37]	N/K	N/K

N/K = no information known to the UK manufacturers   SF = sugar-free

1. Extemporaneously prepared antidepressant liquids need care as most tricyclics have marked local anaesthetic actions.
2. Review of IV antidepressants in *Int Drug Therapy Newsletter* 1981, **16**, 35.
3. Produced by Rosemont Pharmaceuticals, Leeds (address in BNF). Some are 'specials'.
4. IM injections of lorazepam must be diluted with an equal quantity of water or saline and used only where oral or IV routes are not possible. A sub-lingual presentation of lorazepam is available in US (Greenblatt *et al, J Pharmaceut Scin* 1982, **71**, 248–52). Rectal use of lorazepam is possible (*Paediatr Neurol* 1987, **3**, 321–26).
5. 100mg/ml chlorpromazine concentrate is a 'special' from Penn Pharmaceuticals.
6. A clozapine suspension is possible (*Pharm J*, 1996, **257**, 190–91), using Guy's Hospital Paediatric base and stable for up to 18 days.
7. Various strengths of dothiepin are available as a 'special' from Knoll, eg. 25mg, 50mg or 75mg in 5ml or 10ml dose units. Knoll Specials Manufacturing Unit have made suppositories to special order and could provide powder if necessary.
8. Available as diazepam solution ('Valium') and diazepam emulsion ('Diazemuls').
9. Diazepam 5mg/5ml syrup available from Lagap Pharmaceuticals.
10. Paraldehyde can be used as an enema, diluted 50:50 either with arachis oil or water (see entry in *1.17.2*).
11. 'Antabuse' tablets are readily dispersible.
12. Report of valproate suppositories in *Arch Neurol* 1989, **46**, 906–9. 300mg and 100mg suppositories available on named-patient basis from Sanofi Winthrop Ltd, Floats Road, Wythenshawe, Manchester M23 9NF.
13. 2mg/5ml and 20mg/5ml syrups of zuclopenthixol are available in other parts of Europe. Lundbeck's export department in Copenhagen would be able to advise on availability.
14. Vaginal absorption of lithium appears possible (case report Tente *et al, JAMA* 1994, **272**, 1723–24).
15. A rectal gel of carbamazepine has been used (*Clin Pharm* 1990, **9**, 13–14, Storey & Trimble *NEJM* 1992, **327**, 1318–19). Carbamazepine suppositories are available in UK, at 125mg and 250mg. 125mg rectally is equivalent to 100mg orally so increase the oral dose by 25% to convert to rectal, with a maximum rectal dose 250mg qds for 7 days.
16. Special from Penn Pharmaceuticals.
17*. Intranasal midazolam is possible, and as effective as IV diazepam in febrile seizures (n=47, RCT, Lahat *et al, BMJ* 2000, **321**, 83-86) and acute anxiety in children (n=43, Ljungman *et al, Pediatrics* 2000, **105**, 73-78; Wallace, *Lancet* 1997, **349**, 222 editorial). Buccal/sublingual absorption of midazolam is possible as an alternative to rectal diazepam for acute seizures in refractory epilepsy (RCT, Scott *et al, Lancet* 1999, **353**, 623–26, comment by Wiebe, *Evidence-Based Med* 2000, **5**, 20, disputed by Ellis *et al, Lancet* 1999, **353**, 1796).
18. Phenelzine is too unstable in water for even a short-dated liquid to be made.
19. A solution with a seven-day expiry is possible but the very strong local anaesthetic action of mianserin makes this distinctly unpleasant.
20. A commercial nortriptyline syrup was available in the UK at one time and is available in USA at 10mg/5ml.
21. A trazodone injection was once tested some years ago.
22. Amitriptyline is absorbed rectally (*Pharmacotherapy* 1990, **10**, 256) and so suppositories are possible and have been reported to successful (*NEJM* 1982, **306**, 996).
23. Implants of disulfiram can be tried but do not prove to be particularly successful. They are available on a named-patient basis, imported from G Streuli and Co AG (Ltd), Pharmazutika, 8730, Uznach, Switzerland. They consist of 100mg tablets (10+) implanted subcutaneously in the lower left quadrant of the abdominal wall

24. Extemporaneous liquids of clobazam are possible, stable for one month at room temperature. Hoechst UK have a formula.
25. Doxepin has a bitter taste but an extemporaneous preparation has been made for this freely soluble drug (Pfizer have a formula).
26. Gabapentin capsules can be broken open and the contents swallowed but it has an unpleasant taste. The drug itself is soluble, more particularly in acid solution. Rectal absorption of gabapentin has been shown to be poor (n=2, Kriel *et al, Epilepsia* 1997, **38**, 1242–44).
27. An extemporaneous liquid of amitriptyline can be made (*J Clin Pharm* 1976, **1**, 107), which has an eight-week expiry.
28. A small study showed that sub-cutaneous amitriptyline may be possible (*Acta Univ Palacki Olomuc, Fac Med* 1968, **49**, 291–305).
29. Sertraline is poorly soluble and has a particularly unpleasant bitter taste. A suspension in methylcellulose suspending base would be needed but as no stability data exists this would have to have a very short expiry.
30. A perphenazine injection is made by Schering in the USA.
31. The formula for an extemporaneous benzhexol syrup, stable for 4 weeks, is held by Lederle.
32. A levomepromazine syrup has been used at Bangour Hospital, West Lothian, stable for 7 days in a fridge.
33. Valproate solutions of 200mg/ml and 300mg/ml are available in many countries, eg. Austria, Netherlands etc.
34. There is no theoretical reason why a short-expiry suspension of amoxapine could not be made.
35*. A 25mg/ml oral concentrate of loxapine is available in USA (Lederle). An extemporaneous liquid could be made, but needs to be in an acid solution. A 50mg/ml IM injection is also available in the USA (Lederle) and can be used subcutaneously (Saunder *et al, Am J Health-System Pharm* 1999, **56**, 1259-61).
36. Procyclidine injection in glycerin and orange syrup is possible (7 day expiry) for oral use.
37. Tetrabenazine 10mg/ml syrup using 'Nitoman' tablets has been used.
38. Dispersable tablets of 5mg, 25mg and 100mg are available in UK. Rectal absorption of lamotrigine compressed tablets is possible, but is not as quick or complete as when given orally (n=12, RCT, Birnbaum *et al, Epilepsia* 2000, **41**, 850-53).
39. Flupentixol drops containing 100mg/ml or 4mg/ml are available in some European countries. Lundbeck's export department in Copenhagen would be able to advise on availability.
40. Fluvoxamine is not available as a syrup. Duphar state that tablets can be crushed to form a suspension of unknown stability, which needs to be prepared freshly each time.
41. Sachets of pure vigabatrin powder are available from Marion Merrell Dow Ltd. which can be added to a drink immediately before use, or through a nasogastric tube if necessary.
42. A stable oral solution of midazolam is possible (Steedman *et al, Am J Hosp Pharm* 1992, **49**, 615–18, Mehta *et al, Hosp Pharm Pract* 1993, **3**, 224–26), eg. stable for 14 days at 4°C in flavoured liquid gelatin (Bhatt-Mehta, *Am J Hosp Pharm* 1993, **50**, 472–5). Buccal liquid midazolam may be as effective as rectal diazepam for treatment of prolonged seizures, and more socially acceptable and convenient (n=42, RCT, Scott *et al, Lancet* 1999, **353**, 623–26, editorial, *ibid*, 608-9). For midazolam pharmacokinetics following intravenous and buccal administration, see Schwagmeier *et al* (*B J Clin Pharmacol* 1998, **46**, 203–6). Intranasal midazolam have been used for childhood seizures (Lahat *et al. Lancet* 1998, **352**, 620 letter).
43. Rectal doxepin given as capsules has been mentioned (Storey & Trimble, *NEJM* 1992, **327**, 1318–19)
44. Moclobemide tablets can be dispersed in water and the liquid (including sediment) taken.
45. Available as 'Stesolid' (Dumex) and 'Rectubes' (CP). Absorption from 'Stesolid' rectal solution peaks at 15 minutes (Moolenaar *et al, Int J Pharmaceutics* 1980, **5**, 127–37). An unmarketed diazepam rectal gel (Diastat) displays rapid, consistent absorption and is well tolerated. Alterations in cognition were mild and dissipated within 4hr of drug administration and it may offer an easy, safe and bioavailable method to administer diazepam (Cloyd *et al, Epilepsia* 1998, **39**, 520–26, comparison of rectal diazepam gel and placebo for acute repetitive seizures, Dreifuss *et al, NEJM* 1998, **338**, 1869–75).
46. Warner Lambert state that ethosuximide capsules can be cooled until solid and then cut up and mixed with food. Alternatively, the liquid content of 'Zarontin' capsules can be emptied out and mixed with warm water or other drinks. No stability data exists and so these actions should only be done at the time of each dose.
47. Roche have the formula for a chlordiazepoxide 2mg/ml syrup using 'Librium' capsules, which is stable for one week in a fridge.
48. An IV injection of mirtazapine is licensed in Germany.
49*. Absorption of 200mg phenytoin from rectal suppositories with polyethylene glycol base is highly variable, unpredictable and not recommended (n=6, open, Burstein *et al, Pharmacother* 2000, **20**, 562–67), although suggested as possible (Chang *et al, Ann Pharmacother* 1999, **33**, 781–86).
50*. Fluoxetine can be absorbed sub-lingually from the oral liquid to give therapeutic blood levels (n=2, Pakyurek and Pasol, *Am J Psych* 1999, **156**, 1833–34).
51*. A liquid olanzapine has been prepared (Harvey *et al, Pharm J* 2000, **265**, 275–76). Dispersible tablets are also available.
52* Topiramate 'sprinkle' capsules (50mg) are available in UK (*Pharm J* 2000, **265**, 866).
53*. An IV formulation of citalopram has been reported.
    For sources of unlicensed products, see the section near the end of *Chapter 1*.
54* An IM olanzapine injection is close to marketing.

2.4 WEIGHT CHANGES WITH PSYCHOTROPIC DRUGS

Importance

Drug-induced weight gain is a potential threat to health, lowers self-esteem and the social embarrassment caused may lead to non-concordance (and hence risks relapse). The available data is difficult to compare due to the non-equivalence of collection and presentation.

Some body weight gain is common with many psychotropic drugs, and although in most instances the gain is not 'clinically' significant (although it may be significant to the individual), the gain induced by some drugs, such as lithium and atypical antipsychotics, *can* be large and clinically significant. Risk factors for weight increase have not yet been well characterised, although in general drug-induced bodyweight gain is greatest in individuals with a past and/or family history of obesity (Ackerman and Nolan, *CNS Drugs* 1998, **9**, 135–51, 96 refs).

Review: body weight changes with psychotropics (mechanisms and management, Pijl and Meinders, *Drug Safety* 1996, **14**, 329–42).

ANTIPSYCHOTICS

The FDA definition of 'clinically significant' weight gain is 7% or greater increase over baseline weight. Phenothiazines appear to have the most potent appetite stimulating effect and up to 80% of people treated with it gain weight. Most weight is gained in the first 6–12 months of treatment and then stabilises, being maintained for at least two years. Loxapine and weekly pimozide have been reported to induce weight loss, although daily pimozide may cause a gain in weight (Falloon *et al, Psychological Med* 1978, **8**, 59–70). Weight gain is a common side-effect of olanzapine, with many gaining significant amounts. Although the degree of weight gain is probably similar to clozapine, it appears to be at least partly reversible by nutritional advice and exercise (retrospective study, males, n=90, Wirshing *et al, J Clin Psych* 1999, **60**, 358–63), unlike clozapine, where it is greater than the other atypicals and appears to be sustained despite nutritional advice and exercise.

Relative weight gain with antipsychotics (Allison *et al, Am J Psych* 1999, **156**, 1686–96, 96 refs, reviewed by Fenton, *EBMH* 2000, **3**, 58)

	Long-term change *	95% CI	Change at 10/52†
Pimozide	-2.7	-9.3–3.9	–
Placebo	-1	-1.8–0.1	0.4 (-1.3–0.5)
Trifluoperazine	0.3	-0.9–1.5	–
Ziprasidone	0.3	-0.3–0.8	0 (-0.5–0.6)
Haloperidol	0.5	0.2–0.8	0.5 (0.1–1)
Polypharmacy	0.5	0.2–0.7	1.2 (0.4–2.1)
Loxapine	0.7	-2.6–3.9	–
Non-drug controls	0.8	0.1–1.6	1.3 (0.8–1.8)
Fluphenazine	1.1	0.1–2.2	0.4 (-0.7–1.5)
Risperidone	1.7	1.4–2	2 (1.6–2.4)
Quetiapine	2.5	1.5–3.5	–
Thioridazine	2.8	1.6–4	3.4 (1.8–5.2)
Sertindole	2.9	2.7–3.2	3 (1.8–4.1)
Olanzapine	4.2	3.7–4.6	3.5 (3.3–3.7)
Chlorpromazine	4.2	2.9–5.4	2.1 (0.9–3.4)
Clozapine	5.7	4.3–7	4 (2.7–5.3)
Perphenazine	5.8	0.4–11.1	–

* longer-term weight change in kg (random effects model)
† weight change at 10 weeks (fixed effects model)
Please bear in mind that this is aggregated data, so subject to error, weight was often measured at a different time and there may be a dose-relationship.

Numerous mechanisms have been proposed, including:

- Sedation – leading to decreased activity
- Thirst – anticholinergic dry mouth may increase fluid and calorie intake
- Reduced metabolism – fat and carbohydrate oxidation
- Neurotransmitter-mediated increase in appetite, leading to increased food intake. The effect may be via $5-HT_{2C}$ and $5-HT_{2A}$ receptor blockade (rats without a $5-HT_{2C}$ receptor become obese), H1 or H2 receptor affinity (retrospective study, males, n=90, Wirshing *et al, J Clin Psych* 1999, **60**, 358–63) and perhaps D2-blockade and polypeptides such as CCK (review by Stahl, *J Clin Psych* 1998, **59**, 500–1)
- Changes in leptin levels – Leptin is a multifunctional polypeptide produced by fat cells and is thought to signal the size of the adipose tissue to the brain. Weight gain induced by clozapine or olanzapine seems related to an increase in leptin levels (n=44, Kraus *et al, Am J Psych* 1999, **156**, 312–14), and may explain why the gain is seen predominantly around the waist. Other polypeptides, eg. reductin, may also be implicated
- Fluid retention – via peripheral oedema, a minor effect
- Endocrine effects – increased prolactin (which may promote adiposity and is related to weight gain in men, Baptista *et al, Pharmacopsychiatry* 1997, **30**, 250–55), variation in cortisol, altered insulin secretion.

Most weight is gained during the first 12–16 weeks of therapy, although can still continue for 6 months. It can be more marked during in-patient stays, perhaps due to lower physical activity. A large US survey (schizophrenics n=570, non-schizophrenic comparators n=97,819) showed male schizophrenics to be as obese as the general population, but female schizophrenics to be as, or more, obese than the general population, suggesting that weight gain is a significant problem particularly for females taking antipsychotics (Allison *et al, J Clin Psych* 1999, **60**, 215–20).

Reviews*: Taylor and McAskill, *Acta Psych Scand* 2000, **101**, 416–32, 94 refs; Baptista, *Acta Psych Scand* 1999, **100**, 3–16; 163 refs, Allison *et al, Am J Psych* 1999, **156**, 1686–96.

Management

(substantial review by Baptista, *Acta Psych Scand* 1999, **100**, 3–16, 163 refs)

Like all of us, people taking antipsychotics are increasingly aware of the harmful effects of sustained obesity.

1. Routinely take a baseline weight measurement, and warn the patient of the potential for change in weight, difficulty in predicting outcome, plateau effect after several months, need to optimise calorie intake etc.

2. Particularly counsel patients with a higher risk of weight gain, eg. being female, prone to overeat when under stress, narcissistic personality traits, family or personal history of obesity and a greater than 6.5kg difference between adult maximum and minimum weights (Kalucy, *Drugs* 1980, **19**, 268–78).

3. Consult a dietician and seek advice, since most weight is gained in the first few months and it is easier to prevent weight gain than lose it once gained. Moderate physical exercise may be helpful and carbohydrate craving and excessive intake of high calorie fluids avoided.

4. Adjust the dose. The relationship between dose and weight gain is complex, but generally only a major reduction is likely to help. A slower introduction of, eg. olanzapine may reduce final weight gain.

5. Appetite suppressants may exacerbate psychosis or fail to work, although bromocriptine and amantadine may induce weight loss (Correa *et al, J Clin Psychopharmacol* 1987, **7**, 91–95).

6*.Intermittent and low-dose anti-psychotics, although controversial, have been recommended (Buchanan and Carpenter, *CNS Drugs* 1996, **5**, 240–45). For clozapine, adjunctive quetiapine has been used. After 6 months on clozapine (200–800mg/d), patients had 25% dose converted to quetiapine (using ratio 1mg clozapine:2mg quetiapine) for 10 months. The average weight loss was 0.22–10.5kg after one-month, and maintained, with 100% user satisfaction reported (open, 10/12, n=65, Reinstein *et al, Clin Drug Invest* 1999, **18**, 99–104).

7. Two other strategies have been suggested, although neither has been researched in people taking antipsychotics. Metformin may decrease weight and improve endocrine disturbances in primarily obese people (Fontobonne *et al, Diabetes Care* 1996, **19**, 920–26), and may have a role in antipsychotic-induced weight gain. Estrogen (which promotes weight loss by several mechanisms) and tamoxifen show a possible preventative role in animal studies (see Baptista, *Acta Psych Scand* 1999, **100**, 3–16).

ANTIDEPRESSANTS

Weight change in depression is well known and weight loss or gain can be part of the presenting symptoms. Although weight gain with antidepressants may be reversal of a pre-treatment weight loss in some people (although heavier people are more likely to gain weight if they become depressed, n=68, *Psych Res* 1991, **38**, 197–200), the main cause seems to be a decreased metabolic rate (Fernstein *et al, Biol Psych* 1985, **20**, 688–92) rather than improved mood. It is important that this fact is recognised as it is relevant in the management of this adverse effect. There is also an association with tricyclics of strong antihistaminic actions.

SSRIs *

Overall, there is a tendency with SSRIs for weight loss over the first 6 weeks, then gradually to regain this over 6 months, and then many may gain weight over the longer-term (reviewed by Sussman and Ginsberg, *Psych Ann* 1998, **28**, 89–97). In the short-term, SSRIs may increase metabolic rate, suppress appetite, and increase basal body temperature (n=20, *Am J Clin Nutrition* 1995, **61**, 1020). **Fluoxetine** acute therapy is associated with modest weight loss, with any weight gain after that due to recovery from depression, rather than any other mechanism (n=839, Michelson *et al, Am J Psych* 1999, **156**, 1170–76). Pooled data shows that more obese patients tend to lose more weight and weight loss is directly proportional to baseline weight. Underweight people may tend to gain weight (review in *Clin Pharm* 1989, **8**, 727–33). In a trial of obese patients, fluoxetine 60mg/d produced greater weight loss than placebo until 20 weeks, when this tended to wear off and the advantage of fluoxetine over placebo at 52 weeks was not clinically significant (n=458, RCT, Goldstein *et al, Int J Obesity* 1994, **18**, 129–35). **Paroxetine** has a slight clinically insignificant weight loss potential (*J Psychopharmacol* 1990, **4**, 300, n=71, Christiansen *et al, Acta Psych Scand* 1996, **93**, 158–63) although one study showed 30% of 61 patients gained 1–4kg (*Acta Psych Scand* 1992, **86**, 437–44). **Fluvoxamine** causes a non-significant weight loss (*J Psychopharmacol* 1990, **4**, 299) at 100–150mg/d over six months (Harris and Ashford, *B J Clin Res* 1991, **2**, 81–88). **Sertraline** may have a limited weight gain effect. No significant weight changes have been reported with **citalopram** (Milne & Goa, *Drugs* 1991, **41**, 450–77) although 8 of 18 patients treated with citalopram at one clinic showed carbohydrate craving and weight gain, particularly early on in treatment (Bouwer and Harvey, *Int Clin Psychopharmacol* 1996, **11**, 273–78). **Review**: role of serotonin in regulating food intake and food selection (Pijl and Meinders, *J Serotonin Res* 1994, **1**, 21–45).

Tricyclics

Weight gain with tricyclics is well-documented but not as well known or appreciated as it should be. The two main causes are drug-induced carbohydrate craving (Paykel, *B J Psych* 1973, **123**, 501–7) **and** a decreased metabolic rate (Fernstein *et al, Biol Psych* 1985, **20**, 688–92), rather than improved mood.

Little comparative data is available, but weight gain has been reported with **amitriptyline** (89% of patients; see also n=73, Christiansen *et al, Acta Psych Scand* 1996, **93**, 158–63) and nortriptyline (67%) in one of the few comparative studies (Fernstrom and Kupfer, *Psych Res* 1988, **26**, 256–71). With **imipramine** at an average of 215mg/d, less than a 5% weight change occurred in over 50% of people, with 13% gaining more than 10%, most of whom had lost weight before treatment (*J Aff Dis* 1990, **20**, 165–72) and 46% of 57 patients in another study gained 1–6kg with imipramine (*Acta Psych Scand* 1992, **86**, 437–44). With **clomipramine**, 22% of 67 patients gained weight, averaging 1.1kg over 8 months (*B J Psych* 1992, **160**, 519–24).

MAOIs and RIMAs

With the MAOIs, weight gain may be related to reduced blood glucose concentrations stimulating hunger or through central mechanisms. Weight gain is very rare with **tranylcypromine** and weight loss is more likely (*J Clin Psychopharmacol* 1985, **5**, 2–9). **Phenelzine** is the most widely implicated (45 reports, including 32 of over 15lbs added). 15% of 62 patients on **moclobemide** gained weight, although overall there was a mean 0.1kg weight loss in all patients (*B J Psych* 1992, **160**, 519–24).

Other antidepressants

Venlafaxine is usually associated with weight loss (eg. Anon, *J Clin Psych* 1993, **54**, 119–26). Unusual appetite and weight gain has been reported with **mianserin** (Harris and Harper, *Lancet* 1980, **i**, 590). There are no reports of proven weight changes with **trazodone** (Barnett *et al*, *J Clin Psychopharmacol* 1985, **5**, 161–64) nor **reboxetine** (SPC). Increased appetite and weight gain has been reported in patients treated with **mirtazapine**. One study showed increased appetite but without significant weight changes (n=90, Claghorn, *J Aff Dis* 1995, **34**, 165–71) and another showed a slightly higher incidence than with amitriptyline (Smith *et al*, *Psychopharmacol Bull* 1990, **26**, 191–96). Overall, the incidence of weight gain with mirtazapine in all trials combined seems to be about 12%, with weight loss in 3%.

Management

It is always best to anticipate problems before they appear and suggest remedies beforehand. Switching antidepressants is probably the best strategy (see *2.2.5*) since reduced metabolism is the main mechanism. An open trial of naltrexone for tricyclic-induced weight gain (Zimmermann *et al*, *Biol Psych* 1997, **41**, 747–49) showed good improvement in continuous hunger and small weight loss at eight weeks. Anecdotally, **ranitidine**

used at night has abolished the weight gain with mirtazapine, through reduction in 'midnight raids' on the fridge.

LITHIUM *

Weight gain, the second most common reason for non-compliance, is reported to occur in around 33% (up to 65%, *Acta Psych Scand* 1976, **53**, 139–47), of which 25% are probably obese (Sachs and Guille, *J Clin Psych* 1999, **60** (Suppl 21, 16–19). Weight increase occurs predominantly during the first two years of treatment, occurs more often in people already overweight and may be more common in women than men. Increased thirst has been noted in 89% (*Acta Psych Scand* 1976, **53**, 139–47) and strongly correlates with weight gain. Increased hunger/food intake has not been directly shown (*J Psychopharmacol* 1990, **4**, 303) and so the predominant mechanism may thus be due to increased intake of high-calorie drinks. Thyroid status should also be assessed, as a possible contributory cause. Lithium also increases insulin secretion, which may lead to more adipose tissue being produced, and thus may have a contributory effect on BMI gain.

Lithium-induced weight gain has been disputed by Armong (n=42, open, *B J Psych* 1996, **169**, 251–52) in a study that showed no significant weight gain, even if taken with concomitant antipsychotics and antidepressants, a surprising finding. One study using Body Mass Index (n=117, *Acta Psych Scand* 1989, **80**, 538–40) showed a non-significant BMI increase, with 27% actually showing a reduced BMI.

Management

Counselling, eg. use plain/low-calorie beverages, along with normal sodium intake, dietary advice and monitoring, particularly during the first year, may be adequate.

Reviews: general (Baptista *et al*, *Pharmacopsychiatry* 1995, **28**, 35–44) and treatment of lithium-induced weight gain using a calorie and electrolyte controlled diet (*Am J Psych* 1976, **133**, 1082–84; Baptista *et al*, *Pharmacopsychiatry* 1995, **28**, 35–44).

BENZODIAZEPINES

Alprazolam has been reported to cause increased appetite and weight gain in healthy male volunteers (n=17, Haney *et al, Psychopharmacology* 1997, **132**, 311–14).

ANTICONVULSANTS

Carbamazepine *

Studies have show that 43% may gain weight (n=70, Corman *et al, Can J Neurol Sci* 1997, **24**, 240–44) and 8% may gain over 5kg (Mattson *et al, NEJM* 1992, **327**, 765–71), and may be due to increased appetite, reversed by discontinuation but not by dieting (n=4, Lampl *et al, Clin Neuropharmacol* 1991, **14**, 251–55).

Clobazam

Weight gain has been reported during one study (Ananth *et al, Curr Ther Res* 1979, **26**, 119–26).

Gabapentin

In a study of high-dose gabapentin over at least 12 months, 10 patients gained more than 10% of their baseline weight, 15 gained 5% to 10%, 16 had no change and 3 lost 5% to 10%. Weight was gained in months 2 and 3 and tended to stabilise after 6–9 months, although the doses of gabapentin remained unchanged (n=44, DeToledo *et al, Ther Drug Monit* 1997, **19**, 394–96). Mean weight gain of 6.9kg (range 3.2–14.5kg) has been noted (n=11, open, Gidal *et al, Ann Pharmacother* 1995, **29**, 1048).

Oxcarbazepine*

Weight gain has been reported as a relatively frequent side-effect.

Tiagabine *

Adjunctive tiagabine may have no significant effect on body weight (n=349, Hogan *et al, Epilepsy Res* 2000, **41**, 23–28).

Topiramate

Topiramate has been reported to produce weight loss, an advantage as an alternative mood stabiliser, if early promise is confirmed (n=2, Gordon and Price, *Am J Psych* 1999, **156**, 968–69). It is even being investigated as an appetite suppressant (*Pharm J* 1999, **263**, 475). The effect appears dose-related, with average amounts lost ranging from 1.1kg/1.5% (up to 200mg/d) to 5.9kg/7% (800mg/d or above). The effect peaks at 12–15 months, is greater in people with higher starting weights and is at least partially reversible (MI).

Valproate*

Weight gain is recognised as a common ADR. One study indicated that up to 71% gain weight, often sustained and socially significant (n=70, Corman *et al, Can J Neurol Sci* 1997, **24**, 240–44; risk factors in children see Novak *et al, J Child Neurol* 1999, **14**, 490–95), although this may be due to other factors (n=211, Easter *et al, Seizure,* 1997, **6**, 121–25). Higher serum leptin and insulin levels were found in 15 patients becoming obese after one year of valproate, compared to the 25 who did not gain weight (n=40, Verrotti *et al, Neurology* 1999, **53**, 230–33; Demir and Aysun, *Pediatr Neurol* 2000, **22**, 361–64).

Vigabatrin

Weight gain may occur in 5–40% patients prescribed vigabatrin long-term as add-on therapy (Grant and Heel, *Drugs* 1991, **41**, 889–926).

OTHER DRUGS*

No significant weight changes have been seen yet in clinical trials with **acamprosate**. A retrospective study showed that weight loss with **methylphenidate** occurred more with heavier children and recommended that BMI percentile curves are used as the best measure of weight changes (study and review, Schertz *et al, Pediatrics* 1996, **98**, 763–69). Weight loss may occur with **bupropion**, with 28% treated losing greater than 5lb, but weight gain occurred in 9% patients (MI). Carbohydrate craving has also been reported.

2.5 SEXUAL DYSFUNCTION WITH PSYCHOTROPICS

Dysfunction of the three phases of sexual activity (desire, excitement/erection and orgasm) is associated with some psychiatric illnesses, eg. reduced sexual desire/activity in schizophrenia, impotence and loss of libido in depression etc. Drug effects are thus difficult to identify accurately, but seem to be rapidly reversible on discontinuing treatment. Drug effects have been attributed to:

1. Central unspecific actions, eg. sedation.
2. Central specific actions, eg. 5-HT blockade (5-HT may set the threshold for orgasm/ejaculation, and SSRIs may raise this threshold, ie. orgasmic responses/

effects, *J Psychiact Drugs* 1992, **24**, 1–40), DA blockade (dopamine may be involved with arousal, copulation and penile reflexes, ie. libido effects, *Psychopharmacol* 1989, **98**, 363–68), cholinergic or adrenergic blockade. Noradrenaline release may facilitate libido and erections and the facilitatory effects of serotonin on sexual activity may only occur when noradrenaline activity occurs (Fernandex-Guasti *et al, Brain Research* 1986, **377**, 112–18).

3. Peripheral actions, eg. hypotension.

4. Endocrine effects, eg. testosterone, prolactin (may be underestimated as women are often excluded from trials or required to take oral contraceptives, Dickson and Glazer, *Schizo Res* 1999, **35**[Suppl 35], S67–S73).

Only recently has the literature treated this issue systematically, despite great clinical importance. Patients are often unwilling to volunteer or talk about sexual matters. Such side-effects (and fear thereof) will increase the risk of non-concordance/ compliance.

The effects of SSRIs on sexual functioning have received much publicity and seem strongly dose-related and may vary among the group according to serotonin and dopamine reuptake mechanisms, induction of prolactin release, anticholinergic effects, inhibition of nitric oxide synthetase, and propensity for accumulation over time.

Reviews*: SSRI-related sexual dysfunction (Rosen *et al, J Clin Psychopharmacol* 1999, **19**, 67–85), effects of antidepressants on sexual function (Baldwin *et al, Int J Psych Clin Pract* 1997, **1**, 47–58, 67 refs; Seagraves, *J Clin Psych* 1998, **59**[Suppl 4], 48–54), sexual side-effects of new antidepressants (Mir and Taylor, *Psych Bull* 1998, **22**, 438–41), diagnosis, incidence and management (Clayton and Shen, *Drug Saf* 1998, **19**, 299–312), antipsychotics (mentioned in Wirshing *et al, Curr Opin Psych* 2000, **13**, 45–50), counselling advice (Gutierrez and Stimmel, *Pharmacotherapy* 1999, **19**, 823–31, 57 refs).

2.5.1 DESIRE OR LIBIDO

Antidepressants

Since depression is associated with decreased libido and successful treatment associated with a return to normal levels, any associated drug effect is difficult to quantify accurately.

Antidepressants are widely implicated in reduction of libido, eg. **clomipramine** (Steiger, *J Clin Psychopharmacol* 1988, **8**, 349–54), with sedation a possible contributory cause. A retrospective review concluded that libido disturbance occurs in about 45% of women on SSRIs (Aldrich *et al, Clin Drug Invest* 1996, **11**, 353–59). A prospective study has shown that during SSRI treatment, difficulties with desire and arousal in depressed women tend to remit with the illness, whereas in men orgasmic dysfunction appears as an adverse effect (n=225, open, Piazza *et al, Am J Psych* 1997, **154**, 1757–59). Reduced libido and some sexual dysfunction has been reported with **citalopram** in several studies (eg. Michael and Herrod, *B J Psych* 1997, **171**, 90).

Conversely, increased libido has occurred with **imipramine** and **trimipramine** (*J Psychosomat Obstet Gynaecol* 1985, **4**, 125–28) but the incidence is unknown. **Trazodone** improved libido and erections in two-thirds of patients studied (Kurt *et al, J Urology* 1994, **152**, 407–9). For **venlafaxine**, increased libido to above premorbid levels in a male has been reported (n=1, Michael and Owen, *B J Psych* 1997, **170**, 193) with high dose venlafaxine, as has decreased libido (Mir and Taylor, *Psych Bull* 1998, **22**, 438–41). 18% patients in one study showed increased libido with **moclobemide** (Philipp *et al, Int Clin Psychopharmacol* 1993, **7**, 149–53) and hyperorgasmia and hyperarousal has been reported (Lauerma, *Int Clin Psychopharmacol* 1995, **10**, 123–24).

Mirtazapine has been shown to improve the 3 stages of sexual activity, particularly in women (n=25, 12/52, open, Boyarsky *et al, Depr Anx* 1999, **9**, 175–79).

Management of antidepressant-induced loss of libido

1. **Switch antidepressants** – trazodone and bupropion have been associated with increases in libido above levels prior to depression. Mirtazapine, moclobemide and nefazodone are other possible alternatives.

2. **Adjunctive drugs** have been suggested (eg. buspirone, amantadine, cyproheptadine etc, see section *2.5.3*).

Lithium

20% male patients experience reduced libido on lithium, but report preserved pleasure, no distress and it did not cause non-compliance (n=35, open, Aizenberg *et al, Clin Neuropharmacol* 1996, **19**, 515–59). See also next section (*2.5.2*).

Benzodiazepines/anxiolytics/ hypnotics/etc

Bearing in mind the huge number of prescriptions, few reports of problems exist, and those usually only at higher doses, eg. complete loss of libido with short-term oral **lorazepam** at 3mg/d (n=2, *Am J Psych* 1988, **145**, 1313–14), not associated with sedation. In lower doses they may tend to have a helpful effect on anxiety-related problems, such as fear of failure. Their sedative effects may reduce arousal. **Flunitrazepam** has been cited as having a disinhibiting effect and been used as a 'date-rape' drug.

Antipsychotics

Untreated schizophrenics show a decreased sexual desire, and antipsychotics may restore libido but have a deleterious effect on erectile and orgasmic ability and satisfaction (n=122, survey, Aizenberg *et al, J Clin Psych* 1995, **56**, 137–41). There are no systematic investigations.

Anticonvulsants

Barbiturates, phenytoin and **primidone** are reported to decrease libido (Mattson *et al, NEJM* 1985, **313**, 145) but increased libido with **ethosuximide** has been known (SPC). Some 'reawakening of sexual desire' with **lamotrigine** has been reported (Betts, *Seizure* 1992, **1**, 3–6).

Other drugs

Fluctuations in libido have been reported with **acamprosate** (MI).

2.5.2 AROUSAL AND ERECTION/ IMPOTENCE

The evidence linking erectile dysfunction to antidepressants is unclear. Although many cases have been reported, controlled studies have failed to show a clear link.

Tricyclics

Most tricyclics have been reported as causing impotence and many delay or inhibit ejaculation. A negative effect has been implicated in up to 30% of patients (250mg/d **imipramine** by Harrison *et al, J Clin Psychopharmacol* 1986, **6**, 144–49), may be plasma-level or dose-related (eg. *J Clin Psychopharmacol* 1988, **8**, 349–54) but is not inevitable (d/b, p/c, Harrison *et al, J Clin Psychopharmacol* 1986, **6**, 144–49). In an OCD trial, 92% **clomipramine**-treated patients suffered sexual dysfunction, including problems with erection and ejaculation, reversible in all but one when the drug was stopped, did not seem dose-related and tolerance was rare (n=33, *B J Psych* 1987, **151**, 107–12).

SSRIs

The UK post-marketing monitoring service report on **paroxetine** indicates that male sexual dysfunction is more common with paroxetine than fluoxetine or fluvoxamine. The incidence of **fluoxetine**-induced sexual dysfunction ranges from 5% to 8% (Herman *et al, J Clin Psych* 1990, **51**, 225–27). Improved erectile function has also been reported with **fluoxetine** (eg. n=2, Power-Smith, *B J Psych* 1994, **164**, 249–50) and **paroxetine** 20mg/d (MacHale and Phanjoo, *B J Psych* 1994, **164**, 854), which were independent of depression. Impotence was reported with **citalopram** in one study in alcoholics (Naranjo *et al, Clin Pharmacol Ther* 1987, **41**, 266–74).

MAOIs

MAOIs have been implicated in up to 40% of patients, eg. a study with **phenelzine** (*J Clin Psychopharmacol* 1986, **6**, 144–9), with 60–90mg/d causing impotence (*NEJM* 1971, **285**, 987–91), retarded ejaculation (*Am J Psych* 1979, **136**, 1200–1) and loss of libido and anorgasmia (*J Nerv Ment Dis* 1978, **166**, 349–57) in males. Phenelzine had little effect on erectile function in another study (d/b, p/c, Harrison *et al, J Clin Psychopharmacol* 1986, **6**, 144–49). Some stimulation of sexual function has been seen in trials with **moclobemide** (eg. Lingjaerde *et al, Acta Psych Scand* 1995, **92**, 125–31).

Other antidepressants

Erectile failure and impotence (7% incidence) have been reported with **venlafaxine** (Anon, *J Clin Psych* 1993, **54**, 119–26) reduced erection-performance with **mianserin** (*Psychosomatics* 1983, **24**, 1076–81) and spontaneous ejaculations with **nefazodone** 200mg/d (n=1, Michael and Ramana, *B J Psych* 1996, **169**, 672–73). There are no reported problems with **mirtazapine**, with an incidence comparable with placebo. There is a 5% incidence of impotence reported with **reboxetine** (MI), particularly at doses above 8mg/d.

Lithium

Lithium has been reported to have caused impairing of desire and arousal in 31% patients, but did not have a major impact on self-satisfaction and sense of pleasure (n=35 males, survey, Aizenberg *et al, Clin Neuropharmacol* 1996, **19**, 515–59).

Benzodiazepines

There have been some reports of erectile dysfunction, eg. 42% men treated with clonazepam for PTSD (n=43, Fossey and Hamner, *Anxiety* 1994–95, **1**, 233–36) and with alprazolam (*Hum Psychopharmacol* 1990, **5**, 159–63).

Antipsychotics

Although limited evidence is available, antipsychotics can cause impotence and ejaculatory dysfunction (*Am J Psych* 1982, **139**, 633–37), possibly by an effect on prolactin levels. **Thioridazine** may be worse than the other antipsychotics. In one study, 60% of men reported sexual dysfunction (achieving and maintaining erection) with thioridazine (dose 150mg/d or above) but only 25% had the same problem with other antipsychotics (Kotin *et al, Am J Psych* 1976, **133**, 82–85). In a trial of **risperidone** in chronic schizophrenia, erectile dysfunction was seen in 18% on 12mg/d, but less than 11% on other doses (cf. 13% pts with erectile dysfunction on 10mg/d haloperidol) (n=1362, Peuskens *et al, B J Psych* 1995, **166**, 712–26). Butyrophenones (eg. **haloperidol**) and **pimozide** lack the peripheral autonomic effects of the others and rarely seem to cause problems (isolated case of pimozide-induced impotence in *Am J Psych* 1982, **139**, 1374). No problems have been reported yet with **olanzapine**. Impotence can occur in more than 1% of patients with **zotepine**.

Anticholinergics

Anticholinergics prescribed with antipsychotics are likely to potentiate the effect of antipsychotics on erectile function and may in themselves cause impotence (MI).

Anticonvulsants*

Uncontrolled studies have shown reduced sexual activity and impotence in male epileptics on anticonvulsants, probably due to falls in free testosterone levels (*BMJ* 1982, **284**, 85–86). **Carbamazepine** may cause impotence (Mattson *et al, NEJM* 1985, **313**, 145). Impotence due to other AEDs has resolved with lamotrigine (n=3, Husain *et al, South Med J* 2000, **93**, 335–36).

Other drugs

Disulfiram may cause impotence (Snyder, *Biol Psych* 1981, **16**, 399).

Management

The problem seems rapidly reversible if the drug is withdrawn. **Yohimbine** and **pentoxifylline** given 1–2 hours pre-intercourse have been shown to improve antidepressant-induced impotence (Nessel, *Am J Psych* 1994, **151**, 453). Yohimbine PRN (*J Clin Psych* 1992, **53**, 207–9) or 5.4–10.8mg tds have been used successfully (Ashton, *Am J Psych* 1994, **151**, 1397). See also *2.5.3*.

2.5.3 ANORGASMIA (inc. inhibition of ejaculation)

Anorgasmia appears to be dose-related in many cases and patients may suffer with one drug but not with a related drug. The exact incidences are not known but are probably grossly under-reported due to a reluctance, particularly among females, to discuss this with their physicians, especially if they are male, and vice versa.

SSRIs

SSRI-induced anorgasmia may be related to an effect on nitric oxide (Sussman and Ginsberg, *Psych Ann* 1998, **28**, 89–97). Abnormal or delayed ejaculation in men appears to be a dose-dependent effect. A study has also shown the anti-ejaculatory effect from **paroxetine** to be greatest, fluoxetine and sertraline next, with little effect from fluvoxamine, the effect being the same in men with either life-long rapid-ejaculation (<1min) or less-rapid ejaculation (>1 min) (RCT, n=32, Waldinger *et al, J Clin Psychopharmacol* 1998, **18**, 274–81; supported by n=344, open, Montejo-Gonzalez *et al, J Sex Marital Ther* 1997, **23**, 176–94). 8% men (and partners) preferred the effect. As it is dose-related, reducing the dose or discontinuing is effective. **Fluoxetine**-induced anorgasmia in both males and females (including also delayed orgasm and reduced libido) is well-reported (eg. *J Clin Psych* 1991, **52**, 66–68) at therapeutic doses. It may occur in about 8% of patients (*J Clin Psych* 1990, **51**, 25–27) and is more likely in patients with a history of antidepressant anorgasmia. About 17% of patients on **sertraline** report sexual dysfunction, mainly delayed ejaculation (*Clin Pharm* 1992, **11**, 930–57). With **fluvoxamine**, there was a 35% incidence in healthy volunteers (10 male and 10 female) at 150mg/d (Nafziger *et al, J Clin Psych* 1999, **60**, 187–90). Switching to another SSRI may help, as there are cases of **citalopram** treating depression but not causing sexual impairment where other SSRIs had caused it (n=2, Pallanti and Koran, *Am J Psych* 1999, **156**, 796).

Conversely, although delayed orgasm can be a negative effect in women, delayed ejaculation could sometimes be considered as a positive effect in men. **Paroxetine** at 20–40mg/d (or 2–4 hours before sex) has been shown to have a remarkable effect on improving premature ejaculation, starting within a week and improving over six weeks, with libido understandably also improving (n=17, d/b, p/c, Waldinger *et al, Am J Psych* 1994, **151**, 1377–79). There is unpublished evidence for a similar effect from **sertraline** and **fluoxetine** (n=1, Forster and King, *Am J Psych* 1994, **151**, 1523). The effect is evidently so predictable that the SSRIs are now considered the accepted treatment for premature ejaculation (review by Balon, *J Sex Marital Ther* 1996, **22**, 85–96).

Tricyclics

Most tricyclics have been reported to cause anorgasmia and painful ejaculation. In two **clomipramine** trials (n=46, n=33) up to 90% developed total or partial anorgasmia, persisting over at least five months and with men and women equally effected, a serious side-effect. In one of these studies, the effect was reversible in all but one when the drug was stopped, seemed dose-related and tolerance was rare (*B J Psych* 1987, **151**, 107–12).

Anorgasmia has also been reported with **imipramine**, and switching tricyclics may help (n=11, *J Clin Psychopharmacol* 1986, **6**, 144). Painful ejaculation with clomipramine and imipramine has been reported (*J Clin Psych* 1991, **52**, 461–63).

Conversely, there is one case of increased orgasmic capacity with clomipramine, including orgasm with spontaneous yawning (McLean, *Can J Psych* 1983, **28**, 569–70).

Related antidepressants *

Erectile failure, delayed orgasm, and abnormal or painful ejaculation (n=1, Michael, *B J Psych* 2000, **177**, 282–83) have been reported with **venlafaxine** (Anon, *J Clin Psych* 1993, **54**, 119–26), as has anorgasmia with **trazodone** (*Am J Psych* 1988, **145**, 896) and **nefazodone** (0.6%, Reynolds, *J Clin Psych* 1997, **58**, 89). The effect with **mirtazapine** is similar to placebo, but a case has been reported (Berigan and Harazin, *J Clin Psych* 1998, **59**, 319–20). Mirtazapine might be useful in patients who are unable to tolerate SSRIs because of sexual dysfunction and demonstrated no effect on sexual function (n=11, Koutouvidis *et al, Int Clin Psychopharmacol* 1999, **14**, 253–55; n=4, Farah, *J Clin Psych* 1999, **60**, 260–61). 69% of people with SSRI-induced sexual dysfunction had a return to normal (58%) or significant improvement in sexual functioning when switched to mirtazapine (open, 6/52, n=19, Gelenberg *et al, J Clin Psych* 2000, **61**, 356-60). Hyperorgasmia has been reported with **moclobemide** (n=1, Lauerma, *Int Clin Psychopharmacol* 1995, **10**, 123–24) but delayed orgasm or anorgasmia has not been reported.

MAOIs

All MAOIs have been implicated but particularly **phenelzine** (many cases, eg. *Am J Psych* 1979, **136**, 1616–17, 1200) and isolated cases with **tranylcypromine** and **isocarboxazid**. There are some reports of anorgasmia in females (*Am J Psych* 1982, **139**, 1353–54) including normal libido but inhibited orgasmic reflex, and in males (*J Nerv Ment Dis* 1978, **166**, 349–57). This may spontaneously remit and appears dose-dependent.

Antipsychotics

Many drugs have been implicated, but particularly the phenothiazines, with **thi-**

oridazine appeared the worst of the bunch, eg. In up to 30% of males on thioridazine. There are reports with other phenothiazines. There are reports of loxapine not having this problem (eg. *Psychosomatics* 1982, **23**, 959–61). Ejaculatory dysfunction with **risperidone** may occur in 8–18%, peaking at 12mg/d (cf 7% patients with ejaculatory dysfunction on 10mg/d haloperidol, n=1362, Peuskens *et al, B J Psych* 1995, **166**, 712–26). Abnormal ejaculation has been reported rarely with **zotepine**. No problems have been reported yet with **olanzapine** and **quetiapine**.

In women, little other than the above has been reported, but thioridazine and trifluoperazine have been recorded as causing anorgasmia (*Psychosomatics* 1982, **23**, 959–61). It is likely to be more prevalent than reports suggest.

Again the butyrophenones (eg. **halo-peridol**) and **pimozide** lack peripheral autonomic effects and hence rarely seem to cause problems.

Anxiolytics

Few reports of problems exist, and usually only at higher doses. In lower doses they may tend to have a helpful effect on anxiety-related problems such as, in men, fear of failure. The effect on women may be the reverse. The few reports include **diazepam**, **flurazepam**, and **alprazolam**.

Anticonvulsants *

There is a case of **carbamazepine**-induced ejaculatory failure (Leris *et al, B J Urology* 1997, **79**, 485). Reversible ejaculatory failure and anorgasmia (but not libido nor erection) has been reported with **gabapentin** (n=1, Labbate and Rubet, *Am J Psych* 1999, **156**, 972; n=1, Brannon and Rolland, *J Clin Psycho-pharmacol* 2000, **20**, 379–81).

Others*

Bupropion seems to have no effect on subjective nor objective measures of erectile or overall sexual functioning (n=14 men, 10/52, p/c, s/b, Rowland *et al, J Clin Psychopharmacol* 1997, **17**, 350–57; n=364 both sexes, RCT, Coleman *et al, Ann Clin Psychiatry* 1999, **11**, 205–15), and in some (male and female) it may even improve, an effect not related just to the antidepressant effect (n=30, s/b, Modell *et al, J Sex Marital Ther* 2000, **26**, 231–40).

Management

There are a number of strategies which can be used to manage psychotropic-induced anorgasmia (particularly from antidepressants):

1. **Discontinuation:** See *1.14* for treatment duration recommendations and *2.2.5* for discontinuing anti-depressant advice.

2. **Dose adjustment:** SSRI-induced anorgasmia has been treated with 'drug holidays' (antidepressant reduced or omitted Friday, Saturday and Sunday), which resulted in improved sexual function in patients on paroxetine and sertraline but not with fluoxetine, presumably due to fluoxetine's longer half-life (where a sabbatical rather than a holiday would be required). No return of depressive symptoms was noted in this 4-week study (open, n=30, Rothschild, *Am J Psych* 1995, **152**, 1514–16). Care would be needed to avoid the potential for SSRI discontinuation syndromes with omitted doses at weekends (see *2.2.5*). Reduced **fluvoxamine** dose at weekends has been successful and avoids drug discontinuation effects (Nemeth *et al, Am J Psych* 1996, **153**, 1365). Alternatively, if the effect is plasma level related and sexual activity takes place, eg. in the evening, switching a once-daily dose to last thing at night would ensure trough plasma levels at the appropriate time. Reduction of dose to minimum effective dose may also help.

3. **Waiting for spontaneous resolution**, which only works in about a third of patients.

4. **Switching drugs:** Alternate drugs with a low incidence of problems include bupropion, trazodone, nefazodone or mirtazapine.

5. **Use of counter-acting drugs** (all these drug strategies are of highly variable reported efficacy):
   Amantadine – 100mg bd/tds has been used to treat fluoxetine-induced anorgasmia (*J Clin Psych* 1992, **53**, 212–13).
   Bethanechol – taken 1–2hrs prior to intercourse has been claimed to relieve

sexual dysfunction in some patients on tricyclics but may only occasionally be successful (*J Clin Psych* 1990, **51**[Suppl 1], 21–25).

Bupropion – 75–150mg 1–2 hours prior to sexual activity successfully reversed a range of SSRI-induced sexual dysfunction in 66% patients (open trial, n=47, Ashton and Rosen, *J Clin Psych* 1998, **59**, 112–15).

Buspirone – 40% patients taking either citalopram or paroxetine reported sexual problems, of whom 58% improved on buspirone 20–60mg/d, whereas only 30% improved on placebo (n=117, p/c, Landen *et al, J Clin Psychopharmacol* 1999, **19**, 268–71).

Cyproheptadine – 2–4+mg 30–60 minutes before sex (provided they can then stay awake) has been used to treat anorgasmia induced by fluvoxamine (Arnott and Nutt, *B J Psych* 1994, **164**, 838–39), citalopram (Lauerma, *Acta Psych Scand* 1996, **93**, 69–70) and fluoxetine (Segraves, *J Clin Psych* 1993, **11**[Monograph 1], 1–4, 4mg tds, *J Clin Psych* 1992, **53**, 174), although relapse of depression has been reported (see *4.3.2.2*). There is a single case of **citalopram**-induced anorgasmia treated with cyproheptadine 4mg (but not 2mg) the day before intercourse, this being referred to by the male patient as 'the catapult pills' (Lauerma, *Acta Psych Scand* 1996, **93**, 69–70).

Ginkgo biloba* – a small study failed to show any significant reversal of SSRI-induced sexual dysfunction (n=22, open, Ashton *et al, Am J Psych* 2000, **157**, 836–37, letter).

Granisitron — this 5-HT$_3$ antagonist has been used to treat fluoxetine-induced anorgasmia (Nelson *et al, J Clin Psych* 1997, **58**, 496–97).

Imipramine – 25–50mg at night has been used for thioridazine-induced male orgasmic disorder, with 50% improving (n=8, open pilot, Aizenberg *et al, J Sex Marital Ther* 1996, **22**, 225–29).

Nefazodone* – 100–150mg 60 minutes prior to intercourse has been successful for SSRI (sertraline 100mg/d) induced anorgasmia (Reynolds, *J Clin Psych* 1997, **58**, 89; n=1, Michael *et al, B J Psych* 1999, **175**, 491, letter).

Sildenafil (the 'Pfizer Riser') – there are many reported cases of SSRI-induced anorgasmia responding to sildenafil 50–100mg 1 hour pre-sex in both men and women (eg. open study, Fava *et al, Psychother Psychosom* 1998, **67**, 328–31; n=10 females, Nurnberg *et al, Am J Psych* 1999, **156**, 1664)

Stimulants – methylphenidate and dexamfetamine (15–20mg/d) have been used, for antidepressant-induced anorgasmia.

Trazodone* – has reversed fluoxetine-induced dysfunction (Michael and O'Donnell, *Can J Psych* 2000, **45**, 847–48)

Yohimbine – 5.5mg has been used to treat anorgasmia induced by fluoxetine (Segraves, *J Clin Psych* 1993, **11**[Monograph 1], 1–4), sertraline and paroxetine (in men and women, Segraves, *B J Psych* 1994, **165**, 554) and clomipramine (*J Clin Psych* 1990, **51**, 32–33). Yohimbine can cause insomnia, so rolling over and going to sleep afterwards is less of an option.

2.5.4 PRIAPISM

Priapism (persistent painful penile turgidity in the absence of sexual arousal) longer than 4 hours is considered a urological emergency as up to 50% of sufferers become impotent as a result. Men, particularly aged between 30 and 40, should be warned about the possibility of priapism as early treatment may prevent or minimise long-term complications. Treatment within 4–6 hours (before local hypoxemia) reduces morbidity, need for invasive procedures and impotence. Frequent prolonged erections before the onset of priapism may occur and so the reporting of these is essential. Clinical cases report a usual period of 1 day to 9 months between initiation of medication and onset. In a review of psychotropic-induced priapism, the authors conclude that it is not dose-dependent, nor correlated with treatment duration (Weiner and Lowe, *CNS Drugs* 1998, **9**, 371–79).

Priapism may be due to a hypersensitivity reaction (*B J Psych* 1990, **157**, 759–62) or more likely to alpha-adrenergic receptor blockade (*Ann Emerg Med* 1984, **14**, 600–2), by inhibiting sympathetically controlled detumescence via direct alpha-blockade. Risk factors may include blood dyscrasias, sickle cell trait, alcohol, cannabis and previous episodes of delayed penile detumescence, which may have occurred in up to 50% of priapism cases (*J Urol* 1977, **117**, 455–58). Priapism has been reported with many psychiatric drugs. Most reports exist with trazodone and phenothiazines.

Reviews: general (Patel *et al, B J Hosp Med* 1996, **55**, 315–19).

Antidepressants

Trazodone: many cases have appeared in the literature, with a risk estimated to be between 1 in 1000 and 1 in 10,000, the majority occurring at doses of 150mg/d or less (range 50–400mg/d) and within the first 28 days (range single dose through to 18 months) (*J Clin Psych* 1987, **48**, 244–45). No effect has yet been reported with **nefazodone** (review by Baldwin, *J Psychopharmacol* 1996, **10**[Suppl 1], 30–34). There are isolated reports with other antidepressants eg. **sertraline** (Rand, *J Clin Psych* 1998, **59**, 538).

Antipsychotics

Many antipsychotics have been implicated in causing priapism, particularly the phenothiazines. There are isolated reports for **haloperidol**, **clozapine** and **zuclopenthixol** decanoate (case of recurrent priapism, van Hemert *et al, Int Clin Psychopharmacol* 1995, **10**, 199–200). There appear to be few predictive indicators, eg. it has occurred after a single dose and after 10 years.

Other drugs

Other drugs implicated include **diazepam** (*Psychosomatics* 1984, **25**, 629–30), **phenytoin** (*B J Urol* 1988, **61**, 261) and **buspirone** (Coates, *South Med J* 1990, **83**, 983).

Treatment/management

Prompt treatment, within 4 to 6 hours of onset, reduces morbidity and decreases need for surgical intervention. Treatment recommendations include penile aspiration, irrigation, instillation of vaso-active agents and, if necessary, shunting procedures. Patient education is perhaps the most important consideration (Weiner and Lowe, *CNS Drugs* 1998, **9**, 371–79). Symptomatic treatment with ice packs, enemas, medication and anaesthesia is common, although results are not consistent. Intracavernosal injections of **metaraminol**, an alpha adrenergic agonist (*Lancet* 1984, **2**, 220–21) and **amyl nitrate** (short review in *Hospital Pharmacy* 1991, **26**, 343) have been used. Neuroleptic-induced priapism has been managed with **benztropine** 6mg/d, **diphenhydramine** (*Ann Emerg Med* 1984, **14**, 600–2) and abolished by the addition of **atenolol** 75mg/d (*Am J Psych* 1988, **145**, 1480). Painful treatment-resistant priapism has been treated successfully with **ethyl chloride spray** (Bos and Buys, *B J Urology* 1994, **74**, 677–78).

2.5.5 FERTILITY *

It is not thought that fertility in males is directly adversely effected by psychotropics, although there are conflicting reports of anticonvulsant drug effects.

Amenorrhoea is more likely in women on typical antipsychotics, due to the drug-induced rise in prolactin levels via a dopamine blockade of the tuberoinfundibular system. Up to 50–90% can be expected to become amenorrhoeic (Gingell *et al, B J Psych* 1993, **162**, 127). Prolactin levels may rise within days of starting a typical antipsychotic.

Clozapine has a minimal prolactin-raising effect, a lower impact on female fertility and women may thus be more likely to conceive on clozapine than other antipsychotics. It has also been suggested that clozapine may have an effect on improving male fertility (Dickson and Edwards, *Am J Psych* 1997, **154**, 582–83). There have been cases of pregnancy occurring soon after switching to atypicals (short review in Wirshing *et al, Curr Opin Psych* 2000, **13**, 45–50). There may be many reasons for this, eg. restored gonadal function, improved desire and functioning, decreased negative symptoms etc.

Very high doses of chlorpromazine decreased sperm motility by 50%, but the authors thought this unlikely to cause decreased fertility. Diazepam, phenytoin and phenobarbital had no detectable effect (Hong *et al, Eur J Clin Pharmacol* 1982, **22**, 413–16). **Lithium** could possibly inhibit sperm motility (Raoof *et* al, B J Clin Pharmacol 1989, **28**, 715–17) in men but concentrations in the vagina are unlikely to have a clinical effect on inhibiting sperm motility (Salas *et al, B J Clin Pharmacol* 1989, **28**, 715P).

3.1 BREAST-FEEDING

	Lower risk	Moderate risk	High risk
Antipsychotics	Sulpiride [5]	Amisulpride[5] Flupentixol [4] Haloperidol[6] Loxapine?[8] Phenothiazines (low dose only) [7] Zuclopenthixol [4]	Clozapine[3] Olanzapine[2] Phenothiazines [7] Quetiapine [2] Risperidone[1] Zotepine[2]
Antidepressants	Flupentixol LD[4] Moclobemide[16] Tricyclics[12] (most) Tryptophan[16]	Amoxapine[16] Mianserin[16] Mirtazapine[11] St John's wort[16] SSRIs[9] Trazodone[12]	Doxepin?[12] MAOIs[15] Maprotiline[12] Nefazodone[13] Reboxetine[14] Venlafaxine[10]
Anxiolytics + hypnotics	Benzodiazepines LD[17] Chloral[21] Temazepam LD[17] Zolpidem[19]	Benzodiazepines[17] Beta-blockers[20] Clomethiazole[21]	Buspirone[18] Zaleplon[19] Zopiclone[19]
Anticonvulsants	Carbamazepine[22] Phenytoin[24] Valproate [23]	Acetazolamide [28] Benzodiazepines[17] Vigabatrin [27]	Barbiturates[25] Gabapentin[26] Lamotrigine? [26] Levetiracetam [27] Ethosuximide [28] Oxcarbazepine [22] Tiagabine[27] Topiramate[27]
Others		Anticholinergics[30] Disulfiram[31] Methadone[34]	Acamprosate [31] Anticholinesterases [29] Bupropion[36] Lithium[34] Methylphenidate[34] Modafinil [33]

General Principals (adapted from *Maudsley Guidelines*, 2001)

1. All psychotropics pass into the milk, so no decision is risk-free. Breast milk is more acidic than plasma, so basic compounds may be retained and concentrations accumulate. Protein binding may also be a factor (in general, drug binding to milk proteins is less than to plasma proteins).

2. Milk levels are usually around 1% of maternal plasma levels, but there have been few formal studies.

3. Drugs should be avoided if the infant is premature, or has renal, hepatic, cardiac or neurological impairment

4. Avoid drugs with long half-lives, sedating drugs etc.

5. Since nearly all psychotropics can be given as a once daily dose, this should be achieved, as a single daily dose just before the infants longest sleep period feed (eg. peak milk concentrations after oral administration: amitriptyline 1.5hrs, imipramine 1hr, moclobemide <3hrs, sertraline 7–10hrs, chlorpromazine 2hrs, fluvoxamine 4hrs).

6. If a mother was taking a drug during pregnancy, it will not usually be necessary to switch drugs during breast feeding as the amount the infant is exposed to will be less than that exposed to *in utero*.

7. Adverse effects will often be dose related so use the minimum effective maternal dose.

8. Polypharmacy may lead to enhanced adverse effects in the infant.

9. Drug effects on the development of the infant's brain are not clear and so monitor biochemical and behavioural parameters, especially if any infant shows signs of possible psychotropic side-effects (eg. sedation, tremulousness, colic etc.), take appropriate action, eg. dose reduction, drug change, etc.

Reviews: pharmacokinetic overview and therapeutic implications (Spigset and Hagg, *CNS Drugs* 1998, **9**, 111–34), general (McElhatton, *Prescriber* 1999, **10**, 101–17).

3.1.1 Antipsychotics:

Review*: general (Tenyi *et al*, *Paediatr Drugs* 2000, **2**, 23–28, recommending monotherapy at low dose has the lowest risk, polytherapy at higher doses not recommended).

1. The UK SPC for **risperidone** states that women should not breast-feed.
2. **Olanzapine** is excreted in the milk of rats but no human data is available and so patients should not breast-feed while taking this drug (MI). No information is available for **quetiapine** and the SPC recommends avoiding. **Zotepine** and norzotepine may be secreted into breast milk (where milk levels can reach 50% of maternal plasma levels) and is incompatible with breast-feeding mothers (MI).
3. **Clozapine** is contraindicated in breast-feeding as animal studies suggest it is excreted into breast milk and so risks agranulocytosis. In the close study of one mother, there was some accumulation of clozapine in breast milk (possibly due to higher lipid concentrations), and so doses must be kept low if breast-feeding is essential (Barnas, *Am J Psych* 1994, **151**, 945) and the infants plasma monitored. There are reports indicating that babies experience sedation if mothers take clozapine and breast-feed (MI).
4. A study showed that 0.6mcg/kg or 1–2% of the maternal **flupentixol** dose might reach the infant and thus is probably safe at low dose (eg. <2mg/d) (n=6, *Eur J Clin Pharmacol* 1988, **35**, 217–20). Higher doses of **zuclo-penthixol** (*Psychopharmacology* [Berlin] 1986, **90**, 417–18) and flupentixol can produce drowsiness in the child. More studies would be needed at higher doses to confirm safety.
5. A **sulpiride** dose of 100mg/d to the mother is likely to give the child less than 1mg/d. No adverse effects have been reported at higher doses (*BMJ* 1982, **285**, 249–51). There is no information available for **amisulpride**.
6*. **Haloperidol** is excreted into breast milk but levels are probably low (eg. Whalley *et al, BMJ* 1981, **282**, 1746–47), although infant levels may be the same as adults and some element of delayed development has been detected (n=5, Yoshida *et al, Psychol Med* 1998, **28**, 81–91) and so the infant must be monitored carefully (*BMJ* 1981, **283**, 230 + refs).
7*. High doses of **phenothiazines** can produce drowsiness in the infant (review in *Am J Psych* 1978, **135**, 801–5). **Chlor-promazine** has an inconsistent milk/plasma ratio and drowsiness and lethargy are possible but not inevitable (*B J Clin Pharmacol* 1978, **5**, 272–73). With careful monitoring it should be safe. Neonatal exposure to chlorpromazine was shown to have no effect on development up to 5 years of age (*Psychiatr Q* 1957, **31**, 690–95), although some element of delayed development has been suggested (n=3, Yoshida *et al, Psychol Med* 1998, **28**, 81–91). In one case report the amount of **perphenazine** passed to an infant was about 0.1% of the adult dose in terms of mcg/kg body weight (Olesen *et al, Am J Psych* 1990, **10**, 1378–79) and this drug may become 'trapped' in milk due to its physio-chemical properties (*Clin Pharmacokin* 1980, **5**, 1–66).
8. **Loxapine** and its metabolites have been shown to appear in breast milk but no data on the potential effects is known.

3.1.2 Antidepressants:

The data on breast-feeding and antidepressants is relatively limited, with few studies in which infant blood levels have been assessed. The collected data indicates that infants older than 10 weeks are at low risk of adverse events (review by Wisner *et al, Am J Psych* 1996, **153**, 1132).

9*. Treatment with the **SSRIs** citalopram, fluvoxamine, paroxetine or sertraline seems to be compatible with breast-feeding, although fluoxetine should probably best be avoided during lactation, unless used during pregnancy. The limited data indicates that healthy full-term infants are unlikely to be harmed by SSRIs (McElhatton, *Prescriber* 1999, **10**, 101–17). One study and review of the literature concluded that at normal doses, less than 10% of the adult therapeutic dose of **fluoxetine** (on a mg/kg basis) reaches the infant and that this is low enough for women to continue breast-feeding (Nulman and Koren, *Teratology* 1996, **53**, 304–8), with no developmental effects seen (n=4, Yoshida *et al, B J Psych* 1998, **172**, 175–79). Substantial levels of fluoxetine were, however, detectable in the serum at one infant at six weeks, possibly causing colic (Lester *et al, J Am Acad Child Adolesc Psych* 1993, **32**, 1253–55) and in another study, whilst the mean combined fluoxetine/ norfluoxetine dose transmitted to infants via breast milk was generally below a 10% notional level of concern, there was considerable interpatient variability and adverse effects have been observed in breast-fed infants. Considering the potential for accumulation, careful monitoring of the infants is mandatory, especially in neonates exposed to these drugs in utero (n=14, Kristensen *et al, Br J Clin Pharmacol* 1999, **48**, 521–27). **Paroxetine** 10–50mg/d is found in milk, but at highly variable levels (sample n=108, 2–101ng/ml). In one study, a significant gradient effect was seen, with greater concentrations in later portions (hind milk) than earlier portions (fore milk), but no adverse effects in the infants (16 mother and infant pairs, Stowe *et al, Am J Psych* 2000, **257**, 185–89). In a second study, around 0.3–2.2% (mean 1.2%) of weight-adjusted maternal dose appeared in the milk (but no difference between hind and fore milk), with none (n=7) or unquantifiable (n=1) levels in the infant serum and no observed infant adverse effects (n=10, Begg *et al, Br J Clin Pharmacol* 1999, **48**, 142–47). **Fluvoxamine** levels in milk and plasma have been determined in case studies. In one, the estimated daily intake by the infant was about 0.5% of the maternal dose (100 or 200mg/d) and was thought by the authors to be of little risk. The infants showed no adverse effects (n=2, Wright *et al, B J Clin Pharmacol* 1991, **31**, 209) and there were no concerns about development up to 21 months in one (Yoshida *et al, Br J Clin Pharmacol* 1997, **44**, 210–11). In a study using serial levels, milk fluvoxamine levels were found at higher levels than previously reported and roughly paralleled the serum levels, but that the absolute dose received by the infant was low, and that breast-feeding was at an acceptable risk (n=1, Hägg *et al, Br J Clin Pharmacol* 2000, **49**, 286–88). The data indicates low levels of **sertraline** and metabolite in the infant, which are unlikely to cause any significant adverse effects (n=8, Kristensen *et al, Br J Clin Pharmacol* 1998, **45**, 453–57). Doses of up to 200mg/d may produce sertraline (and almost undetectable desmethyl-sertraline) in the milk, peaking at 7–10 hours post-last dose, with no reported adverse effects (n=12, Stowe *et al, Am J Psych* 1997, **154**, 1255–60). Higher levels have been reported rarely (one of 9 had much higher levels) (Wisner *et al, Am J Psych* 1998, **155**, 690–92), and withdrawal reactions in breast-fed children after the mother has abruptly stopped sertraline have been reported (Kent and Laidlaw, *B J Psych* 1995, **167**, 412–13), implying that sertraline may appear in breast-milk at levels sufficient to suppress withdrawal after birth. This does not seem to be a common problem (Ratan and Friedman, *B J Psych* 1995, **167**, 824; Altshuler *et al, J Clin Psych* 1995, **56**, 243–45). A small single-dose study showed that **citalopram** is excreted into breast milk at about the same level as fluoxetine, and the infant might receive around 1.8% of the weight-adjusted maternal dose, or 4–17mcg/kg/d (n=2, Spigset *et al, Br J Clin Pharmacol* 1997, **44**, 295–98). A second single patient study showed peak citalopram milk concentrations 3–9 hours after last dose, the infant receiving 5% of maternal dose, and no signs of effect on the infant were seen (Jensen *et al, Ther Drug Monit* 1997, **19**, 236–39).

10. The total dose of **venlafaxine** and O-desmethylvenlafaxine (OMV) ingested by breast-fed infants can be as high as 9.2% of the maternal intake. Measurable concentrations of OMV in the infants' plasma have been shown, although the infants were healthy and showed no acute effects, but exposed infants should be observed closely (n=3, Ilett *et al, Br J Clin Pharmacol* 1998, **45**, 459–62). Animal studies have indicated some non-specific foetal developmental delay and decreased weight.

11. **Mirtazapine** is excreted only in small amounts in breast milk, but use cannot yet be actually formally recommended.

12*. **Tricyclic** antidepressants should be used with care, but it does not seem warranted to recommend that breast-feeding should be discontinued completely, as significant tricyclic levels have not been detected in neonatal serum (except for doxepin and maprotiline). One study has indicated about 1% of maternal dose/kg reaching the infant, minute amounts in the infant serum, no acute toxic effects and no evidence of developmental delay (n=10, Yoshida *et al, J Aff Disord* 1997, **43**, 225–37). For **imipramine**, a milk/plasma ratio of 0.05–0.08, based on high dose samples, would lead to 0.1% of the maternal daily dose appearing in milk. **Amitriptyline**/nortriptyline levels were undetectable in the serum of a breast-fed infant whose mother took 75mg/d of amitriptyline for three weeks (Brixen-Rasmussen *et al, Psycho-pharmacology* 1982, **76**, 94–95). The E-10-hydroxy-nortriptyline metabolite of amitriptyline is also excreted in breast milk but not at a greater level than amitriptyline or nortriptyline (Breyer-Pfaff, *Am J Psych* 1995, **152**, 812–13). Two studies, including 12 mother-baby pairs, showed no detectable **nortriptyline** in the infant serum, despite some unusually high maternal plasma levels, although two infants had low levels of 10-hydroxy metabolites. None of the infants showed any adverse effects and so the risk could be considered very low (Wisner and Perel, *Am J Psych* 1996, **153**, 295). **Maprotiline** has a long half-life and is present in milk in significant amounts so should not be used (*Drug & Ther Bull* 1983, **21**, 48). In two studies of children who had received **dothiepin/dosulepin** via breast milk, no detectable adverse effects on cognitive development were detected (compared to a variety of controls, Buist and Janson, *B J Psych* 1995, **167**, 370–73) and the drug is unlikely to be a significant hazard for the infant (Ilett *et al, B J Clin Pharmacol* 1992, **33**, 635–39). Case reports suggest that the infant may receive only up to 3.7% of the mother's **clomipramine** dose (n=1, Pons *et al, Clin Pharmaco-kinetics* 1994, **27**, 270–89) and with no adverse effects (n=4, Wisner *et al, J Clin Psych* 1995, **56**, 17–20). **Doxepin**, however, has a longer-acting metabolite

N-desmethyldoxepin which may accumulate in breast-fed infants, causing severe drowsiness and respiratory depression (near fatal case at 75mg/d in 8-week-old baby reported by Matheson *et al, Lancet* 1985, **ii**, 1124), and adverse effects have been reported in a newborn infant breast-fed by a mother treated with doxepin (Frey *et al, Ann Pharmacother* 1999, **33**, 690–93). Another report failed to detect any effects in the infant at a maternal doxepin dose of 150mg (Kemp *et al, Br J Clin Pharmacol* 1995, **20**, 497–99; Wisner *et al, Am J Psych* 1996, **153**, 1132) and so metabolic differences could explain these. If the former is accepted and extrapolated to other tricyclics, the general advice is to observe the child carefully for sedation and respiratory depression. A tricyclic with a short half-life for itself (and any active metabolites) would appear to be the better option.

It has been recommended that amitriptyline and imipramine are the preferred tricyclic antidepressants (review by Duncan and Taylor, *Psych Bull* 1995, **19**, 551–52).

13. With **trazodone**, a 50mg single-dose study showed that 1% passed into the milk (n=6, *B J Clin Pharmacol* 1986, **22**, 367–70). More information on, eg. metabolites, is needed but it would appear to be of low risk. There is no published data on excretion of **nefazodone** in breast milk and so caution is advised.

14. **Reboxetine** is excreted in milk in rats but no human data exists so the drug should be avoided (SPC).

15. Minimal data is available for the **MAOIs**. **Tranylcypromine** is excreted in breast milk but levels are not thought to be significant (*Am J Hosp Pharm* 1974, **31**, 844–54). Some sources state that MAOI levels in milk are too small to affect the child (*Am J Psych* 1978, **135**, 417–18) but this has not been supported by any studies other than with tranylcypromine.

16. In 6 lactating women, 0.06% of a single dose of **moclobemide** was excreted unchanged in the milk. It would seem unlikely this amount would produce adverse effects in the baby (Pons *et al, B J Clin Pharmacol* 1990, **29**, 27–31). Two

women taking **mianserin** 60mg/d and 40mg/d have been studied. Mianserin levels were 22 and 25mcg/l in maternal plasma and 80 and 20mcg/l in milk. These are low levels and the infants showed no untoward effects (Buist *et al, B J Clin Pharmacol* 1993, **36**, 133–34). **Amoxapine** appears in human milk, probably at low levels (*J Nerv Mental Dis* 1979, **165**, 635). Lack of toxicity data means **St. John's wort** should best be avoided in breast-feeding. There are no known problems with **tryptophan**.

3.1.3 Anxiolytics and hypnotics:

17. The CSM has noted that since **benzodiazepines** are excreted in breast milk, they should not be given to lactating mothers (*Curr Prob* 1997, **23**, 10). Repeated doses of long-acting benzodiazepines can produce lethargy and weight loss but low and single doses are probably of low risk provided the infant is monitored for drowsiness. Oxazepam seems to be preferable to diazepam in lactating women, but with all anxiolytic benzodiazepines, infants should be observed for signs of sedation and poor suckling. **Diazepam, oxazepam, lorazepam, lormetazepam, nitrazepam** and **flunitrazepam** have all been shown in breast milk. **Temazepam** levels have been reported to be below detection levels at doses of 10–20mg/d and no adverse effects have been seen (*B J Clin Pharmacol* 1992, **33**, 204–5).

18. **Buspirone** should be avoided, based on excretion studies in rats, although there is no specific human data to show adverse effects.

19*. **Zaleplon** is excreted in breast milk, and should not be administered to breast-feeding mothers, although the actual amount likely to be transferred may be very low, eg. 0.017% of maternal dose (n=5, Darwish *et al, J Clin Pharmacol* 1999, **39**, 670–74). **Zopiclone** is contraindicated in breast-feeding as it is excreted in appreciable amounts (up to 50% of maternal levels, see *B J Clin Pharmacol* 1990, **30**, 267–71). Single occasional doses of 7.5mg are probably of low risk as accumulation is unlikely. The American Academy of Pediatrics considers **zolpidem** compatible

with breast-feeding, as it is found only in minute amounts in milk due to its low lipophilic properties and rapid onset and excretion. One study of zolpidem in five lactating women taking a (high) stat dose of 20mg showed that 0.76–3.88mg of zolpidem was excreted into breast milk, nearly all within 3 hours of a dose (Pons *et al, Eur J Clin Pharmacol* 1989, **37**, 245–48). A low dose at bedtime and avoiding breast-feeding for the next few hours would minimise the (unknown) potential effect on an infant.

20. The amounts of **beta-blockers** in milk are probably too small to effect the baby (less than 0.1% of maternal doses) but could produce bradycardia and hypoglycaemia in high doses (*Ther Drug Monit* 1983, **5**, 87–93).

21. **Clomethiazole** is excreted in insignificant amounts based on IV and oral studies in pre-eclampsia (*Acta Psych Scand* 1986, **73** [Suppl 329], 185–88). An infant might ingest active amounts and although the sedative effects of this could be relevant they are unlikely to be harmful. **Chloral** is excreted in breast milk and the sedation caused in the infant makes this a precaution although only minimal sedation after large feeds has been reported (*Adv Drug React Bull* 1976[Dec] 212). The American Academy of Pediatrics recommends that it can safely be used in lactating mothers, as do the authorities in many European countries.

3.1.4 Anticonvulsants*:

All anticonvulsants are excreted in breast milk but at much lower levels than in maternal plasma and so 'sub-therapeutic' doses only are received by the infant (*Clin Pharmacokinetics* 1982, **7**, 508–43). Breast-feeding should be encouraged as bonding is especially important in epileptic mothers (*Lancet* 1990, **336**, 426–27). An extensive review (Hägg and Spigset, *Drug Safety* 2000, **22**, 425–40, 88 refs) of anticonvulsant use during lactation concluded that:

● Carbamazepine, valproate and phenytoin are compatible

● Ethosuximide, phenobarbital and primidone should be regarded as potentially unsafe and close clinical monitoring of the infant is recommended

● Data on the newer drugs is too sparse for reliable recommendations

● Occasional or short-term treatment with benzodiazepines could be considered as compatible with breast-feeding, although maternal diazepam treatment has caused sedation in suckling infants after short-term use. During long-term use of benzo-diazepines, infants should be observed for signs of sedation and poor suckling.

Review*: general (Bar-Oz *et al, Paediatr Drugs* 2000, **2**, 113–26).

22*. **Carbamazepine** has been classified by the American Academy of Pediatrics Committee on Drugs as compatible with breast-feeding, as levels have been found to be relatively low but this is based on case reports in epilepsy, with only two so far when used as mood stabiliser. The half-life is longer in infants, with levels in milk ranging from 7% to 95% of the mother's serum, probably usually around 10%. There are two cases of adverse effects in the infant (n=1, Merlob *et al, Ann Pharmacother* 1992, **26**, 1563–65; n=1, Frey *et al, Eur J Pediatr* 1990, **150**, 136–38) and several cases of poor feeding. Data is often from the first few days of life so the safety of carbamazepine is not well-proven and may need to be re-assessed. The mother should be informed of the potential signs of hepatic dysfunction and CNS effects (review, Chaudron and Jefferson, *J Clin Psych* 2000, **161**, 79–90). **Oxcar-bazepine** is excreted into breast milk, the breast milk/plasma ration for drug and metabolite being about 0.5, similar to carbamazepine (n=1, Bulau *et al, Eur J Clin Pharmacol* 1988, **34**, 311–13), and it is contraindicated in the UK.

23*. **Valproate** has been classified by the American Academy of Pediatrics Committee on Drugs as compatible with breast-feeding, based on case reports in epilepsy. Infant serum levels range from undetectable (n=16, van Unruh *et al, Ther Drug Monit* 1984, **6**, 272–76) to 40% mother's serum level, 5–12%

being common, with a wide variation mainly because of the low number of patients studied. There is a reported adverse (haematological) event (Stahl *et al, J Pediatr* 1997, **130**, 1001–3). In 6 mother-infant pairs where infant exposure was exclusively during breast-feeding, mothers had valproate levels in the usual range for bipolar (39–79 mcg/mL) but infants had low levels (0.7–1.5mcg/mL), thus presenting a relatively low risk compared to the risk of relapse in the mother (n=6, Piontek *et al, J Clin Psych* 2000, **61**, 170–72). Valproate thus appears relatively safe, but with the risk of haematological effects. Care and careful counselling is needed for higher doses (review, Chaudron and Jefferson, *J Clin Psych* 2000, **161**, 79–90).

24. Small quantities of **phenytoin** are excreted in breast milk, peaking at 3 hours, and have been considered clinically safe (*Adv Drug React Ac Pois Rev* 1982, **1**, 255–87).

25. Larger doses of **phenobarbital** and **primidone** may accumulate in breast milk. This may cause unacceptable drowsi-ness and lead to the need to stop or at least reduce breast-feeding.

26*. Extensive passage of **lamotrigine** into breast milk occurs, and with a slow elimination in the newborn, concen-trations in the infant may reach levels at which pharmacological effects can be expected. In one report, the milk to maternal serum ratio was a consistent 0.6, with infant serum levels of 23–33% of the maternal serum levels. This is probably of low risk provided all remain alert to the potential for life-threatening rashes (n=3, Ohman *et al, Epilepsia* 1998, **39**[Suppl 2], 21; review, Chaudron and Jefferson, *J Clin Psych* 2000, **161**, 79–90). **Gabapentin** crosses into breast milk. The manufacturers have data on 6 cases, where gabapentin levels in milk were equal to plasma levels, with no reports of infant levels (review, Chaudron and Jefferson, *J Clin Psych* 2000, **161**, 79–90).

27*. A small study suggested that the quantity of **vigabatrin** ingested through milk is small, at around 1–3% of the daily dose (n=2, Tran *et al, Br J Clin Pharmacol* 1998, **45**, 409–11), but information is contradictory. **Topiramate** and **tiagabine** are not recommended as no human information is currently available. Animal studies indicate **levetiracetam** is excreted into breast milk and so breast-feeding is not recommended.

28. **Ethosuximide** is excreted in breast milk, with detectable infant levels. It might still be wise to monitor levels if possible. Very low doses of **acetazolamide** were transferred by breast-feeding in one reported case (Soderman *et al, Br J Clin Pharmacol* 1984, **17**, 599–600).

3.1.5 Others:

29*. There is no information available on **donepezil, galantamine** and **rivastigmine,** so should not be used in breast-feeding mothers (SPC).

30. There is no data on **anticholinergics** in breast milk.

31. No information is available to date on **disulfiram** in breast milk and so use must be with great caution. There is the possibility of interactions with paediatric medicines (see *4.7.1).* **Acamprosate** is excreted in the milk of lactating animals and so the UK SPC states that use in breast-feeding is a contraindication. No human data proving safety exists.

32*. **Lithium** has been classified by the American Academy of Pediatrics Committee on Drugs as contraindicated in breast-feeding since 1989. Breast milk levels are approximately 40% (range 24–72%), with infant serum having levels 5–200% of the mother's serum concentrations, with 2 case reports of adverse events (eg. hypotonia and lethargy) attributed to lithium (n=1, Tunnessen and Hertz, *J Pediatr* 1972, **81**, 804–7; n=1, Skausig and Schou, *Ugeskr Laeger* 1977, **139**, 400–1),

although the latter was probably multifactorial. The recommendation to contraindicate lithium in breast-feeding is thus based on limited evidence. Informed choice, with careful monitoring of the infant (considering poorer renal excretion and fluid balance/ electrolytes), use of low doses, may help if the risk of relapse is high if stopping. **Reviews***: Chaudron and Jefferson, *J Clin Psych* 2000, **161**, 79–90; Amanth, *Lithium* 1993, **4**, 231–37; Llewellyn *et al, J Clin Psych* 1998, **59**[Suppl 6], 57–64.

33. **Modafinil** is contraindicated in breast-feeding (MI).

34. No information is available for **methylphenidate** (SPC) so do not use.

35. **Methadone** at maintenance doses reduces the risk of poor quality street drugs being used and has been used successfully in breast-feeding. A 12-mother study showed that the amount of methadone in breast milk was measurable but low (insufficient to prevent the development of a neonatal absence syndrome in 7 infants), infant plasma levels were below the limit of detection in seven infants, and no adverse effects attributable to methadone were noted. The conclusion was that breast-feeding should not be discouraged in women on a methadone maintenance programme (Wojnar-Horton *et al, Br J Clin Pharmacol* 1997, **44**, 543). Stopping opiates is also dangerous as withdrawal reactions can damage the foetus more than methadone (for effect on the child in the first year, see *Arch Dis Childhood* 1989, **64**, 235–45).

36*. **Bupropion** and metabolites accumulate in breast milk at higher levels than plasma, although one report indicated that these were not detectable in the infants plasma (n=1, Briggs *et al, Ann Pharmacother* 1993, **27**, 431–33).

3.2 CARDIOVASCULAR DISEASE

	Lower risk	Moderate risk	Higher risk
Antipsychotics	Amisulpride [5] Flupentixol [4] Olanzapine [2] Quetiapine [2] Risperidone [1] Sulpiride [5] Zuclopenthixol [4]	Haloperidol[6] Loxapine[8] Phenothiazines[7] Risperidone[1]	Clozapine [3] Pimozide [8] Thioridazine [7] Zotepine [2]
Antidepressants	Mianserin[16] Mirtazapine [11] SSRIs[9] Trazodone[13] Tryptophan[16]	MAOIs[15] Moclobemide[16] Nefazodone [13] Reboxetine [14] Venlafaxine[10]	Tricyclics[12]
Anxiolytics + hypnotics	Benzodiazepines[17] Buspirone[18] Zopiclone [19] Zaleplon [19] Zolpidem [19]	Beta-blockers[20] Chloral[21] Clomethiazole[21]	
Anticonvulsants	Benzodiazepines[17] Gabapentin[26] Lamotrigine[26] Tiagabine[27] Topiramate[27] Valproate[23] Vigabatrin[27]	Barbiturates [25] Carbamazepine [22] Paraldehyde [28] Phenytoin[2] Oxcarbazepine [22]	Fosphenytoin[24]
Others	Acamprosate[31]	Anticholinergics[30] Anticholinesterases [29] Bupropion[36] Dexamfetamine[34] Lithium[32] Modafinil[33]	Disulfiram[31]

General Principals (adapted from *Maudsley Guidelines*, 2001)

1. Polypharmacy should be avoided where possible, particularly with drugs likely to effect cardiac rate and electrolyte balance.
2. Awareness of QT prolongation is increasing, and so care is essential. A QTc prolonged to about 450ms is considered of some concern, and above about 500/520ms to be of risk of leading to Torsade de Pointes, which may be fatal.
3. Avoid drugs specifically contra-indicated eg. thioridazine, pimozide etc.
4. Start low and go slow is, as ever, good advice. Rapid dose escalation should be avoided.

Angina

Avoid drugs causing orthostatic hypotension, which may exacerbate angina. Avoid drugs causing tachycardia, eg. phenothiazines, clozapine, risperidone etc. Trazodone, nefazodone and tricyclics are best avoided, although most other antidepressants are thought to be of relatively low risk.

Arrhythmias

SSRIs are first choice antidepressants for depression with arrhythmias, and are preferred to tricyclic antidepressants because of their lack of antiarrhythmic/proarrhythmic potential (*Drugs & Ther Perspect* 1998, **11**, 11–13). Avoid phenothiazines, butyrophenones and pimozide. Sulpiride and olanzapine seem of low risk.

Heart failure (HF)

For chronic stable heart failure, avoid beta-blockers and take care with drugs causing orthostatic hypotension, eg. phenothiazines, clozapine, risperidone, tricyclics etc. For acute HF, the cause will indicate which drugs are safer to use. Remember that lithium and diuretics need extra care.

Hypertension

Drugs causing orthostatic hypotension should be monitored closely. Avoid MAOIs. Hypertension can occur with venlafaxine (high dose), clozapine and sometimes with tricyclics and antipsychotics.

Myocardial infarction (MI)

If essential, use SSRIs (except perhaps fluvoxamine), trazodone or mianserin. Avoid high-dose antipsychotics, phenothiazines and pimozide. Butyrophenones, thioxanthenes and benzamides are safer.

3.2.1 Antipsychotics:

1. **Risperidone** should be used with caution due to orthostatic hypotension,

low doses slightly dropping bp and increasing heart rate. It is best to introduce it slowly over several weeks.

2*. Postural hypotension has been seen infrequently with **olanzapine**. Blood pressure monitoring is recommended periodically in patients over 65. An increase in the QTc interval has been seen rarely. One study showed that olanzapine (mean 14mg/d) produced fasting triglyceride levels raised by a mean of 60mg/dL (37%) (n=25, 12/52, Osser *et al, J Clin Psych* 1999, **60**, 767–70), which since triglycerides are a significant risk factor for exacerbation of CHD, needs care (Grundy, *Am J Cardiol* 1998, **81**(4A), 18B–25B). The SPC for **quetiapine** recommends caution with drugs known to prolong the QTc interval and in patients with cardiovascular disease or conditions predisposing to hypotension. Trials did not show sustained changes in the QTc interval. Orthostatic hypotension is more common in the elderly. **Zotepine** causes a dose-related QTc interval prolongation and caution is necessary in patients with CHD and with other drugs known to cause QTc prolongation. Increased heart rate can occur so care in angina pectoris is necessary, and orthostatic hypotension can occur initially in treatment, so bp measuring is recommended. Caution is necessary in severe hypertension.

3*. **Clozapine** has cardiac side-effects, eg. tachycardia and postural hypotension (particularly early in treatment). A recent study showed that 13% had cardiac abnormalities before and 31% after starting clozapine. Risk factors included increased age (but less so if there was a normal ECG with other antipsychotics). Prolonged QTc was dose-dependent, often corrected itself with time, was mostly during the initial stages of treatment, mostly benign and pathological prolongation of QTc was rare (n=61, Kang *et al, J Clin Psych* 2000, **61**, 441–46). Clozapine has also been associated with potentially fatal myocarditis (n=15, 5 occurring within 5 weeks of starting) and cardiomyopathy (n=8) in physically healthy young adults (from Australian database of 8000, Kilian *et al, Lancet* 1999, **354**, 1841–45). Regular ECG monitoring, especially at higher doses, may be very valuable.

4. Cardiac disease is a UK SPC

precaution for **flupentixol** and **zuclopenthixol**.

5. No changes in ECG status have been reported in short and long-term studies of **amisulpride**. There are no specific problems reported with **sulpiride** (SPC).

6*. **Haloperidol** may have the risk of occasional arrythmias and so the use of high dosage with non-responders is cautioned. Prolonged QT-interval has been reported with both haloperidol and **droperidol** (n=596, Reilly *et al, Lancet* 2000, **35**, 1048–52).

7*. Some ECG abnormalities have been reported with **phenothiazines**, eg. tachycardia, T-wave abnormalities, ST depression, QT prolongation and right bundle branch block. **Thioridazine** is now contraindicated in patients with a history of cardiac arrhythmias or at risk of problems. Dose-related increases in risk of lengthened QT-interval have been reported, detectable at doses as low as 10mg/d (n=596, Reilly *et al, Lancet* 2000, **355**, 1048–52). **Levomepromazine** (methotrimeprazine) causes orthostatic hypotension which can, on occasion, be prolonged and profound. Sudden death has also been reported.

8. **Loxapine** can increase pulse rate and produce transient hypotension. With **pimozide**, the UK CSM has had many reports of serious or fatal cardiac reactions to pimozide. They recommend:

i. Start at 2–4mg/d. Increase by 2–4mg/d weekly (max. 20mg/d).

ii. Perform ECG pre-treatment. C/I if a prolonged QT interval or a history of arrhythmia is noted.

iii. Repeat ECG annually. Review if QT interval is lengthened.

iv. Avoid concurrent treatment with other antipsychotics (including depots), tricyclics and other QT interval-prolonging drugs (eg. some anti-malarials, antiarrhythmics, terfenadine, astemizole and diuretics). For CSM advice, see *Curr Prob* 1995, **21**, 2.

3.2.2 Antidepressants*:

Depressed patients are at greater risk of myocardial infarction and vice versa, and, during the first six months post-infarction, patients who become depressed have a five-fold increase in mortality (Frazure-Smith *et al, JAMA* 1999, **270**, 1819–25). Depressed patients are less likely to follow recommendations to reduce cardiac risk during recovery from a myocardial infarction (n=204, survey, Ziegelstein *et al, Arch Int Med* 2000, **160**, 1818–23). Treatment of depression in this group is thus of singular importance. There is a strong association between the use of tricyclic anti-depressants, but not with the use of selective serotonin reuptake inhibitors (SSRIs), and the risk of myocardial infarction (Cohen *et al, Am J Med* 2000, **108**, 2–8).

Reviews*: general (Roose and Spatz, *Drug Safety* 1999, **20**, 459–65, 25 refs).

9*. Despite some reported cases of car-diac effects, the SSRIs are generally considered safer to use in cardiac diseases (eg. n=456, Guy and Silke, *J Clin Psych* 1990, **51**[Suppl 13], 37–39; Glassman *et al, JAMA* 1993, **269**, 2673–75), but the evidence for this is claimed by some to be inconclusive. A naturalistic study in severely ill (sub-acute cardiac rehabilitation unit) elderly cardiac patients showed that **paroxetine**, **sertraline** and **fluoxetine** had little adverse effect on cardiac state and appeared relatively safe and effective, but care was needed with drug inter-actions (n=17, Askinazi, *Am J Psych* 1996, **153**, 135–36). Several open trials have indicated **fluoxetine** up to 60mg/day to have no significant adverse cardiac effects in patients with pre-existing CHF, conduction disease and/or ventricular arrhythmia (n=27, open, 7/52, average age 73, Roose *et al, Am J Psych* 1998, **155**, 660–66). In another, fluoxetine 20mg/d produced a modest reduction in bp, and patients with pre-existing, stable cardiovascular disease (including hypertension) showed no significant bp change (n=796, 12/52, Amsterdam *et al, J Clin Psychopharmacol* 1999, **19**, 9–14). Rare cases of, eg. atrial fibrillation, bradycardia and syncope have been reported. **Citalopram** has no significant reported effect on blood pressure, cardiac

conduction nor heart rate (Milne & Goa, *Drugs* 1991, **41**, 450–77), but exacer-bation of pre-existing bradycardia has been reported (eg. Nyth *et al, Acta Psych Scand* 1992, **86**, 138–45), as has occasional postural dizziness (review of citalopram cardiac safety: Rasmussen *et al, J Clin Psychopharmacol* 1999, **19**, 407–15).

Review: safety of SSRIs in CHD (Sheline *et al, Am J Med* 1997, **102**, 54–59).

10. **Venlafaxine** has a dose-dependent effect on supine diastolic blood pressure, clinically significant at high doses (>200–300mg/d), probably as a result of noradrenergic potentiation (3% incidence at less than 100mg/d, 7% for 150–200mg/d and 13% above 300mg/d). Increased heart rate, serum lipids (eg. rises in cholesterol of 2–3mg/dL) and palpitations (Khan *et al, Psychopharmacol Bull* 1991, **27**, 141–44) have been reported and so caution is required for patients with pre-existing cardiovascular disease, recent myocardial infarction or hyper-lipidaemia (Anon, *J Clin Psych* 1993, **54**, 119–26). It may not adversely effect control of blood pressure in people with pre-existing hypertension (meta-analysis, n=3744, Thase, *J Clin Psych* 1998, **59**, 502–8). People who get this effect may be CYP2D6 deficient, which might help predict future side-effects and drug responses (case and review, Blythe and Hackett, *Hum Exp Toxicol* 1999, **18**, 309–13). Blood pressure monitoring at doses above 200mg/d is recommended.

11. Although hypertension, hypotension and tachycardia have been reported with **mirtazapine**, the incidences of 6%, 4% and 2% respectively are the same as placebo (Smith *et al, Psychopharmacol Bull* 1990, **26**, 191–6). No ECG changes have been observed in reported trials, nor bp and heart rate changes in a six-week depressed inpatient trial (n=251, RCT, Zivkov and Jongh, *Human Psycho-pharmacol* 1995, **10**, 173–80). Mild dizziness and vertigo (described as postural hypotension but with no measurement of parameters) was noted in two patients in one trial, although

treatment continued (van Moffaert *et al, Int Clin Psychopharm* 1995, **10**, 3–9). Mirtazapine would seem to be relatively safe.

12. **Tricyclics** produce orthostatic hypotension (and hence occasional myocardial infarction), have antiarrhythmic actions (quinidine-like) in high dose and antimuscarinic actions (raising heart rate). Thus, tricyclics should only be used with caution in patients with ischaemic heart disease and/or ventricular arrhythmia. SSRIs are generally considered safer. In patients with recurrent chest pain but normal coronary angiograms, imipramine therapy over 9–33 months produced no symptoms of a proarrhythmic effect, a slightly prolonged corrected QT interval and reduced chest pain (n=58, Cannon *et al, NEJM* 1994, **330**, 1411–17). Conversely, in 24 patients with major depression compared with 24 controls, 150mg/d of amitriptyline increased heart rate from 78bpm to 93bpm and all other heart rate analysis parameters significantly worsened (Rechlin *et al, Psychopharmacology* 1994, **116**, 110–14). Care is needed in:

Angina pectoris: use an SSRI.

Arrhythmias: Tricyclics are contraindicated if severe cardiac conduction disorders (eg. 2° or 3° atrioventricular block or right bundle branch block) exist (quinidine-like effect) although there should be no problem if a pacemaker is fitted. If only a minor disorder (eg. isolated left or right bundle branch block) then no antidepressant is contraindicated. Tricyclics (especially imipramine) have a quinidine-like action which may, in fact, be useful, but it is generally considered safer to use a newer antidepressant and treat the arrhythmia with a specific drug.

Heart failure: Care is needed, especially as orthostatic hypotension can be a major problem.

Hypertension: Lower tricyclic doses tend to raise blood pressure, higher doses tend to lower blood pressure. Care is also needed in orthostatic hypotension.

Myocardial infarction: Avoid all antidepressants for the first two months, if possible, as all have some undesirable cardiovascular effects, eg. increased heart rate, postural hypotension, quinidine-like activity etc.

13. One case of reversible ventricular tachycardia (*Chest* 1990, **98**, 247–48) and QT prolongation has been reported with **trazodone** overdose (Levenson, *Am J Psych* 1999, **156**, 929–70) but is generally considered of low risk. There is no published evidence of cardiac problems with **nefazodone**, but, then again, no systematic studies have been carried out. Reduced doses may be needed if used with antihypertensive drugs and there is an alleged potential for interaction with other cardiovascular drugs (see *4.3.3.4*). Nefazodone may have a reduced incidence of orthostatic hypotension in the elderly (MI).

14. **Reboxetine** increased baseline heart rate in 20% of patients in short-term trials. Orthostatic hypotension occurs with increasing frequency at higher doses.

15*. **Isocarboxazid, phenelzine** and **tranylcypromine** are contraindicated in severe cardiac disease.

16*. Many cases of hypertension have been reported with **moclobemide** (eg. Boyd, *Lancet* 1995, **346**, 1498) so monitoring bp may be useful. Occasional hypertension with tyramine in patients with pre-existing labile hypertension has also occurred (*Acta Psych Scand* 1990, **360** [Suppl], 69–70) and so caution in cardiac disease would be sensible. There are no apparent problems with **mianserin** and **tryptophan**.

3.2.3 Anxiolytics and hypnotics:

17. **Benzodiazepines** are relatively safe but contraindicated in acute pulmonary insufficiency. One study in 12 elderly patients showed that temazepam (up to 30mg/d) caused a fall in systolic blood pressure and an increase in heart rate (Ford, *B J Clin Pharmacol* 1990, **29**, 61–67).

18*. **Buspirone** may have some cardiac effects, eg. rare cases of hypertension and tachycardia.

19*. There are no apparent problems with **zaleplon, zolpidem** and **zopiclone**.

20. The use of **beta-blockers** would depend upon the nature of the cardiac disease.

21. **Clomethiazole** is contraindicated in acute pulmonary insufficiency and should be used with care in chronic pulmonary insufficiency. **Chloral** is contraindicated in severe cardiac disease.

3.2.4 Anticonvulsants:

22*. Cardiovascular effects from **carbamazepine** are uncommon but cardiac conduction changes (*Ann Neurol* 1987, **22**, 280), hypertension and atrio-ventricular block (*Am J Psych* 1992, **149**, 572–73) have been reported. There is a case of a patient with a permanent dual-chamber pacemaker, where carbamazepine elevated ventricular and atrial thresholds, thus making the pacemaker ineffective (Ambrosi *et al*, *Lancet* 1993, **342**, 365). Patients on **oxcarbazepine** with cardiac insufficiency and secondary heart failure should have regular weight measurements to determine the occurrence of fluid retention (SPC).

23*. There are some reports of cardiac effects with **valproate**, but no specific cautions.

24*. **Phenytoin** has many cardiac effects and is a useful third-line treatment in cardiac arrhythmias. It is, however, contraindicated in sinus bradycardia, sino-atrial block, second and third degree A-V block and patients with Adams-Stokes syndrome. Severe cardiovascular ADRs have been reported with **fosphenytoin** IV, including asystole, VF and cardiac arrest, mostly within 30mins of an injection. The CSM thus recommend (*Curr Prob Pharmacovigilance* 2000, **26**[May], 1):

• Try to monitor heart rate, bp and respiration during the infusion

• Observe for at least 30 minutes after the infusion ends

• As hypotension may occur at recommended doses and rates, dose or rate reduction may be necessary

• Reduce the loading dose and/or infusion rate by 10-25% in elderly or those with hepatic or renal impairment .

25. IV **barbiturates** can cause hypotension.

26. There is no evidence of any problems with **gabapentin** in cardiac disease. ECG monitoring is recommended in cases of **lamotrigine** overdose (Buckley *et al, Lancet* 1993, **342**, 1552–53).

27. There is no evidence to date of cardiac adverse effects from **vigabatrin**. No significant changes in ECG, blood pressure or heart rate have been noted in initial clinical trials with **topiramate** (MI) and **tiagabine** (MI).

28. There have been reports of hypotension and tachycardia in young children given IV **paraldehyde** (Sinal and Crowe, *Pediatrics* 1976, **57**, 158).

3.2.5 Others:

29*. Anticholinesterases may cause bradycardia so care is needed with the use of **donepezil** in patients with sick sinus syndrome or other conduction conditions (MI). Heart block has been reported with donepezil, and so the SPC has recommended to consider this before prescribing (*Curr Prob Pharmacovig* 1999, **25**, 7). Rare cases of syncope and angina pectoris have been noted in **rivastigmine** trials (MI). **Galantamine** should be used with caution in people with cardiovascular conditions, eg. sick sinus syndrome or other supraventricular cardiac conduction disturbances (SPC). Syncope and severe bradycardia have been reported.

30. **Anticholinergics** should be used with caution, particularly in those with a tendency to tachycardia. Sinus bradycardia has been reported with **benztropine** (*Am J Psych* 1992, **149**, 711) and **benzhexol** (trihexyphenidyl) (*Drug Intell Clin Pharm* 1986, **20**, 786–87).

31. **Disulfiram** is contraindicated in the presence of cardiac failure, coronary artery disease, previous history of CVA and hypertension. The Antabuse-alcohol reaction can cause cardiac arrest even in healthy adults. There are no known problems with **acamprosate** (MI).

32*. **Lithium** rarely causes clinical problems although cardiac failure and sick sinus syndrome are contraindications Usually benign cardiovascular side-effects may occur in 20–30% patients. The main problems with lithium can be T-wave flattening (or possibly inversion), ventricular ectopics, congestive myopathy (reviewed by O'Shea, *Irish Med J* 1985, **78**, 222–24), bradycardia (Farag *et al, Lancet* 1994, **343**, 1371), ECG changes and conduction disturbances, eg. sinus node dysfunction (Terao *et al, Acta Psych Scand* 1996, **93**, 407–8). An analysis, however, of 827 patients by Ahrens *et al* (*J Aff Dis* 1995, **33**, 67–75) showed that deaths from cardiac-related causes are no different in people taking lithium than the general population and so, despite the above reported problems, lithium can be considered not to have a significant risk in this situation (reviewed by Ananth *Lithium* 1993, **4**, 167–79). A pre-treatment ECG is very useful, especially in elderly people.

33*. **Modafinil** is contraindicated in severe hypertension and arrhythmia and used with caution in patients with concurrent heart disease. Monitor heart rate and blood pressure if used in moderate hypertension (MI; discussion by Heitmann *et al, Clin Pharmacol & Therap* 1999, **65**, 328–35).

34*. The manufacturers caution to monitor bp in hypertensive patients with **methylphenidate**.

35. There is little evidence of developing hypertension with **dexamfetamine**, although regular bp testing has been recommended (ASDA, *Sleep* 1994, **17**, 348–51).

36*. **Bupropion** may cause small rises in supine blood pressure (RCT, n=58, Kiev *et al, Ann Clin Psychiatry* 1994, **6**, 107–15), but tends not to cause significant conduction complications, nor exacerbate ventricular arrhythmias and has a low rate of orthostatic hypotension (n=36, open trial in patients with depression and pre-existing heart disease, Roose *et al, Am J Psych* 1991, **148**, 512–16). Infrequent occurrences of orthostatic hypotension, tachycardia, stroke and vasodilation have been reported with bupropion. Significant cardiac conduction prolongation does not seem to occur (Wenger and Stern, *J Clin Psych* 1983, **44**, 176–82; review Roose, *Am Heart J* 2000, **140**[4 Suppl], 84–88).

3.3 DIABETES

	Lower risk	Moderate risk	High risk
Antipsychotics	Amisulpride[5] Butyrophenones[6] Loxapine[8] Risperidone[1] Sulpiride[5] Thioxanthenes[4]	Clozapine[3] Phenothiazines[7] Quetiapine[2] Zotepine[12]	Olanzapine?[2]
Antidepressants	Moclobemide[16] Nefazodone[13] Reboxetine[14] SSRIs[9] Trazodone[13] Tryptophan[16] Venlafaxine[10]	Fluoxetine[9] Mianserin[16] Mirtazapine[11] Tricyclics[12]	MAOIs[15]
Anxiolytics and hypnotics	Benzodiazepines[17] Buspirone[18] Chloral[21] Clomethiazole[21] Zaleplon[19] Zolpidem[19] Zopiclone[19]	Beta-blockers[20]	
Anticonvulsants	Acetazolamide[28] Barbiturates[25] Benzodiazepines[17] Carbamazepine[22] Ethosuximide[28] Gabapentin[26] Oxcarbazepine[22] Vigabatrin[27]	Phenytoin[24] Tiagabine[27] Topiramate?[27] Valproate[23]	
Others	Acamprosate[31] Anticholinergics[30] Anticholinesterases[29] Lithium[32] Methylphenidate[22] Modafinil[33]	Bupropion[34] Disulfiram[31]	

3.3.1 Antipsychotics:

1. There is no evidence from the manufacturers of any effect of **risperidone** on blood biochemistry etc.

2*. Hyperglycaemia with **olanzapine** occurs in 1/100 to 1/1000 (Bettinger *et al, Ann Pharmacother* 2000, **34**, 865–67), may need insulin to manage (eg. n=1, *J Clin Psych* 1998, **12**, 687–88) and may severely exacerbate diabetic control (n=1, Ober *et al, Am J Psych* 1999, **156**, 970). One study showed that olanzapine (mean 14mg/d) produced fasting triglyceride levels raised by a mean of 60mg/dL (37%) (n=25, 12/52, Osser *et al, J Clin Psych* 1999, **60**, 767–70), which needs care since triglycerides are a risk factor for precipitation or exacerbation of diabetes (Grundy, *Am J Cardiol* 1998, **81**(4A), 18B–25B). Occasional hypo- and hyperglycaemia has been reported with **zotepine** (MI). There is no data yet with **quetiapine**.

3*. Elevated insulin levels have been shown with **clozapine** (Melkersson *et al, J Clin Psych* 1999, **60**, 783–91), and a dose-related effect noted, indicating a probable influence on insulin secretion. There is also a study showing a non-significant increase in the number of people having or developing type 2 diabetes mellitus and/or impaired glucose tolerance on clozapine compared to depot antipsychotics (n=130, Hagg *et al, J Clin Psych* 1998, **59**, 294–99). There have also been case reports of high-dose clozapine causing severe hyperglycaemia, requiring insulin (Kamran *et al, Am J Psych* 1994, **151**, 1395). Thus, additional glucose monitoring is strongly indicated in diabetics on clozapine. In addition, a study has indicated that patients on clozapine experience significant weight gain and lipid abnormalities (eg. raised serum triglycerides) and have an increased risk (52% over 5 years) of hyperglycaemia and of diagnosed diabetes mellitus (37% over 5 years). Weight increase, surprisingly, was not a significant risk factor for developing diabetes (n=82, naturalistic, 5 years, Henderson *et al, Am J Psych* 2000, **157**, 975–81, including lengthy discussion of possible mechanisms, similar findings of raised triglycerides in a similar study: n=222, Gaulin *et al, Am J Psych* 1999, **156**, 1270–72). Addition of quetiapine has been suggested as a possible management option (n=65, open, 10/12, Reinstein *et al, Clin Drug Invest* 1999, **18**, 99–104).

4*. Lack of relationship between serum levels of **zuclopenthixol** (n=9) and plasma insulin has been shown (Melkersson *et al, J Clin Psych* 1999, **60**, 783–91). The UK SPC for **flupen-thixol** notes that control of diabetes may be impaired.

5*. There are no apparent problems with **sulpiride** and **amisulpride**.

6*. There are no apparent problems with **haloperidol**.

7*. The 22 diabetics in a large study of **chlorpromazine** did not show any significant modifications to blood sugar levels. Five patients developed diabetes but all five appeared prone to diabetes, eg. overweight, family history etc (n=850, *Am J Psych* 1968, **125**, 253–55). Lack of relationship between serum levels of **perphenazine** (n=12) and plasma insulin has been shown (Melkersson *et al, J Clin Psych* 1999, **60**, 783–91).

8*. There are no apparent problems with **pimozide** nor **loxapine**.

3.3.2 Antidepressants:

Depression in diabetics may be as common as 27% and, in a review of the treatment of depression in diabetes, sertraline was recommended as the drug of choice and the SSRIs being generally preferred to tricyclics and MAOIs (Goodnick *et al, J Clin Psych* 1995, **56**, 128–36). SSRIs may decrease serum glucose levels by up to 30% and cause anorexia (reducing body weight), and may enable diabetics to control hunger and eating better, via their serotonergic effects, unlike the tricyclics, which often have an appetite-raising effect.

9*. No dose changes are recommended with **citalopram**. It has been used to help treat diabetic neuropathy (Sindrup *et al, Clin Pharmacol Ther* 1992, **52**, 547–52) and no changes in glycaemic control were noticed during this trial. There have been no major reports of problems with **sertraline**, including the 16 patients with diabetes mellitus receiving this drug in early clinical trials. One review recommended sertraline as the drug of choice in diabetes (Goodnick *et al, J Clin Psych* 1995, **56**, 128–36). There is, however, a case of hypo-glycemia associated with high doses of sertraline in non-insulin-dependent diabetes mellitus (n=1, Takhar and Williamson, *Can J Clin Pharmacol* 1999, **6**, 12–14). Little is reported with **paroxetine**. Diabetics may become hypoglycaemic during **fluoxetine** treatment (*Drug & Ther Bull* 1990, **28**, 33) and its side-effects, eg. tremor, nausea, sweating and anxiety may be mistaken for hypoglycaemia (case and discussion in *Lancet* 1992, **339**, 1296). Most problems have been reported with the more common non-insulin dependent diabetes mellitus (NIDDM, type 2 disease, adult-onset) rather than the insulin dependent form (IDDM, type 1 disease, juvenile-onset). Fluoxetine enhances the action of insulin in NIDDM irrespective of any effect on reducing weight (Kutnowski *et al, Int J Obesity* 1992, **16**[Suppl 4], 63–66, Potter van Loon *et al, Int J Obesity* 1992, **16**[Suppl 4], 55–61). If fluoxetine is used, counsel about this effect, note a possible loss of hypoglycemic awareness (n=1, Sawka *et al, J Ped* 2000, **136**, 394–96) and regularly check serum glucose levels (review by Salmon, *Psych Bull* 1995, **19**, 553–54).

10. There is no published evidence of problems with **venlafaxine**.

11. The manufacturers of **mirtazapine** recommend care although there are no reports of problems and this is purely a 'class labelling' precaution.

12*. **Tricyclics** may adversely affect diabetic control as they increase serum glucose levels by up to 150%, increase carbohydrate craving and reduce meta-bolic rate but are generally considered safe unless the diabetes is very brittle. Hypoglycemia has been associated with maprotiline (n=1, Isotani and Kameoka, *Diabetes Care* 1999, **22**, 862).

13. There is a single case of **nefazodone** producing rapid and wide fluctuations in blood sugar levels in a diabetic woman

(Warnock, *Am J Psych* 1997, **154**, 288–89). There are no apparent problems with **trazodone**.

14. There are no apparent problems with **reboxetine**.

15. **MAOIs** may decrease serum glucose levels by up to 35% due to a direct influence on gluconeogenesis (Goodnick *et al*, *J Clin Psych* 1995, **56**, 128–36). Diabetes is a UK SPC precaution, eg. **isocarboxazid**.

16. There is a case of **mianserin** dose-related hyperglycaemia in a non-diabetic woman (Marley and Rohan, *Lancet* 1993, **342**, 1430–31). **Moclobemide** 600mg/d did not modify the effect of glibenclamide on plasma glucose and insulin levels in healthy individuals (Amrein *et al*, *Psychopharmacology* 1992, **106**, S24–S31).

3.3.4 Anxiolytics and hypnotics

17*. There is a case of a diabetic presenting with a reduction in insulin requirements after discontinuing **clonazepam** (n=1, Wagner *et al*, *Diabetes Care* 1999, **22**, 2099).

18*. There are no apparent problems with **buspirone**.

19*. There are no apparent problems with **zaleplon**, **zolpidem** and **zopiclone**.

20. **Propranolol** may prolong the hypoglycaemic response to insulin and may effect hypoglycaemic episodes.

21*. There are no apparent problems with **clomethiazole** or **chloral**.

3.3.4 Anticonvulsants:

22. There is an isolated report of **carbamazepine**-induced urinary retention in 2 diabetic patients, where withdrawal improved the condition (Steiner and Birman, *Neurology* 1993, **43**, 1855–56). There are no apparent problems with **oxcarbazepine**.

23. **Valproate** may give false positives in urine tests for diabetes. Protein binding of valproate may be lower in diabetes (Doucet *et al*, *E J Clin Pharmacol* 1993, **45**, 577–79).

24. Hypoglycaemia has been reported with **phenytoin** and glucose metabolism can be affected. Protein binding of phenytoin may be lower in diabetes (Doucet *et al*, *E J Clin Pharmacol* 1993, **45**, 577–79).

25. There are no apparent problems with the **barbiturates**.

26. There are no apparent problems with **lamotrigine**. Blood glucose fluctuations have been reported with **gabapentin** (SPC).

27. No information is available on **topiramate** and **tiagabine**.

28*. There are no apparent problems with **ethosuximide**. Hyperglycaemia has been reported with **acetazolamide** in diabetics and prediabetics, but probably not normal patients, so some care may be necessary.

3.3.5 Others:

29*. There are no apparent problems with **donepezil** nor **galantamine**, but diabetes mellitus is a precaution for **rivastigmine**.

30. There are no known problems with the **anticholinergic** agents.

31. The UK SPC for **disulfiram** recommends caution in diabetes mellitus. There are no apparent problems with **acamprosate**.

32. There is no problem with **lithium** in diabetes, but many patients on lithium develop polyuria and polydipsia, a diabetes insipidus-like syndrome via an effect on cAMP and vasopressin. This can be controlled by ensuring an adequate fluid and salt intake. Lithium may also increase insulin secretion.

33*. There are no apparent problems with **methylphenidate**. A transient loss of appetite may occur. There are no apparent problems with **modafinil**.

34*. Animal studies suggest some risks with **bupropion**, and hyper- and hypoglycemia have been reported and so caution should be utilised with type II diabetics (El-Dakhakhny *et al*, *Arzneimittelforschung* 1996, **46**, 667–69).

3.4 EPILEPSY

	Lower risk	Moderate risk	High risk
Antipsychotics	Amisulpride [5] Haloperidol [6] Pimozide [8] Quetiapine[2] Risperidone?[1] Sulpiride[5] Zuclopenthixol[4]	Olanzapine [2] Phenothiazines (most) [7]	Chlorpromazine[7] Clozapine [3] Loxapine[8] Zotepine[2]
Antidepressants	MAOIs [15] Moclobemide?[16] Reboxetine[14] SSRIs[9] Tryptophan[16]	Mianserin [16] Mirtazapine [13] Nefazodone[13] Trazodone[13] Tricyclics (most)[12] Venlafaxine[10]	Amoxapine[12] Maprotiline[12]
Anxiolytics and hypnotics	Benzodiazepines[17] Beta-blockers[20] Chloral[21] Clomethiazole[21] Zaleplon[19] Zolpidem[19] Zopiclone[19]	Buspirone [18]	
Others	Acamprosate [24] Anticholinergics[23] Modafinil[26]	Disulfiram[24] Anticholinesterases [22] Lithium[25] Methylphenidate [26]	Bupropion [27]

Review: psychotropic-induced reductions in seizure threshold (Stimmel and Dolpheide, *CNS Drugs* 1996, **5**, 37–50).

3.4.1 Antipsychotics:

General principals

1. Keep the daily dose as low as possible – the effect may be dose-related.
2. Take extra care with risk factors including head trauma, previous seizure history and concomitant drugs (especially other antipsychotics). The most susceptible patients are those with a history of epilepsy, a condition that predisposes to epilepsy and those withdrawing from central depressants, eg. benzodiazepines, alcohol, barbiturates etc.
3. Use lowest risk drugs unless essential.
4. Use a slow rate of introduction and withdrawal. Anticonvulsant cover may be appropriate.
5. Dose changes should be small and gentle.
6. Avoid antipsychotics having more antihistaminic, antiserotonergic, sedative and antiadrenergic effects, which may have a greater seizure threshold lowering effect (Marks and Luchins, *Psychiat Med* 1991, **9**, 37–52).

Reviews: antipsychotics in epilepsy (McConnell *et al, Psych Bull* 1997, **21**, 642–45; Ring, *Progress Neurol Psych* 1998, **2**, 29–32).

1. There is little information about

risperidone. Pre-marketing trials showed a seizure incidence of 0.3% (n=2607).

2. The SPC for **olanzapine** states that it should be used cautiously with patients with a history of seizures. Unexplained (ie. patients without reported risk factors) seizures occurred in up to 0.88% patients during pre-marketing trials (n=2500). There may be a slightly higher risk of seizures in people over 65 (MI). The incidence of seizures during **quetiapine** trials has been equivalent to placebo (MI). **Zotepine** has an established dose-related pro-convulsive effect. It should not be used in patients with a personal or family history of epilepsy. The risk of seizures is dose-related and rises above 300mg/d (open, n=129, Hori *et al, Jpn J Psychiatry Neurol* 1992, **46**, 161–67).

3. **Clozapine** can cause seizures, the risk rising from 1% (<300mg/d), through 2.7% (300–600mg/d) to 4.4% (>600mg/d). EEG changes occur in 75% people on clozapine, with up to 40% having paroxysmal discharges (reviewed by Pacia and Devinsky, *Neurology* 1994, **44**, 2247–49). A more rapid dose-titration increases the risk. Many centres use valproate as routine anticonvulsant cover at higher doses of clozapine. See also *4.2.2*.

4. **Zuclopenthixol** may have only mild to moderate effects, with few reports, and may be one of the drugs of choice.

5. There are no known problems with

amisulpride, but a spontaneously resolving generalised convulsion occurred after a 3g overdose (Tracqui *et al, Hum Exp Toxicol* 1995, **14**, 294–98). **Sulpiride** may be a reasonable choice, as only a few cases of convulsions have been reported and it has only shown minimal EEG effects, although care is recommended in patients with unstable epilepsy.

6. **Haloperidol** (*Gen Hosp Psych* 1987, **9**, 135–41) may have only mild to moderate effects, and may be a suitable drug.

7. **Thioridazine** may have a low effect as, although it may enhance spike activity at low dose, it may not do so at higher dose (Oliver *et al, Arch Gen Psych* 1982, **39**, 206–9). **Fluphenazine** may also be low (*JAMA* 1980, **244**, 1460–63). The incidence of seizures with **chlorpromazine** may be 9% at doses above 1g/d and 0.5% at less than 1g/d and is best avoided.

8. **Pimozide** may have a low effect as, although it may enhance spike activity at low dose, it may not do so at higher dose (Oliver *et al, Arch Gen Psych* 1982, **39**, 206–9). **Loxapine**, however, lowers the seizure threshold and can cause convulsions even at normal doses.

3.4.2 Antidepressants:

Unless a large scale trial is carried out (unlikely), the best antidepressant in epilepsy will remain unknown. All patients will require individual assessment of risk factors and recognition that there is a dose-dependent relationship between antidepressants and seizures. A **slow rate of introduction** reduces the risk.

Reviews*: Duncan and Taylor *Psych Bull* 1995, **19**, 355–57 and correspondence; Curran and de Pauw, *Drug Safety* 1998, **18**, 125–33, 60 refs; Pisani *et al, Epilepsia* 1999, **40**[Suppl 10] S48–56.

9. Serotonin function is unlikely to be of major importance in the genesis of seizures and so **SSRIs** are likely to have a low pro-convulsive effect. **Fluvoxamine** has a low pro-convulsive effect (*Neuropsychobiology* 1984, **12**, 249–54) although findings of a lack of epileptogenic effect (*Lancet* 1990, **336**, 386) have been disputed (*Lancet* 1990, **336**, 947) and there have been some CSM reports of fits. **Fluoxetine** has a probable seizure incidence of 0.2%, similar to other antidepressants (MI), although it has been reported to be associated with more seizures than other SSRIs (Ware and Stewart, *DICP Ann Pharmacother* 1989, **23**, 428). Conversely, in an open study of 17 patients with complex partial seizures (with and without secondary generalisation), the addition of fluoxetine in six resulted in disappearance of seizures and a 30% reduction in the other 11 (Favale *et al, Neurology* 1995, **45**, 1926–27). **Paroxetine** appears to have a minimal potential for producing seizures at clinically useful doses (*J Psychopharmacol* 1987, **1**, 31–34). Seizures have occurred rarely in trials and no cause-effect relationship has been proven (Milne & Goa, *Drugs* 1991, **41**, 450–77). With **sertraline**, seizures occurred in early clinical trials at a similar frequency to placebo and only in people with a history of seizures (MI). **Citalopram** has not been reported to interact with anticonvulsants nor have a proconvulsive effect.

10. Seizures have been reported in 0.26% of patients treated with **venlafaxine** during clinical trials and so a slow introduction and withdrawal is recommended.

11. One grand mal seizure has been reported in a patient with a history of seizures receiving **mirtazapine** at a high dose of 80mg/d during a trial. More definite information would be needed before a cause-effect link could be made. Care and monitoring would thus be standard.

12. All **tricyclics** seem to lower the seizure threshold, **amitriptyline** is reputed to be probably the most pro-convulsive antidepressant, with **doxepin** possibly of lowest risk. TDM of tricyclics reduces the risk of tricyclic-induced seizures by indicating when dosage adjustments are required (literature review by Preskorn and Fast, *J Clin Psych* 1992, **53**, 160–62). There is a high incidence of CSM reports of convulsions with **maprotiline** (*Lancet* 1979, **ii**, 1368) plus some EEG abnormalities (*Am J Med Genetics* 1988,

31, 369–73). A slow rate of introduction reduces the risk (*Psychol Med* 1977, **7**, 265–70).

13. There is no published evidence of problems with **nefazodone** but the SPC naturally recommends use only with caution. The SPC for **trazodone** was recently changed to include care in epilepsy, and to avoid abrupt changes in dose.

14. **Reboxetine** may be particularly useful in epilepsy as the spontaneous incidence of seizures is <0.2% (n=1500), with no seizures (even minor) in overdose and minimal interaction potential.

15. **MAOIs** are generally not considered epileptogenic at therapeutic doses (Rabkin *et al, J Clin Psychopharmacol* 1984, **4**, 270–78). The adverse reactions of myoclonic jerks (Lieberman *et al, J Clin Psychopharmacol* 1985, **5**, 221–28) and serotonin syndrome can occasionally be interpreted as seizures.

16*. There have been no reports of problems with **moclobemide** nor **tryptophan** in epilepsy to date. **Mianserin** is often quoted as being relatively safe in epilepsy (*B J Clin Pharmacol* 1983, **15**, 290S–311S). One study of 84 overdoses of 1g or more showed no convulsions (*Curr Med Res Opin* 1980, **6**, 44). There is one case of depression in an 83-year-old woman which resolved completely following a GTC seizure induced by mianserin (Rosenthal *et al, Int J Ger Psych* 1995, **10**, 415–18). Seizures have been reported at therapeutic doses of **amoxapine** (*J Clin Psych* 1984, **45**, 358–59) although the UK SPC states that this only occurs outside the recommended dosage range.

3.4.3 Anxiolytics and hypnotics:

17. For **benzodiazepines**, see *1.17*.

18. Animal studies show **buspirone** to be inactive in attenuating drug-induced seizures. No anticonvulsant activity is expected. The UK SPC states buspirone to be contraindicated in epilepsy

but there is no evidence yet that it is actually epileptogenic (*Psychopathology* 1984, **17**[Suppl 3], 69–78).

19. A weak anticonvulsant activity for **zopiclone** has been shown (*Pharmacol Biochem Behav* 1985, **23**, 653–59). **Zolpidem** is not reported to have any anticonvulsant activity. There is no data on **zaleplon**.

20. There are no apparent problems with the **beta-blockers**.

21. For **chloral** and **clomethiazole**, see *1.17.1* and *1.17.2*.

3.4.4 Others:

22*. Cholinomimetics may have some potential for causing seizures so care is needed with **donepezil** in pre-existing seizure activity (MI). Care should be exercised with the use of **rivastigmine** in patients predisposed to seizures (MI). There has been no increase in the incidence of convulsions with **galantamine** in clinical trials (SPC).

23. There are no problems reported with the **anticholinergic** agents.

24. The UK SPC for **disulfiram** recommends caution in epilepsy. The manufacturers report no known problems with **acamprosate** in epilepsy.

25. **Lithium** has a marked epileptogenic activity (*JAMA* 1980, **244**, 1460–63) in overdose, but probably has no effect at standard dose. **Carbamazepine** and **valproate** may be suitable alternatives.

26*. **Methylphenidate** is not associated with significant risk at therapeutic doses (mentioned in Zaccara *et al, Drug Saf* 1990, **5**, 109–51), but the UK SPC suggests caution. There are no apparent problems with **modafinil**.

27*. **Bupropion** has some epileptogenic activity. Doses should not exceed 450mg/d, no single dose should be above 200mg and doses should not be increased at more than 150mg/d (MI). The risk of seizures is about 4 in 1000 and there appears to be correlation between plasma concentration and the risk for seizures.

3.5 GLAUCOMA (angle-closure)

	Lower risk	Moderate risk	Higher risk
Antipsychotics	Butyrophenones[2] Risperidone[3] Sulpiride[3] Thioxanthenes[2]	Clozapine[2] Loxapine[2] Phenothiazines[1] Zotepine[3]	Olanzapine[3]
Antidepressants	Flupentixol[5] MAOIs[5] Mirtazapine[5] Moclobemide[5] Nefazodone[5] Trazodone[5] Tryptophan[5] Venlafaxine[5]	SSRIs[5]	Tricyclics[4]
Others	Acamprosate[6] Benzodiazepines[6] Caffeine[8] Clomethiazole[6] Disulfiram[6] Gabapentin[6] Lithium[6] Lofexidine[6] Naltrexone[6] Phenobarbital[6] Phenytoin[6] Tiagabine[6] Topiramate[6] Valproate[6] Vigabatrin[6]	Carbamazepine[6]	Anticholinergics[10] Dexamfetamine[7] Methylphenidate[9]

Angle-closure glaucoma (short review, Khaw, *Prescribers' J* 1997, **37**, 34–39) occurs in eyes with a narrow anterior chamber angle, where drainage of the aqueous fluid through the anterior chamber angle is reduced or blocked. Drugs with anticholinergic properties have the potential to either induce angle-closure glaucoma or to worsen it. Although the degree of anticholinergic effect of a drug is of relevance, the individual's susceptibility to those effects is of greater importance.

General advice: Patients with shallow anterior chamber and/or narrow angles or with previously diagnosed glaucoma may be treated with drugs with anticholinergic properties **provided** intraocular pressure is monitored, an ophthalmologist is involved and information given on the symptoms of acute-angle closure, with advice to stop the drug and seek medical attention immediately should those symptoms occur. In a patient with a shallow anterior chamber and narrow angles an ophthalmologist would normally perform an iridotomy or some type of drainage surgery to allow drug use. Treatment with miotic therapy, eg. pilocarpine may not necessarily protect the patient with narrow angles against drug-induced angle closure. Indeed, pilocarpine itself has been reported to rarely cause pupillary block (Zimmerman *et al, Ophthalmology* 1981, **88**, 85–88).

The main symptoms of acute angle-closure glaucoma are blurred vision, 'coloured haloes' around bright lights, intense pain, lacrimation, lid oedema, red eye, nausea and vomiting (review by Oshika, *Drug Safety* 1995, **12**, 256–63). The incidence rises with age due to the aging process, eg. thickening of the lens. Emotional effects may also play a part (eg. Croll and Croll, *Am J Ophthalmol* 1960, **49**, 297–305). The peak effect from a drug on intraocular pressure can occur within 5–24 hours (or sooner) (Lieberman and Stoudemire, *Psychosomatics* 1987, **28**, 145–48).

3.5.1 Antipsychotics:

1. **Phenothiazines** are weak anticholinergics so some potential for problems exists. Screening for glaucoma has been recommended before initiating therapy (Reid *et al, Int Pharmacopsych* 1976, **11**, 163–74), although several studies have shown no detectable angle-closure glaucoma in, eg. 100 patients taking thioridazine, 98 on fluphenazine and 99 on chlorpromazine (Applebaum, *Arch Ophthalmol* 1963, **69**, 578–80). Other large studies have shown similar results although Bock & Swain (*Am J Ophthalmol* 1963, **56**, 808–10) noted 2 patients with borderline increased intraocular pressure among 27 patients taking chlorpromazine. Thus, there is need for routine care (see introduction).

There are a few case reports of stat high-dose iv or im chlorpromazine producing a transient decrease in intraocular pressure (mentioned in review by Bristow and Hirsch, *Drug Safety* 1993, **8**, 136–48, 76 refs).

2. Other antipsychotics with similar anticholinergic effects would include **clozapine, loxapine, flupentixol** and **zuclopenthixol**. **Zotepine** has anticholinergic effects and should be used with caution in narrow angle glaucoma.

3. Antipsychotics with little or no anticholinergic effect must still be considered to have a potential for problems, albeit probably at a low level, eg. **sulpiride, haloperidol** and **risperidone**. **Olanzapine**, is, however, contraindicated in angle-closure glaucoma in the UK.

3.5.2 Antidepressants:

4. **Tricyclics** have a greater anticholinergic effect than phenothiazines. If patients are at risk of angle-closure glaucoma, pre-treatment examination by an ophthalmologist is recommended. Patients with a narrow anterior chamber angle who are receiving glaucoma treatment or who have had laser treatment should have few problems provided care (see introduction) is taken (Oshika, *Drug Safety* 1995, **12**, 256–63). There is a report of four patients with narrow angles all developing acute-angle closure glaucoma with imipramine (Ritch *et al, Arch Ophthalmol* 1994, **112**, 67–68), with clomipramine, exacerbated by postural hypotension (Schlingemann *et al, Lancet* 1996, **347**, 465) and acute exacerbation with maprotiline in a woman already being treated for angle-closure glaucoma (Yamada and Higashi, *Jpn J Clin Ophthalmol* 1991, **45**, 953–55). The effect can be made worse with MAOIs (Goldberg, *JAMA* 1964, **190**, 456–62). A survey by Reid & Blouin (*Psychosomatics* 1976, **17**, 83–85) showed no abnormal intraocular pressures in patients taking tricyclics, even in combination with pheno-thiazines, but a postal survey of ophthalmologists and psychiatrists indicated that occasional, probably drug-induced, cases had been seen, most frequently associated with amitriptyline (Review by Lieberman and Stoudemire, *Psychosomatics* 1987, **28**, 145–48). See general advice.

5*. Antidepressants which can cause dilation of the pupil include the **SSRIs, mirtazapine, moclobemide, trazodone, nefazodone** and **MAOIs**. There is a possible case with **fluoxetine** in a patient sensitive to anticholinergic effects and with a positive family history (Ahmad, *DICP Ann Phar macother* 1991, **25**, 436). Acute angle-closure glaucoma associated with **paroxetine** has been reported (n=7, Eke and Bates, *BMJ* 1997, **314**, 1387). There is limited experience with **reboxetine** but the SPC recommends close supervision. Raised intraocular pressure or narrow-angle glaucoma is a **venlafaxine** UK SPC warning (12.99).

3.5.3 Others:

6. There are no reported problems with any of the **anticonvulsants, mood stabilisers, anxiolytics** nor **hypnotics**.

7. **Amfetamine** causes a transient rise in intraocular pressure but which is not associated with closure of the angle.

8. **Caffeine** has been reported to cause a transient rise in intraocular pressure but which is not associated with closure of the angle, but this has now been disproven as it was probably due to daily fluctuations in intraocular pressure.

9. **Methylphenidate** causes a transient rise in intraocular pressure but which is not associated with closure of the angle. There is a single case of uneventful use of methylphenidate in a 55-year-old male with ADHD and primary open-angle glaucoma well-controlled by pilocarpine and betaxolol (Bartlik *et al, Arch Gen Psych* 1997, **54**, 188–89).

10. **Anticholinergics** are contraindicated in angle-closure glaucoma.

3.6 LIVER DISEASE

	Lower risk	Moderate risk	High risk
Antipsychotics	Amisulpride[5] Flupentixol[4] Haloperidol[6] Pimozide[8] Sulpiride[5] Zuclopenthixol[4]	Clozapine[3] Loxapine[8] Olanzapine[2] Phenothiazines[7] Quetiapine[2] Risperidone[1]	Zotepine[2]
Antidepressants	Mianserin[16] Paroxetine[9] Tryptophan[16]	Mirtazapine[11] Moclobemide[16] Nefazodone[13] Reboxetine[14] SSRIs[9] Trazodone[13] Tricyclics[12] Venlafaxine[10]	Lofepramine[12] MAOIs[15]
Anxiolytics and hypnotics	Lorazepam LD[17] Oxazepam LD[17] Temazepam LD[17]	Buspirone[18] Clomethiazole[21] Propranolol LD[20] Zaleplon[19] Zolpidem[19] Zopiclone[19]	Benzodiazepines (esp LA)[17] Chloral[21] Propranolol HD[20]
Anticonvulsants	Carbamazepine[22] Ethosuximide[28] Gabapentin[26] Topiramate?[27] Vigabatrin[27]	Acetazolamide[28] Benzodiazepine[17] Lamotrigine[27] Levetiracetam[27] Oxcarbazepine[22] Paraldehyde[28] Tiagabine[27]	Barbiturates[25] Phenytoin[24] Valproate[23]
Others	Donepezil[29] Lithium[32]	Acamprosate[31] Anticholinergics[30] Bupropion[35] Disulfiram[31] Galantamine[29] Methylphenidate[34] Modafinil[33] Rivastigmine[29]	

LD	=	low dose.
HD	=	high dose
SA	=	short-acting.
LA	=	long-acting.

General Principals (adapted from *Maudsley Guidelines*, 2001)

1. The greater the degree of hepatic impairment, the greater the degree of impaired drug metabolism, the greater the risk of drug toxicity, the lower should be the starting and final dose. People may be more sensitive to common or predictable side-effects.
2. LFTs do not necessarily correlate well with metabolic impairment, although give a reasonable indication.
3. Care is needed with drugs with a high first-pass clearance effect.
4. In severe liver disease, avoid drugs with marked side-effects of sedation and constipation.
5. Start low, go slow, monitor LFTs regularly (eg weekly).

3.6.1 Antipsychotics:

1. Unbound **risperidone** increases in liver disease and so initial doses and dose increments should be halved in patients with liver impairment (SPC), and a dose of 4mg/d not exceeded. Risperidone-induced jaundice has been reported (n=1, Oyewole *et al, Int J Ger Psych* 1996. **11**, 179), as has rapid onset risperidone-induced hepatotoxicity (Phillips *et al, Ann Pharmacother* 1998, **32**, 843).
2. A lower **olanzapine** starting dose of 5mg/d may be appropriate (MI). Transient, asymptomatic elevations in ALT and AST have been noted and monitoring of these in patients with risk factors (eg. hepatic impairment, concomitant hepatotoxic drugs) may be appropriate. A single-dose study with **quetiapine** showed some reduced clearance compared to controls so the starting dose should be 25mg/d, with dose increments of 25–50mg/d (eg. Thyrum *et al, Prog Neuropsychopharmacol Biol Psych* 2000, **24**, 521–33). **Zotepine** levels may be 2–3 times higher in patients with liver impairment. Start at 25mg bd up to maximum of 75mg bd and measure LFTs weekly for the first three months of therapy for patients with hepatic impairment (MI).

3. Severe hepatic disease is a contra-indication for **clozapine**, and so lower doses and regular plasma level monitoring would be necessray if used. There are reported cases of toxic hepatitis associated with clozapine at 300–400mg/d, with AST levels dramatically raised, an eosinophilia developing early and full LFT normalisation within 4–5 weeks of clozapine stopping (Kellner *et al, Am J Psych* 1993, **150**, 985–86; Thatcher *et al, Am J Psych* 1995, **152**, 296–97).

4*. No dosage adjustments are necessary for **flupentixol** (Jann *et al, Clin Pharmacokinet* 1985, **10**, 315–33) nor **zuclopenthixol** although both undergo hepatic metabolism and so some caution would be wise in significant hepatic impairment.

5. **Sulpiride** and **amisulpride** are virtually unmetabolised with little or no bilary excretion. There is a low incidence of liver toxicity reported, with a transient rise in serum transaminase the only reported effect (*Acta Psych Scand* 1984, **69**[Suppl 311], 7–41). Dosage adjustments are thus unnecessary (SPC).

6*. There are no apparent problems with **haloperidol**, although the UK SPC states liver disease to be a caution.

7. **Phenothiazines** may cause hepato-canalicular cholestasis and there have been suggestions of possible immunological liver damage. Onset is usually during the first month of therapy. They may precipitate coma due to increased cerebral neurone sensitivity. **Chlorpromazine** is particularly hepatotoxic.

8. No specific problems are known in liver damage with **loxapine**, but due to extensive metabolism of the drug, use in severe liver disease is likely to be of a higher risk.

3.6.2 Antidepressants:

9. In hepatic impairment, alternate day-dosing of **fluoxetine** is recommended. Cirrhotic patients show higher plasma levels of fluoxetine and norfluoxetine and lengthened half-lives, and a 50% reduction in dose is recommended, especially if a low albumin is present

(n=14, Schenker *et al, Clin Pharmacol Ther* 1988, **44**, 353–59). **Citalopram** is metabolised extensively by the liver, with three major metabolites. Doses at the lower end of the therapeutic range should be used (Milne & Goa, *Drugs* 1991, **41**, 450–77). No liver enzyme abnormalities were noted in that paper, reviewing 1000 patients treated with citalopram. **Sertraline** is extensively metabolised by the liver and there is insufficient evidence in significant hepatic dysfunction for use to be other than a contraindication. One study showed a 2.5-fold increase in half-life and a 1.6-fold increase in sertraline/desmethylsertraline peak levels in 10 patients with stable chronic cirrhosis (cf 10 controls, Demolis *et al, Br J Clin Pharmacol* 1996, **42**, 394–97). **Paroxetine** appears to be the safest option, using doses at the lower end of the therapeutic range. There is a case of biopsy-confirmed chronic active hepatitis that was probably attributable to paroxetine (Benbow and Gill, *BMJ* 1997, **314**, 1387). **Fluvoxamine** should be started at 50mg/d and monitored carefully, as raised hepatic enzymes have been reported.

10. **Venlafaxine** clearance is reduced by about 35% in mild to moderate hepatic impairment and so doses should be reduced by about 25–50% respectively, although there is much inter-patient variability in liver damage (Anon, *J Clin Psych* 1993, **54**, 119–26). It is not recommended in severe hepatic impairment.

11*. **Mirtazapine** clearance was reduced by 33% in moderate hepatic impairment in a single dose study (n=16, Murdoch *et al, B J Clin Pharmacol* 1993, **35**, 76P) and so dosage reduction may be necessary. Transient asymptomatic raised liver enzymes (eg. SGTP) have been noted in a few patients in early clinical trials.

12. Most **tricyclics** have a high first-pass clearance by the liver, and so lower starting doses are necessary. Increased sedation with tricyclics is likely due to decreased metabolism eg. **amitriptyline** has been reported to have doubled or tripled plasma levels in patients with

cirrhosis (eg. Hrdina *et al, Can J Psych* 1985, **30**, 111–12) and should be avoided. Increased blood levels may also be caused by reduced plasma protein binding if albumin levels are lower, as with many tricyclics protein binding is high. Particular care is obviously needed if albumin levels are low. SSRIs such as paroxetine would appear to be easier to use than tricyclics in liver disease. Cholestatic jaundice has occasionally been noted with tricyclics. **Lofepramine** is contraindicated.

13*. **Nefazodone** is metabolised to three metabolites; OH-nefazodone, desethyl-hydroxy-nefazodone and mCPP. Accumulation can thus occur in liver impairment, eg. increased half-life, and so doses in the lower end of the range should be used. Nefazodone-induced liver failure has been reported, two cases requiring transplantation (n=3, Aranda-Micahel *et al, Ann Int Med* 1999, **130**, 285–88). **Trazodone** should be used with care in severe hepatic impairment.

14*. **Reboxetine** half-life and plasma levels appear to rise in severe hepatic insufficiency and dose adjustment may be necessary. A starting dose of 2mg bd is recommended (n=12, Tran *et al, Clin Drug Invest* 2000, **19**, 473–77).

15. **MAOIs** are hepatotoxic and may precipitate coma. Patients may also be more sensitive to side-effects (Morgan & Read, *Gut* 1972, **13**, 697–701). If essential, start with a low dose, increase gradually and observe carefully. **Isocarboxazid** is contraindicated with any degree of impaired hepatic function.

16. **Moclobemide** clearance can be reduced and half-life increased in cirrhosis and so doses should be reduced by a half or third to avoid accumulation (Stoeckel *et al, Acta Psych Scand* 1990, **360**[Suppl], 94–97). There are no apparent problems with **mianserin** and **tryptophan**.

3.6.4 Anxiolytics and hypnotics:

17. The metabolism of **diazepam** and **chlordiazepoxide** is impaired in liver disease. The half-lives of the metabolites desmethylchlordiazepoxide and demoxepam are reported to be prolonged to up to 346hrs and 150hrs respectively (*Med Tox* 1989, **4**, 73–76) and may be detectable two months after stopping treatment in patients with hepatic encephalopathy (*Gastroenterology*, 1991, **101**, 274–75) and which may induce coma. Impaired metabolism has been reported with **alprazolam, clobazam** and **midazolam** (significantly impaired in cirrhosis, as it is metabolised by at least 3 different P450 enzymes, Wandel *et al, B J Anaesthesia* 1994, **73**, 658–61). The metabolism of **lorazepam, temazepam** and **oxazepam** is unchanged and these are probably the benzodiazepines of choice in low dose (reviewed by Peppers, *Pharmacotherapy* 1996, **16**, 49–58).

18. **Buspirone** plasma levels have been shown to be higher in patients with hepatic failure, with a good correlation between steady-state buspirone levels and serum albumin (Barbhaiya *et al, E J Clin Pharmacol* 1994, **46**, 41–47). Caution is recommended with a history of hepatic impairment and not used in severe hepatic disease.

19*. Elimination of **zopiclone** can be reduced with hepatic dysfunction producing enhanced adverse effects (*B J Clin Pharmac* 1983, **16**, 259). A lower dose of 3.75mg to 7.5mg (but no higher) can be used with caution in hepatic disease. Plasma protein binding of **zolpidem** is reduced in hepatic impairment (Pacifici, *Int J Clin Pharmacol Ther Toxicol* 1988, **26**, 439–43). Zolpidem is contraindicated in severe hepatic insufficiency and reduced doses are recommended in cirrhosis and other hepatic impairment due to increases in half-life (up to 10 hours in cirrhosis) and peak plasma concentrations. Hepatoxicity has been associated with zolpidem (n=1, Karsenti *et al, BMJ* 1999, **318**, 1179). **Zaleplon** is contraindicated in severe hepatic insufficiency and the dose should be reduced to 5mg in patients with mild to moderate hepatic impairment.

20. The metabolism of **propranolol** is impaired in decompensated liver disease and by portal systemic shunting. High doses are potentially toxic and so reduced oral doses are needed. Propranolol may

increase the risk of developing hepatic encephalopathy.

21. Due to increased availability and reduced clearance, higher blood levels of **clomethiazole** occur in severe liver disease (perhaps a ten-fold increase) and so reduced oral doses are needed, eg. a third of normal (*BMJ* 1978, **ii**, 861) and sedation can mask the onset of liver coma. **Chloral** is contraindicated in marked hepatic impairment.

3.6.4 Anticonvulsants:

22*. Serious hepatic disorders from **carbamazepine** are rare, but jaundice, hepatitis and liver function disorders have been reported, and so use should be with caution. Although **oxcarbazepine** is rapidly and extensively metabolised, no dose adjustments are generally needed in mild to moderate hepatic impairment. Oxcarbazepine has not been studied in severe hepatic impairment (SPC).

23. **Valproate** is contraindicated in active liver disease, as it can be hepatotoxic and liver failure can occur in about 1 in 10,000 cases. The risk is higher early on in therapy and lessens after a couple of months (review in *Med Tox* 1988, **3**, 85–106). Electron-microscopy shows lipid droplets and a scarcity of cytoplasmic cells and normal mitocondria (Caparros-Lefebvre *et al, Lancet* 1993, **341**, 1604). Hepato-toxicity occurs mostly in children and presents as worsening epilepsy, drowsiness and with biochemical and/or clinical evidence of liver failure. Some fatal cases have been reported. Care needs to be taken if valproate is used in children, especially if used with other anticonvulsants.

24*. **Phenytoin** is highly protein bound and extensively metabolised. Accumulation and toxicity of phenytoin may thus occur in severe liver disease. Use reduced doses and monitor for toxicity. In uraemia, protein binding may be reduced but active/free levels remain unchanged. Therapeutic control may then be possible at plasma levels below the usual range. Severe cardiovascular ADRs have been reported with **fosphenytoin** IV (see *3.2.4*) and a reduction in loading dose and/or infusion rate by 10–25% is recommended in hepatic impairment.

25. Increased cerebral sensitivity and the impaired metabolism of **barbiturates** may precipitate coma. Plasma albumin-binding may be reduced but this may have no clinical effect.

26*. **Gabapentin** is virtually un-metabolised and so dose adjustments are unnecessary. Initial and maintenance doses of **lamotrigine** should be reduced by 50% in moderate (Child-Pugh grade B) hepatic impairment, and by 75% in severe (Child-Pugh grade C) impairment.

27*. **Vigabatrin** can cause decreased LFT levels but there is no evidence of hepatic toxicity. **Topiramate** is not extensively metabolised. About 60% is excreted unchanged via the kidneys. In moderate-to-severe liver disease, clearance is reduced by about 26% although the resultant changes in plasma levels have been considered clinically insignificant by the manufacturers. **Tiagabine** is metabolised by the liver. Initial doses in mild to moderate hepatic impairment should be lower. Use in severe hepatic impairment is not recommended (Lau *et al, Epilepsia* 1997, **38**, 445–51). No dose adjustment is needed with **levetiracetam** in mild to moderate hepatic impairment, but a 50% dose reduction is recommended in severe impairment due to concomitant renal impairment (see SPC).

28*.There are no apparent problems with **ethosuximide**. **Acetazolamide** should be used with caution. **Paraldehyde** elimination is slowed in hepatic failure and so lower doses may be needed.

3.6.5 Others:

29*.No change in dose is necessary with **donepezil** in mild to moderate hepatic impairment (MI). **Rivastigmine** is contraindicated in severe liver impairment (MI). In moderate to severe impaired hepatic function, start with **galantamine** 4mg/d, increasing slowly to a maximum of 8mg bd, as the half-life may be increased by about 30%. In severe (Childs-Pugh >9) impairment, galantamine is contraindicated (due to current lack of safety data). No dosage reduction is necessary for mild impairment (SPC).

30. The UK SPCs for the **anticholinergics** all urge some caution in hepatic disease.

31. The UK SPC for **disulfiram** recommends caution in liver disease. Although some evidence of further raised LFTs was noted, an open trial showed disulfiram was safe in patients with elevated LFTs and/or evidence of Hepatitis C virus, provided LFTs were monitored regularly (n=57, Saxon *et al, J Clin Psych* 1998, **59**, 313–16). The UK SPC for **acamprosate** states that use in severe hepatic failure (Child-Pugh grade C) is a contraindication but the pharmacokinetics are not altered by mild to moderate hepatic dysfunction.

32. There are no problems with **lithium** in liver disease.

33. The maximum **modafinil** dose of 400mg/d should only be used in the absence of hepatic impairment (MI).

34. There is no data on **methylphenidate**.

35*. **Bupropion** is extensively metabolised and there are rare reports of abnormal LFTs, liver damage and hepatotoxicity, with some metabolite half-lives prolonged in cirrhosis. Reduced initial doses and close monitoring is required, as a prolonged half-life has been reported in hepatic failure (DeVane *et al, J Clin Psychopharmacol* 1990, **10**, 366–73).

3.7 OLD AGE

	Lower risk	Moderate risk	Higher risk
Antipsychotics	Amisulpride [5] Risperidone? [1] Sulpiride[5]	Butyrophenones [6] Loxapine [8] Olanzapine? [2] Phenothiazines[7] Quetiapine[2] Thioxanthenes[4]	Clozapine[4] Thioridazine[7] Zotepine[2]
Antidepressants	Lofepramine[12] Mirtazapine[11] Moclobemide[16] SSRIs[9] Tryptophan[16] Venlafaxine[10]	Flupentixol[4] MAOIs[15] Mianserin[16] Nefazodone[13] Nortriptyline[12] Reboxetine[14] Trazodone	Tricyclics (most)[12]
Anxiolytics &hypnotics	Alprazolam[17] Buspirone[18] Clobazam[17] Lorazepam[17] Oxazepam[17] Oxprenolol[20] Zaleplon[19] Zopiclone[19]	Clomethiazole[21] Flunitrazepam[17] Flurazepam[17] Propranolol[20] Temazepam[17] Zolpidem[19]	Benzodiazepines long-acting[21]
Anticonvulsants[7]	Carbamazepine [22] Clobazam[17] Oxcarbazepine[22] Tiagabine[27] Topiramate? [27]	Barbiturates[25] Clonazepam[17] Gabapentin[26] Lamotrigine[26] Levetiracetam[27] Piracetam? [27] Valproate[23]	Acetazolamide [28] Benzodiazepines (most)[17] Fosphenytoin [24] Paraldehyde [28] Phenytoin [24] Vigabatrin [27]
Others	Anticholinesterases [29] Bupropion [35] Modafinil [33]	Anticholinergics [29] Lithium [32]	Acamprosate? [31] Methylphenidate [34]

In the elderly, drug absorption and distribution are altered, metabolism, cardiac output and renal perfusion are reduced and tissue sensitivity is usually increased.

General Principals (adapted from *Maudsley Guidelines*, 2001)

1. Increased sensitivity to drugs occurs due to age-related changes in pharmacokinetics (ADME and protein binding) and pharmacodynamics (neuronal changes, receptor binding etc). The over 70s have about twice as many ADRs as under 50s, eg. postural hypotension with antipsychotics, longer sedation with hypnotics, increased sensitivity to anticholinergic side-effects of drugs etc.

2. Hepatic changes (eg. reduced metabolism) and reduced renal clearance will affect many drugs.

3. The lowest effective dose should be used, so '**start low and go slow**', avoid polypharmacy (see below) and monitor effects (both positive and negative) regularly and frequently.

4. Avoid drugs with sedative and hypotensive effects, which can increase the under-rated risks of falls. A meta-analysis concluded that psychotropics are associated with a small increase in falls (Leipzig *et al, J Am Ger Soc* 1999, **47**, 30–39; reviewed by Shorr, *EBMH* 1999, **2**, 95).

5. Use drugs only when necessary, decide a treatment aim, keep therapy simple, use the smallest effective doses and discontinue gradually if no apparent benefit can be seen.

6. Most drugs are highly lipophilic and an increased fat to lean body mass ratio, in addition to decreased metabolism and excretion, means that half-lives usually increase.

7. Consider other factors, eg. potential poor compliance due to social or physical reasons, or use of OTC medicines.

Review*: geriatric psychopharmacology (Zubenko and Sunderland, *Harvard Rev Psych* 2000, **7**, 311–33, 202 refs).

3.7.1 Antipsychotics:

Antipsychotics can relieve psychotic symptoms in older adults but frequent assessments for side-effects are very useful before treatment, and then every 3–6 months. Side-effects (eg postural hypotension, anticholinergic effects, Parkinsonism) are common. Single daily doses are usually appropriate once stable (as indeed they are in younger adults).

Doses should be reviewed regularly, and periodic reduction in dose (eg. by 10–25% every four weeks) for some patients may be indicated (Eimer, *Consult Pharm* 1992, **7**, 921–33).

Reviews*: general (Phanjoo (*Adv Psych Treat* 1996, **2**, 133–39; Sciolla and Jeste, *Int J Psych Clin Prac* 1998, **2**, S27–34, 55 refs), atypicals in elderly (Yiu-Chung *et al, Pharmacotherapy* 1999, **19**, 811–22; Jeste *et al, Am J Geriatr Psychiatry* 1999, **7**, 70–76).

1. **Risperidone** is partially metabolised to an active metabolite (Nyberg *et al, Psychopharmacology* 1993, **110**, 265–72) and so lower doses may be needed only if hepatic impairment is present (see *3.6.1*). It has been reported that decreased clearance in the elderly lengthens the half-life of risperidone, but the significance of this is not known (Cohen, *Pharmacotherapy* 1994, **14**, 71–76). The UK SPC now states that risperidone is well tolerated in the elderly when used with a starting dose of 0.5mg bd or lower and adjusted up to 2mg bd.

2. A lower **olanzapine** starting dose of 5mg/d is not routinely recommended but may be appropriate in some patients as the mean elimination half-life is 50% longer and clearance slightly reduced in healthy elderly patients. Blood pressure monitoring is recommended periodically and there may be a slightly higher risk of seizures in people over 65 (MI). Transient sedation and somnolence were more marked in the elderly in pre-marketing trials. The mean clearance of **quetiapine** in elderly patients was 30–50% lower than healthy adults so the starting dose should be 25mg/d, with dose increments of 25–50mg/d and the final dose is likely to be less than in younger patients (Thyrum *et al, Psychopharmacol Bull* 1996, **32**, 524, abstract). An open trial showed quetiapine to be well tolerated and clinically effective in elderly patients, with somnolence (32%), dizziness (13%) and postural hypotension (13%) the most common side-effects (n=151, 12/52, McManus *et al, J Clin Psych* 1999, **60**, 292–98). Orthostatic hypotension is more common in the elderly. **Zotepine** levels may be 2–3 times higher in elderly patients. Start at 25mg bd up to a maximum of 75mg bd for elderly patients.

3*. **Clozapine** may be safe, well-tolerated and effective in the elderly (n=133, Barak *et al, Comp Psych* 1999, **40**, 320–25) at doses as low as 50–100mg, but as there may be an increased incidence of agranulocytosis, great care should be taken.

4. **Zuclopenthixol** and **flupentixol** should be used with caution in renal disease. Lower doses of flupentixol may be needed due to changed kinetics (*Jann et al, Clin Pharmacokinet* 1985, **10**, 315–33), and, as with other anti-psychotics, the elderly suffer more side-effects (Balant-Gorgia and Balant, *Clin Pharmacokinet* 1987, **13**, 65–90).

5. Single doses of **amisulpride** are well tolerated and show a similar pharma-cokinetic profile in healthy elderly and young subjects (n=20, Hamon-Vilcot *et al, Eur J Clin Pharmacol* 1998, **54**, 405–9).

6. For the **butyrophenones**, an increased severity of side-effects including oversedation, hypotension and respiratory depression may occur (eg. Holloway, *Drug Intell Clin Pharm* 1974, **8**, 623–42) and so lower starting doses are indicated.

7*. It is generally recommended that one half to one third the adult dose of **pheno-thiazines** should be used for elderly patients, who are more susceptible to Parkinsonian side-effects (n=120, Caligiuri *et al, J Clin Psychopharmacol* 1999, **19**, 322–28), and which are often then harder to manage. **Thioridazine** may cause orthostatic hypotension and QT prolongation and so should be avoided (Cohen and Sommer, *J Clin Psychopharmacol* 1988, **8**, 336–39). **Chlorpromazine**, except in very low dose, should be avoided **Levomepro-mazine** is not recommended for use in people over 50 unless the risk of hypotensive reaction has been assessed (MI).

8. Doses of **loxapine** of around 40mg/d have been used successfully in the elderly (Branchey *et al, J Am Ger Soc* 1978, **26**, 263–67).

3.7.2 Antidepressants:

Drugs with anticholinergic side-effects may further harm an already compromised cholinergic system.

9*. SSRIs have obvious benefits in the elderly (fewer anticholinergic effects, a benign cardiovascular profile, ease of use and safety in overdose) but some unappreciated risks, including falls, hyponatraemia, weight loss, sexual dysfunction and drug interactions (Herrmann, *Can J Clin Pharmacol* 2000, **7**, 91–95). The half-life of **fluoxetine** appears not significantly different in the elderly (Lemberger *et al, J Clin Psych* 1985, **46**, 14–19) and when compared to doxepin was as effective but produced less side-effects in the elderly (Feighner and Cohn, *J Clin Psych* 1985, **46**, 20–25). In an open study of 20 depressed and physically ill hospitalised elderly patients with multiple pathology and poly-pharmacy, fluoxetine was claimed to be a safe and effective antidepressant in this difficult to treat cohort (Evans and Lye, *J Clin Exp Gerontol* 1992, **14**, 297–307). No pharmacokinetic differences have been seen with **fluvoxamine** in the elderly and so no dose alterations are necessary (de Vries *et al, Ther Drug Monitor* 1992, **14**, 493–98). **Sertraline** clearance may be reduced by up to 40% and half-life increased by 40% in elderly volunteers, but this does not seem to warrant dosage adjustment (Warrington, *Int Clin Psychopharmacol* 1991, **6**[Suppl 2], 11–21). A study of younger (18–45) and older (over 65) volunteers (n=22 for each group) showed a similar sertraline half-life (32–27 hours) in all groups except younger men, where the half-life was 22 hours (Ronfeld *et al, Clin Pharmacokin* 1997, [Suppl 1], 22–30). Initially, lower doses of 10mg are recommended for **paroxetine**, as blood levels with 20mg/d in the elderly can be similar to those of 30mg/d in younger people (Bayer *et al, Acta Psych Scand* 1989, **80**[Suppl 350], 85–86; Lundmark *et al, Acta Psych Scand* 1989, **80**[Suppl 350], 76–80, review of paroxetine in old age Holliday and Plosker, *Drugs and Aging* 1993, **3**, 278–99). A prolonged **citalopram** half-life (up to 3.8 days) and raised steady-state plasma levels in the elderly may be due to reduced meta-bolism. Dose reduction (by up to 50%) has been suggested but normal adult doses have been used in some studies with no apparent problem (eg. Bouchard *et al, Acta Psych Scand* 1987, **76**, 583–92). The manufacturers recommend a starting dose of 20 mg/d in all patients.

10. **Venlafaxine** clearance is reduced by about 15% in the elderly, probably due to reduced renal function, but dosage adjustment is not generally considered necessary (Anon, *J Clin Psych* 1993, **54**, 119–26). Postural hypotension may be more common.

11. **Mirtazapine** dosage is the same in the elderly as younger adults, although the manufacturers' recommend care with dosage increments. In an elderly patient trial, mirtazapine 15–45mg/d was shown to have equivalent efficacy, but relatively fewer cardiac effects compared with sub-therapeutic amitriptyline 30–90mg/d (n=115, d/b, Hoyberg *et al, Acta Psych Scand* 1996, **93**, 184–90).

12. Reduced initial doses of **tricyclics** are recommended, with perhaps slightly lower final doses, depending upon toler-ance, as cognitive and central effects are enhanced in the elderly. Higher serum levels occur with standard doses (reviewed by Hicks *et al, J Clin Psych* 1981, **42**, 374–85) with reduced clearance and doubled half-life shown with **imipramine** (Benetello *et al, Int J Clin Pharmaco Res* 1990, **10**, 191–95). Single night-time doses of **dothiepin/ dosulepin** have been used in the elderly with no increase in side-effects (Khan, *J Int Med Res* 1981, **9**, 108–12). Elderly patients may respond to lower doses of **lofepramine** but in a trial of depressed elderly inpatients, low dose lofepramine (70mg/d) was no better than placebo, indicating that full, or at least higher, doses are necessary (n=63. 4/52, Tan *et al, B J Clin Pharmacol* 1994, **37**, 321–24). **Nortriptyline** kinetics appear the same in the elderly as the young (Katz *et al, Neuro-psychopharmacology* 1989, **2**, 229–36) although individual variation is high and the elderly may respond to lower doses (Kanba *et al, Prog Neuro-Psychopharmacol Biol Psychiatr* 1992, **16**, 301–9). ECG changes

may occur so care is needed in cardio-vascular disease. Anti-cholinergic side-effects are also more common. It has been noted that when tricyclic non-response has occurred in an elderly person, response to an alternative antidepressant, eg. MAOI etc may take up to 5–6 weeks, rather than the 3–4 weeks normally expected (Flint and Rifat, *J Aff Dis* 1996, **36**, 95–105) so do not give up too soon.

13. Single daily dosing of **trazodone** may not be appropriate in the elderly, and reduced doses may be appropriate, eg. one study showed 150mg/d to be the optimum in the elderly (Mukherjee and Davey, *J Int Med Res* 1986, **14**, 279–84). Half-life is increased in elderly men, but not women (Greenblatt *et al, Clin Pharmacol Ther* 1987, **42**, 193–200). Increased plasma concentrations of **nefazodone** can occur, especially in older women, so it is best to start with a lower dose and assess the dose titration carefully. A trial designed to assess the effect of various antidepressants on driving, cognitive function and daytime sleepiness showed that elderly people do not have an increased sensitivity to the effects of nefazodone (n=12, d/b, c/o, van Laar *et al, J Clin Psychopharmacol* 1995, **15**, 30–40).

14*. The incidence of side-effects with **reboxetine** is no greater in the elderly than in younger people, although the half-life is doubled in the elderly (Holm and Spencer, *CNS Drugs* 1999, **12**, 65–83). A delayed lowering of potassium levels has been reported (SPC) and some treatment-emergent tachycardia (SPC). Frail elderly may need dose reductions. The UK SPC had the recommendation for use in the elderly removed in November 1997, for lack of positive information rather than the presence of negative information.

15*. Although **MAOIs** are often considered as more toxic to the elderly, mainly due to postural hypotension and dizziness, they can be highly effective in resistant depression in the elderly (reviewed by Volz and Gleiter, *Drugs & Aging* 1998, **13**, 341–55).

16. **Moclobemide** is considered to be safe, effective and having a seemingly beneficial effect on cognitive functions (use in the elderly reviewed by Nair *et al, Acta Psych Scand* 1995, **91** [Suppl 386], 28–35) and a trial in elderly depressed and/or demented patients showed it to cause no cognitive impairment, if not a slight improvement (n=694, d/b, p/c, Roth *et al, B J Psych* 1996, **168**, 149–57). **Mianserin** elimination is highly variable and often prolonged in the elderly (Begg *et al, B J Clin Pharmacol* 1989, **27**, 445–51). Doses may need to be adjusted, although reduced receptor sensitivity may not necessarily lead to increased side-effects. There are no apparent problems with **tryptophan**.

3.7.3 Anxiolytics and hypnotics:

Reviews*: hypnotics in the elderly (Woodward, *CNS Drugs* 1999, **11**, 263–79), sleep in the elderly (Asplund, *Drugs & Aging* 1999, **14**, 91–103).

17*. All **benzodiazepines** should be used with care in the elderly, as side-effects are likely to be enhanced. Disturbances in gait have been reported to be more common in people over 60 with **clonazepam** (Court and Kase, *J Neurol Neurosurg Psych* 1976, **39**, 297). The half-lives of **clobazam** and **alprazolam** may be longer in elderly men, but not in women, and so reduced doses are recommended in the former (Greenblatt *et al, B J Clin Pharmac* 1981, **12**, 631–36). Increased therapeutic effects and significant individual variation has been reported in elderly people with **flunitrazepam**, although pharmacokinetic variables appear the same in the young and old (Davis and Cook, *Clin Pharmacokinet* 1986, **11**, 18–35). Lower doses of **flurazepam** are recommended, as with other longer-acting **benzodiazepines**. Reduced doses of **temazepam** are usually recommended as the half-life can reach 24hrs in elderly people and one study in 12 elderly patients showed that temazepam (up to 30mg/d) caused a fall in systolic blood pressure and an increase in heart rate (Ford, *B J Clin Pharmacol* 1990, **29**, 61–67). Reduced doses are recommended. An extended half-life and a high tissue compartment uptake mean reduced doses are necessary if **nitrazepam** is essential. A steady state can be reached in 4–5 days in the elderly. Increased daytime cognitive impairment and CNS side-effects have been shown at 5mg/d (Morgan, *Psychopharmacology* 1985, **86**, 209–11). **Chlordiazepoxide** and **clorazepate** doses should be reduced by about a half in the elderly (Ochs *et al*, *Clin Pharmacol Ther* 1987, **41**, 562–70), as with all longer-acting and multiple metabolite benzodiazepines. Reduced doses of **diazepam** should be used in the elderly, due to variable responses, eg. diazepam 2.5mg produced significant memory impairment, reduced psychomotor performance and sedation in the elderly (Pomara *et al*, *J Clin Psych* 1985, **46**, 185–87). Lower doses of **midazolam** are needed in the elderly, possibly due to decreased metabolism (n=18, Albrecht *et al*, *Clin Pharmacol & Therap* 1999, **65**, 630–39). Normal adult doses of **oxazepam** can be used as there are apparently no clinically significant pharmacokinetic changes in the elderly (Dreyfuss *et al*, *J Clin Psych* 1986, **47**, 511–4). Minimal accumulation, compared to diazepam, may occur and oxazepam may be a drug of choice in the elderly (Salzman *et al*, *Arch Gen Psych* 1983, **40**, 293–97). If used as a hypnotic, **lorazepam** doses should probably be slightly reduced.

18. There do not appear to be any significant changes in the pharmacokinetics of **buspirone** in the elderly and so dose adjustments are not considered necessary (Gammans *et al*, *J Clin Pharmacol* 1989, **29**, 72–78).

19. Normal adult doses of **zopiclone** can be used (Goa and Heel, *Drugs* 1986, **32**, 48–65). One study in 30 elderly people showed **zolpidem** at 5mg to be an effective hypnotic dose with no consistent memory or performance effects nor daytime drowsiness, with doses of 10mg or above reducing REM sleep slightly (Scharf *et al*, *J Clin Psych* 1991, **52**, 77–83). Another study showed similar efficacy and lack of adverse effects in an elderly population (n=221, Roger and Attali, *Clin Therap*

1993, **15**, 127–36). A 5mg dose of zolpidem (half the healthy adult dose) is recommended. There appears to be no problem with **zaleplon** in the elderly.

20. Increased **propranolol** side-effects have been reported in the elderly and so reduced initial doses are generally recommended. Unlike propranolol, dosing adjustments for **oxprenolol** are not considered necessary.

21. **Clomethiazole** doses should be reduced, as the half-life can be at least doubled and plasma levels up to five times normal can occur (Dehlin, *Acta Psych Scand* 1986, **73**[Suppl 329], 112–15).

3.7.4 Anticonvulsants:

For **anticonvulsants**, it is best to avoid renally excreted drugs (eg. **vigabatrin** and **gabapentin**) as, for example, the renal excretion of vigabatrin may be reduced in the elderly to one sixth compared with younger people. Hepatically metabolised drugs, eg. **carbamazepine** and **lamotrigine** are not influenced by age, rather by genetic factors and are to be preferred.

Review: epilepsy in old age (Bene, *Prescriber* 1997, **8**, 31–36).

22*. No significant changes have been shown with **carbamazepine** in the elderly (eg. n=10, Read *et al*, *Seizure* 1998, **7**, 159–62) and so doses are likely to be the same in the elderly, although they may be more susceptible to cardiac arrhythmias associated with carbamazepine (Richens, *Pharm J* 1993, **251**, 50). Although the AUC with **oxcarbazepine** may be 30–60% higher in the elderly, no dose recommendations exist, other than gradual dose titration (n=48, van Heiningen *et al*, *Clin Pharmacol Ther* 1991, **50**, 410–19), and any dose adjustment recommended if the patient has compromised renal function (SPC).

23. The half-life of **valproate** may be doubled in old age, possibly via reduced metabolism (Bryson *et al*, *B J Clin Pharmacol* 1983, **16**, 104–5) but total blood levels are similar to younger adults (Bauer *et al*, *Clin Pharmacol Ther* 1985, **37**, 697–700). A naturalistic retrospective study of valproate in elderly patients showed a 62% response

rate, no LFT abnormalities and was well tolerated (n=35, Kando *et al, J Clin Psych* 1996, **57**, 238–40). The proportion of free drug may be increased via reduced protein binding but, overall, the effect is likely to be of low significance. Compared to younger adults, valproate for mania may have a different therapeutic window (65–90mcg/mL) in the elderly (n=59, retrospective, Chen *et al, J Clin Psych* 1999, **60**, 181–86).

24. Reduced doses of **phenytoin** may be needed with the elderly. Great care in monitoring is necessary, especially in those with hypoalbuminaemia or renal disease as these may have an increased level of side-effects and toxicity (Hayes *et al, B J Clin Pharmacol* 1975, **2**, 73). In people aged from 60 to 80, doses 20% lower will maintain blood levels, compared to younger adults (study by Bauer and Blouin, *Clin Pharmacol* 1982, **31**, 301–4). It may be that reduced doses are only needed with monotherapy, as opposed to anticonvulsant polypharmacy (review by Bachmann and Belloto, *Drugs & Aging* 1999, **15**, 235–50). The elderly may also be more susceptible to cardiac arrhythmias associated with phenytoin (Richens, *Pharm J* 1993, **251**, 50). Severe cardiovascular ADRs have been reported with **fosphenytoin** IV (see *3.2*), and a reduction in the loading dose and/or infusion rate by 10–25% in the elderly is recommended.

25. The half-lives of **phenobarbital** and **primidone** are longer in the elderly due to reduced metabolism and so reduced doses should be used (reviewed by Hicks *et al, J Clin Psych* 1981, **42**, 374–85).

26. **Lamotrigine** is hepatically metabolised and this is influenced by genetic factors rather than by age. An increased volume of distribution in the elderly has been shown to increase the half-life of lamotrigine thus increasing the chance of side-effects, and so, reduced doses may be needed. One study, however, showed that the half-life does not appear to be increased in the elderly (Betts, *Seizure* 1992, **1**, 3–6). **Gabapentin** clearance is reduced in old age, probably via reduced renal clearance (Boyd *et al, Pharm Res* 1990, **7**[Suppl], S215).

27*. **Vigabatrin** is renally excreted and this may be reduced in the elderly to one sixth compared to younger people. Reduced doses have been recommended in people with a creatinine clearance of less than 60 ml/min (Grant and Heel, *Drugs* 1991, **41**, 889–926) and some have recommended that it should be avoided in the elderly (eg. Richens, *Pharm J* 1993, **251**, 50). No age-related changes in pharmacokinetics have been detected with **topiramate**. The half-life of **piracetam** is extended in the elderly (Platt *et al, Arzneimittel Forschung* 1985, **35**, 533–35). There is no need to adjust the dose of **tiagabine** on the basis of age, although slightly higher plasma levels of tiagabine may occur in the elderly (n=24, Snel *et al, J Clin Pharmacol* 1997, **37**, 1015–20). Since renal impairment may occur, reduced doses of **levetiracetam** are recommended (see renal), as the half-life may increase by about 40%.

28. Lower **acetazolamide** doses are indicated (Chapron *et al, J Clin Pharmacol* 1989, **29**, 348–53). Deaths have been reported in debilitated patients given only 8ml **paraldehyde** and so use should be with the utmost caution (Baratham and Tinckler, *Med J Aust*, 1964, **51**, 877).

3.7.5 Others:

29*. There are no specific problems with **donepezil** and **rivastigmine**, provided the dose titration guidelines are followed. **Galantamine** levels are about 30-40% higher in elderly patients than healthy young individuals.

30. An initial low dose is usually recommended for **benzhexol** (trihexyphenidyl). Clearance of **procyclidine** may be reduced in the elderly and so twice daily dosing may be more appropriate than thrice daily dosing (Whiteman *et al, Eur J Clin Pharmacol* 1985, **28**, 73–78). No significant pharmacokinetic changes occur with **orphenadrine** in the elderly and so no specific dose adjustments are necessary. Confusion can be induced in the elderly by further compromising brain cholinergic activity.

31. The UK SPC for **acamprosate** states that it should not be used in the elderly,

due more to lack of data rather than specific reported problems.

32*. Reduced **lithium** clearance in the elderly through reduced renal function and increased volume of distribution (review by Sproule *et al, Drugs Aging* 2000, **16**, 165–77) mean that doses reduced by as much as 50% may be necessary (Hardy *et al, J Clin Psychopharmacol* 1987, **7**, 153–58). The elderly may also develop symptoms of lithium toxicity at standard therapeutic blood levels (Nakra and Grossberg, *J Geriatr Drug Ther* 1987, **2**, 47–63). However, lithium can be safely used in the elderly if monitored closely and frequently. Hypothyroidism can also occur.

33. In the elderly, a **modafinil** starting dose of 100mg/d is recommended (MI).

34. There is no data for **methylphenidate**.

35*. **Bupropion** appears well tolerated in the elderly, although some accumulation and greater side-effects might occur (Branconnier *et al, Psychopharmacol Bull* 1983, **19**, 658–62). There has been successful use for depression in elderly (RCT, n=100, Weihs *et al, J Clin Psych* 2000, **61**, 196–202).

3.8 PREGNANCY

	Lower risk (FDA=A)	Moderate risk (FDA = B or C)	Higher risk (FDA = D or X)
Antipsychotics		Butyrophenones[6] Clozapine[3] Loxapine[8] Olanzapine?[2] Phenothiazines[7] Quetiapine[2] Risperidone[1] Sulpiride[5] Thioxanthenes[4]	Zotepine[2]
Antidepressants	Flupentixol?[4] Tryptophan?[16]	MAOIs[15] Mianserin[16] Mirtazapine[11] Moclobemide[16] Nefazodone[13] SSRIs[9] St John's wort[16] Trazodone[13] Tricyclics[12] Venlafaxine[10]	
Anxiolytics and hypnotics		Beta-blockers[20] Buspirone[18] Chloral[21] Clomethiazole[21] Clonazepam[17] Promethazine[21] Zaleplon[19] Zopiclone[19]	Alprazolam[17] Chlordiazepoxide[17] Lorazepam[17] Oxazepam[17] Temazepam[17] Zolpidem[19]
Anticonvulsants[9]		Acetazolamide[28] Carbamazepine[22] Clonazepam?[17] Ethosuximide[28] Gabapentin[25] Lamotrigine[25] Oxcarbazepine[22] Paraldehyde[28] Tiagabine[27]	Benzodiazepines[17] Phenobarbital[25] Phenytoin[24] Topiramate[27] Valproate[23] Vigabatrin[27]
Others		Anticholinergics[34] Anticholinesterases[29] Bupropion[35] Dexamfetamine[42] Disulfiram[38] Lithium[36] Methadone LD[35] Methylphenidate[36]	Acamprosate[31] Lithium[32] Methadone HD[34] Modafinil?[33]

The FDA has established five categories to indicate a drugs potential for teratogenicity, and, where known, these classifications are noted in the text:

A – Controlled studies in women fail to show a risk in the first trimester and the risk of foetal harm seems remote.

B – *Either* animal tests do not show a risk but there are no human studies *or* animal studies show a risk but human studies have failed to show a risk to the fetus.

C – *Either* animal studies show teratogenic or embryocidal effects but there are no controlled studies in women *or* there are no studies in either animals or humans.

D – Definite evidence of a risk to the foetus exists but the benefits in certain circumstances (eg. life-threatening situations) may make use acceptable.

X – Foetal abnormalities have been shown in animals or humans or both and the risk outweighs any possible benefits.

Further information should be sought on individual drugs to balance the risk-benefit ratio in a particular individual patient. For the record, spontaneous major or gross malformations (usually defined as incompatible with life or requiring surgical correction) occur in 2–4% of pregnancies and spontaneous abortions in about 10–20% of clinically recognised pregnancies. In the first trimester, teratogenicity is the main drug risk, in the 2–3rd, growth retardation and neurological damage may occur and after birth, drug withdrawal effects may occur.

Although there are a few reports that pregnancy may protect against the risk of, eg. bipolar disorder, other papers show increased risk (reviewed by Viguera and Cohen, *Psychopharmacol Bull* 1998, **34**, 339–46).

In the UK, a National Teratology Information Service is available (reminder from Bateman and McElhatton, *BMJ* 1997, **314**, 1414–15) and would be delighted to answer all your questions (0191-232-1525). NTIS carries out individual risk assessments for pregnant women exposed to drugs or chemicals and offers pre-conceptual advice, research and follow-up information.

Assessing risk: Recent retrospective studies are more useful pointers to risk than the length of time a drug has been on the market or anecdotal case reports.

General Principals (adapted from *Maudsley Guidelines*, 2001)

Pre-conception:

1. For planned conception, discuss the risks and benefits of discontinuing or continuing medication, eg. relapse, teratogenicity etc, the unpredictability of the pre-conceptual duration, and that no decision is risk-free. Avoiding all drugs during the first trimester is the ideal.

2. Consider the risk of pregnancy even if not currently planned, eg. carry out a pregnancy test before starting teratogenic drugs in a woman of child-bearing age. As up to 50% of pregnancies are unplanned, document the patient's birth control method, document potential risks for pregnancy exposure to drug(s), encourage proper nutrition, exercise and vitamin supplementation, note any other substances taken, eg. excess caffeine, alcohol, natural products etc and educate about the potential risks and inquire about any pregnancy plans and emphasise the need for pre-pregnancy consultation.

3. For drugs of known significant risk or where there is little data, consider switching to a lower-risk drug before conception.

Pregnancy:

1. Avoid all drugs during the first trimester if possible. The maximum teratogenic potential is from days 17–60 after conception, and decisions must balance the relative *vs* absolute risk.

2. Behavioural teratogenesis and subtle functional disturbances (eg. learning difficulties, neurological deficits, developmental delay etc), and an effect on labour and delivery may occur in the second and third trimesters.

3. Use the lowest possible (maintenance) dose and monitor effects (adverse and desired) carefully.

4. In many cases, the risk of relapse (and subsequent higher dose drug use) will be higher than the risk of foetal damage.

5. Avoid polypharmacy, as synergistic teratogenicity can occur (up to 16% with multiple AEDs, n=172, Kaneko *et al, Epilepsia* 1988, **29**, 459–67).

6. The pharmacokinetics of drugs may change during pregnancy and so doses may need to be adjusted (see, eg. lithium, tricyclics).

7. Discontinuation effects have been reported in the newborn (see benzodiazepines, tricyclics, SSRIs etc) and these psychotropics should, if possible, be gradually reduced or withdrawn over the weeks before delivery is due.

Reviews: *Drugs in Pregnancy and Lactation: A Reference Guide to Fetal and Neonatal Risk*, by Briggs *et al*, Williams and Wilkins, Baltimore, MD, study from 1988–90 in 22 countries by Marchetti *et al*, general (*E J Clin Pharmacol* 1993, **45**, 495–501; Koren *et al, NEJM* 1998, **338**, 1128–37, 95 refs; McElhatton, *Prescriber* 1999, 10, 101–17), longer-term studies in children (*JAMA* 1990, **263**, 1844), general review of psychopharmacology in pregnancy (Miller, *Prim Care Update Ob Gyn* 1996, **3**, 79–86), pharmacokinetic changes during pregnancy and their clinical relevance to specific drugs (Loebstein *et al, Clin Pharmacokinet* 1997, **33**, 328–43).

3.8.1 Antipsychotics:

Reviews: Trixler and Tenyi (*Drug Safety* 1997, **16**, 403–10, 67 refs) and Pinkofsky (*Ann Clin Psychiatry* 1997, **9**, 175–79).

1. **Risperidone** (FDA=C) has no reported teratogenicity in animal tests but no human data is available as yet.

2. No adequate information is available yet with **olanzapine** (FDA=C) and so use should only be when the potential benefit outweighs the potential risk (MI), although no teratogenic effects have been seen in animal studies. Four human cases (3 normal births and one miscarriage) were unremarkable. No information is available for **quetiapine** (FDA=C) and the SPC recommends using only if the

benefits justify the risk. **Zotepine** crosses the placenta and although there are no indications of teratogenicity (Fukuhara *et al, Arzneimittelforschung* 1979, **29**, 1600–6), there is insufficient data in humans and the drug is contraindicated in pregnancy.

3. Women are more likely to conceive on **clozapine** (FDA = B) than most other antipsychotics due to the relative lack of effect of clozapine on prolactin. In the close study of one patient, there was clear accumulation of clozapine in the infant (possibly due to higher albumin concentrations) (Barnas, *Am J Psych* 1994, **151**, 945). Of 84 reports of pregnancy with clozapine with known outcomes, there were 51 births, 7 miscarriages and 14 elective terminations, of which one was due to known abnormalities (patient taking clozapine 25mg/d plus lithium). Of the 51 births, 43 were born healthy and normal and 8 had abnormalities, ranging from low glucose levels through to malformations. Clozapine is known to pass the placental barrier in animals and is assumed to do so in humans. Novartis has full details and should be approached before decisions about use in pregnancy are taken. No clear conclusion can be drawn from this, although combined with animal studies it would appear clozapine is not a major teratogen. The manufacturers do not recommend it.

4. **Thioxanthenes:** (no FDA classification as not available in US).

Flupentixol passes across the placenta and foetal levels are about a quarter of the mother's (Kirk and Jorgensen, *Psychopharmacology* 1980, **72**, 107–8). There is no positive evidence of teratogenicity although Lundbeck do not recommend its use. Studies in 3 species have not shown malformations. A total of fifteen cases of variable birth defects have been reported. With **zuclopen-thixol**, few birth defects have been recorded, at a rate consistent with the spontaneous levels of malformations.

5. **Sulpiride** has been used as an antinauseant in pregnancy. There are no published reports of abnormalities in animals or humans (*Int J Res Preg* 1982, **3**, 173–77, + MI). (FDA N/A).

6. **Butyrophenones**:

The safety of **haloperidol** (FDA=C) in pregnancy has not been established although it was once used in hyperemesis gravidarum and the drug passes into the foetus (Uematsu *et al, Ther Drug Monit* 1991, **13**, 183–87). There are isolated cases of alleged teratogenicity with haloperidol (eg. unproven limb malformations) but no cause-effect relationship has been established and there are no reports of haloperidol alone causing abnormalities (MI).

7. **Phenothiazines:** (FDA: Chlorpromazine = C, levomepromazine = C, promazine = C, thioridazine = C, trifluoperazine = C, others N/A)

The teratogenicity of phenothiazines has been investigated in some studies, although most of the data is based on low dose use and thus not necessarily applicable to higher dose use. The phenothiazines are considered by some as of lowest risk, although the potential for hypotension, sedation and anticholinergic effects means that any use must be with extreme care. Severe congenital abnormalities were not significantly different in the studies of 543 women taking low-dose phenothiazines, other than **prochlorperazine** (FDA=C) for nausea (Milkovich and van den Berg, *Am J Obstet Gynecol* 1976, **125**, 244–48) and in 1309 mothers, mostly taking prochlorperazine (Slone *et al, Am J Obstet Gynecol* 1977, **128**, 486–8). The largest study, of 315 pregnancies, where phenothiazines were taken in the first trimester, showed a statistically significant difference in malformation rate of 3.5% in the aliphatic (**chlorpromazine** and **promazine**) phenothiazine-treated group (11 malformed infants) compared with 1.6% in the control group. There was no apparent trend in the type of abnormality and the risk is still considered low (*Adv Drug React Bull* 1983 [Aug] 372). There was no difference with the other phenothiazines, which appear to have an incidence of malformations similar to the background incidence (*Teratology* 1977, **15**, 57–64). Although **levomepromazine** (methotrimeprazine) is an aliphatic phenothiazine, it has generally been considered safe for both mother and foetus if used occasionally in low dose, later in pregnancy. A follow-up of **trifluoperazine** pregnancies showed no teratogenic effects (Moriarity, *Can Med Assoc J* 1963, **88**, 97). There are also reports of extrapyramidal symptoms (Hill *et al, J Pediatr* 1966, **69**, 589–95) and neonatal jaundice. In the neonate, lethargy and extrapyramidal symptoms have been reported, as has respiratory depression when given in high dose (above 500mg chlorpromazine equivalents) close to term. In the longer term, a lack of impaired mental or physical development has been shown at 2 and 7 years in a 16-child follow-up study (Ayd, *Int Drug Ther Newsletter* 1976, **11**, 5). See also a short comment about 'Is fluphenazine a teratogen?' (Merlob *et al, Am J Med* Genet 1994, **52**, 231–32).

8. The safety of **loxapine** (FDA = C) in pregnancy is unknown. There are two reports of gastrointestinal malformations in infants whose mothers took loxapine throughout pregnancy but no similar cases are reported elsewhere.

3.8.2 Antidepressants:

There is little data on the newer drugs so the lowest risk in the first trimester would appear to be to use either imipramine, amitriptyline or an SSRI, none of which have data suggesting a significant risk. A study (*NEJM* 1997, **336**, 258–62) indicates that if women take anti-depressant drugs during their pregnancy, there seems to be no effect on the neurological development or intelligence of their children (see 20 below).

Review: depression during pregnancy and postpartum (Dwight and Walker, *Curr Opin Psych* 1998, **11**, 85–88).

9. **SSRIs**: (FDA: Citalopram = C, fluoxamine = B, fluvoxamine = C, paroxetine = B, sertraline = B).

In a prospective, multicentre cohort study of 267 women exposed to an SSRI antidepressant (fluvoxamine, sertraline or paroxetine) during pregnancy and 267 controls, exposure to SSRIs at recommended doses did not appear to be associated with increased teratogenicity (relative risk 1.06, 95% CI, 0.43–2.62)

or higher rates of miscarriage, stillbirth, or prematurity. Gestational ages and birth weights were similar amongst off-spring of both groups of women (Kulin *et al, JAMA* 1998, **279**, 609–10).

No embryotoxic or teratogenic effects have been seen in animals with **paroxetine** (*Acta Psych Scand* 1989, **80** [Suppl 350], 37–39) and, in the limited human data available, no abnormalities have been seen yet. In a woman taking 30mg/d paroxetine, the child showed an increased respiratory rate, muscle tone and jitteriness over first few days, resolving over 4 days. Infant serum levels peaked at 75nmol/l at day two (cf 185nmol/l in the mother's serum). A withdrawal syndrome seems likely and so gradual dose reduction before delivery should be considered (Dahl *et al, B J Psych* 1997, **171**, 391–92). Information is available on over 2000 **fluoxetine**-exposed pregnancies, reported in 3 prospective cohort-controlled studies and 4 prospective surveys. Based on published studies, there is no increased risk of mal-formations occuring in women exposed to fluoxetine and no evidence of teratogenicity (eg. study and review, Nulman and Koren, *Teratology* 1996, **53**, 304–8). There is an absence of perinatal sequelae and no evidence of increase in major malformations, spontaneous abortion, poor perinatal state or neurodevelopmental delay. A prospective study on first-trimester exposure involved 128 women taking fluoxetine, 110 taking no known teratogen and 74 taking a tricyclic. No statistical differences in pregnancy outcome, age or weight were shown, but a slight tendency to miscarriage in both drug groups (SSRI 14.8%, TCA 12.2%, no drug 7.8%). The authors concluded that fluoxetine was unlikely to be a major teratogen but further work on miscarriage and any potential developmental effects was needed (Pastuszak *et al, JAMA* 1993, **269**, 2246–48). Of 544 reported cases in the USA of fluoxetine taken during preg-nancy, 91 were electively terminated and there were 72 (15.9%) spontaneous abortions, 13 (3.4%) perinatal major malformations and 7 post-perinatal malformations reported. These rates have been concluded as being similar to the unexposed population (Goldstein and Marvel, *JAMA*, 1993, **270**, 2177–78) but this has been disputed as the previous study (Pastuszak *et al, JAMA* 1993, **269**, 2246–48) showed similar miscarriage rates which were double that in the control group. Chambers *et al* (*NEJM* 1996, **335**, 1010–15, n=228) could not show increased miscarriage rates nor major foetal abnormalities or a consistent pattern of events suggesting teratogenicity, although there was a higher rate of having three or more minor anomalies and no account was taken of the severity of maternal depression (see Dwight and Walker, *Curr Opin Psych* 1998, **11**, 85–88). A careful prospective study of children (assessed between 18 and 86 months) whose mothers had taken either **fluoxetine** (55 children) or no drug (84) showed fluoxetine to have no effect on global IQ, language development or behavioural development (Nulman *et al, NEJM* 1997, **336,** 258–62). The SPC naturally states caution and use should only be if clearly needed. There is no information available for **sertraline** at present nor **citalopram**.

10. There is no further evidence available at the moment for **venlafaxine**. It is contraindicated in the UK in pregnancy (FDA = C).

11. Animal tests do not show **mirtazapine** (FDA=C) to be teratogenic nor cause foetal harm. The one human case was unremarkable.

12. **Tricyclic antidepressants:**

(FDA: amitriptyline = D, amoxapine = C, clomipramine = C, desipramine = C, doxepin = C, maprotiline = B, nortriptyline = D, protriptyline = C, trimipramine = C)

Evidence from studies shows no increase in spontaneous abortions, malformations nor pattern of defects from tricyclics (reviewed by Goldberg *et al, Int J Psych in Med* 1994, **24**, 129–47). A meta-analysis of the use of tricyclics in pregnancy, reviewing over 300,000 live births including 414 first trimester exposures, failed to show a significant association between tricyclics and congenital malformations, although

withdrawal symptoms were noted (Altshuler *et al, Am J Psych* 1996, **153**, 592–605). The metabolism of tricyclics in the neonate is much slower, so anticholinergic and other side-effects are more marked. Amitriptyline and imipramine are considered the tricyclics of choice, based on cumulative data on their relative safety.

Discontinuation effects have been noted, sometimes requiring active treatment, eg. withdrawal symptoms from clomipramine in the neonate have been reported widely, eg. jittery/twitchy infants which resolved upon introduction of the drug in the child, either via a drip or via breast milk (Schimmel *et al, Clin Toxicol* 1991, **29**, 479–84), lethargic and cyanotic babies who had abnormal movements and feeding difficulties where symptomatic treatment was successful (n=2, Cowe *et al, Pediatrics* 1982, **69**, 233–34; *BMJ* 1982, **284**, 1837–38) and foetal seizures unresponsive to phenobarbital and phenytoin, which settled with clomipramine, in a mother who took up to 150mg/d clomipramine and stopped abruptly (child was born prematurely 4 days later, Bromiker and Kaplan, *JAMA* 1994, **272**, 1722–23). In pregnancy, mild toxicity in the infant has been seen with imipramine, eg. respiratory distress, hypotonia, irritability, tremors, convulsions, jerky movements etc. (eg. Ware and DeVane, *J Clin Psych* 1990, **51**, 482–84). Phenobarbital can improve these symptoms, which can persist for a total duration of up to two weeks.

Postnatal development:

A careful study of children (assessed between 18 and 86 months) whose mothers had taken either a tricyclic (n=84) or no drug (n=80) showed tricyclics to have no effect on global IQ, language development or behavioural development compared to no drug (Nulman *et al, NEJM* 1997, **336**, 258–62).

13. For **trazodone** (FDA = C) at very high doses (15+ times the maximum human dose), there appears to be some foetal resorption and congenital abnormalities but little human data exists to support this. There is no published evidence of problems with **nefazodone** (FDA=C) but

the UK SPC naturally recommends use only if clearly needed.

14. No teratogenic effects have been noted with **reboxetine** in animal studies but little human data exists so the drug should be avoided in pregnancy (SPC).

15. **MAOIs:** (FDA: isocarboxazid = C, phenelzine = C, tranylcypromine = C). There are no reports of human teratogenicity with **phenelzine** nor **tranylcypromine**, although it has been suggested that the risk of teratogenic problems may be roughly doubled if tranylcypromine is taken in the first trimester (Segal *et al, Pediatrics* 1982, **69**, 241–43). (See also Briggs *et al, Drugs in Pregnancy and Lactation,* Williams and Wilkins). Growth retardation and foetal toxicity have been reported. MAOIs should be avoided if at all possible due to maternal toxicity and lack of published safety data. **MAOIs** may interact with drugs used in labour (see pethidine under MAOIs in *4.3.4*).

16. There is no evidence of teratogenicity with **mianserin** in animals except at toxic doses (Brogden *et al, Drugs* 1978, **16**, 273–301) but no human data is available (FDA = N/A). No data is available yet on the use of **moclobemide** in pregnancy. No human data is available for **tryptophan**. Early animal tests showed some adverse effects (Meier and Wilson, *Life Sci* 1983, **32**, 1193–96). Slight in-vitro uterotonic activity has been reported and the lack of safety and toxicity data suggests that **St. John's wort** is currently best avoided in pregnancy.

3.8.3 Anxiolytics and hypnotics

For a review of the treatment of anxiety during pregnancy see McGrath *et al,* (*Drug Safety* 1999, **20**, 171–86).

17. **Benzodiazepines:**(FDA: alprazolam = D, chlordiazepoxide = D, clonazepam = C, diazepam = D, lorazepam = D, oxazepam = D, temazepam = X, others not available) Assessment of 104,000 births in the USA has shown a higher incidence of teratogenicity in women taking benzodiazepines but multiple alcohol and illicit substance exposure could account for this (Bergman *et al, Lancet* 1992, **340**, 694–96). With **alprazolam**

there are no formal reports of teratogenicity. With **chlordiazepoxide**, an increased risk of teratogenicity has been suggested if chlordiazepoxide is taken during the first 42 days of pregnancy (11.4 per 100 live births) compared to after 42 days (3.6 per 100 live births, 175 studied — Milkovich and van den Berg, *NEJM* 1974, **291**, 1268–71) although later Hartz *et al* (*NEJM* 1975, **292**, 726) were unable to find significant differences when 800 patients were studied. **Clobazam** is known to pass the placenta and benzodiazepine withdrawal symptoms in the neonate have been suggested. For **diazepam**, studies show a varying risk of oral clefts, with the worst case scenario bringing the risk to 7 in 1000. In late pregnancy, doses of 30mg or more of diazepam IM or IV during the last 15 hours of labour can induce neonatal respiratory depression and feeding problems. 10mg given IV within 10 minutes of birth has been shown not to affect Apgar scores (McAllister, *B J Anaesth* 1980, **52**, 423–27). As with other benzodiazepines, withdrawal symptoms in the neonate have been seen (Rementeria and Bhatt, *J Pediatr* 1977, **90**, 123). As **lorazepam** crosses the placenta, the floppy baby syndrome and respiratory depression can occur, especially if IV doses are used close to birth. Oral use during later pregnancy may show delayed feeding in full-term infants but premature infants may have lower Apgar scores and respiratory depression (Whitelaw *et al, BMJ* 1981, **282**, 1106–8). **Clorazepate** also passes the placenta. Animal studies have not shown teratogenicity although some cognitive impairment was indicated. In 1997, the UK CSM restated the danger of high doses and use during pregnancy or labour due to the effects on the neonate such as hypothermia, hypotonia, respiratory depression and withdrawal symptoms (*Curr Prob* 1997, **23**, 10). Shorter-acting benzodiazepines on a 'when required' basis may be acceptable later in pregnancy, but the first trimester should be avoided if possible.

After birth, benzodiazepine withdrawal symptoms have been noticed in the neonate with many benzodiazepines (Athinarayanan *et al, Am J Obstet Gynae* 1976, **124**, 212). The 'floppy baby' syndrome, as it is often termed, includes facial features and CNS dysfunction and can occur particularly with higher doses (eg. >30mg diazepam equivalent per day) of longer-acting benzodiazepines (*J Pediatrics* 1989, **114**, 126–31), eg. **nitrazepam** (*Lancet* 1977, **ii**, 878).

18. There is no evidence of a teratogenic effect from **buspirone** (FDA=B) but some effects on survival and weights has been noted in some, but not all, animal tests. This is a UK SPC contraindication.

19. **Zopiclone** has not been contra-indicated in pregnancy. Animal tests have shown no abnormalities and the limited human data is unremarkable. Little information is currently available on **zolpidem** (FDA=B) and **zaleplon** (FDA=C). Until more is known, they should be avoided in pregnancy, especially during the first trimester.

20. **Beta-blockers:** (FDA: propranolol = C, oxprenolol = C)

Beta-blockers are not generally considered teratogens but a connection between **propranolol** use in pregnancy and tracheosophageal fistulas (Campbell, *NEJM* 1985, **313**, 518) and intrauterine growth retardation has been proposed. Direct effects of beta-blockade on the foetus would also occur, eg. bradycardia etc. (for reviews etc. see Livingstone *et al, Clin Exp Hypertens* 1983, **2**, 341–50; O'Connor *et al, Lancet* 1981, **2**, 1168). Use in the second and third trimesters may aggravate or produce neonatal hypoglycaemia. Foetal and neonatal bradycardia may occur especially in pregnancies already complicated by placental insufficiency (eg. severe maternal hypertension). Due to direct cardiac effects, hypoglycaemia, apnoea etc; it may be prudent to discontinue treatment 1–2 weeks before delivery.

21. Maternally administered **chloral** (FDA=C) lowers bilirubin concentrations in the infant (*J Pediat* 1976, **89**, 657). No increase in congenital anomalies was seen in a study of 71 women who took chloral in the first 4 months of pregnancy or to 358 women who took chloral at some time in pregnancy (Heinonen *et al, Birth Defects and Drugs in Pregnancy*, Publishing Sciences Group 1977, 336–37). The UK manufacturers state that **clomethiazole** should not be used, particularly in the first and third trimesters, although it has been used widely for pre-eclampsia. Adverse effects of platelet aggregation in the neonate have been reported with **promethazine** (FDA=C) (Corby and Schulman, *J Pediatr* 1971, **79**, 307), although overall promethazine may be safe and appropriate as a hypnotic.

3.8.4 Anticonvulsants*

Pregnant women with epilepsy are at increased risk of seizures and complications, with increased seizures in about 25–33%. One of the main reasons for this increase is the marked alterations in plasma protein binding of drugs as pregnancy progresses, resulting in declining plasma levels.

A prospective study of 211 women with epilepsy treated with anti-convulsants showed that the risk of abnormal outcomes (10.7%) was three times that of controls (3.4%), with phenobarbital showing the highest risk (Waters *et al, Arch Neurol* 1994, **51**, 250–53). The main malformations include dysmorphic features (see below), haemorrhagic disorders (due to Vitamin K-dependent clotting factor deficiency) and spina bifida (review by Yerby, *Epilepsia* 1992, **33**[Suppl 1], S23–27). A retrospective study of 151 pregnancies in 124 women with epilepsy showed that most have an uncomplicated pregnancy and normal healthy offspring. Maternal treatment with phenytoin might be associated with congenital mal-formations but no other risk factors could be identified (Sabers *et al, Acta Neurol Scand* 1998, **97**, 164–70). A retrospective cohort study of children born to epileptic mothers showed that most antiepileptic drugs were associated with an increased risk of major congenital abnormalities, in particular valproate, carbamazepine, benzodiazepines, caffeine and pheno-barbital (n=1411, Samren *et al, Ann Neurol* 1999, **46**, 739–44). A review of anticonvulsants in pregnancy (Malone and D'Alton, *Semin Perinatol* 1997, **21**,

114–23), concluded that the lowest dose of one of the major drugs probably has less risk than that of recurrent seizures. Smoking and anticonvulsants may increase the risk of pre-term delivery, lower birthweight, length and head circumference (n=193, controls n=24,094, Hvas *et al, B J Obs Gynaecol* 2000, **107**, 896–902).

A recent survey has suggested that children exposed to anticonvulsants during pregnancy have a higher frequency of educational needs statements (10.3% drug exposed cf. 5.7% non-drug-exposed). The figure for valproate (30%), and possibly also polypharmacy, were much higher, again suggesting a drug effect. Prospective studies are needed to confirm this (n=400 school-age children: 150 exposed to monotherapy, 74 to polytherapy and 176 to none, Adab *et al, J Neurol Neurosurg Psychiatry* 2001, **70**, 15–21).

Summary of the risks of pregnancy in women with epilepsy:

- 25–33% increase in maternal seizure frequency
- 10% risk of vaginal bleeding
- 7% risk of neonatal haemorrhage if no vitamin K is given
- 10% risk of infant facial dysmorphism
- 4–6% risk of major malformations (30% of which are oral facial defects)
- 1–2% risk of spina bifida with valproate
- 0.5–1% risk of spina bifida with carbamazepine.

(Yerby, *Epilepsia* 1992, **33**[Suppl 1], S23–27).

Summary of risk minimisation strategies*:

Evidence suggests that recent literature has been slow to influence clinical practice (Wiebe, *BMJ* 2000, **320**, 3–4, editorial).

1. Pre-conception:

- Education of the patient as to the risks and benefits of continued treatment
- Adequate Oral Contraceptive dosage (see interactions, *4.5*) until conception is planned, eg. 50–75microg of ethinyloestradiol

- Regular multivitamins with folate before oral contraceptives are stopped, to reduce the chance of spina bifida
- Seizure control with the lowest dose monotherapy targeted
- Diagnosis verified and the need for anticonvulsants confirmed.

2. After conception:

- Education of the patient about risk minimisation.

3. Seizure control without toxicity:

- Do not change drugs if the patient is stabilised
- Multivitamins with folate continued
- Frequent monitoring of free anticonvulsant concentrations and dose adjustment if necessary
- Monotherapy continued if possible
- Vitamin K given during last week of pregnancy if possible (Deblay *et al, Lancet* 1982, **1**, 1247)
- Ultrasound and AFPs carried out.

Facial dysmorphism has been described in uncontrolled seizure patients, as well as with phenytoin, phenobarbital, primidone, valproate, benzodiazepines and carbamazepine. All appear quite similar and not really drug-specific and some effects, especially digital, appear to resolve with age.

Reviews*: general (Leppik *et al, CNS Drugs* 1999, **11**, 191–206; Chang and McAuley, *Ann Pharmacother* 1998, **32**, 794–801, 63 refs; Nulman *et al, Drugs* 1999, **57**, 535–44, 75 refs; Simar, *CNS Drugs* 1999, **12**, 451–70), advice to patients (Yerby, *Epilepsia* 1997, **38**, 957–58), long-term outcomes (Koch *et al, Epilepsia* 1999, **40**, 1237–43).

22*. Carbamazepine (FDA=C) has been considered by many to be the anti-convulsant of choice in epilepsy, with some studies showing no teratogenicity (Nakane *et al, Epilepsia* 1980, **21**, 663–80). However, an association with malformations, particularly spina bifida (1% incidence, Rosa, *NEJM* 1991, **324**, 674–77, *BMJ* 1991, **303**, 651), and a pattern of minor problems, such as craniofacial defects (11%), fingernail hypoplasia (27%) and developmental delay (20%) has been made (Jones *et al, NEJM* 1989, **320**, 1661–66, +

correspondence in *NEJM*, 1989, **321**, 1480–81). All of these cases were in women on polytherapy and so an interaction effect is possible, and the effect of the epilepsy itself is not known (letters in *NEJM* 1991, **325**, 664–65). However, when compared to matched controls, 47 children born to mothers taking carbamazepine monotherapy during pregnancy showed a 'carbamazepine syndrome' (facial dysmorphic features) and mild mental retardation, unrelated to dose or maternal convulsions (Ornoy and Cohen, *Arch Dis Child* 1996, **75**, 517). In monotherapy, carbamazepine may have a negative influence on body dimensions (n=963, Wide *et al, Epilepsia* 2000, **41**, 854–61). The CSM recommends the need for counselling and screening for neural tube defects (*Curr Problems* 1993, **19**, 8), which can detect 90–95% of neural tube defects if carried out with AFP levels at 16–18 weeks. One study showed no long-term effects from carbamazepine (Van der Pol *et al, Am J Obstet Gynecol* 1991, **164**, 121–28). In late pregnancy, routine vitamin K to mothers and the neonates is usually recommended. For a review of carbamazepine teratogenicity see *Lancet* 1991, **337**, 1316–17 (editorial) and comment that seizures pose a greater overall risk than properly used anticonvulsants.

In a controlled study of *in utero* exposure, 36 children born to mothers taking carbamazepine were compared to matched controls. Allowing for variables, the carbamazepine children had similar IQs and language abilities to controls (n=36, Scolnik *et al, JAMA* 1994, **271**, 767), suggesting the lack of a clinically important adverse effect on cognitive development.

Oxcarbazepine (FDA = C) is closely related to carbamazepine. The placenta may contribute to the metabolism of oxcarbazepine (Pienimaki *et al, Epilepsia* 1997, **38**, 309–16) and the UK SPC mentions that data indicates that oxcarbazepine may cause serious birth defects.

23*. **Valproate** (FDA = D) crosses the placenta easily (Bailey and Pool, *BMJ* 1983, **286**, 190) and teratogenicity,

especially spina bifida, has been strongly linked. UK rates with valproate are stated to be about 1%, which is 50 times the spontaneous rate. The CSM recommends counselling and screening for neural tube defects (*Curr Problems* 1993, **19**, 8). This should take place in a specialist centre with high resolution ultrasound and experienced technicians. Amniocentesis should be carried out if plasma AFP levels are raised or ultrasound unclear (*BMJ* 1986, **293**, 1485–88; *BMJ* 1991, **302**, 56 + 1262. See also *Drug & Ther Bull* 1990, **28**, 59–60). In a small study of 17 infants born to 17 mothers on valproate during pregnancy, 11 were admitted to a neurological unit, 9 with neurological problems (including seizures) and 2 with major malformations. A 'foetal valproate syndrome' was proposed, presenting as congenital heart defects and a withdrawal syndrome of irritability, jitteriness, hypotonia and feeding problems. The authors related the former to valproate in the first trimester and the withdrawal syndrome to higher doses (Thisted and Ebbesen, *Arch Dis Child* 1993, **69**, 288–91). The UK SPC now states that there have been rare reports of haemorrhagic syndrome in neonates whose mothers took valproate in pregnancy. This has been a suggestion that *in utero* exposure to valproate may lead to a higher than expected incidence of education needs statements, although a prospective study would be needed to confirm this (n=400 school-age children: 150 exposed to monotherapy, 74 to polytherapy and 176 to none, Adab *et al, J Neurol Neurosurg Psychiatry* 2001, **70**, 15–21). Dividing daily doses and using SR preparations to reduce the peak levels may be wise. Folic acid supplementation at 4mg/d before and during pregnancy has also been recommended.

Reviews*: valproate disposition in pregnancy (Omtzigt *et al, Eur J Clin Pharmacol* 1992, **43**, 381–88), valproate in women of reproductive age (Piontek and Wisner, *J Clin Psych* 2000, **61**, 161–63).

24. **Phenytoin** (FDA = D) crosses the placenta freely and teratogenicity is well established, particularly the 'foetal

hydantoin syndrome'. This syndrome includes growth retardation, micro-cephaly, mental retardation, facial defects including cleft lip and/or palate, digit and nail hypoplasia, rib anomalies, hirsuitism, low hairlines and inguinal hernia, plus cardiovascular gastro-intestinal or genitourinary anomalies (2 cases and review by Ozkinay *et al, Turk J Pediatr* 1998, **40**, 273–78). The full syndrome occurs in about 8–10% of children born to mothers who took phenytoin in the first trimester (Witter *et al, Obstet Gynecol* 1981, **58**, 100S–105S; n=88, Rodriguez-Palomares *et al, Arch Med Res* 1995, **26**, 371–77) and a part syndrome in a further 30% of children (Seeler *et al, Pediatrics* 1979, **63**, 524–27; see also controlled prospective study, n=34, Nulman *et al, Am J Med Genet* 1997, **68**, 18–24). It appears not to be dose-related (n=88, Rodriguez-Palomares *et al, Arch Med Res* 1995, **26**, 371–77). Prediction of the teratogenic risk may be possible by measuring microsomal epoxide hydrolase activity (*NEJM* 1990, **332**, 1567–72). It has also been noted that epileptic fathers taking phenytoin have increased rates of malformed children (Friis, *Acta Neurol Scand* 1983, **94**[Suppl], 39–43).

The syndrome may be related to phenytoin-induced reduction in GSH levels, enhancing peroxidative damage to the foetus via the placental circulation (Lui *et al, Human Toxicol* 1997, **16**, 177–81). Phenytoin also inhibits the synthesis of Vitamin K-dependent clotting factors and neonatal haemorrhage may occur. Vitamin K deficiency may also be the cause of abnormal facial development, via abnormal development of the cartilaginous nasal septum. Early Vitamin K supplementation in at-risk pregnancies is thus recommended (n=10, Howe *et al, Am J Med Genet* 1995, **58**, 238–44) and to the neonate after birth (Yerby, *Epilepsia* 1987, **28**[Suppl 3], S29–S36).

The kinetics of phenytoin change in pregnancy, elimination increases (single dose study, n=5, Dickinson *et al, B J Clin Pharmacol* 1989, **28**, 17–27) and plasma levels fall steadily as the pregnancy progresses, with possible change in seizure frequency (45% increase, Knight and Rhind, *Epilepsia* 1975, **16**, 99–110; no significant change, Tomson *et al, Epilepsia* 1994, **35**, 122–30). Bound levels may be reduced with free (ie. active) levels unchanged in pregnancy and so care with plasma level interpretation is needed (review of phenytoin disposition and metabolism in pregnancy, Eadie *et al, Eur J Clin Pharmacol* 1992, **43**, 389–92; for 'Guidelines for the care of epileptic women of child-bearing age' see *Epilepsia* 1989, **30**, 409–10).

Risk reduction with phenytoin:

The general consensus seems to be that where documented seizures are proven to be controlled by phenytoin, then the risks of withdrawal are probably greater than with the continued use of pheny-toin, with the following precautions:

1. Use of minimal effective doses. At least monthly blood level monitoring both during pregnancy, and for up to six months after, are essential to avoid toxi-city and an increased teratogenic risk (see above, noting relevance of free levels).

2. Use of folic acid 5mg/d from before conception. One study resulted in **no** birth defects in the 33 mothers who took folic acid from before conception or immediately upon becoming pregnant but there were 10 children with malformations from the 66 born to mothers who did not take folic acid, a significant and **highly important** difference (Biale and Lewenthal, *Eur J Obstet Gynecol Reprod Biol* 1984, **18**, 211). The neural tube closes around the time of the first missed period and so folic acid supplements need to be started before pregnancy is detected.

3. Vitamin K supplementation (see above).

After birth, a withdrawal syndrome, including irritability and haemorrhage has been reported (Hill *et al, Am J Dis Child* 1974, **127**, 645–53). One study has indicated a negative neuro-developmental effect from phenytoin. In a controlled study of *in utero* exposure, 34 children born to mothers taking phenytoin and 36 children born to mothers taking carbamazepine were compared to matched controls.

Allowing for other variables, the phenytoin children had a significantly lower mean IQ and language ability, the carbamazepine children being similar to controls (Scolnik *et al, JAMA* 1994, **271**, 767). This strongly suggests a clinically important adverse effect in the long-term. Developmental impairment and reduced growth and head circumference has been reported at 7 years (Gal and Sharpless, *Drug Intell Clin Pharm* 1984, **18**, 186–201). Reports of malignancies in the infant have probably been disproven (Koren *et al, Teratology* 1989, **40**, 157–62).

25*. **Phenobarbital** (FDA = D) has been implicated as a teratogen, although many cases that have occurred have been as part of combination therapy. Minor digital deformities (finger-like thumbs, rudimentary or missing nails) as well as hip and facial abnormalities have been reported. In the longer-term, a smaller head circumference and an impaired cognitive development was suggested in two studies (n=122, van der Pol *et al, Am J Obstet Gynecol* 1991, **164**, 121–28). Prenatal exposure to combined phenobarbital and phenytoin (n=172) compared to controls (n=168) produced smaller head size at birth and persistent learning problems (12%) compared to controls (1%) (Dessens *et al, Acta Paediatrica* 2000, **89**, 533–41; see also *JAMA* 1990, **263**, 1844). There is some evidence of a direct neurotoxic effect by phenobarbital on developing foetal neurones, which may be responsible for some cognitive or CNS abnormalities (Neale *et al, Pediatr Neurol* 1985, **1**, 143–50). Withdrawal symptoms, such as seizures and irritability have occurred in the neonate, some delayed by up to two weeks after birth. Neonatal bleeding in the first 24 hours has been reported, as has respiratory depression.

26*. Although there is little data on **lamotrigine** (FDA=C), it appears to have pharmacokinetic and pharmaco-dynamic properties that suggest a safer outcome with its use in pregnancy compared with older AEDs (Lilly and Kaplan-Machlis, *J Pharm Tech* 1999, **15**, 75–77). Lamotrigine plasma levels may decrease

significantly as pregnancy progresses, to such a degree that dose adjustments may be indicated (n=1, Tomson *et al, Epilepsia* 1997, **38**, 1039–41). No human data is available on **gabapentin** (FDA=C)

27*. **Vigabatrin** is contraindicated due to a slight increase in the incidence of cleft palate at high doses in one animal test. One small study suggested that slow placental transfer of vigabatrin occurs (n=2, Tran *et al, Br J Clin Pharmacol* 1998, **45**, 409–11). No human data is available on **tiagabine** (FDA=C) in pregnancy and so use should only be where clearly indicated. **Topiramate** (FDA=C) has shown some teratogenicity in mice, rats and rabbits at high dose (Mendez *et al, Epilepsia* 1995, **36**[Suppl 3], 1073–77), similar to acetazolamide (MI). It should not be used in pregnancy unless the benefit clearly outweighs the risk. Some animal studies show animal reproductive toxicity, and so **levetiracetam** (FDA=C) should not be used unless clearly necessary (MI).

28. For **acetazolamide** (FDA = C), animal tests indicate that it is teratogenic and can increase miscarriages at toxic doses, and two probable human cases exist (Worsham *et al, JAMA* 1978, **240**, 251–52). If use is essential, maternal electrolyte balance should be monitored. There are reported cases of malformations with **ethosuximide** (FDA=C) alone and about 35 when combined with other drugs but no cause-effect relationship has been proven. Although animal studies in rats have raised some concerns, no systematic human data is available. **Paraldehyde** FDA=C.

3.8.5 Others*:

29*. Very high doses of **donepezil** (FDA=C) may have some minor effects in pregnancy but no teratogenicity has been detected (MI). The safety of **rivastigmine** (FDA=C) in pregnancy has not been established (MI). There is no data on **galantamine** in pregnancy, although animal studies show a slight delay in foetal and neonatal development (SPC).

30. **Anticholinergics:** (FDA: benzhexol/ trihexyphenidyl = C, benztropine = C, procyclidine = C)

There is little data available on these drugs. A 'small left colon syndrome' has been reported in two children born to mothers who took benztropine and other psychotropic drugs late in pregnancy (Falterman and Richardson, *J Paediatr* 1980, **92**, 308–10) although a cause-effect relationship was not established.

31. For **disulfiram** (FDA = C) there have been isolated reports of congenital abnormalities (eg. Gardner and Clarkson, *NZ Med J* 1981, **93**, 184–86), although other drugs were often taken and the symptoms were similar to the foetal alcohol syndrome. In animals, disulfiram has been shown to be embryotoxic. The risk-benefit ratio for the risks of alcoholism against disulfiram for the foetus must be assessed carefully. The UK SPC for **acamprosate** states that use in pregnancy is a contraindication. Animal studies have not shown any evidence of teratogenicity.

32. **Lithium** (FDA = D) readily crosses the placenta and cases of cardiac arrhythmia, hypotonia and hypo-thyroidism have been reported (full review by Schou, *J Clin Psych* 1990, **51**, 410–13). Studies show that congenital malformation rates with lithium (2.8%) are similar to control rates (2.4%) and suggest that lithium is not an important human teratogen, if used with adequate screening (including level II ultrasound and foetal echocardiography) to detect Ebstein's anomaly (n=148, *Lancet* 1992, **339**, 530–33; *Lancet* 1992, **339**, 869). The malformation risk in the first trimester is of the order of 4–12% and hence still greater than the general population. The risk of Ebstein's anomaly (a rare congenital downward displacement of the tricuspid valve into the right ventricle) exists if the drug is taken during weeks 2 to 6 post-conception. Ebstein's anomaly is 20 times more common with lithium, but the risk rises from 1 in 20K to 1 in 1K, and must be weighed against the 50% chance of relapsing if the drug is stopped (Cohen *et al, JAMA* 1994, **271**, 146–50; *Pharm J* 1994, **252**, 119; review by

Amanth, *Lithium* 1993, **4**, 231–37). The CSM has, however, stated lithium to be a 'commonly recognised' teratogen (*Curr Prob* 1997, **23**, 11).

A recent study (n=101, retrospective, Viguera *et al, Am J Psych* 2000, **157**, 179–84) has noted that:

● The heart is formed very early, so stopping lithium when pregnancy is confirmed is too late

● The relapse rates at 40 weeks after lithium discontinuation were similar for pregnant (52%) and non-pregnant (58%) women, but much higher than the year before discontinuation (21%), so pregnancy is relatively 'risk neutral'

● Women who remained stable over the first 40/52 since lithium discon-tinuation were 2.9 times more likely to relapse than non-pregnant women during weeks 41–62 (70% *vs* 24%)

● The rates are higher in rapid rather than gradual discontinuation

● The 50% relapse rate within 35 weeks is high, and the risk from consequentially needed drugs is high

● There were no major malformations in the children born to the women (n=9) who continued lithium throughout pregnancy

● An unstudied option might be to stop lithium gradually as soon as pregnancy is known, then reintroduce in the third trimester.

During pregnancy, thyroid suppression may also produce neonatal goitre and cardiac arrhythmias. Neonatal lithium toxicity is usually associated with poor maternal control, as renal clearance is increased during pregnancy and so higher doses are needed. Lithium clearance changes markedly near end of term and the dose may need to be reduced by up to 30–50% in the last few weeks, so measure plasma levels carefully and frequently.

A study of 60 healthy children born to mothers who took lithium during the first trimester did not reveal any increased frequency of physical or mental anomalies among the lithium children compared to their non-lithium exposed siblings over 5–10 years (n=60,

Schou, *Acta Psych Scand* 1976, **54**, 193–97).

Reviews: Llewellyn *et al, (J Clin Psych* 1998, **59**[Suppl 6], 57–64), Yonkers *et al* (*CNS Drugs* 1998, **9**, 261–69), guidelines on use in pregnancy (Cohen *et al, JAMA* 1994, **271**, 146–50).

33*. **Modafinil** (FDA=C) is contra-indicated in pregnancy (MI). Pre-clinical studies have shown no teratogenicity but more information is required.

34*. **Methadone** (FDA: B, or D if used in high dose or for prolonged periods) at maintenance doses has been used successfully, does not appear to be overtly teratogenic and reduces the risk of poor quality street drugs being used. With potential illicit drug-using mothers, teratogenicity with methadone will obviously be very difficult to ascertain but there does not appear to be a clear association with malformations (eg. study by Newman *et al, Am J Obstet Gynecol* 1975, **121**, 233–37; Newman, *NY J Med* 1974, **74**, 52). Predictably, a foetal withdrawal syndrome, occurring within the first 24 hours has been seen. Symptoms include tremor, irritability, hyperactivity, jitteriness, shrill cry, vomiting, diarrhoea and convulsions. Stopping opiates abruptly is dangerous as withdrawal reactions can damage the foetus more than methadone. Long-term developmental outcome seems unaffected (Kaltenbach and Finnegan, *Neurotoxicol Teratol* 1987, **9**, 311–13. For effect on child in first year see *Arch Dis Childhood* 1989, **64**, 235–45). There have also been numerous reports of sudden death, reduced body weight and head circumference etc. but these are virtually all in uncontrolled situations and so other effects can not be excluded. In a study of methadone maintenance in pregnancy, head circumference and birth weight were slightly lower with methadone compared to controls (n=32, Brown *et al, Am J Obs Gynecol* 1998, **179**, 459–63). Slow-release morphine is no better at reducing neonatal withdrawal symptoms than methadone (n=48, Fischer *et al, Addiction* 1999, **94**, 231–39).

35. No teratogenic effects have been reported in patients who took **dexamfetamine** (FDA=C) before knowing they were pregnant (Guilleminault, *Sleep* 1993, **16**, 199–201).

36*. There is little information available for **methylphenidate** (FDA=C), and the few reported cases are unremarkable, but the UK SPC advises caution.

37. **Bupropion** (FDA=B) Animal studies have shown no definitive evidence of teratogenicity nor impaired fertility (Briggs *et al*, 1992).

3.9 RENAL IMPAIRMENT (see also BNF)

	Lower risk	Moderate risk	Higher risk (greater care needed)
Antipsychotics	Loxapine[8]	Butyrophenones[6] Clozapine[3] Olanzapine[2] Phenothiazines[7] Quetiapine[2] Thioxanthenes[4]	Amisulpride[5] Risperidone[1] Sulpiride[5] Zotepine[2]
Antidepressants	Mianserin[16] Moclobemide[16] Tricyclics[12] Trazodone[13] Tryptophan[16]	MAOIs[15] Mirtazapine[11] Nefazodone[13] Reboxetine[14] SSRIs[9]	Fluoxetine[9] Venlafaxine[10]
Anxiolytics and hypnotics	Zaleplon[19] Zopiclone[19]	Benzodiazepines[17] Beta-blockers[20] Clomethiazole[21] Zolpidem[19]	Buspirone[18] Chloral[21]
Anticonvulsants	Phenytoin[24] Tiagabine[27]	Barbiturates[25] Benzodiazepines[17] Carbamazepine[22] Ethosuximide[28] Fosphenytoin[24] Lamotrigine[26] Piracetam[27] Topiramate[27]	Gabapentin[26] Levetiracetam[27] Midazolam[17] Oxcarbazepine[22] Valproate[23] Vigabatrin[27]
Others	Anticholinesterases[29]	Anticholinergics[30] Bupropion[34] Disulfiram[31] Modafinil[33]	Acamprosate[31] Lithium[32]

Grade	GFR ml/min.	Serum Creatinine micromol/L
Mild	20–50	150–300
Moderate	10–20	300–700
Severe	<10	>700

General Principals (adapted from *Maudsley Guidelines*, 2001)

1. Renal impairment will lead to accumulation of drugs – the greater the impairment, the greater the potential for accumulation.

2. Serum creatinine may not be raised in the elderly, although renal impairment may be present.

3. Care is needed with drugs or active metabolites predominantly cleared by the kidney, eg. antidepressants and antipsychotics (except substituted benzamides).

4. Start low and go slow, adjusting doses to tolerance.

5. Adverse effects such as postural hypotension, sedation and confusion may be more common.

6. Care is needed with drugs with marked anticholinergic activity, which may cause urinary retention and interfere with U&E measurements.

3.9.1 Antipsychotics:

Lower doses of all antipsychotics should be used as increased cerebral sensitivity and EPSEs may occur.

1. **Risperidone** elimination is reduced in renal disease and so initial doses and dose increments should be halved, up to about 4mg/d.

2. **Olanzapine** is excreted primarily (57%) via the renal pathway and 30% in faeces. A lower olanzapine starting dose of 5mg/d may be appropriate in renal impairment (review: Callaghan *et al, Clin Pharmacokinetics* 1999, **37**, 177–93). If creatinine clearance is <10ml/min, there is only a slight (11%) increase in half-life and 17% reduction in clearance. Eight patients with severe renal impairment given **quetiapine** showed some reduced clearance compared to controls so the starting dose should be 25mg/d, with dose increments of 25–50mg/d (eg. Thyrum *et al, Prog Neuropsychopharmacol Biol Psych* 2000, **24**, 521–33). 17% of a dose of **zotepine** is excreted through the kidneys and levels may be 2–3 times higher in patients with renal impairment. Start at 25mg bd up to a maximum of 75mg bd.

3. **Clozapine** is contraindicated in severe renal disease. In mild to moderate renal failure, start at 12.5mg/d and increase slowly.

4*. **Zuclopenthixol** and **flupentixol**

should be used with caution in renal impairment (SPC), as some accumulation of metabolites has been reported. No dosage adjustment of flupentixol is usually necessary (Jann *et al, Clin Pharmacokinet* 1985, **10**, 315–33).

5. **Sulpiride** is mainly cleared by the kidneys and its half-life can range from 6–25hrs, depending upon renal function. Reduce the dose by 35–70% or extend the dosage interval by a factor of 1.5 to 3 if necessary (*Clin Pharmacokinet* 1989, **17**, 367–73). **Amisulpride** is principally cleared unchanged through the kidneys, so care is needed in moderate to severe renal insufficiency (GFR 10–30ml/min). It is not appreciably removed during haemodialysis.

6*. There are no apparent problems with **haloperidol**, and it is less sedative and causes little postural hypotension. The UK SPC recommends caution as some accumulation might occur.

7. There is little information on phenothiazines, but excretion may be slower and accumulation may occur, causing sedation, postural hypotension etc. **Levomepromazine** (methotrimeprazine) should be used with care in renal disease, and **chlorpromazine** and **thioridazine** avoided.

8. **Loxapine** is 70% excreted via the kidneys and 30% via faeces. No specific problems in renal damage are known.

3.9.2 Antidepressants:

9. If the GFR is less than 10ml/min do not use **fluoxetine**, unless the patient is on dialysis. If the GFR is 10–50ml/min. the manufacturers suggest alternate day dosing, with care. In moderate renal impairment, reduce the initial dose of **paroxetine** to 10mg/d, and increase only if necessary. Data from early **citalopram** trials showed that renal clearance accounts for about 20% total citalopram elimination, and although half-life increases slightly, no reduction of citalopram dosage is warranted in patients with moderately impaired renal function. In severe renal failure, a lower dosage of citalopram may be appropriate (Joffe *et al, Eur J Clin Pharmacol* 1998, **54**, 237–42). Use of **sertraline** is not

recommended by the manufacturers although they have 'data on file' of a single dose study which showed no significant changes in sertraline kinetics in mild, moderate or severe renal failure. **Fluvoxamine** should be used with care, starting at 50mg/d and increasing only slowly. An unpublished report indicated that fluvoxamine does not accumulate at 100mg/d in renal impairment.

10. About 1–10% of a **venlafaxine** dose is cleared unchanged by the kidney and 30% renally excreted as the major metabolite. Total clearance is reduced by about 35% in mild to moderate renal impairment (GFR 10–30ml/min) and so doses should be reduced by about 25–50% respectively, although there is much inter-patient variability in renal impairment (Anon, *J Clin Psych* 1993, **54**, 119–26). An open study of 36 subjects (12 with renal impairment, 8 on dialysis and 18 matched controls) showed that clearance was reduced by about 55% in moderate to severe renal disease, and the authors suggested a 50% reduction in venlafaxine dose, given once a day, where GFR was less than 30ml/min (Troy *et al, Clin Pharmacol Therapeut* 1994, **56**, 14–21). Single daily dosing is thus appropriate, with daily doses also reduced by 50% in dialysis and doses separated from dialysis itself. It is not recommended in severe renal failure but has been used in haemodialysis, with the dose reduced by 50% and withheld until after dialysis is complete.

11*. **Mirtazapine** clearance is reduced by 33% in moderate renal failure and by 50% in severe but not in mild renal failure in a single dose study (n=40, Bengtsson *et al, Hum Psychopharmacol* 1998, **13**, 357–65), and so care with higher doses is recommended.

12. **Tricyclics** should be started at low dose and increased slowly, with divided doses. Avoid lofepramine in severe renal impairment, as 50% is renally excreted.

13*. Accumulation of **nefazodone** and its metabolites could occur in renal impairment and so lower doses should be used in severe renal impairment. No dosage adjustment is necessary for

trazodone (Catanese *et al, Boll Chim Farm* 1978, **117**, 424–27).

14*. **Reboxetine** half-life and plasma levels appear to rise (up to two-fold), particularly in severe renal impairment where dose adjustment may be necessary. After a single-dose reboxetine study, a reduction in starting dose to 2mg BD in patients with moderate to severe renal dysfunction has been suggested (n=18, Coulomb *et al, J Clin Pharmacol* 2000, **40**, 482–87).

15*. No dosage adjustments are usually necessary for the **MAOIs**, although **isocarboxazid** should be used with caution with impaired renal function to prevent accumulation (SPC).

16. Dosage adjustments in renal disease are not necessary for **moclobemide** (*Acta Psych Scand* 1990, **360** [Suppl], 94–97), **mianserin** nor **tryptophan**.

3.9.3 Anxiolytics and hypnotics:

17. Low dose anticonvulsant use of **benzodiazepines** may be acceptable as higher doses produce an increase in CNS side-effects. **Chlordiazepoxide** can be given in normal doses and is not affected by haemodialysis (*Am J Kidney Dis* 1983, **3**, 155). In severe renal failure, doses of **oxazepam** should be reduced to 75% (*Am J Kidney Dis* 1983, **3**, 155). In a case report of one patient with end stage renal failure and haemodialysis, **clobazam** and metabolite concentrations were measured and were no different to those with normal renal function. The authors recommended that there is no need to change clobazam doses in any degree of renal failure or in haemodialysis (Roberts and Zoanetti, *Ann Pharmacother* 1994, **28**, 966–67). Accumulation of metabolites of **midazolam** may be responsible for prolonged sedation (*Lancet* 1995, **346**, 145) and there has been a report of 5 patients with severe renal failure suffering prolonged sedation with midazolam, not reversible by flumazenil (Bauer *et al, Lancet* 1995, **346**, 145–47).

18. **Buspirone** plasma levels have been shown to be higher in patients with renal failure, with a good correlation between steady-state buspirone levels and serum albumin (Barbhaiya *et al, E J Clin Pharmacol* 1994, **46**, 41–47). It is contraindicated in moderate or severe renal impairment.

19*. Plasma protein binding of **zolpidem** is reduced in renal failure (Pacifici, *Int J Clin Pharmacol Ther Toxicol* 1988, **26**, 439–43). The half-life may be doubled but no dosage adjustments are recommended by the manufacturers in mild renal dysfunction. The pharmacokinetics of **zaleplon** and **zopiclone** are not significantly different in renal insufficiency, and so dose alteration is not required.

20. In severe renal disease plasma levels of **beta-blockers** may be higher and so starting doses should be lower. Beta-blockers may also reduce renal blood flow and adversely affect renal function.

21. Caution is needed with **clomethiazole** in chronic renal disease. **Chloral** is contraindicated in moderate to marked renal impairment (*Am J Kidney Dis* 1983, **3**, 155).

3.9.4 Anticonvulsants:

22. **Carbamazepine** rarely causes renal disturbances although it has been suggested that doses should be reduced by 25% in severe renal failure (*Am J Kidney Dis* 1983, **3**, 155). For **oxcarbazepine** in renal impairment (creatinine clearance less than 30ml/min), start at half the usual dose (300mg/day), increasing at no more frequently than weekly intervals. In patients with pre-existing renal conditions associated with low sodium or in patients treated concomitantly with sodium-lowering drugs (eg, diuretics, desmopressin) as well as NSAIDs, serum sodium levels should be monitored (see SPC).

23. **Valproate** is eliminated mainly through the kidneys and the UK SPC now states that it may be necessary to decrease the dosage in renal insufficiency.

24*. No specific dose adjustments are required, but **phenytoin** protein binding is altered in uraemia which can be problematic in accurately assessing serum levels. Severe cardiovascular ADRs have been reported with **fosphenytoin** IV (see *3.2*) and so a reduced loading dose and/or infusion rate by 10–25% in renal impairment is recommended.

25. High-dose **phenobarbital**, in particular, causes increased sedation and the dosage interval should be increased to at least 12–16 hours in severe renal failure (*Am J Kidney Dis* 1985, **3**, 155). Large doses of **primidone** should be avoided. Active metabolites of **amylobarbital** accumulate in severe renal disease.

26*. Most of a dose of **gabapentin** is excreted unchanged in the urine (Hooper *et al, B J Clin Pharmacol* 1991, **31**, 171–74). The UK manufacturers recommend dose reductions as follows:

Creatine clearance	Dosage and frequency
60–90ml/min	400mg tds
30–60ml/min	300mg bd
15–30ml/min	300mg/d
<15ml/min	300mg alternate days

Patients undergoing haemodialysis should receive a loading dose of 400mg and 200–300mg for every four hours of dialysis. Alternatively, a single-dose study of gabapentin 400mg in adults with varying degrees of renal function (but none on dialysis) showed that clearance correlated well with creatinine clearance, with increased half-life with poorer renal function. The authors suggested normal gabapentin doses for creatinine clearance of 60ml/min, 600mg/d for 30–59ml/min, 300mg/d for 15–29ml/min and 150mg/d for CLcr less than 15ml/min (n=60, open, Blum *et al, Clin Pharmacol Therapeut* 1994, **56**, 154–59). A reduced maintenance dose of **lamotrigine** is usually recommended in severe renal impairment, but the dose probably needs little adjustment in mild to moderate impairment (n=21, Wootton *et al, B J Clin Pharmacol* 1997, **43**, 23–27) and even in end stage renal failure (SPC), although the major glucuronide metabolite levels may increase eight-fold due to reduced renal clearance.

27*. **Vigabatrin** is excreted by the kidneys and so reduced doses are recommended with a creatinine clearance of <60mL/min. About 60% of a **topiramate** dose is excreted unchanged via the kidneys. Time to

steady state may be 10–15 days in severe renal impairment instead of 4–8 days with normal renal function. Dose titration may thus need to be more careful. Supplemental doses of 50% of the daily dose should be given on haemodialysis days. There is an increased risk of renal stone formation, via its carbonic anhydrase inhibition, carbonic anhydrase being a known inhibitor of renal crystallisation. Care is needed to ensure adequate fluid throughput, especially in patients with known disposition to this problem (Wasserstein *et al, Epilepsia* 1995, **36**[Suppl 3], S153). **Piracetam** is excreted unchanged via the kidneys and dose adjustments may be needed in renal impairment (Tacconi and Wurtman, *Adv Neurol* 1986, **43**, 675–85). There are no apparent problems with **tiagabine** (n=25, Cato *et al, Epilepsia* 1998, **39**, 43–47).

Since 66% of a dose of **levetiracetam** is excreted unchanged in the urine, dose reductions are necessary in impaired renal function:

Renal function	Creatinine clearance	Dosage and frequency
Normal	>80ml/min	500–1500mg bd
Mild	50–79ml/min	500–1000mg bd
Moderate 30–49ml/min	250–750mg bd	
Severe	<30ml/min	250–500mg bd
End-stage renal disease, undergoing dialysis	–	50–100 bd

Following dialysis, a 250–500mg supplemental dose is recommended.

28. **Ethosuximide** doses should be reduced by 25% in severe renal failure (*Am J Kidney Dis* 1983, **3**, 155).

3.9.5 Others:

29*. No change in dose is necessary with **donepezil** in mild to moderate renal impairment (MI). There are no reported problems with **rivastigmine** (MI). No dosage reduction of **galantamine** is necessary for creatinine clearance greater than 9ml/min. In severe impairment (<9ml/min) galantamine is contraindicated (due current to lack of safety data) (SPC).

30. The UK SPCs recommend some caution in renal disease with the **anticholinergics**.

31. The UK SPC for **disulfiram** recommends caution in renal disease. The UK SPC for **acamprosate** states that use in renal insufficiency (serum creatinine >120micromol/L) is a contraindication.

32. **Lithium** is contraindicated in severe renal impairment. If lithium use is unavoidable, use alternate day dosing, use very low doses (25–75% normal) and frequent level estimating. There is a case of lithium augmentation being used successfully in a 78-year-old woman with borderline impaired renal function, using 125mg on alternate days, with the above-mentioned close monitoring (Gash *et al, J Aff Dis* 1995, 51–53). For a review of lithium and the kidney, see Gitlin (*Drug Safety* 1999, **20**, 231–43, 77 refs).

33. The maximum **modafinil** dose of 400mg/d should only be used in the absence of renal impairment (MI).

34*. **Bupropion** and metabolites are almost exclusively (85%) excreted through the kidneys and so, in renal failure, the initial dose should be reduced and close monitoring for toxicity carried out.

Full reviews, assessments and references for most of these interactions can be found in standard reference books. Resources include *Drug Interactions* by Ivan Stockley (Blackwell Scientific, Oxford), or *Drug Interactions in Psychiatry*, edited by Ciraulo, Shader, Greenblatt and Creelman (Williams & Wilkins, Maryland)

Absolute classification of interactions is impossible. Many factors, eg. age, concurrent illness, P450 status etc. are important. Single case reports merely suggest a possible interaction, and more structured formal studies may show the probable likelihood of an interaction. In order to give some guidance, interactions with the drugs in **CAPITAL LETTERS** are those which could be:

● Potentially hazardous
● Where a dosage adjustment is likely to have to be made
● Well-established and documented
● Of clinical significance
● Rare but important.

How to use this section:
1. Look up the psychiatric drug or group.
2. Look up the drug group of the interacting drug.
3. If no entry there, look up the actual drug.
4. If still no entry, little or nothing has been reported to date.

4.1 ANXIOLYTICS & HYPNOTICS

4.1.1 BENZODIAZEPINES

Benzodiazepines are mainly metabolised by CYP2C and CYP3A3/4.

Review:* Clinically significant pharmacokinetic drug interactions with benzodiazepines (Tanaka, *J Clin Pharm & Therapeut* 1999, **24**, 347).

Acamprosate + benzodiazepines
See acamprosate (*4.6.1*).

Acetazolamide + benzodiazepines
A theoretical and clinically insignificant interaction.

ALCOHOL + BENZODIAZEPINES
See alcohol (*4.7.1*).

Amfetamines + benzodiazepines
Animal studies have shown a clinically insignificant interaction.

Amiodarone + clonazepam
Clonazepam toxicity at low dose caused by amiodarone has been reported (n=1, Witt *et al, Ann Pharmacother* 1993, **27**, 1463–64).

Antacids + benzodiazepines
Diazepam and chlordiazepoxide absorption is slightly delayed by antacids (*Clin Pharmacol Ther* 1978, **24**, 600–9) but total absorption remains the same.

Anticholinergics + benzodiazepines
Benzodiazepine absorption may be delayed by anticholinergics, but the amount absorbed remains unchanged.

Anticoagulants + benzodiazepines
Lack of an interaction has been demonstrated (eg. Orme *et al, BMJ* 1972, **3**, 611) and benzodiazepines are a suitable alternative to chloral. Three isolated cases of adverse reactions have been reported (*NZ Med J* 1974, **85**, 305).

Antihistamines + benzodiazepines
Enhanced sedation is possible.

Antihypertensives+benzodiazepines
Enhanced hypotension is possible.

Antipsychotics + benzodiazepines
See antipsychotics (*4.2.1*).

Atropine + benzodiazepines
No interaction is thought to occur (*Br J Anaes* 1982, **54**, 1231–34).

Baclofen + benzodiazepines
Enhanced sedation can occur.

Barbiturates + benzodiazepines
Enhanced sedation and increased benzodiazepine clearance may occur via CYP3A4 induction (*Clin Pharmacol Ther* 1979, **26**, 103). Dose adjustment may be necessary.

Beta-blockers + benzodiazepines *
Propranolol and metoprolol produce a small but significant reduction in diazepam clearance (*Clin. Pharmacol & Therapeutics* 1984, **36**, 451–54) and patients may become more 'accident-prone' on the combination. In a small study, propranolol and labetolol had no effect on oxazepam pharmacokinetics (n=6, Sonne *et*

al, B J Clin Pharmacol 1990, **29**, 33–37), but some effect on reaction times was seen. Metoprolol appears not to interact significantly with lorazepam (n=12, open, Scott *et al, Eur J Clin Pharmacol* 1991, **40**, 405–9).

Buprenorphine + flunitrazepam *

Buprenorphine does not inhibit the metabolism of flunitrazepam and so any interaction is likely to be pharmacodynamic rather than metabolic (Kilicarslan and Sellers, *Am J Psych* 2000, **157**, 1164–66).

Buspirone + benzodiazepines

See buspirone (*4.1.2*).

CALCIUM-CHANNEL BLOCKERS + BENZODIAZEPINES *

Both diltiazem and verapamil significantly raise midazolam levels and half-life, via 3A4 induction, increasing sedative side-effects. A 50% midazolam dose reduction has been suggested (Backman *et al, B J Clin Pharmacol* 1994, **37**, 221–25).

Cannabis + benzodiazepines

See cannabis (*4.7.2*).

Carbamazepine + benzodiazepines

See carbamazepine (*4.5.1*).

Charcoal, activated + diazepam

25g activated charcoal given 30 minutes after diazepam 5mg reduced diazepam AUC by 27%, but not peak levels. Concurrent gastric lavage does not provide any additional reductions (n=9, RCT, Lapatto-Reiniluoto *et al, Br J Clin Pharmacol* 1999, **48**, 148–53).

Citalopram + triazolam *

See citalopram (*4.3.2.1*).

Clarithromycin + midazolam

Higher dose clarithromycin (2.5g/d) may increase the availability of midazolam, probably via CYP3A4 competition (n=16, Gorski *et al, Clin Pharmacol Ther* 1998, **64**, 133–43).

CLOZAPINE + BENZODIAZEPINES

See clozapine (*4.2.2*).

Cyclophosphamide + benzodiazepines

Increased cyclophosphamide toxicity has been proposed (*J Pharm Dyn* 1983, **6**, 767–72).

Dehydroepiandrosterone + alprazolam *

Alprazolam rapidly and significantly increases dehydroepiandrosterone concentrations (n=38, Kroboth *et al, J Clin Psychopharmacol* 1999, **19**, 114–24).

Dextropropoxyphene + alprazolam

Increased sedation can occur with alprazolam (*Br J Clin Pharmac* 1985, **19**, 51–57).

Digoxin + benzodiazepines

Lack of interaction has been shown (*Clin Pharmacol Ther* 1985, **38**, 595).

Diflunisal + benzodiazepines

Diflunisal may reduce the effect of some benzodiazepines (lorazepam, temazepam and oxazepam) by increasing metabolism (Van Hecken *et al, B J Clin Pharmacol* 1985, **20**, 225).

Disulfiram + benzodiazepines

See disulfiram (*4.6.6*).

Ethambutol + diazepam

No interaction is thought to occur (n=6, Ochs *et al, Clin Pharmacol Ther* 1981, **29**, 671–78).

Fluoxetine + benzodiazepines

See fluoxetine (*4.3.2.2*).

Fluvoxamine + benzodiazepines

See fluvoxamine (*4.3.2.3*).

Food + benzodiazepines

Food delays the absorption of benzodiazepines, only significant if a rapid onset of action is needed.

Gabapentin + clonazepam

See gabapentin (*4.5.3*).

Grapefruit juice + triazolam *

200ml normal-strength grapefruit juice increases plasma triazolam levels, and repeated consumption produces a greater increase (n=12, RCT, Lilja *et al, Eur J Clin Pharmacol* 2000, **56**, 411–15).

H2-blockers + benzodiazepines

Cimetidine inhibits the metabolism of long-acting benzodiazepines via CYP3A4 but not lorazepam, oxazepam and temazepam. Only a few patients experience increased side-effects and the clinical effect is probably negligible. The other H-2 blockers do not interact this way (eg. ranitidine, Klotz *et al, J Clin Pharmacol* 1987, **27**, 210), although ranitidine may slightly reduce the absorption of diazepam.

Heparin + benzodiazepines

A transient rise in benzodiazepine levels could occur (n=5, Routledge *et al, B J Clin Pharmacol* 1980, **9**, 171).

Indometacin + diazepam

Increased dizziness may occur (*Pharmacol Toxicol* 1988, **62**, 293–97).

Isoniazid + benzodiazepines

Isoniazid reduces the clearance of diazepam but not of oxazepam (n=9, Ochs *et al, Clin Pharmacol Ther* 1981, **29**, 671–78).

Itraconazole + benzodiazepines

Increased midazolam oral bio-availability occurs in patients on itraconazole and ketoconazole (Olkkola *et al, Clin Pharmacol Ther* 1994, **55**, 481–85). Midazolam levels were significantly higher with itraconazole 200mg/d for 4 days, the effect being detectable up to four days after cessation of treatment (n=9, Backman *et al, Eur J Clin Pharmacol* 1998, **54**, 53–58).

Ketoconazole + benzodiazepines

An increase in the effect of chlordiazepoxide can occur with oral ketoconazole and up to a 6-fold increase in midazolam levels can occur (Olkkola *et al, Clin Pharmacol Ther* 1994, **55**, 481–85).

Lamotrigine + clonazepam

See lamotrigine (*4.5.4*).

LEVODOPA + BENZODIAZEPINES

Levodopa can be antagonised by diazepam, nitrazepam and chlordiazepoxide (Yousselson *et al, Ann Int Med* 1982, **96**, 259), much reducing its effect, so observe for worsening parkinsonian symptoms.

Lithium + benzodiazepines

See lithium (*4.4*).

MAOIs + benzodiazepines

See MAOIs (*4.3.4*).

Methadone + diazepam

Enhanced sedation may occur (*Drug Alc Dep* 1986, **18**, 195–202).

Metronidazole + benzodiazepines

Lack of an interaction has been reported (*Clin Pharmacol Ther* 1986, **39**, 181).

Mianserin + benzodiazepines

See mianserin (*4.3.3.1*).

Mirtazapine + benzodiazepines

See mirtazapine (*4.3.3.2*).

Moclobemide + benzodiazepines

See moclobemide (*4.3.3.3*).

Muscle relaxants + benzodiazepines*

Variable relatively minor effects have been reported (n=113, Driessen *et al, Acta Anaesthesiol Scand* 1986, **30**, 642–46). Diazepam may hasten the onset and prolong the duration of vecuronium (n=20, RCT, Yuan *et al, Chung Hua I Hsueh Tsa Chih (Taipei)* 1994, **54**, 259–64), but midazolam appears not to do this (n=10, Husby *et al, Acta Anaesthesiol Scand* 1989, **33**, 280–82). Diazepam may reduce succinylcholines side-effects (*Clin Pharmacol Ther* 1979, **26**, 395), probably of very limited significance.

Narcotic analgesics/opioids + benzodiazepines

Synergism (eg. Kissin *et al, Anesth Analg* 1990, **71**, 65) and changes in haemodynamic status (Heikkila *et al, Acta Anesthesiol Scand* 1984, **28**, 683) have been reported.

NEFAZODONE + BENZODIAZEPINES

See nefazodone (*4.3.3.4*).

Nimodipine + benzodiazepines

Lack of a clinically significant interaction during chronic oral administration has been reported (n=24, Heine *et al, B J Clin Pharmacol* 1994, **38**, 39–43).

Olanzapine + benzodiazepines

See olanzapine (*4.2.3*).

Ondansetron + temazepam

Lack of interaction has been shown (n=24, Preston *et al, Anaesthesia* 1996, **51**, 827–30).

Oral contraceptives + benzodiazepines

OCs may increase the effects of longer-acting benzodiazepines (Stoehr *et al, Clin Pharmacol Ther* 1984, **36**, 683–90), not thought to be of clinical significance.

Paraldehyde + benzodiazepines

Enhanced sedation would be expected.

Paroxetine + benzodiazepines

See paroxetine (*4.3.2.4*).

Phenobarbital + benzodiazepines

See barbiturates + benzodiazepines in this section.

Phenytoin + benzodiazepines

See phenytoin (*4.5.8*).

Physostigmine + benzodiazepines*

Physostigmine may reverse diazepam-induced sleep (*J Neurochem* 1980, **34**, 856) and midazolam-induced somnolence (Ho *et al, Ma Tsui Hsueh Tsa Chi* 1991, **29**, 643–47).

Progabide + clonazepam

Lack of interaction has been reported (*Epilepsia* 1987, **28**, 68–73).

Propofol + midazolam *

Propofol decreases the clearance of midazolam by 37% and increases half-life by 61%, probably by inhibiting CYP3A4 (n=24, RCT, Hamaoka *et al, Clin Pharmacol & Ther* 1999, **66**, 110–17).

Proton-pump inhibitors + benzodiazepines*

Omeprazole, but not pantoprazole (Steinijans *et al, Int J Clin Pharmacol Ther* 1996, **34**, S31–S50), can reduce diazepam clearance by up to 50% (Andersson *et al, Eur J Clin Pharmacol* 1990, **39**, 51), probably by a P450 mechanism (Zomorodi and Houston, *Br J Clin Pharmacol* 1996, **42**, 157–62).

Quetiapine + benzodiazepines

See quetiapine (*4.2.4*).

Reboxetine + benzodiazepines

See reboxetine (*4.3.3.5*).

Rifampicin + benzodiazepines

Much increased diazepam clearance can occur via 3A4 induction (Ohnhaus, *Clin Pharmacol Ther* 1987, **42**, 148). Midazolam levels were significantly reduced by rifampicin 600mg/d for 5 days in another study, the effect lasting well over four days (n=9, Backman *et al, Eur J Clin Pharmacol* 1998, **54**, 53–58).

Ritonavir + benzodiazepines *

Extensive impairment of triazolam and alprazolam clearance by short-term low-dose ritonavir may occur (Greenblatt *et al, J Clin Psychopharmacol* 1999, **19**, 293–96, editorial).

Rivastigmine + benzodiazepines

See rivastigmine (*4.6.3.3*).

Sertraline + benzodiazepines

See sertraline (*4.3.2.5*).

Smoking + benzodiazepines

See smoking (*4.7.4*).

Tiagabine + benzodiazepines

See tiagabine (*4.5.10*).

Tricyclics + benzodiazepines

Enhanced sedation has been reported and would be expected. Reduced hydroxylation of clomipramine has been

reported and dose reduction may be necessary (*Pharmaceutisch Weekblad* 1992, **14**[4] Suppl D, D3).

Valproate + benzodiazepines *

Valproate displaces diazepam from plasma protein-binding sites (*B J Clin Pharmacol* 1982, **13**, 553) and so doses may need to be reduced. Valproate increases lorazepam levels by up to 40% (Anderson *et al, Epilepsia* 1994, **35**, 221–25; n=16, RCT, Samara *et al, J Clin Pharmacol* 1997, **37**, 442–50) but lorazepam has no effect on valproate kinetics. Concurrent valproate and clonazepam is alleged to cause absence seizures and clobazam may increase valproate levels.

Venlafaxine + benzodiazepines

See venlafaxine (*4.3.3.8*).

Warfarin + benzodiazepines *

An interaction is unreported but theoretically possible (mentioned in Sayal *et al, Acta Psych Scand* 2000, **102**, 250–55).

Xanthines + benzodiazepines *

Xanthines, eg. theophylline, aminophylline and caffeine antagonise the sedative (and possibly anxiolytic) effects of benzodiazepines (eg. midazolam 12mg is moderately antagonised by 250mg caffeine, n=114, Mattila *et al, Int J Clin Pharmacol Ther* 2000, **38**, 581–87). This can be very useful in the treatment of benzodiazepine overdose but care must be taken if a patient on a benzodiazepine has theophylline stopped, as respiratory depression can then occur.

Zotepine + benzodiazepines

See zotepine (*4.2.6*).

4.1.2 BUSPIRONE

Buspirone may be metabolised by CYP3A4.

Alcohol + buspirone

See alcohol (*4.7.1*).

Benzodiazepines + buspirone

Two studies with diazepam have shown only a minimal enhanced sedation (eg. Mattila *et al, Clin Pharmacol Ther* 1986, **40**, 620–26). Alprazolam appears not to interact with alprazolam (n=12, Buch *at el, J Clin Pharmacol* 1993, **33**, 1104–9).

Calcium channel blockers + buspirone

80mg verapamil or 60mg diltiazem increase buspirone plasma concentrations 3-fold and 5-fold respectively, peak plasma levels also being raised, probably by CYP3A4 inhibition, potentially enhancing the therapeutic and side-effects of buspirone (n=9, Lamberg *et al, Clin Pharmacol Ther* 1998, **63**, 640–45).

Cimetidine + buspirone *

Lack of interaction has been reported (n=10, open, Gammans *et al, Pharmacotherapy* 1987, **7**, 72–79).

Citalopram + buspirone

See citalopram (*4.3.2.1*).

Clozapine + buspirone

Near fatal gastrointestinal bleeding and hyperglycaemia occurring one month after buspirone was added to a stable clozapine regimen has been reported, but no firm explanation found (n=1, Good, *Am J Psych* 1997, **154**, 1473).

Erythromycin + buspirone

Erythromycin and itraconazole increased plasma buspirone levels dramatically in one study, probably via CYP3A4 inhibition, with increased buspirone side-effects noted (n=8, Kivisto *et al, Clin Pharmacol Ther* 1997, **62**, 348–54).

Fluvoxamine + buspirone *

Fluvoxamine 100mg/d raises buspirone levels, probably via CYP3A4 inhibition. No impaired psychomotor performance occurs and so is probably of limited significance (RCT, n=10, Lamberg *et al, Eur J Clin Pharmacol* 1998, **54**, 761–66).

Fluoxetine + buspirone

Reduced anxiolytic effect, dystonia, akathisia (n=1, *Can J Psych* 1990, **35**, 722–23) and anorgasmia (Jenike *et al, J Clin Psych* 1991, **52**, 13–14) have been reported.

Grapefruit juice + buspirone

200ml double-strength grapefruit juice raised peak buspirone plasma levels 4-fold, probably via CYP3A4 inhibition or delayed gastric emptying. Concomitant buspirone and at least large amounts of grapefruit juice should be avoided or dose adjustments made

(n=10, RCT, Lilja *et al, Clin Pharmacol Ther* 1998, **64**, 655–60).

Itraconazole + buspirone

See erythromycin + buspirone.

MAOIs + BUSPIRONE

See MAOIs (*4.3.4*).

NSAIDs + buspirone

GI side-effects and headache may be slightly more common with the combination (n=150, Kiev and Domantay, *Curr Ther Res* 1989, **46**, 1086–90).

Phenytoin + buspirone

Buspirone does not appear to displace phenytoin from plasma binding sites (Gammans *et al, Am J Med* 1985, **80**[Suppl 3B], 41–51).

Propranolol + buspirone

Buspirone appears not to displace propranolol from plasma binding sites (Gammans *et al, Am J Med* 1985, **80**[Suppl 3B], 41–51).

Rifampicin + buspirone

Rifampicin may reduce the peak plasma levels of buspirone, probably via CYP3A4 induction. Significant changes in psychomotor tests have been noted and so dose adjustment may be necessary (n=10, Lamberg *et al, Br J Clin Pharmacol* 1998, **45**, 381–85).

Trazodone + buspirone

There are some isolated reports of raised SGPT/ALT levels and a case of serotonin syndrome (Goldberg and Huk, *Psychosomatics* 1992, **3**, 235).

Warfarin + buspirone

Buspirone does not appear to displace warfarin from plasma binding sites (Gammans *et al, Am J Med* 1985, **80**[Suppl 3B], 41–51).

Zudovidine + buspirone

The combination has been used safely (n=2, Batki, *J Clin Psychopharmacol* 1990, **10**[Suppl 3], 111S–15S).

4.1.3 CHLORAL

ALCOHOL + CHLORAL

See alcohol (*4.7.1*).

Fluvoxamine + chloral

See fluvoxamine (*4.3.2.3*).

Furosemide (frusemide) + chloral

Diaphoresis, facial flushing and agitation occurred with chloral and IV furosemide, which stopped when the chloral was discontinued (Dean *et al*, *Clin Pharm* 1991, **10**, 385–87).

MAOIs + chloral

See MAOIs (*4.3.4*).

Phenytoin + chloral

See phenytoin (*4.5.8*).

Nicoumalone + chloral

An enhanced anticoagulant effect can occur. See also warfarin + chloral.

Warfarin + chloral

The anticoagulant effects of warfarin are increased slightly by chloral, probably by plasma protein displacement (*NEJM* 1972, **286**, 53–55). This can be important if chloral is given as a PRN hypnotic.

4.1.4 ZALEPLON

Zaleplon is primarily metabolised by aldehyde oxidase and a small amount by CYP3A4 to inactive metabolites. As with other such drugs, use with CNS-depressants needs care.

Alcohol + zaleplon

Not recommended due to the risk of enhanced sedation.

Antipsychotics + zaleplon *

Additive psychomotor effects may occur with the combination of zaleplon and thioridazine (n=12, RCT, Hetta *et al*, *Eur J Clin Pharmacol* 2000, **56**, 211–17).

Carbamazepine + zaleplon

Co-administration may reduce zaleplon efficacy through CYP3A4 induction.

Cimetidine + zaleplon

Riased zaleplon levels can occur with cimetidine, via aldehyde oxidase and 3A4 inhibition.

Digoxin + zaleplon *

Lack of interaction has been shown (n=18, Sanchez-Garcia *et al*, *Am J Health Syst Pharm* 2000, **15**, 2267–70).

Erythromycin + zaleplon

Raised zaleplon levels can occur, via 3A4 inhibition.

Ibuprofen + zaleplon *

Lack of significant interaction has been shown (n=17, open, Sanchez-Garcia *et al*, *Am J Health Syst Pharm* 2000, **57**, 1137–41).

Ketoconazole + zaleplon

Raised zaleplon levels can occur, via 3A4 inhibition.

Narcotics + zaleplon

Enhanced euphoria is possible.

Rifampicin + zaleplon

A four-fold reduction in zaleplon levels can occur, via CYP3A4 induction.

Phenobarbital + zaleplon

Reduced zaleplon levels can occur, via CYP3A4 induction.

Warfarin + zaleplon

No interaction (MI).

4.1.5 ZOLPIDEM

Enhanced sedation would be expected with concurrent use of zolpidem with any CNS depressant.

Alcohol + zolpidem

See alcohol (*4.7.1*).

Antipsychotics + zolpidem

Excessive sedation has been reported with chlorpromazine (Desager *et al*, *Psychopharmacol* 1988, **96**, 63–66).

Bupropion + zolpidem *

See bupropion (*4.6.4*).

Caffeine + zolpidem

In a parallel group study, 300mg caffeine did not antagonise the sedative effects of zolpidem 10mg given during the day (Mattila *et al*, *Eur J Clin Pharmacol* 1998, **54**, 421–25).

Fluconazole + zolpidem *

See ketoconazole + zolpidem.

Food + zolpidem

The rate of absorption of zolpidem is slowed significantly by food.

H2-blockers + zolpidem

Lack of a significant interaction has been shown with both cimetidine and ranitidine (Hulhoven *et al*, *Int J Clin Pharmacol Res* 1988, **8**, 471–76).

Ketoconazole + zolpidem *

Ketoconazole lengthens the half-life of zolpidem by about 25% (RCT, n=12, Greenblatt *et al*, *Clin Pharmacol Ther* 1998, **64**, 661–71).

Itraconazole + zolpidem *

Single doses of itraconazole or fluconazole lengthen the half-life of zolpidem, but not significantly (RCT, n=12, Greenblatt *et al*, *Clin Pharmacol Ther* 1998, **64**, 661–71). Itraconazole 200mg/d for 4 days had no marked effect on the pharmacokinetics of zolpidem, although the central effects of zolpidem were slightly increased (n=10, Luurila *et* *al, Eur J Clin Pharmacol* 1998, **54**, 163–66).

Rifampicin + zolpidem

A study showed rifampicin to significantly reduce zolpidem plasma levels and therapeutic effect, via enhanced CYP3A4 metabolism (RCT, n=8, Villikka *et al, Br J Clin Pharmacol* 1997, **43**, 629–34).

SSRIs + zolpidem

SSRIs may enhance zolpidem-associated hallucinations (n=5, Elko *et al, J Toxicol Clin Toxicol* 1998, **36**, 195–203). A study showed minimal pharmacokinetic interaction between fluoxetine 20mg/d and regular zolpidem 10mg/d in healthy women, with no significant psychomotor function changes, although zolpidem half-life increased slightly (n=29, 5/52, Allard *et al, Drug Metab Dispos* 1998, **26**, 617–22).

4.1.6 ZOPICLONE

Alcohol + zopiclone

See alcohol (*4.7.1*).

Aspirin + zopiclone

Lack of interaction has been shown (MI).

Atropine + zopiclone

See metoclopramide + zopiclone below.

Caffeine + zopiclone *

Caffeine has been reported to moderately antagonise the psychomotor impairment caused by zopiclone (Mattila *et al, Pharmacol Toxicol* 1992, **70**, 286–89).

Erythromycin + zopiclone

500mg erythromycin accelerates zopiclone absorption, leading to a more rapid onset, which could be clinically significant in the elderly (n=10, Aranko *et al, B J Clin Pharmacol* 1994, **38**, 363–67).

Itraconazole + zopiclone

Itraconazole significantly increased zopiclone plasma levels by 28% and half-life by 40% but had no clinical significance in the young volunteers (n=10, d/b, p/c, c/o, Jalava *et al, Eur J Clin Pharmacol* 1996, **51**, 331–34).

Metoclopramide + zopiclone

Zopiclone levels are significantly increased by metoclopramide but decreased by atropine (*B J Clin Pharmacol* 1986, **21**, 615).

Ranitidine + zopiclone

Lack of interaction has been shown (MI).

Rifampicin + zopiclone

Rifampicin significantly reduces zopiclone plasma levels and therapeutic effect, via enhanced CYP3A4 metabolism (RCT, n=8, Villikka *et al, Br J Clin Pharmacol* 1997, **43**, 471–74).

Tricyclics + zopiclone

One study showed decreased levels of trimipramine and zopiclone, of doubtful significance (n=10, RCT, Caille *et al, Biopharm Drug Dispos* 1984, **5**, 117–25).

4.2 ANTIPSYCHOTICS — see also clozapine *(4.2.2)*, olanzapine *(4.2.3)*, risperidone *(4.2.4)*, quetiapine *(4.2.5)* and zotepine *(4.2.6)*.

4.2.1 General

There are few specific interactions reported for some antipsychotics, other than additive sedation.

Reviews: interactions with antihypertensive durgs (Markowitz *et al, Ann Pharmacother* 1995, **29**, 603–9).

ACE inhibitors + antipsychotics

An enhanced hypotensive effect can occur, with severe postural hypotension with chlorpromazine and other antipsychotics, eg. captopril plus chlorpromazine (White, *Arch Int Med* 1986, **146**, 1833–34).

Activated charcoal + phenothiazines

Decreased antipsychotic absorption is likely.

ALCOHOL + ANTIPSYCHOTICS

See alcohol (*4.7.1*).

Amfetamines + antipsychotics

The antipsychotic effects of phenothiazines can be antagonised by amfetamines although haloperidol can be used to treat amfetamine-induced psychosis.

Amiodarone + phenothiazines

The BNF notes an increased risk of ventricular arrhythmias with phenothiazines.

Antacids + antipsychotics

Antacids may reduce chlorpromazine and possibly haloperidol serum levels. Sulpiride absorption may be reduced by sucralfate or aluminium containing antacids (*Int J Pharmaceut* 1984, **22**, 257–63). Any problem can be minimised by separating doses by a couple of hours.

Anticholinergics + antipsychotics

Anticholinergics may reduce the improvement in positive symptoms produced by antipsychotics (*Lancet* 1988, **ii**, 199–25), probably by lowering the serum levels of oral and depot antipsychotics (*B J Psych* 1986, **149**, 726–33), but not by increased clearance (Chetty *et al, Eur J Clin Pharmacol* 1994, **46**, 523–26). Additive anticholinergic effects may also occur (see also *1.20.1*).

ANTICONVULSANTS + ANTIPSYCHOTICS

Antipsychotics lower the seizure threshold and may thus antagonise anticonvulsant actions. See also individual anticonvulsants (*4.5*).

Antihypertensives + phenothiazines

A combined hypotensive effect can cause dizziness etc.

Antimalarials + chlorpromazine

One study showed markedly increased chlorpromazine levels with anti-malarials, eg. chloroquine and 'Fansidar' (*Trop Geogr Med* 1988, **40**, 31–33).

Ascorbic acid + fluphenazine

An isolated case exists of reduced fluphenazine levels (*JAMA* 1979, **241**, 2008) with 1g/d of ascorbic acid.

Astemizole + antipsychotics

See terfenadine + antipsychotics.

BARBITURATES + ANTIPSYCHOTICS

Additive sedative effects can occur acutely with this combination, eg. death following IM injection of haloperidol and phenobarbital has been recorded (*J Clin Psych* 1978, **39**, 673). Phenobarbital administration may lower the plasma levels of some antipsychotics, eg. haloperidol by 40–75% and thioridazine by 25–30% (Gay *et al, Neurology* 1983, **33**, 1631–32). Antagonism of the anticonvulsant effects may also occur.

Benzodiazepines + antipsychotics

Enhanced sedation and impaired psychomotor function can occur (see *1.1*).

Beta-blockers + antipsychotics *

Generally, raised plasma levels of the antipsychotic occur, of possible clinical significance, eg. chlorpromazine levels may rise by up to 100–500% with propranolol (Peet *et al, Lancet* 1980, **ii**, 978), although pindolol has no significant effect on haloperidol levels (Greendyke and Guyla, *J Clin Psych* 1988, **49**, 105–7). See also review by Markowitz *et al* (*Ann Pharmacother* 1995, **29**, 603–9). Thioridazine is now contraindicated with propranolol due to QTc prolongation.

Betel nut + antipsychotics *

Betel nut (Areca catechu), which contains a cholinergic alkaloid, arecoline, has been reported to cause rigidity, bradykinesia, tremor, stiffness and akathisia with flupentixol and fluphenazine (Deahl, *Mov Disord* 1998, **4**, 330–33).

Bromocriptine + antipsychotics

A predictable reversal of the antipsychotic effect may occur. Antipsychotics may also antagonise the hypoprolactinaemic and antiparkinsonian effects of bromocriptine.

Calcium-channel blockers + antipsychotics

An increased antipsychotic concentration or enhanced hypotension could be predicted (review by Markowitz *et al, Ann Pharmacother* 1995, **29**, 603–9).

Cannabis + antipsychotics

See cannabis (*4.7.2*).

CARBAMAZEPINE + ANTIPSYCHOTICS

See carbamazepine (*4.5.1*).

Cimetidine + antipsychotics

Chlorpromazine levels may be reduced by 30% by cimetidine (*J Clin Pharmacol* 1983, **24**, 99–102) and ranitidine is a suitable alternative.

Citalopram + antipsychotics

See citalopram (*4.3.2.1*).

CLARITHROMYCIN + ANTIPSYCHOTICS *

The BNF notes an increased risk of arrhythmias with phenothiazines and recommends avoiding the combination. Death has been reported when clarithromycin was added to pimozide in a young man with a documented prolonged QT interval (n=1, Flockhart *et al, J Clin Psychopharmacol* 2000, **20**, 317–24).

Clonidine + antipsychotics

Animal studies have shown phenothiazines and haloperidol (but not pimozide) to antagonise the hypotensive effect of clonidine. Case reports exist of severe hypotension (Frunicillo *et al, Am J Psych* 1985, **142**, 274) and of delirium (review by Markowitz *et al, Ann Pharmacother* 1995, **29**, 603–9).

Clozapine + antipsychotics
See clozapine (*4.2.2*).

Cocaine + antipsychotics
See cocaine (*4.7.3*).

Desferrioxamine + prochlorperazine
Prolonged unconsciousness may occur (MI).

Diazoxide + chlorpromazine
Enhanced hypoglycaemic effects have been reported (n=1, *Lancet* 1975, **2**, 658).

Disopyramide + antipsychotics
Increased anticholinergic effects may occur.

Disulfiram + antipsychotics
See disulfiram (*4.6.6*).

Domperidone + antipsychotics
There is an enhanced risk of EPSEs.

Donepezil + antipsychotics
See donepezil (*4.6.3.1*).

Erythromycin + antipsychotics
See clarithromycin + antipsychotics.

FLUOXETINE + ANTIPSYCHOTICS
Severe EPSEs have been reported with fluoxetine and haloperidol (n=1, Tate, *Am J Psych* 1989, **146**, 399–400), dystonia with fluphenazine 2.5mg (n=1, *Am J Psych* 1993, **150**, 836–37), stupor and confusion with pimozide 8mg/d (n=1, Hansen-Grant *et al, Am J Psych* 1993, **150**, 1750–51), and of severe bradycardia and drowsiness in an elderly patient, reversed when the pimozide was stopped. The probable mechanism is CYP2D6 inhibition leading to raised levels. The combination should thus be avoided if possible (Ahmed *et al, Can J Psych* 1993, 62–63). Citalopram and sertraline would be suitable alternatives.

Fluvoxamine + antipsychotics
See fluvoxamine (*4.3.2.3*).

Ginseng + haloperidol
Ginseng may potentiate the general effects of haloperidol (Mitra *et al, Indian J Exp Biol* 1996, **34**, 41–47).

GUANETHIDINE + ANTIPSYCHOTICS
Reduced hypotensive effects may occur if possible.

Hydroxyzine + phenothiazines
The antipsychotic effect of phenothiazines may be decreased (*Dis Nerv Syst* 1970, **31**, 412).

Hypoglycaemics + chlorpromazine
Chlorpromazine 100mg or more can induce hyperglycaemia and upset the control of diabetes with oral hypoglycaemics (*Am J Psych* 1968, **125**, 253).

Indometacin + haloperidol
One study showed profound drowsiness and confusion on the combination (Bird *et al, Lancet* 1983, **i**, 830–31).

Itraconazole + haloperidol *
Itraconazole 200mg/d for 7 days significantly increases haloperidol and metabolite levels, leading to increased side effects, presumably due to CYP3A4 inhibition (n=13, Yasui *et al, J Clin Psychopharmacol* 1999, **19**, 149–54).

LEVODOPA + ANTIPSYCHOTICS
The therapeutic effect of levodopa is antagonised by antipsychotics and vice versa. Levodopa may worsen anti-psychotic-induced EPSEs.

Lithium + antipsychotics
See lithium (*4.4*).

Loratadine + antipsychotics
See terfenadine + antipsychotics.

MAOIs + antipsychotics
See MAOIs (*4.3.4*).

Methyldopa + haloperidol
Pseudo-dementia with haloperidol and methyldopa has been reported (n=3, Nadel and Wallach, *B J Psych* 1979, **135**, 484). There is also an enhanced risk of EPSEs and postural hypotension.

Metirosine + antipsychotics
An enhanced risk of EPSEs exists.

Metoclopramide + antipsychotics
An enhanced risk of EPSEs exists.

Minocycline + phenothiazines
There is a single reported case of pigmented galactorrhoea on the combination (*Arch Dermatol* 1985, **121**, 417).

Naltrexone + phenothiazines
Severe drowsiness may occur with thioridazine (Maany *et al, Am J Psych* 1987, **144**, 966) or chlorpromazine.

Nefazodone + antipsychotics
See nefazodone (*4.3.3.4*).

Olanzapine + haloperidol
See olanzapine (*4.2.3*).

Oxcarbazepine + antipsychotics *

See oxcarbazepine (*4.5.6*).

Paroxetine + antipsychotics

See paroxetine (*4.3.2.4*).

Pethidine + phenothiazines

Increased CNS toxicity and hypotension can occur (n=10, Stambaugh and Wainer, *J Clin Pharmacol* 1981, **21**, 140–46).

Phenylpropanolamine+thioridazine

A single fatal case of arrhythmia exists (*Can Med Ass J* 1978, **119**, 729).

PHENYTOIN + ANTIPSYCHOTICS

Phenytoin may reduce haloperidol levels by 40–75%, probably via enzyme induction (n=30, Linnoila *et al, Am J Psych* 1980, **137**, 819). Chlorpromazine may increase phenytoin levels by up to 50% (Sands *et al, Drug Intell Clin Pharm* 1987, **21**, 267–72) although other studies show a nil or opposite effect. Antipsychotics lower the seizure threshold and may antagonise the anticonvulsant effect of phenytoin.

Piperazine + chlorpromazine *

The validity of a single case of convulsions with the combination has been queried by a small study (*NEJM* 1970, **282**, 149; see also Sturman, *B J Pharmacol* 1974, **50**, 153–55).

Polymyxin + phenothiazines

The neuromuscular blocking effects of polypeptide antibiotics may be increased by phenothiazines with prolonged respiratory depression possible (*JAMA* 1966, **196**, 181).

Procarbazine + antipsychotics

Enhanced sedation is possible (MI).

Quetiapine + other antipsychotics

See quetiapine (*4.2.4*).

Ranitidine + antipsychotics

See cimetidine + antipsychotics.

Reboxetine + antipsychotics

See reboxetine (*4.3.3.5*).

Rifampicin + haloperidol *

Rifampicin may reduce the serum levels of haloperidol by a third (n=17, Kim *et al, J Clin Psychopharmacol* 1996, **16**, 247–52), a clinically significant effect. Care would also be needed if rifampicin were stopped.

Smoking + antipsychotics

See smoking (*4.7.4*).

Succinylcholine + promazine

A single case of prolonged apnoea in a patient has been reported.

Sucralfate + antipsychotics

See antacids + antipsychotics.

Tea or coffee + antipsychotics

Typical antipsychotics precipitate out of solution to form a tannin complex with tea and coffee (*Lancet* 1979, **ii**, 1130–31). The clinical significance is thought to be minimal (*Lancet* 1981, **i**, 1217–18).

TERFENADINE + ANTIPSYCHOTICS

There is an increased risk of cardiovascular side-effects (such as syncope, prolonged QT interval and ventricular arrhythmias) with terfenadine and astemizole, and it should not be used with other potentially arrhythmogenic drugs such as antipsychotics, a 1993 CSM warning. Terfenadine is metabolised by CYP2D6 only, but loratadine by CYP2D6 and CYP3A4, allowing alternate pathways to be used if one is inhibited. Loratadine and chlorphenamine are currently considered suitable, although there are three unproven reports of arrhythmia with loratadine.

Tetrabenazine + antipsychotics

Only a single case of enhanced EPSEs in a Huntington's patient exists (*Can J Psych* 1986, **31**, 865–66) although it would be a predictable effect.

Thiazide diuretics + antipsychotics

Although no case reports exist, enhanced thioridazine cardiotoxicity has been suggested (Thornton and Pray, *Am J Nurs* 1976, **76**, 245–46).

Trazodone + antipsychotics

See trazodone (*4.3.3.6*).

Tricyclics + antipsychotics

See tricyclics (*4.3.1*).

Valproate + antipsychotics *

Chlorpromazine may inhibit the metabolism of valproate and so monitoring of valproate levels may be appropriate (*J Clin Psychopharmacol* 1984, **4**, 254–61). In a study of the effects of valproate on **haloperidol** plasma levels and outcome in schizophrenia, valproate had no significant effect on either plasma levels or on psychopathology (n=27, 4/52, Hesslinger *et al, J Clin Psychopharmacol* 1999, **19**, 310–15). There are cases of dose-related generalised oedema with **risperidone** and valproate (n=2, Sanders and Lehrer, *J Clin Psych* 1998, **59**, 689–90), although valproate has no significant effect on plasma levels of risperidone and 9-hydroxyrisperidone (n=33, Spina *et al, Ther Drug Monit* 2000, **22**, 481–85). Two studies have shown that valproate produces a non-clinically significant rise in **clozapine**, but lower nor-clozapine, levels (n=37+6, Facciola *et al, Ther Drug Monit* 1999, **21**, 341–45). Antipsychotics lower the seizure threshold and may antagonise the anticonvulsant effect of valproate.

Venlafaxine + antipsychotics

See venlafaxine (*4.3.3.8*).

Warfarin + antipsychotics *

An interaction is theoretically possible (mentioned in Sayal *et al, Acta Psych Scand* 2000, **102**, 250–55).

Zaleplon + antipsychotics

See zaleplon (*4.1.4*).

Zolpidem + antipsychotics

See zolpidem (*4.1.5*).

Zotepine + antipsychotics

See zotepine (*4.2.6*).

4.2.2. ANTIPSYCHOTICS — CLOZAPINE (see also *4.2.1* for other, more general, interactions)

The major metabolic route of clozapine is to norclozapine, which is more stable but more toxic to stem cells (Gerson *et al, B J Haematology* 1994, **86**, 555–61). CYP1A2 is the major metabolising enzyme, with 2D6 and 3A4 possibly having an effect, as well as many other P450 and FMO enzymes involved.

Reviews:* clozapine interactions (Taylor, *B J Psych* 1997, **171**, 109–12, 46 refs), general (Linnet *et al, Drug Metab Dispos* 1997, **25**, 1379–82; Chang *et al, Prog Neuropsychopharmacol Biol Psychiatry* 1998, **22**, 723–39).

ACE inhibitors + clozapine

Clozapine plus diltiazem or enalapril (Aronowitz *et al, J Clin Psycho-pharmacol* 1994, **14**, 429–30) has been reported to produce additional hypotension.

Alcohol + clozapine

See antipsychotics + alcohol (*4.7.1*).

ANTIBIOTICS + CLOZAPINE

Antibiotics reported to cause leucopenia/neutropenia might enhance the likelihood of clozapine-induced neutropenia and hence should be avoided if possible.

1. **LESS likely to cause neutropenia (safer to use)**: penicillins (all except benzyl-penicillin G), all tetracyclines, amino-glycosides, macrolides, clarithromycin, some anti-TBs (ethambutol, pyrazina-mide, streptomycin), clofazimide, hexa-mine, sodium fusidate, spectinomycin, colistin, polymyxin B and cycloserine.

2. **MORE likely/CAN** cause leuco-penia and/or neutropenia (**less safe to use**): cephalosporins and cephamycins, clindamycin, lincomycin, sulphon-amides and trimethoprim, some anti-TBs (capreomycin, isoniazid, rifampicin), dapsone, metronidazole, tinidazole, the 4-Quinolones (ciprofloxacin, nalidixic acid etc), nitrofurantoin, chloram-phenicol, vancomycin and telcoplanin.

Chose antibiotics from the *first list as first choice* where possible and be aware of the potential for problems if drugs from the second list must be used (full details in *Clozaril newsletter*, Spring 1994, 5). See also individual drugs for other interactions.

Anticholinergics + clozapine

See antipsychotics (*4.2.1*).

Antihypertensives + clozapine

Potentiation of the antihypertensive effects may occur. This can be particularly important during the upward dose titration period.

Antipsychotics (other) + clozapine

There is an enhanced risk of agranulo-cytosis (MI) which would additionally be complicated by the long-term nature of any drug given as a depot.

BENZODIAZEPINES + CLOZAPINE

There are cases of severe hypotension and respiratory depression (eg. n=3, Finkel *et al, NEJM* 1991, **325**, 518) sudden death after IV lorazepam (n=1, Klimke & Klieser, *Am J Psych* 1994, **151**, 780), and of lorazepam and clozapine developed toxic effects, eg. sedation etc (n=2, *Am J Psych* 1991, **148**, 1606–7). Monitor for enhanced sedation and take particular care when a clozapine dose is being increased.

Buspirone + clozapine

See buspirone (*4.1.2*).

Caffeine + clozapine *

Caffeine and clozapine are both metabolised by CYP1A2 and so some competitive inhibition of metabolism may occur. Caffeine in doses of 400–1000mg inhibits the metabolism of clozapine to an extent that might be significant in some people (n=12, open RCT, Hagg *et al, Br J Clin Pharmacol* 2000, **49**, 59–63). Drowsiness and sialorrhoea occurred with the combination, with clozapine levels halving when caffeine was stopped (n=1, Odom-White and de Leon, *J Clin Psych* 1996, **57**, 175–76).

CARBAMAZEPINE + CLOZAPINE

See antipsychotics + carbamazepine (*4.5.1*).

Chloramphenicol + clozapine

There is an enhanced risk of agranulocytosis.

Ciprofloxacin + clozapine

There is a case of clozapine levels falling by nearly 50% when ciprofloxacin was stopped, probably due to CYP1A2 inhibition (Markowitz *et al, Am J Psych* 1997, **153**, 881).

Clonidine + clozapine

See clonidine + antipsychotics (*4.2.1*).

Cimetidine + clozapine

Clozapine levels rose by over 50% in one case with cimetidine (Czymanski *et al, J Clin Psych* 1991, **52**, 21). There is no evidence that ranitidine interacts and so use that instead.

Cocaine + clozapine *

See cocaine (*4.7.3*).

Co-trimoxazole + clozapine

There is an enhanced risk of agranulocytosis (mandatory precaution in the UK SPC).

Cytotoxic agents + clozapine

There is an enhanced risk of agranulocytosis (mandatory precaution in the UK SPC).

Digoxin + clozapine

The UK SPC for clozapine advises caution with highly bound drugs, which would include digoxin. Monitor for adverse effects and adjust doses as necessary.

Erythromycin + clozapine

Raised clozapine levels have been reported, with seizures seven days after erythromycin 250mg/d was added to clozapine 800mg/d with levels falling by 50% when the erythromycin was stopped (Funderburg *et al, Am J Psych* 1994, **151**, 1840) and increased toxicity, eg. somnolence and leukocytosis (n=1, Cohen *et al, Arch Int Med* 1996, **156**, 675–77). Reduced clozapine metabolism via CYP1A2 is the probable mechanism

FLUOXETINE + CLOZAPINE

Fluoxetine produces significant increases in plasma clozapine and norclozapine levels, with some inter-individual variation (n=80, Centorrino *et al, Am J Psych* 1996, **153**, 820–22), with several case reports (eg. n=6, Centorrino *et al, Am J Psych* 1994, **151**, 123–25), including death (n=1, Ferslew *et al, J Forensic Sci* 1998, **43**, 1082–85). Uncontrollable myoclonic jerks have been reported (n=1, Kingsbury and Puckett, *Am J Psych* 1995, **152**, 473–72). The mechanism is possibly CYP2D6 inhibition. The risk of clozapine toxicity must be considered carefully and measuring clozapine levels may be useful.

FLUVOXAMINE + CLOZAPINE

Clozapine plasma levels may rise up to 9-fold with the addition of fluvoxamine 100–200mg/d (eg. n=3, Dumortier *et al, Am J Psych* 1996, **153**, 738–39; n=2, Dequardo and Roberts, *Am J Psych* 1996, **153**, 840–41; n=1, Armstrong and Stephans, *J Clin Psych* 1997, **58**, 499), probably by CYP1A2 inhibition. So predictable is the effect that fluvoxamine has been used to counteract CYP1A2 induction by smoking which can lead to clozapine non-response (n=3, Bender and Eap, *Arch Gen Psych* 1998, **55**, 1048–50) in CYP1A2 rapid metabolisers. Close pharmacokinetic monitoring is necessary as the effect can be dramatic over a few days in some patients even with very low doses.

Itraconazole + clozapine

Itraconazole 200mg/d over 7 days had no effect on plasma clozapine and norclozapine levels (RCT, n=7, Raaska and Neuvonen, *Eur J Clin Pharmacol* 1998, **54**, 167–70).

Lithium + clozapine

See antipsychotics + lithium (*4.4*).

MAOIs + clozapine

Enhanced sedation may occur with all CNS depressants (MI).

PAROXETINE + CLOZAPINE

Paroxetine produces significant increases in plasma clozapine and norclozapine levels (n=60, Centorrino *et al, Am J Psych* 1996, **153**, 820–22) and so the risk of clozapine toxicity must be considered carefully.

Penicillamine + clozapine

There is an enhanced risk of agranulo-cytosis (mandatory precaution in the UK SPC).

Phenobarbital + clozapine

Elevated plasma clozapine levels (requiring dose reduction) have been reported after discontinuation of pheno-barbital, presumably from removal of CYP1A2 induction (n=1, Lane *et al, J Clin Psych* 1998, **59**, 131–33).

Phenylbutazone + clozapine

There is an enhanced risk of agranulo-cytosis (mandatory precaution in the UK SPC).

PHENYTOIN + CLOZAPINE

Serum concentrations of clozapine may be markedly reduced by phenytoin (n=2, Miller *et al, J Clin Psych* 1991, **52**, 23) via CYP1A2 induction, so monitor for reduced effect.

Pyrazolone analgesics + clozapine

There is an enhanced risk of agranulo-cytosis (mandatory precaution in UK SPC).

Rifampicin + clozapine

There is a single case of a 600% reduction in clozapine levels 2–3 weeks after rifampicin was started, probably via 1A2 and 3A4 induction (Joos *et al, J Clin Psychopharmacol* 1998, **18**, 83–85).

RISPERIDONE + CLOZAPINE

There have been two cases of raised clozapine levels with this combination, eg. levels rose by 73% in a schizo-affective on 600mg/d clozapine when risperidone 2mg/d was added (Tyson *et al, Am J Psych* 1995, **152**, 1401–2) and a patient quite suddenly developed an agran-ulocytosis six weeks after risperidone 6mg/d was added to a stable clozapine

regimen of 900mg/d (Godleski and Sernyak, *Am J Psych* 1996, **153**, 735). The mechanism may be via CYP2D6 and so care with this combination is essential.

Sertraline + clozapine

Sertraline produces significant increases in plasma clozapine and norclozapine levels, with some interindividual variation (n=80, Centorrino *et al, Am J Psych* 1996, **153**, 820–22). The risk of clozapine toxicity must be considered carefully.

Smoking + clozapine

See antipsychotics + smoking (*4.7.4*).

Sulphonamides + clozapine

There is an enhanced risk of agranulo-cytosis (MI).

Tricyclics + clozapine

See antipsychotics + tricyclics (*4.3.1*)

Valproate + clozapine

Although valproate is often used as anti-convulsant cover for higher dose clozapine, a careful study showed valproate to produce a 15% drop in clozapine levels and a 65% drop in norclozapine levels (n=7, Longo and Salzman, *Am J Psych* 1995, **152**, 650), although raised clozapine levels have been reported (n=1, Costello and Suppes, *J Clin Psychopharmacol* 1995, **15**, 139–41). Clozapine may of course also lower the seizure threshold and antagonise the anticonvulsant effect of valproate.

Venlafaxine + clozapine

See venlafaxine (*4.3.3.8*).

Warfarin + clozapine *

The UK SPC for clozapine advises caution with highly bound drugs, which would include warfarin. There are no case reports, although caution is still needed (mentioned in Sayal *et al, Acta Psych Scand* 2000, **102**, 250–55). Monitor carefully for an enhanced warfarin effect and adjust doses as necessary.

4.2.3 ANTIPSYCHOTICS — OLANZAPINE (see also *4.2.1* for other, more general, interactions)

Olanzapine is metabolised by CYP1A2 and CYP2D6, with little or no effect on CYP1A2, 2D6, 2C19, 2C9 and 3A at normal doses. It is highly bound to albumin (90%) and alpha 1-acid glycoprotein (77%) and interactions may be possible through this mechanism. The metabolic pathways of olanzapine also include N-glucuronidation, reducing its overall sensitivity to drugs that might induce or inhibit its own metabolism via CYP or flavin-containing mono-oxygenase (FMO) systems. Olanzapine is approximately 60% excreted in urine and 30% in faeces. Fixed doses appear to give higher levels in women.

Review:* extensive, of pharmacokinetics and pharmacodynamics (Callaghan *et al, Clin Pharmacokinetics* 1999, **37**, 177–93, 56 refs).

Alcohol + olanzapine

See antipsychotics + alcohol (*4.7.1*).

Aminophylline + olanzapine *

Lack of interaction has been shown with aminophylline and theophylline (n=16, Macias *et al, Pharmacotherapy* 1998, **18**, 1237–48).

Antacids + olanzapine

There is no effect on olanzapine bioavailability (MI).

Benzodiazepines + olanzapine

Single dose studies showed no effect of olanzapine on the metabolism of diazepam. Mild increases in heart rate, sedation and dry mouth were noted with the combination, but no dose adjustment deemed necessary (MI).

Biperiden + olanzapine

Lack of interaction has been reported (MI).

Carbamazepine + olanzapine

Carbamazepine increases olanzapine clearance by 44% and reduces half-life by 20%, but dose adjustment is not needed as olanzapine has a wide therapeutic index (n=11, Lucas *et al, Eur J Clin Pharmacol* 1998, **54**, 639–43). The mechanism is probably CYP1A2 induction by carbamazepine.

Charcoal (activated) + olanzapine

Activated charcoal reduces olanzapine bioavailability by 50–60% (MI).

Cimetidine + olanzapine

There is no effect on olanzapine bioavailability (MI).

Ciprofloxacin + olanzapine

Raised olanzapine levels have been reported, possibly caused by ciprofloxacin (n=1, Markowitz and DeVane, *J Clin Psychophamacol* 1999, **19**, 289–91, letter).

Fluoxetine + olanzapine *

Melancholic depression has been reported with the combination, possibly due to CYP2D6 inhibition (n=1, Nelson and Swartz, *Ann Clin Psychiatry* 2000, **12**, 167–70).

Haloperidol + olanzapine *

An interaction has been suggested (Gomberg, *J Clin Psychopharmacol* 1999, **19**, 272–73).

Lithium + olanzapine

See antipsychotics + lithium (*4.2.1*).

Smoking + olanzapine

See antipsychotics + smoking (*4.7.4*).

Theophylline + olanzapine*

See aminophylline and olanzapine.

Tricyclics + olanzapine *

Single dose studies show no effect of olanzapine on the metabolism of imipramine (n=9, open, Callaghan *et al, J Clin Pharmacol* 1997, **37**, 971–78) and desipramine (MI). Seizures have been reported with olanzapine and clomipramine (Deshauer *et al, J Clin Psychopharmacol* 2000, **20**, 283–84).

Warfarin + olanzapine *

Single dose studies show no effect of olanzapine on the metabolism of warfarin (MI) although it could be possible (mentioned in Sayal *et al, Acta Psych Scand* 2000, **102**, 250–55).

4.2.4 ANTIPSYCHOTICS — QUETIAPINE (see also *4.2.1* for other, more general, interactions)

Quetiapine is metabolised primarily by the CYP3A4 enzyme. Most information is currently from the manufacturers.

Alcohol + quetiapine

See alcohol (*4.7.1*).

Antipsychotics (other) + quetiapine

Haloperidol and risperidone had no effect on quetiapine but thioridazine reduced quetiapine levels, probably by enzyme induction (MI).

Barbiturates + quetiapine

Lower levels of quetiapine would be expected, due to enzyme induction by barbiturates.

Benzodiazepines + quetiapine

Single doses of lorazepam and diazepam were unaffected by quetiapine.

Carbamazepine + quetiapine

Lower levels of quetiapine would be expected, due to CYP3A4 induction by carbamazepine.

Cimetidine + quetiapine

No interaction occurs.

Erythromycin + quetiapine

Raised quetiapine levels are likely via CYP3A4 inhibition.

Ketoconazole + quetiapine

Raised quetiapine levels are likely via CYP3A4 inhibition.

Lithium + quetiapine

Slightly increased lithium levels may occur.

Phenytoin + quetiapine

Lower levels of quetiapine would be expected, due to CYP3A4 induction by phenytoin.

Rifampicin + quetiapine

Lower levels of quetiapine would be expected, due to CYP3A4 induction by rifampicin.

SSRIs + quetiapine

No interaction with fluoxetine has been shown.

Tricyclics + quetiapine

No interaction with imipramine has been shown.

Warfarin + quetiapine *

No interaction is likely to occur (mentioned in Sayal *et al, Acta Psych Scand* 2000, **102**, 250–55), but an isolated case has been reported (n=1, Rogers *et al, J Clin Psychopharmacol* 1999, **19**, 382–83).

4.2.5 ANTIPSYCHOTICS — RISPERIDONE (see also *4.2.1* for other, more general, interactions)

CARBAMAZEPINE+RISPERIDONE *

See antipsychotics + carbamazepine (*4.5.1*).

CLOZAPINE + RISPERIDONE

See clozapine (*4.2.2*).

Donepezil + risperidone

Severe EPSEs have been reported (n=1, Magnuson *et al, Am J Psych* 1998, **155**, 1459).

Lithium + risperidone

See antipsychotics + lithium (*4.4*).

Mirtazapine + risperidone

See mirtazapine (*4.3.3.2*).

Phenytoin + risperidone *

Severe EPSEs have been reported (n=1, Sanderson, *J Clin Psych* 1996, **57**, 177).

Tricyclics + risperidone

See antipsychotics + tricyclics (*4.3.1*).

Valproate + risperidone *

See antipsychotics (*4.2.1*).

4.2.6 ZOTEPINE

Zotepine is metabolised by CYP1A2 and CYP3A4 to norzotepine and both have a plasma protein binding of 97%, making protein-displacement interactions unlikely. Zotepine has no significant effect on CYP2D6.

Alcohol + zotepine

Zotepine should not be used in people with alcohol intoxication (MI).

Anticonvulsants + zotepine

Zotepine lowers the seizure threshold.

Anticholinergics + zotepine

Biperiden had no effect on zotepine kinetics, side-effects or efficacy in one study (n=21, Otani *et al, B J Psych* 1990, **157**, 128–30).

Anticoagulants + zotepine

The Japanese SPC notes that zotepine has been reported to enhance the risk of bleeding when given with anti-coagulants, eg. with nicoumalone, dicoumarol and warfarin, possibly via a change in protein binding.

Antipsychotics (other) + zotepine

Co-prescribing other antipsychotics with zotepine can raise the incidence of seizures.

Benzodiazepines + zotepine

Diazepam increases zotepine levels by 10% (higher in Japanese patients) and doubles norzotepine levels (n=17, Kondo *et al, Psychopharmacol (Berl)* 1996, **127**, 311–14), possibly via CYP3A4 inhibition.

Carbamazepine + zotepine

See antipsychotics+carbamazepine (*4.5.1*).

Clonidine + zotepine

The Japanese SPC notes that zotepine has alpha-1-adrenergic antagonistic properties which may decrease the hypotensive actions of clonidine.

Hypotensive drugs + zotepine

Zotepine has alpha-1 blocking activity and care is needed with other hypotensive agents.

Phenytoin + zotepine

The Japanese SPC notes that zotepine may increase phenytoin plasma levels, so more frequent monitoring is required.

Smoking + zotepine

See antipsychotics + smoking (4.7.4).

SSRIs + zotepine

Fluoxetine increases zotepine levels by 10% and doubles norzotepine levels (MI). Deep vein thrombosis possibly linked to concurrent paroxetine and zotepine has been reported (n=2, Pantel et al, Pharmacopsychiatry 1997, **30**, 109–11).

Tricyclics + zotepine

Desipramine does not seem to affect zotepine levels (MI).

4.3 ANTIDEPRESSANTS

4.3.1 TRICYCLIC ANTIDEPRESSANTS

Tricyclics are metabolised by a range of P450 enzymes, eg. CYP1A2, CYP2D6 and CYP3A3/4. Some tricyclics have several metabolic routes, which may vary with concentration and where inhibition of one route may switch another on.

Acamprosate + tricyclics

See acamprosate (4.6.1).

Acetazolamide + tricyclics

An interaction is unlikely to occur.

ALCOHOL + TRICYCLICS

See alcohol (4.7.1).

Amiodarone + tricyclics

The BNF notes an increased risk of ventricular arrhythmias with tricyclics.

Anaesthetics + tricyclics

Halothane and pancuronium (or gallamine) should be used with care with tricyclics with strong anticholinergic actions. Enflurane may be a safer alternative.

Anticholinergics + tricyclics

Enhanced anticholinergic effects may occur, especially in the elderly.

Antihistamines + tricyclics

Enhanced sedation and anticholinergic effects are possible.

Antipsychotics + tricyclics *

Tricyclic levels may be up to twice as high if **haloperidol** is taken concurrently, eg. with desipramine (Nelson et al, Am J Psych 1980, **137**, 1232–34), nortriptyline and imipramine. Tricyclic levels may

also rise with phenothiazines (eg. Siris et al, Am J Psych 1982, **143**, 104–6) giving enhanced side-effects, eg. **perphenazine** increases plasma nortriptyline levels by about 25%, probably by inhibition of CYP2D6 (n=25, Mulsant et al, J Clin Psychopharmacol 1997, **17**, 318–21). **Thioridazine** increased imipramine levels to toxic levels in a paediatric patient, and also interfered with the HPLC assay of imipramine levels resulting in a falsely high level (Maynard and Soni, Ther Drug Monit 1996, **18**, 728–31). No significant interaction has been reported with the thioxanthenes (BMJ 1972, **i**, 463), although raised imipramine levels with flupentixol have occurred (n=1, Cook et al, Can J Psychiatry 1986, **31**, 235–37). Up to 100mg/d amitriptyline had no effect on **risperidone** (n=12, open, Sommers et al, Int Clin Psychopharmacol 1997, **12**, 141–45). Antidepressants may also be counter-productive in psychosis (mentioned in Drug Dev Res 1988, **12**, 259–66).

Baclofen + tricyclics

A patient with multiple sclerosis lost muscle tone when nortriptyline and imipramine were added to baclofen (n=1, JAMA 1981, **246**, 1659).

BARBITURATES + TRICYCLICS

Barbiturates can reduce the serum levels of amitriptyline, desipramine, protriptyline (Eur J Clin Pharmacol 1977, **11**, 51) and nortriptyline by 14–60% via CYP3A4 induction. Pentobarbital may affect nortriptyline metabolism within 2 days, both starting (induction) and on discontinuation (n=6, von Bahr et al, Clin Pharmacol Ther 1998, **64**, 18–26). Use an alternative to barbiturates or monitor tricyclic levels.

Benzodiazepines + tricyclics

See benzodiazepines (4.1.1).

Beta-blockers + tricyclics

Enhanced maprotiline toxicity has been reported (Neurobehav Toxicol Teratol 1985, **7**, 203–9), labetolol may decrease the clearance of imipramine (increasing plasma levels by 28%, Hermann et al, J Clin Pharmacol 1992, **32**, 176) and there are two uncertain cases of propranolol possibly raising imipramine levels in children (Gillette and Tannery, J Am Acad Child Adolesc Psych 1994, **33**,

223–4), possibly via 2D6 inhibition. This would appear to be a rare but possible interaction.

Buprenorphine + amitriptyline

No enhanced CNS depressant or respiratory effects have been seen (*Eur J Clin Pharmacol* 1987, **33**, 139–46).

Bupropion + tricyclics *

See bupropion (*4.6.4*).

Cannabis + tricyclics

See antidepressants + cannabis (*4.7.2*).

Calcium-channel blockers + tricyclics

Amitriptyline clearance was reduced by diltiazem and verapamil one study, with adverse effects increased (n=32, Hermann *et al, J Clin Pharmacol* 1992, **32**, 176). There is a case of increased nortriptyline concentrations with diltiazem (Krahenbuhl *et al, Eur J Clin Pharmacol* 1996, **49**, 417–19). Enhanced cardiac side-effects are also possible.

CARBAMAZEPINE + TRICYCLICS

See carbamazepine (*4.5.1*).

Charcoal, activated + tricyclics

5–10g may reduce absorption of tricyclics by up to 75% if given within 30 minutes and may be an effective treatment for overdose even up to two hours after the overdose was taken (Dawling *et al, Eur J Clin Pharmacol* 1978, **14**, 445).

Cholestyramine + doxepin

A case report exists of plasma levels of doxepin reduced to a third by cholestyramine (Geeze *et al, Psychosomatics* 1988, **29**, 233–35).

Citalopram + tricyclics

See citalopram (*4.3.2.1*).

CLONIDINE + TRICYCLICS

Tricyclics can be expected to antagonise the hypotensive effects of clonidine (eg. *J Am Ger Soc* 1983, **31**, 164–65).

Cocaine + tricyclics

See antidepressants + cocaine (*4.7.3*).

Co-trimoxazole + tricyclics

Five cases of relapse when co-trimoxazole was added to antidepressant therapy have been reported (*L'Encephale* 1987, **8**, 123–26).

Dextropropoxyphene + doxepin

Doxepin plasma levels were raised by 150% in one elderly patient when dextropropoxyphene was added (*Clin* *Pharmacol Ther* 1982, **31**, 199) via 2D6 inhibition.

Dicoumarol + tricyclics

An enhanced dicoumarol half-life is possible (Veseil *et al, NEJM* 1970, **283**, 1484), shown with amitriptyline and nortriptyline (Pond *et al, Clin Pharmacol Ther* 1975, **18**, 191).

Disopyramine + tricyclics

Increased anticholinergic effects may be seen (*Clin Pharmacol Ther* 1974, **15**, 551) and the BNF notes an increased risk of ventricular arrhythmias.

Disulfiram + tricyclics

Amitriptyline may enhance the effects of disulfiram (*Lancet* 1969, **i**, 313 + 735) and tricyclic levels may be increased by about 30% by enzyme inhibition (n=2, Ciraulo *et al, Am J Psych* 1985, **142**, 1373–74).

Fibre + tricyclics

There are several cases of a high fibre diet reducing tricyclic levels by up to a third (and hence to inactive levels), eg. with doxepin (*J Clin Psychopharmacol* 1992, **12**, 438). This might explain non-response in some patients.

Fluconazole + nortriptyline

A case of inhibition of CYP3A4 by fluconazole has resulted in elevated, toxic nortriptyline levels (Gannon, *Ann Pharmacother* 1992, **26**, 1456–57).

FLUOXETINE + TRICYCLICS

See fluoxetine (*4.3.2.2*).

FLUVOXAMINE + TRICYCLICS

See fluvoxamine (*4.3.2.3*).

Glyceryl trinitrate + tricyclics

See nitrates + tricyclics.

GUANETHIDINE + TRICYCLICS

The hypotensive effects of guanethidine and similar drugs are antagonised by tricyclics.

H2-blockers + tricyclics

CYP1A2 inhibition by cimetidine may decrease the metabolism and increase half-life and blood levels of tricyclics, eg. amitriptyline (by 37–80%, Curry *et al, Eur J Clin Pharmacol* 1985, **29**, 42–43), doxepin (by 30%, *J Clin Psychopharmacol* 1986, **6**, 8–12), imipramine (by over 100%, *Eur J Clin Pharmacol* 1986, **31**, 285–90) and nortriptyline (by 20%, *Clin Pharmacol Ther* 1984, **35**, 183–87). Other H2-blockers, eg.

ranitidine, do not appear to interact this way (Sutherland *et al, Eur J Clin Pharmacol* 1987, **32**, 159).

Hypoglycaemics + tricyclics

There are two isolated cases of enhanced hypoglycaemia with doxepin and nortriptyline (*Am J Psych* 1987, **144**, 1220–21) so monitor blood glucose regularly.

Levodopa + tricyclics

A small reduction in the effect of levodopa may be seen (*Neurology* 1975, **25**, 1029) but is of low clinical significance.

Levothyroxine + tricyclics

This is usually a synergistic interaction (see depression, *1.14*) but a few isolated cases of tachycardia and hypothyroidism have been reported.

Lithium + tricyclics

The combination is well used (see depression, *1.14*) but some adverse reactions have been reported, eg. myoclonus (Devan and *et al, J Clin Psychopharmacol* 1988, **8**, 446) and neurotoxicity with motor symptoms and seizures (eg. Austin *et al, J Clin Psych* 1990, **51**, 344).

MAOIs + TRICYCLICS

See MAOIs (*4.3.4*).

Methadone + tricyclics

A small study showed desipramine blood levels can double with methadone (n=5, Maany *et al, Am J Psych* 1989, **146**, 1611–13).

Methyldopa + desipramine

The hypotensive effect of methyldopa may be decreased, with possible tachycardia and CNS stimulation (Van Spanning *et al, Int J Clin Pharmacol Biopharm* 1975, **9**, 120).

Methylphenidate + tricyclics

Methylphenidate may inhibit the metabolism of tricyclics producing up to a four-fold increase in levels (eg. *J Dev Behav Pediatrics* 1986, **7**, 265–67).

Mirtazapine + tricyclics

See mirtazapine (*4.3.3.2*)

Moclobemide + tricyclics

See moclobemide (*4.3.3.3*).

Modafinil + tricyclics

See modafinil (*4.6.7*).

Morphine + tricyclics

Tricyclics such as amitriptyline and clomipramine increase the bio-

availability of morphine and potentiate the analgesic effect, a usually beneficial effect (*Lancet* 1987, **i**, 1204).

Nefazodone + tricyclics

See nefazodone (*4.3.3.4*).

Nitrates (sublingual) + tricyclics

Dry mouth may reduce the dissolution of sublingual nitrates.

Olanzapine + tricyclics

See olanzapine (*4.2.3*).

Oral Contraceptives/estrogens + tricyclics

Akathisia (n=3, Krishnan *et al, Am J Psych* 1984, **141**, 696–97), reduced tricyclic effectiveness and enhanced tricyclic toxicity (*JAMA* 1973, **222**, 702) have all been reported. Best to monitor the tricyclic closely.

PAROXETINE + TRICYCLICS

See paroxetine (*4.3.2.4*).

Phenindione + tricyclics

An enhanced risk of bleeding may occur with this combination.

Phenylbutazone + tricyclics

Tricyclic absorption may get delayed or reduced by phenylbutazone (*Eur J Pharmacol* 1970, **10**, 239).

PHENYTOIN + TRICYCLICS

See phenytoin (*4.5.8*).

Quetiapine + tricyclics

See quetiapine (*4.2.4*).

Quinine and quinidine + tricyclics

Studies have shown a much reduced clearance of nortriptyline with quinidine (*Br J Clin Pharmac* 1988, **25**, 140–41) and quinine (*Clin Pharmacol Ther* 1988, **43**, 577–81), via 2D6 inhibition. Best to monitor tricyclic levels.

Reboxetine + tricyclics

See reboxetine (*4.3.3.5*).

Sertraline + tricyclics

See sertraline (*4.3.2.5*).

Smoking + tricyclics

See smoking (*4.7.4*).

St. John's wort + tricyclics

See St. John's wort (*4.3.3.9*).

Sucralfate + amitriptyline

One small study showed a marked reduction in amitriptyline absorption (*Fed Proc* 1986, **45**, 205).

Tea or coffee + tricyclics

Studies have shown that some tricyclics (eg. amitriptyline and imipramine) precipitate out of solution to form a tannin complex with tea and coffee (*J Pharm Sci* 1984, **73**, 1056–58). The clinical significance is thought to be minimal (*Lancet* 1981, **i**, 1217–18).

TERFENADINE + TRICYCLICS

There is an increased risk of cardiovascular side-effects (such as syncope, prolonged QT interval and ventricular arrhythmias) with terfenadine and astemizole, and this should not be used with other potentially arrhythmogenic drugs such as tricyclics, a 1993 UK CSM warning. Cetirizine, loratadine and chlorphenamine are currently considered suitable.

Valproate + tricyclics

See valproate (*4.5.12*).

VASOCONSTRICTOR SYMPATHO-MIMETICS + TRICYCLICS

A greatly enhanced response, eg. hypertension and arrhythmias, to norepinephrine and phenylephrine in patients taking tricyclics has been shown in many reports. Doxepin and maprotiline may have a lesser effect. Local anaesthetics with adrenaline appear safe. Moderate doses of cold cures containing sympathomimetics should present little risk in healthy patients.

Warfarin + tricyclics *

Normally there is no problem but occasional control problems have been reported with lofepramine (mentioned in Sayal *et al, Acta Psych Scand* 2000, **102**, 250–55 and Duncan *et al, Int Clin Psychopharmacol* 1998, **13**, 87–94).

Yohimbine + tricyclics *

Tricyclics can potentiate the blood pressure changes caused by yohimbine, especially if blood pressure is already raised (mentioned in Fugh-Berman, *Lancet* 2000, **355**, 134–38).

Zopiclone + tricyclics

See zopiclone (*4.1.6*).

Zotepine + tricyclics

See zotepine (*4.2.6*).

4.3.2 SSRIs (Selective Serotonin Reuptake Inhibitors)

Drug interactions involving the P450 system have been described for all SSRIs but there are significant differences in the isoenzymes inhibited and the degree of

inhibition (review by van Harten, *Clin Pharmacokinet* 1993, **24**, 203–20).

The most well-known is CYP2D6. *In vitro* inhibition on a molar basis is: paroxetine (most potent), norfluoxetine, fluoxetine, sertraline, fluvoxamine, citalopram (least potent). *In vivo* is probably broadly similar. Fluoxetine and paroxetine are probably similar in 2D6 inhibition, but with some variation (RCT, n=31, using multiple-dose fluoxetine 60mg/d, fluvoxamine 100mg/d, paroxetine 20mg/d, or sertraline 100mg/d, Alfaro *et al, J Clin Psychopharmacol* 1999, **19**, 155–63). There are few other controlled trials; evidence is mainly from case studies and so firm conclusions on the relative merits of SSRIs for interactions with, eg. tricyclics are difficult to make.

Reviews: overview and review of SSRI interactions and P450 effects (Preskorn, *Clin Pharmacokinet* 1997, [Suppl 1], 1–21, 143 refs), clinically significant SSRI interactions (Mitchell, *Drug Safety* 1997, **17**, 390–406, 163 refs) and clinically significant SSRI-CNS interactions (Sproule *et al, Clin Pharmacokinet* 1997, **33**, 454–71, 106 refs).

4.3.2.1 CITALOPRAM

Citalopram is a weak inhibitor of CYP2D6 (Baettig *et al, Eur J Clin Pharmacol* 1993, **44**, 403–5) and metabolised by CYP3A4.

Alcohol + citalopram

See alcohol (*4.7.1*).

Alimemazine (trimeprazine) + citalopram

See antipsychotics + citalopram in this section.

Antipsychotics + citalopram

Levomepromazine and alimemazine may both increase plasma levels of citalopram by about a third (Milne & Goa, *Drugs* 1991, **41**, 450–77), possibly via enzyme inhibition and of minimal clinical significance. There has been no detectable effect from citalopram on the plasma levels of other antipsychotics (n=90, d/b, Syvalahti *et al, J Int Med Res* 1997, **25**, 24–32), eg. citalopram 40mg/d had no effect over 8 weeks on the plasma levels of clozapine (n=8, 200–400mg/d), risperidone (n=7, 4–6mg/d) and their active metabolites in patients with chronic schizophrenia (Avenoso *et* *al, Clin Drug Investigation* 1998, **16**, 393–98).

Benzodiazepines + citalopram *

No pharmacokinetic interaction could be demonstrated between citalopram and the CYP3A4 substrate triazolam (n=18, open, Nolting and Abramowitz, *Pharmacother* 2000, **20**, 750–55).

Buspirone + citalopram

Hyponatraemia and serotonin syndrome has been reported with the combination (Spigset and Adielsson, *Int Clin Psychopharmacol* 1997, **12**, 61–63).

Charcoal, activated + citalopram

25g activated charcoal given 30 minutes after citalopram reduced citalopram AUC by 51%, and peak levels by over 50%. Concurrent gastric lavage did not provide any additional reductions (n=9, RCT, Lapatto-Reiniluoto *et al, Br J Clin Pharmacol* 1999, **48**, 148–53).

Donepezil + citalopram

See SSRIs + donepezil (*4.6.3.1*).

Lithium + citalopram

See lithium (*4.4*).

MAOIs + citalopram

See MAOIs (*4.3.4*).

Oxcarbazepine + citalopram *

See oxcarbazepine (*4.5.6*).

Selegiline + citalopram

A study showed the lack of a clinically significant interaction (n=18, RCT, Laine *et al, Clin Neuropharmacol* 1997, **20**, 419–33).

St. John's wort + citalopram

See SSRIs + St. John's wort (*4.3.3.9*).

Sumatriptan + citalopram

The BNF notes an increased risk of CNS toxicity and recommends avoiding the combination. See also sumatriptan + fluoxetine (*4.3.2.2*).

Sympathomimetics + citalopram

Augmentation of amfetamines is theoretically possible (see also sympathomimetics + fluoxetine).

Tricyclics + citalopram *

Citalopram had no effect on amitriptyline levels (n=3), clomipramine (n=1) and maprotiline (n=1) (Baettig *et al, Eur J Clin Pharmacol* 1993, **44**, 403–5). One small study indicated that citalopram raised desipramine, but not imipramine, levels when added to imipramine (Gram *et al, Ther Drug Monit* 1993, **15**, 18–24)

and lack of interaction between desipramine and citalopram (but not when paroxetine was used) has been reported (n=1, Ashton, *J Clin Psych* 2000, **61**, 144).

Warfarin + citalopram *

Citalopram 40mg/d may produce a small increase in prothrombin time (n=12, Preskorn *et al, Br J Clin Pharmacol* 1997, **44**, 199), but this is probably clinically insignificant (Sayal *et al, Acta Psych Scand* 2000, **102**, 250–55).

Zolpidem + citalopram

See SSRIs + zolpidem (*4.1.5*).

4.3.2.2 FLUOXETINE

Fluoxetine substantially inhibits CYP2D6 and probably CYP2C9/10, moderately inhibits CYP2C19 and weakly inhibits CYP3A3/4. Norfluoxetine is a potent CYP3A4 inhibitor and appears a moderately potent inhibitor of CYP2D6. Fluoxetine may have a higher incidence of interactions with drugs metabolised by these enzymes.

Review: Preskorn, *Int Clin Psychopharmacol* 1994, **9**(Suppl 3), 13–19.

Alcohol + fluoxetine

See alcohol (*4.7.1*).

Amfetamines + fluoxetine

See sympathomimetics + fluoxetine.

ANTIPSYCHOTICS + FLUOXETINE

See antipsychotics (*4.2.1*) and olanzapine (*4.2.3*).

Beta-blockers + fluoxetine

Bradycardia may occur in people taking fluoxetine and metoprolol, possibly due to 2D6 inhibition. Atenolol or sotalol may be suitable alternatives to metoprolol (n=2, Proudlove, *Lancet* 1993, **341**, 967).

Benzodiazepines + fluoxetine

Fluoxetine may slightly increase the plasma levels of some benzodiazepines (eg. diazepam in Lemberger *et al, Clin Pharmacol Ther* 1988, **43**, 412). Desmethyldiazepam levels may be lower, which may explain the lack of additive psychomotor impairment (Ciraulo and Shader, *J Clin Psychopharmacol* 1990, **10**, 213–17). Increased alprazolam levels with fluoxetine are due to decreased clearance (Greenblatt *et al, Clin Pharmacol Ther* 1992, **52**, 479–86) but this does not seem to occur with clonazepam. The clinical significance is minor.

Bupropion + fluoxetine *

See bupropion (*4.6.4*).

Buspirone + fluoxetine

See buspirone (*4.1.2*).

Calcium-channel blockers + fluoxetine

Oedema, weight gain and headache have occurred with verapamil and fluoxetine (n=2, *J Clin Psychopharmacol* 1991, **11**, 390). Lowering doses is recommended if an interaction is suspected.

Cannabis + fluoxetine

See cannabis (*4.7.2*).

Carbamazepine + fluoxetine

Two studies have shown that fluoxetine and its metabolite inhibit carbamazepine metabolism, increasing levels by up to 25% (n=14, Gidal *et al, Ther Drug Monit* 1993, **15**, 405–9). One small study, however, showed fluoxetine 20mg/d to have no effect on carbamazepine levels (n=8, open, Spina *et al, Ther Drug Monit* 1993, **15**, 247–50). A toxic serotonin syndrome has also been reported (n=1, Dursun *et al, Lancet* 1993, **342**, 442–43).

Clarithromycin + fluoxetine

Acute delirium has been reported when clarithromycin was added to fluoxetine (eg. n=1, Tracy and Johns Cupp, *Ann Pharmacother* 1996, **30**, 1199–200), probably via CYP3A4 inhibition.

CLOZAPINE + FLUOXETINE

See clozapine (*4.2.2*).

Cocaine + fluoxetine

See antidepressants + cocaine (*4.7.3*).

Cyclosporin + fluoxetine

Cyclosporin plasma concentrations were nearly doubled by fluoxetine 20mg/d in one case, probably by CYP3A4 inhibition (Holton and Bonser, *BMJ* 1995, **311**, 422).

Cyproheptadine + fluoxetine

Three patients treated with cyproheptadine for fluoxetine-induced anorgasmia relapsed (*J Clin Psych* 1991, **52**, 163–64). There is a case report of interaction in a bulimic patient (*J Clin Psych* 1991, **52**, 261–62).

Dextromethorphan + fluoxetine

Visual hallucinations lasting 6–8hrs occurred in one patient taking fluoxetine 20mg/d who also took a cough mixture containing dextromethorphan (Achamallah, *Am J Psych* 1992, **149**, 1406).

Donepezil + fluoxetine

See SSRIs + donepezil (*4.6.3.1*).

Lithium + fluoxetine *

See lithium (*4.4*).

LSD + fluoxetine

GTC convulsions occurred in one patient who took a double dose of LSD while on fluoxetine 20mg/d, having previously taken single doses of LSD uneventfully (*Am J Psych* 1992, **149**, 843–44).

Mirtazapine + fluoxetine

See fluoxetine (*4.3.3.2*).

Moclobemide + fluoxetine

See SSRIs + moclobemide (*4.3.3.3*).

MAOIs + FLUOXETINE

See MAOIs (*4.3.4*).

Nefazodone + fluoxetine *

Fluoxetine may increase the plasma levels of nefazodone (BNF), and a serotonin syndrome has been reported (n=1, Smith and Wenegrat, *J Clin Psych* 2000, **61**, 146).

Olanzapine + fluoxetine

See fluoxetine (*4.2.3*).

Pentazocine + fluoxetine

Rapid toxicity has been reported, although an interaction was not proven (n=1, *Am J Psych* 1990, **147**, 949–50).

PHENYTOIN + FLUOXETINE *

See phenytoin (*4.5.8*).

Quetiapine + fluoxetine

See SSRIs + quetiapine (*4.2.4*).

Reboxetine + fluoxetine *

See reboxetine (*4.3.3.5*).

Rivastigmine + fluoxetine

See rivastigmine (*4.6.3.3*).

Selegiline + fluoxetine

Three cases exist of toxic reactions, eg. hypomania, hypertension and shivering (*Can J Neurol Sci* 1990, **17**, 352), ataxia in a complex regimen (*Ann Pharmacother* 1992, **26**, 1300) and hypertension (Montastruc *et al, Lancet* 1993, **341**, 555). Discontinue one or both drugs if an adverse reaction occurs.

Sertraline + fluoxetine
See sertraline (*4.3.2.5*).

St. John's wort + fluoxetine
See SSRIs + St. John's wort (*4.3.3.9*).

Sumatriptan + fluoxetine
Lack of significant interaction has been reported (n=14, Blier and Bergeron, *J Clin Psychopharmacol* 1995, **15**, 106–9) although post-marketing surveillance in Canada indicated that a serotonin-like syndrome may occur rarely with the combination (n=22, Joffe and Sokolov, *Acta Psych Scand* 1997, **95**, 551–52). The BNF notes an increased risk of CNS toxicity and recommends avoiding the combination.

Sympathomimetics + fluoxetine
An interaction has been suggested by reports of extreme restlessness, agitation and psychotic symptoms, apparently caused by fluoxetine-augmentation of amfetamines (n=2, Barrett *et al, B J Psych* 1996, **168**, 253). Amfetamine is partly metabolised by CYP2D6, so this interaction probably occurred via inhibition of CYP2D6 (Blue, *B J Psych* 1996, **168**, 653).

Terfenadine + fluoxetine
There are reports of cardiac toxicity with fluoxetine and terfenadine (eg. Swims, *Ann Pharmacother* 1993, **27**, 1404–5), probably by inhibition of CYP3A4 metabolism of terfenadine, resulting in enhanced terfenadine cardiac toxicity, eg. prolonged QT interval. However, one study showed that fluoxetine 60mg/d did not inhibit the (3A4) metabolism of terfenadine and is thus unlikely to affect the (adverse) effects of terfenadine (n=12, Bergstrom *et al, Clin Pharmacol Ther* 1997, **62**, 643–51).

Tolterodine + fluoxetine *
Fluoxetine has been shown to inhibit the metabolism of tolterodine (Brynne *et al, B J Clin Pharmacology* 1999, **48**, 553–63).

Tramadol + fluoxetine *
Serotonin syndrome has been reported with fluoxetine and tramadol (n=1, Kesavan and Sobala, *J Roy Soc Med* 1999, **92**, 474–75).

Trazodone + fluoxetine
Trazodone toxicity may occur with the combination (eg. Neirenberg *et al, J Clin Psych* 1992, **53**, 83).

TRICYCLICS + FLUOXETINE *
Tricyclic levels may double or triple (Bergstrom *et al, Clin Pharmacol Ther* 1992, **51**, 239–48) when fluoxetine is added to:

Amitriptyline (n=1, Muller *et al, Drug Ther Monit* 1991, **13**, 533–36; fatality reported by Preskorn and Baker, *JAMA* 1997, **277**, 1682; study by Vandel *et al, Pharmacol Res* 1995, **31**, 347–53).

Clomipramine – a significant rise in tricyclic levels may occur (n=4, Vandel *et al, Neuropsychobiology* 1992, **25**, 202–7), and severe toxicity (n=1, Balant-Gorgia *et al, Pharmacopsychiatry* 1996, **29**, 38–41) and serotonin syndrome presenting with migraine-like stroke has occurred (n=1, Molaie, *Adv Drug React & Tox Rev* 1997, **16**, 257–58).

Desipramine – fluoxetine 20mg/d was shown to increase desipramine 50mg/d peak plasma levels by 100% and AUC by 480%, with elevated levels persisting for up to three weeks after the fluoxetine was stopped (n=18, RCT, Preskorn *et al, J Clin Psychopharmacol* 1994, **14**, 90–98).

Imipramine (Leroj and Walenty-nowicz, *Can J Psychiatry* 1996, **41**, 318–19; *DICP Ann Pharmacother* 1991, **25**, 1273–74).

Nortriptyline (eg. Aranow *et al, Am J Psych* 1989, **146**, 911–13).

Potentiation may occur even if the tricyclic is used after an interval (*Am J Psych* 1991, **148**, 1601–2). The mechanism is CYP2D6 inhibition (Bergstrom *et al, Clin Pharmacol Ther* 1992, **51**, 239–48). It has been suggested that tricyclic dosage should be reduced by 75% when fluoxetine is added (Westermeyer, *J Clin Pharmacol* 1991, **31**, 388–92). The combination can be also used with care (see *1.14*).

Tryptophan + fluoxetine
Central toxicity has been reported (n=5, Steiner and Fontaine, *Biol Psych* 1986, **21**, 1067–71).

Valproate + fluoxetine *
Valproate levels may rise by up to 50% if fluoxetine is added, although the mechanism is not established (eg. Lucena *et al, Am J Psych* 1998, **155**, 575) and reduced valproate levels have been reported (Droulers *et al, J Clin Psychopharmacol* 1997, **17**, 139–40).

Venlafaxine + fluoxetine

Serotonin syndrome has been reported when venlafaxine was started immediately after fluoxetine was discontinued (n=1, Bhatara *et al, Ann Pharmacother* 1998, **32**, 432–36) and severe anticholinergic side-effects may occur during combined fluoxetine 20mg/d and venlafaxine 37.5mg/d (n=4, Benazzi, *J Clin Psychopharmacol* 1999, **19**, 96–98, letter).

WARFARIN + FLUOXETINE *

An *in vitro* study indicated fluoxetine has a potentially potent effect on warfarin (Schmider *et al, B J Clin Pharmacol* 1997, **44**, 495–98). Raised INR has been reported, within ten days of starting fluoxetine (n=2, *BMJ* 1993, **307**, 241) and in patients on warfarin with stable INRs who experienced dramatic increases in INR when fluoxetine 20mg/d was added (n=2, Hanger and Thomas, *NZ Med J* 1995, **108**, 157). There is also a case report of an elderly man prescribed warfarin, diazepam and fluoxetine who developed an elevated INR and died from a cerebral haemorrhage (Dent and Orrock, *Pharmacotherapy* 1997, **17**, 170–72).

Zolpidem + fluoxetine

See SSRIs + zolpidem (*4.1.5*).

Zotepine + fluoxetine

See SSRIs + zotepine (*4.2.6*).

4.3.2.3 FLUVOXAMINE

Fluvoxamine strongly inhibits CYP1A2, CYP2D6, CYP3A and CYP2C19 activity and may have a high incidence of interactions with drugs metabolised by these enzymes, which may have serious implications for a variety of drugs (n=20, *Clin Pharmacol Ther* 1998, **64**, 257–68).

Alcohol + fluvoxamine

See alcohol (*4.7.1*).

Antipsychotics + fluvoxamine *

Seizures have been reported with levomepromazine (methotrimeprazine) and fluvoxamine (Grinshpoon *et al, Int Clin Psychopharmacol* 1993, **8**, 61–62). Thioridazine is now contraindicated with fluvoxamine due to QTc prolongation. See also clozapine.

Astemizole + fluvoxamine

This is a possible contraindication because of the risk of fatal ventricular arrhythmias via inhibition of CYP3A4.

Benzodiazepines + fluvoxamine

Plasma concentrations of bromazepam are doubled by fluvoxamine, but lorazepam is unaffected (van Harten *et al*, mentioned in *Clin Pharmacokinet* 1993, **24**, 203–20). A study showed that fluvoxamine 100mg/d increased alprazolam plasma levels by 100% and so reduced doses of alprazolam should be used (n=60, Fleishaker and Hulst, *E J Clin Pharmacol* 1994, **46**, 35–39).

Beta-blockers + fluvoxamine

Lack of significant interaction has been shown with atenolol (Benfield and Ward, *Drugs* 1986, **32**, 481–508). Propranolol plasma levels can be raised by fluvoxamine by up to 500% but without major clinical effect (reviewed by Benfield and Ward, *Drugs* 1988, **32**, 313–34).

Buspirone + fluvoxamine

See buspirone (*4.1.2*).

Caffeine + fluvoxamine

Fluvoxamine inhibits caffeine metabolism and half life may rise from 5hrs to 22hrs (Slaughter and Edwards, *Ann Pharmacother* 1995, **29**, 619–24), so an enhanced effect is possible, although one study indicated that the effect was likely to be minimal (n=10, Spigset, *Eur J Clin Pharmacol* 1998, **54**, 665–66).

Carbamazepine + fluvoxamine

One small study showed no effect on carbamazepine levels from fluvoxamine 100mg/d (Spina *et al, Ther Drug Monit* 1993, **15**, 247–50) although several cases exist of fluvoxamine increasing carbamazepine levels and toxicity (eg. Martinelli *et al, B J Clin Pharmacol* 1993, **36**, 615–16).

Chloral + fluvoxamine

Lack of interaction has been reported (Wagner *et al, Adv Pharmacother* 1986, **2**, 34–56).

CLOZAPINE + FLUVOXAMINE

See clozapine (*4.2.2*).

Cyclosporine + fluvoxamine

There is a case report of cyclosporine levels elevated by the introduction of fluvoxamine to a cyclosporine-treated allograft recipient, probably via CYP3A4 inhibition. Intensive monitoring of the serum creatinine and cyclosporine level was indicated, along with appropriate dose reductions (Vella and Sayegh, *Am J Kidney Dis* 1998, **31**, 320–23).

Digoxin + fluvoxamine

Lack of interaction has been reported (d/b, Ochs *et al, J Clin Pharmacol* 1989, **29**, 91–95).

Donepezil + fluvoxamine

See SSRIs + donepezil (*4.6.3.1*).

Lithium + fluvoxamine

Although lack of interaction has been reported (Hendrickx and Floris, *Curr Ther Res* 1991, **49**, 106–10), serotonin syndrome (n=1, Ohman and Spigset, *Pharmacopsychiatry* 1993, **26**, 263–64) and irresistible somnolence have been reported (n=1, Evans and Marwick, *B J Psych* 1990, **156**, 286).

MAOIs + FLUVOXAMINE

See MAOIs (*4.3.4*).

Melatonin + fluvoxamine *

Fluvoxamine 50mg inhibits the metabolism of oral melatonin 5mg, increasing plasma levels (n=5, Hartter *et al, Clin Pharmacol & Therap* 2000, **67**, 1–6), supported by a further case, where combining the treatments improved sleep (n=1, Grozinger *et al, Arch Gen Psych* 2000, **57**, 812–13).

Methadone + fluvoxamine *

Fluvoxamine has been reported to increase methadone levels (n=1, DeMaria and Serota, *J Addict Dis* 1999, **18**, 5–12).

Metoclopramide + fluvoxamine

Acute dystonia has been associated with the combination (Palop *et al, Ann Pharmacother* 1999, **33**, 382, letter).

Moclobemide + fluovoxamine

See SSRIs + moclobemide (*4.3.3.3*).

NICOUMALONE + FLUVOXAMINE

The anticoagulant effects may be enhanced by fluvoxamine.

Pipamperone + fluvoxamine *

Electrocardiographic alterations as a result of acute overdose with fluvoxamine and pipamperone (Gallerani *et al, Clin Drug Investigat* 1998, **15**, 64–68).

Quinidine + fluvoxamine *

Fluvoxamine significantly inhibits the clearance of quinidine, probably by 3A4 inhibition (n=6, open, Damkier *et al, Eur J Clin Pharmacol* 1999, **55**, 451–56).

Reboxetine + fluvoxamine

See reboxetine (*4.3.3.5*).

St. John's wort + fluvoxamine

See SSRIs + St. John's wort (*4.3.3.9*).

Sumatriptan + fluvoxamine

The BNF notes an increased risk of CNS toxicity and recommends avoiding the combination. See also fluoxetine (*4.3.2.2*).

Sympathomimetics + fluvoxamine

Augmentation of amfetamines is theoretically possible (see also fluoxetine, *4.3.2.2*).

Tacrine + fluvoxamine *

Fluvoxamine is a potent inhibitor of tacrine metabolism *in vivo* (Teilmann Larsen *et al, Eur J Clin Pharmacol* 1999, **55**, 375–82).

TERFENADINE + FLUVOXAMINE

This is a contraindication because of the risk of fatal ventricular arrhythmias via inhibition of CYP3A4.

THEOPHYLLINE + FLUVOXAMINE

Several cases of theophylline toxicity have been reported (eg. *Pharm J* 1992, **249**, 137; Devane *et al, Am J Psych* 1997, **154**, 1317–18), probably via CYP1A2 inhibition. The UK CSM recommends avoiding the combination (*Curr Prob* 1994, **20**, 12).

TRICYCLICS + FLUVOXAMINE

Fluvoxamine has been shown to increase amitriptyline, clomipramine (Bertschy *et al, Eur J Clin Pharmacol* 1991, **40**, 119–20) and imipramine levels (*Am J Psych* 1993, **150**, 1566), but not with desipramine (Spina *et al Ther Drug Monit* 1993, **15**, 243–46). Fluvoxamine may inhibit both hydroxylation and N-demethylation, indicating a dual effect on tricyclic metabolism (Hartter *et al, Psychopharmacology* 1993, **110**, 301–8).

Tryptophan + fluvoxamine

Central toxicity has been suggested with fluvoxamine (n=5, Steiner and Fontaine, *Biol Psych* 1986, **21**, 1067–71).

Valproate + fluvoxamine

Augmentation of fluvoxamine has been seen with valproate (Corrigan, *Biol Psych* 1992, **31**, 1178–79).

WARFARIN + FLUVOXAMINE *

An *in vitro* study indicated fluvoxamine has the most potent effect on warfarin of the SSRIs (Schmider *et al, B J Clin Pharmacol* 1997, **44**, 495–98). Fluvoxamine can increase warfarin levels by up to 65%, increasing prothrombin time (*Drugs* 1986, **32,** 313–14), and elevated INR has occurred up to two weeks after fluvoxamine was stopped, a prolonged effect (n=1, Yap and Low, *Singapore Med J* 1999, **40**, 480–82).

Zolpidem + fluvoxamine

See zolpidem (*4.1.5*).

Zotepine + fluvoxamine

See zotepine (*4.2.6*).

4.3.2.4 PAROXETINE

Paroxetine is probably the most potent SSRI inhibitor of CYP2D6 but does not appear to inhibit any other CYP enzyme. It may thus have a higher incidence of interactions with drugs metabolised by this enzyme. The main metabolite has approximately one third the CYP2D6 inhibition potency of paroxetine.

Alcohol + paroxetine

See alcohol (*4.7.1*).

Amylobarbital + paroxetine

No interaction occurs (Cooper *et al, Acta Psych Scand* 1989, **80**[Suppl 350], 53–55).

Anticholinergics + paroxetine

See SSRIs + anticholinergics (*4.6.2*).

Antipsychotics + paroxetine

Lack of interaction between haloperidol and paroxetine has been shown (Cooper *et al, Acta Psych Scand* 1989, **80**[Suppl 350], 53–55). Paroxetine (3-day course) had no detectable effect on thiothixene (a thioxanthene) pharmacokinetics in a small study (n=10, Guthrie *et al, J Clin Pharm Ther* 1997, **22**, 221–16).

Benzodiazepines + paroxetine

Lack of interaction has been shown (Boyer and Blumhardt, *J Clin Psych* 1992, **53**[Suppl 2], 132–24), eg. with oxazepam (Cooper *et al, Acta Psych Scand* 1989, **80**[Suppl 350], 53–55). A case of serotonin syndrome has been reported in a person taking maintenance paroxetine after a single dose clonazepam (Rella and Hoffman, *J Toxicol Clin Toxicol* 1998, **36**, 257–58).

Beta-blockers + paroxetine *

Paroxetine 20mg/d increases the effects of metoprolol 100mg stat, leading to accumulation of S-metoprolol, and so reduced metoprolol levels might be needed (n=8, open, Hemeryck *et al, Clin Pharmacol & Therapeut* 2000, **67**, 283–91).

Carbamazepine + paroxetine

No significant interaction has been found (Mikkelsen *et al, Psychopharmacol* 1991, **103**, B13, Andersen *et al, Epilepsy Res* 1991, **10**, 201–4).

Cimetidine + paroxetine

Cimetidine may inhibit the first-pass metabolism of paroxetine, increasing bioavailability by up to 50% (Bannister *et al, Acta Psych Scand* 1989, **80**[Suppl 350], 102–6) so use ranitidine instead.

CLOZAPINE + PAROXETINE

See clozapine (*4.2.2*).

Dextromethorphan + paroxetine

Paroxetine would be expected to increase dextromethorphan levels by CYP2D6 inhibition (see reported case with fluoxetine, *4.3.2.2*).

Digoxin + paroxetine

Lack of interaction has been shown (Boyer & Blumhardt, *J Clin Psych* 1992, **53**[Suppl 2], 132–34).

Donepezil + paroxetine

See SSRIs + donepezil (*4.6.3.1*).

Galantamine + paroxetine *

See galantamine (*4.6.3.2*).

Interferon alpha + paroxetine *

Previous good response to paroxetine and trazodone was reversed in one woman by interferon alpha, which has anti-serotonergic actions (n=1, McAllister-Williams *et al, B J Psych* 2000, **176**, 93).

Lithium + paroxetine

See SSRIs + lithium (*4.4*).

Mirtazapine + paroxetine

See mirtazapine (*4.3.3.2*).

Moclobemide + paroxetine

See moclobemide + SSRIs (*4.3.3.3*).

MAOIs + PAROXETINE

See MAOIs (*4.3.4*).

Oral contraceptives + paroxetine

Lack of interaction has been shown (Boyer and Blumhardt, *J Clin Psych* 1992, **53**[Suppl 2], 132–34).

Phenytoin + paroxetine

Paroxetine bioavailability may be decreased slightly (Andersen *et al, Epilepsy Res* 1991, **10**, 201–4).

Phenobarbital + paroxetine

Paroxetine bioavailability may be decreased slightly, resulting in a 25% decrease in plasma concentrations (Bannister *et al, Acta Psych Scand* 1989, **80**[Suppl 350], 102–6).

Pindolol + paroxetine

Raised paroxetine levels after the addition of pindolol has been reported, probably via 2D6 inhibition (n=1, Olver and Burrows, *Int J Psych Clin Pract* 1998, **2**, 225–27).

St. John's wort + paroxetine

See SSRIs + St. John's wort (*4.3.3.9*).

Sumatriptan + paroxetine

The BNF notes an increased risk of CNS toxicity and recommends avoiding the combination. See fluoxetine (*4.3.2.2*).

Sympathomimetics + paroxetine

Augmentation of amfetamines is theoretically possible (see sympathomimetics + fluoxetine *4.3.2.2*).

TRICYCLICS + PAROXETINE

CYP2D6 inhibition reduces the metabolism of amitriptyline, imipramine (eg. Skjelbo & Brosen, *B J Clin Pharmacol* 1992, **34**, 256–61) and desipramine (Brosen *et al, Eur J Clin Pharmacol* 1993, **44**, 349–55), resulting in enhanced tricyclic toxicity. Plasma concentrations of tricyclics will be significantly increased by paroxetine, so great care is needed.

Valproate + paroxetine

No significant interaction occurs (Mikkelsen *et al, Psychopharmacol* 1991, **103**, B13, Andersen *et al, Epilepsy Res* 1991, **10**, 201–4).

Warfarin + paroxetine *

An *in vitro* study indicated that all SSRIs have an effect on warfarin (Schmider *et al, B J Clin Pharmacol* 1997, **44**, 495–98), and there are case reports, eg. an up to a 3 point rise in INR has been reported in several patients (mentioned by Askinazi, *Am J Psych* 1996, **153**, 135–36).

Zolpidem + paroxetine

See SSRIs + zolpidem (*4.1.5*).

Zotepine + paroxetine

See SSRIs + zotepine (*4.2.6*).

4.3.2.5 SERTRALINE

Sertraline produces a dose-related inhibition of CYP2D6 but has little, if any, effect on CYP1A2, CYP2C9/10, CYP2C19 or CYP3A3/4. It appears less potent in inhibiting CYP2D6 than most other SSRIs (Baettig *et al, Eur J Clin Pharmacol* 1993, **44**, 403–5) and has, at 50–100mg/d, a low incidence of interactions with drugs metabolised by 2D6.

Alcohol + sertraline

See alcohol (*4.7.1*).

Anticholinergics + sertraline

See SSRIs + anticholinergics (*4.6.2*).

Atenolol + sertraline *

No pharmacodynamic interaction has been found (Warrington, *Int Clin Psychopharmacol* 1991, **6**[Suppl 2], 11–21; RCT, n=10, Ziegler and Wilner, *J Clin Psych* 1996, **57**[Suppl 1], 12–15).

Benzodiazepines + sertraline

A study in male volunteers showed no sertraline effect on diazepam and suggests no effect on the CYP2C and CYP3A4 enzymes (RCT, Gardner *et al, Clin Pharmacokinetics* 1997 [Suppl 1], 43–49), but a slight decrease in plasma levels by 13% may occur (Warrington, *Int Clin Psychopharmacol* 1991, **6**[Suppl 2], 11–21).

Carbamazepine + sertraline *

Lack of significant significant interaction has been reported, but there are cases where sertraline 100mg/d increased carbamazepine (600mg/d) plasma levels, probably via 3A4 inhibition (d/b, p/c, Job, *N Z Med J* 1994, **107**, 43; Lane, *N Z Med J* 1994, **107**, 209), and where non-response to sertraline was due to low plasma levels associated with carbamazepine use, possibly via CYP3A4 induction (n=2, Khan *et al, J Clin Psych* 2000, **61**, 526–27).

Clozapine + sertraline

See clozapine (*4.2.2*).

Digoxin + sertraline

No interaction has been noted (Forster *et al, Biol Psych* 1991, **29**, 355S).

Donepezil + sertraline

See SSRIs + donepezil (*4.6.3.1*).

Erythromycin + sertraline *

There is a case of serotonin syndrome in a child associated with erythromycin and sertraline, possibly via CYP3A4 inhibition (Lee and Lee, *Pharmacother* 1999, **19**, 894–96).

Fluoxetine + sertraline

A possible serotonin syndrome has been reported (see switching antidepressants in *2.2.5*).

Lamotrigine + sertraline

See lamotrigine (*4.5.4*).

Lithium + sertraline

See lithium (*4.4*).

Mirtazapine + sertraline

See SSRIs + mirtazapine (*4.3.3.2*).

Moclobemide + sertraline

See SSRIs + moclobemide (*4.3.3.3*).

MAOIs + SERTRALINE

See MAOIs (*4.3.4*).

Phenytoin + sertraline

Lack of significant interaction has been shown (n=30, RCT, Rapeport *et al, J Clin Psych* 1996, **57**[Suppl 1], 24–28), but dramatically raised phenytoin levels have been reported after the addition of sertraline (n=2, Haselberger *et al, J Clin Psychopharmacol* 1997, **17**, 107–9), so monitoring levels would seem sensible.

St. John's wort + sertraline

See SSRIs + St. John's wort (*4.3.3.9*).

Sumatriptan + sertraline

The BNF notes an increased risk of CNS toxicity and recommends avoiding the combination. See also fluoxetine (*4.3.2.2*).

Sympathomimetics + sertraline

Augmentation of amfetamines is theoretically possible (see sympathomimetics + fluoxetine, *4.3.2.2*).

Terfenadine + sertraline

Current data suggests there is no interaction (*Curr Prob Pharmacovigilance* 1998, **24**, 4).

Tolbutamide + sertraline

In a parallel-group study, 200mg/d sertraline produced a 16% decrease in tolbutamide clearance, possibly via inhibition of CYP2C9 (n=25, RCT, Tremaine *et al, Clin Pharmacokinet* 1997, [Suppl 1], 31–36). A slight decrease in plasma levels by 16% has been reported (n=25, RCT, Warrington, *Int Clin Psychopharmacol* 1991, **6**[Suppl 2], 11–21).

Tramadol + sertraline

Serotonin syndrome has been reported when a tramadol dose was increased with concomitant sertraline (n=1, Mason and Blackburn, *Ann Pharmacother* 1997, **31**, 175–77).

Tricyclics + sertraline

Sertraline probably has a dose-dependent effect on tricyclics, eg. 50mg/d added to desipramine 250mg/d produced only a 60% increase in desipramine levels (letter in *Am J Psych* 1993, **150**, 1125–26) and 50mg/d increased desipramine 50mg/d peak plasma levels by 31% and AUC by 23% (cf. 400% and 480% for fluoxetine 20mg/d, trial by Preskorn *et al, J Clin Psychopharmacol* 1994, **14**, 90–98). However, sertraline 150mg/d increased desipramine levels by 70%, with a 200–300% increase in 4 patients (Zussman *et al, Br J Clin Pharmacol* 1995, **39**, S530–S551; see also n=12, open, Kurtz *et al, Clin Pharmacol Ther* 1997, **62**, 145–56). The mechanism is probably by CYP2D6 inhibition, and lower doses of tricyclics may need to be used. Serotonin syndrome has been reported with sertraline-amitriptyline (letters from Alderman *et al, Ann Pharmacother* 1996, **30**, 1499–500).

Venlafaxine + sertraline

Acute liver damage possibly related to sertraline and venlafaxine ingestion has been reported (Kim *et al, Ann Pharmacother* 1999, **33**, 381–82, letter).

Warfarin + sertraline *

An *in vitro* study indicated that, of the SSRIs, sertraline had the least potent effect on warfarin (Schmider *et al, B J Clin Pharmacol* 1997, **44**, 495–98). It may produce only a modest increase in prothrombin time, considered clinically insignificant by the authors (n=12, RCT, 22/7, Apseloff *et al, Clin Pharmacokinet* 1997, [Suppl 1], 37–42). However, prothrombin time can be increased by 9% (Wilner *et al, Biol Psych* 1991, **29**, 354S–355S) and up to a 3 point rise in INR has been reported in several patients (mentioned by Askinazi, *Am J Psych* 1996, **153**, 135–36).

Zolpidem + sertraline

See SSRIs + zolpidem (*4.1.5*).

Zotepine + sertraline

See zotepine (*4.2.6*).

4.3.3 OTHER ANTIDEPRESSANTS

4.3.3.1 MIANSERIN
ALCOHOL + MIANSERIN
See alcohol (*4.7.1*).

Benzodiazepines + mianserin
Enhanced sedation may occur.

Carbamazepine + mianserin*
Plasma levels of mianserin and enantiomers may be halved by carbamazepine, probably via 3A4 induction (n=12, Eap *et al, Ther Drug Monit* 1999, **21**, 166–70).

Warfarin + mianserin *
There is normally no problem but occasional control problems have been experienced with mianserin (Warwick and Mindham, *B J Psych* 1983, **143**, 308).

4.3.3.2 MIRTAZAPINE
Mirtazapine does not inhibit CYP2D6, CYP1A2 and CYP3A and so interactions via these enzymes are unlikely. Mirtazapine appears mainly metabolised by CYP2D6 and CYP1A2 (Montgomery, *Int Clin Psychopharmacol* 1995, **10**[Suppl 4], 37–45) and if one enzyme is inhibited, the other takes over, so mirtazapine appears less susceptible to P450 interactions. It has linear kinetics from 15–75mg/d, with 100% excreted via the urine and faeces
Review*: Clinical pharmacokinetics (Timmer *et al, Clin Pharmacokinet* 2000, **38**, 461–74).

Alcohol + mirtazapine *
See alcohol (*4.7.1*).

Benzodiazepines + mirtazapine
The combination of diazepam and mirtazapine, not surprisingly, produced an additive sedative effect (Mattila *et al, Pharmacol Toxicol* 1989, **65**, 81–88) and so anyone on the combination should be warned about driving etc.

Carbamazepine + mirtazapine *
Carbamazepine produces a 60% decrease in mirtazapine plasma levels, probably by CYP3A4 induction, and so raised mirtazapine doses might be needed (Ebes *et al*, Organon data on file).

Cimetidine + mirtazapine *
Mirtazapine had no effect on cimetidine but mirtazapine levels were higher (probably by CYP3A4 inhibition by cimetidine), but not enough to require dose reduction (n=12, d/b, p/c. c/o, Sitsen *et al, Eur J Clin Pharmacol* 2000, **56**, 389–94).

Fluoxetine + mirtazapine *
Fluoxetine 20–40mg/d caused a clinically insignificant 32% increase in mirtazapine (15mg/d) plasma levels after an abrupt switch (n=40, Preskorn *et al, Biol Psych* 1997, **41**, 96S).

Lithium + mirtazapine *
There was no pharmacokinetic interaction detected between lithium 600mg/d and mirtazapine 30mg (n=12, 10/7, Sitsen *et al, J Clin Psychopharmacol* 2000, **14**, 172–76).

MAOIs + mirtazapine
The manufacturers cautiously recommend a two-week gap between stopping an MAOI and starting mirtazapine.

Paroxetine + mirtazapine *
Paroxetine 40mg/d caused a clinically insignificant 17% increase in mirtazapine (30mg/d) plasma levels (n=24, Van Lookeren-Campagne *et al*, Organon data on file, mentioned in Timmer *et al, Clin Pharmacokinet* 2000, **38**, 461–74).

Risperidone + mirtazapine *
Mirtazapine 30mg/d had no effect on risperidone 2–6mg/d kinetics in a short trial (n=6, open, Loonen *et al, Eur Neuropsychopharmacol* 1999, **10**, 51–57).

Sertraline + mirtazapine
Hypomania associated with mirtazapine 15mg/d augmentation of sertraline 250mg/d has been reported (n=1, Soutullo *et al, J Clin Psych* 1998, **59**, 320).

Tricyclics + mirtazapine *
Amitriptyline 75mg/d caused clinically irrelevant changes in the kinetics of mirtazapine 30mg/d, and *vice versa* (n=24, Mink *et al*, mentioned in Timmer *et al, Clin Pharmacokinet* 2000, **38**, 461–74).

Warfarin + mirtazapine *
No interaction is known or suspected, but there is insufficient information to

confirm this at present (Sayal *et al, Acta Psych Scand* 2000, **102**, 250–55).

4.3.3.3 MOCLOBEMIDE

Moclobemide is metabolised by 2C19, and inhibits 2D6, 2C19 and 1A2.

Reviews: general (Livingstone, *Lancet* 1995, **345**, 533–34; Berlin and Lecrubier, *CNS Drugs* 1996, **5**, 403–13).

Alcohol + moclobemide

See alcohol (*4.7.1*).

Benzodiazepines + moclobemide

No significant interaction occurs (*Acta Psych Scand* 1990, **360**[Suppl], 844–46).

Bupropion + moclobemide *

See MAOIs + bupropion (*4.6.4*).

CIMETIDINE + MOCLOBEMIDE

Cimetidine may reduce the clearance and prolong the half-life of moclobemide so start with lower doses and monitor closely (Schoerlin *et al, Clin Pharmacol Ther* 1991, **49**, 32–38).

Digoxin + moclobemide

Lack of interaction has been reported (Berlin and Lecrubier, *CNS Drugs* 1996, **5**, 403–13).

Ibuprofen + moclobemide

Moclobemide is alleged to potentiate the effect of ibuprofen (MI), but lack of interaction has been reported (Berlin and Lecrubier, *CNS Drugs* 1996, **5**, 403–13).

Metoprolol + moclobemide

Concurrent metoprolol and moclobemide results in further lowering of blood pressure although postural hypotension was not reported (*Acta Psych Scand* 1990, **360**[Suppl], 84–86).

Nifedipine + moclobemide

No significant interaction occurs, apart from some slight reduction in blood pressure (*Acta Psych Scand* 1990, **360**[Suppl], 84–86).

Opiates + moclobemide

Moclobemide is alleged to potentiate the effect of opiates (MI) and dose reductions of morphine and fentanyl may be considered necessary.

Oral contraceptives + moclobemide

No significant interaction has been detected (*Acta Psych Scand* 1990, **360**[Suppl], 84–86).

Rizatriptan + moclobemide *

Moclobemide may significantly potentiate the effects of rizatriptan and the combination is not recommended (n=12, RCT, Van Haarst *et al, B J Clin Pharmacol* 1999, **48**, 190–96).

SELEGILINE + MOCLOBEMIDE

Selegiline is an MAO-B inhibitor and if combined with an MAO-A inhibitor, such as moclobemide, could produce full MAO inhibition (albeit reversible). The combination is not recommended but if the two need to be used together then full MAOI dietary precautions might be required.

SSRIs + moclobemide

Excitation, insomnia and dysphoria have been reported with fluvoxamine and moclobemide in refractory depression (Ebert, *Psychopharmacology* 1995, **119**, 342–44), as have headaches and fatigue (open, Dingemanse, *Int Clin Psychopharmacol* 1993, **7**, 167–80). The serotonin syndrome would also be a possibility with the combination and the UK SPC for moclobemide contra-indicates the combination. A fatal case, following overdose of paroxetine and moclobemide and subsequent serotonin syndrome, has been reported (Singer and Jones, *J Anal Toxicol* 1997, **21**, 518–20). However, in a study where up to 600mg/d moclobemide was added to established fluoxetine therapy, there was no change in the number, intensity, or type of adverse events. Fluoxetine markedly inhibited the metabolism of moclobemide but did not lead to excessive accumulation. The authors conclude that combination treatment with fluoxetine and moclobemide did not provide any indication of development of the 'serotonin syndrome' (Dingemanse *et al, Clin Pharmacol Ther* 1998, **63**, 403–13).

Sumatriptan + moclobemide

The BNF notes an increased risk of CNS toxicity with the combination, although a small study suggested combined use was safe with care (Blier and Bergeron, *J Clin Psychopharmacol*, 1995, **15**, 106–9).

Sympathomimetics + moclobemide

The UK SPC recommends avoiding this combination. Phenylephrine may slightly raise blood pressure in people taking high dose (600mg/d) moclobemide (Amrein *et al, Psychopharmacology* 1992, **106**, S24–S31) and ephedrine produces a greater rise in bp (Dingemanse, *Int Clin Psychopharmacol* 1993, **7**, 167–80). Another study noted no clinically significant interaction, although the pressor effect may be slightly enhanced (*Acta Psych Scand* 1990, **360**[Suppl], 84–86).

Tricyclics + moclobemide

A rapid and fatal serotonin syndrome has been caused by moclobemide-clomipramine overdose (Ferrer-Dufol *et al, J Toxicol Clin Toxicol* 1998, **36**, 31–32, letter).

Tyramine + moclobemide

Moclobemide does not appear to significantly potentiate the pressor effects of tyramine. Dietary restrictions are generally not required but it is recommended that patients should avoid eating excessive amounts of tyramine containing foods, especially if they have pre-existing hypertension. Minor pressor effects are not seen until about 100mg tyramine (*Acta Psych Scand* 1990, **360**[Suppl], 84–86). Even 150mg tyramine is suggested by some as being safe (*Acta Psych Scand* 1990, **360**[Suppl], 78–80). The use of this combination has, however, been used to treat severe postural hypotension (eg. n=1, *Lancet* 1994, **344**, 1263) and in counteracting clozapine-induced hypotension, allowing dose increases to an active therapeutic level (n=1, Taylor *et al, B J Psych* 1995, **167**, 409–10).

Tricyclics + moclobemide

The UK SPC contraindicates the combination if the tricyclic (or metabolite) is a serotonin reuptake inhibitor, eg. clomipramine, amitriptyline or imipramine. Serotonin syndrome has been reported with moclobemide and clomipramine, imipramine (Brodribb *et al, Lancet* 1994, **343**, 475–76) or an SSRI (eg. *BMJ* 1993, **306**, 248, review of syndrome in *Am J Psych* 1991, **148**, 705–13), and after moclobemide plus either citalopram or clomipramine overdoses (n=5, fatal, Neuvonen *et al, Lancet* 1993, **342**, 1419). Aggressive therapy is needed if

taken in overdose with serotonergic agents (Neuvonen *et al, Lancet* 1993, **342**, 1419). Lack of interaction has been noted with desipramine (*Acta Psych Scand* 1990, **360**[Suppl], 84–86) and amitriptyline 150mg/d (eg. n=21, Amrein *et al, Psychopharmacology* 1992, **106**, S24–S31).

Venlafaxine + moclobemide

See venlafaxine (*4.3.3.8*).

Warfarin + moclobemide *

No interaction is reported, but moclobemide inhibits CYP1A2 and 2C19 and so some potential exists (Sayal *et al, Acta Psych Scand* 2000, **102**, 250–55).

Zolmitriptan + moclobemide *

The BNF notes an increased risk of CNS toxicity with the combination, and that a lower dose of zolmitriptan should be used (review by Rolan, *Cephalalgia* 1997, **17**[Suppl 18], 21–27; Morales Asin, *Neurologia* 1998, **13**[Suppl 2], 25–30).

4.3.3.4 NEFAZODONE

Nefazodone is 99% protein bound but has not been shown to alter *in vitro* binding of other highly protein-bound drugs. Nefazodone may be metabolised by CYP3A4 but this is yet to be established. It is a potent inhibitor of CYP3A4 and weak CYP1A2 inhibitor.

Alcohol + nefazodone

See alcohol (*4.7.1*).

Antihypertensives + nefazodone

The UK SPC states that reduced nefazodone doses may be needed and that there is a potential for interaction with other cardiovascular drugs. It is unclear exactly what this means in clinical practice.

Antipsychotics + nefazodone

Caution is recommended with haloperidol as haloperidol bioavailability may be increased. Chlorpromazine protein binding is unaffected *in vitro* by nefazodone.

Astemizole + nefazodone

This is a possible contraindication because of the risk of fatal ventricular arrhythmias via inhibition of CYP3A4.

BENZODIAZEPINES+NEFAZODONE

Combined psychomotor impairment can occur. Diazepam protein binding is unaffected *in vitro* by nefazodone. Nefazodone is a potent CYP3A3/4 inhibitor and so levels of triazolobenzodiazepines, eg. alprazolam and midazolam can be raised significantly.

CARBAMAZEPINE + NEFAZODONE

Carbamazepine toxicity induced by nefazodone, requiring a 40% reduction in carbamazepine dose has been reported (Ashton and Wolin, *Am J Psych* 1996, **153**, 733). The mechanism could be CYP3A4 inhibition, or displacement of protein-bound drug.

Cimetidine + nefazodone *

No clinically significant interaction has been reported (n=18, RCT, Barbhaiya *et al, B J Clin Pharmacol* 1995, **40**, 161–65) .

Cyclosporine + nefazodone

There are case reports of cyclosporine levels elevated by the introduction of nefazodone, probably via CYP3A4 inhibition. Intensive monitoring of serum creatinine and cyclosporine level was indicated, along with appropriate dose reductions (eg. Vella and Sayegh, *Am J Kidney Dis* 1998, **31**, 320–23).

Digoxin + nefazodone *

Nefazodone may increase digoxin levels by up to 29% (n=18, RCT, Dockens *et al, J Clin Pharmacol* 1996, **36**, 160–67).

Fluoxetine + nefazodone *

See fluoxetine (*4.3.2.2*).

Lithium + nefazodone

Nefazodone increases slow-wave sleep when added to lithium (Sharpley *et al, J Psychopharmacol* 1996, **10** [Suppl 1], 26–29). An open prospective study also showed that when lithium is added to nefazodone (up to 400mg/d), tremor, dry mouth, tiredness, headache and dyspepsia commonly occur, but the combination to be safe and tolerable (n=14, Hawley *et al, Int J Clin Pract* 1998, **2**, 251–54). The UK SPC for nefazodone recommends caution with the combination.

Lidocaine (lignocaine) + nefazodone

Lidocaine protein binding is unaffected *in vitro* by nefazodone.

MAOIs + nefazodone

See MAOIs (*4.3.4*).

Phenytoin + nefazodone

See phenytoin (*4.5.8*).

Pravastatin + nefazodone *

Asymptomatic CK elevation has been reported (Alderman, *Ann Pharmacother* 1999, **33**, 871) but has been strongly disputed as being significant (Bottorf, *Ann Pharmacother* 2000, **34**, 538–39).

Prazosin + nefazodone

Prazosin protein binding is unaffected *in vitro* by nefazodone.

Propranolol + nefazodone

Propranolol protein binding is unaffected *in vitro* by nefazodone.

Sildenafil + nefazodone *

Since nefazodone inhibits CYP3A4, which metabolises sildenafil, raised sildenafil levels could enhance the cardiovascular risk and other ADRs, so care is needed (letter, Pies, *J Clin Psych* 1999, **60**, 792).

Terfenadine + nefazodone

This is a possible contraindication because of the risk of fatal ventricular arrhythmias via inhibition of the CYP3A4 metabolism of terfenadine. As nefazodone is a moderately weak *in vitro* inhibitor of terfenadine metabolism, a clinically significant interaction of terfenadine is more likely with nefazodone than sertraline or fluoxetine, since therapeutic plasma levels of nefazodone are comparatively higher (Jurima-Romet *et al, B J Clin Pharmacol* 1998, **45**, 318–21).

Tricyclics + nefazodone

Desipramine protein binding is unaffected *in vitro* by nefazodone.

Warfarin + nefazodone *

Warfarin protein binding is unaffected *in vitro* by nefazodone, shown in a volunteer study (RCT, Salazar *et al, J Clin Pharmacol* 1995, **35**, 730–38).

Verapamil + nefazodone

Verapamil protein binding is unaffected *in vitro* by nefazodone.

4.3.3.5 REBOXETINE *

Reboxetine is extensively (97%) bound to plasma proteins (particularly the alpha-1 acid glycoprotein fraction) and may interact with drugs with a high affinity for this fraction, eg. dipyridamole, propranolol, methadone, imipramine, chlorpromazine and local anaesthetics. Concomitant tricyclics, SSRIs, MAOIs and lithium have not been assessed. It is not thought to inhibit the CYP system, and has no effect on CYP2D6 (Avenoso *et al, Ther Drug Monit* 1999, **21**, 577). It is metabolised by CYP3A4 but there is a wide safety margin.

Alcohol + reboxetine
See alcohol (*4.7.1*).

Antipsychotics + reboxetine
An interaction is possible (see above).

Benzodiazepines + reboxetine
Lack of interaction has been reported (SPC), although some mild to moderate drowsiness and transient increases in heart rate were noted.

Dipyridamole + reboxetine
An interaction is possible (see above).

Disopyramide + reboxetine
The manufacturers of reboxetine advise caution with the combination (BNF).

Diuretics + reboxetine
There may be an increased risk of hypokalaemia with loop diuretics or thiazides (BNF).

Erythromycin + reboxetine
The manufacturers of reboxetine advise avoiding the combination (BNF).

Flecainide + reboxetine
The manufacturers of reboxetine advise avoiding the combination (BNF).

Fluoxetine + reboxetine *
There are no statistically significant effects of reboxetine on fluoxetine or norfluoxetine pharmacokinetics, and a minimal clinical impact is suggested (n=30, RCT, d/b, p/c, 8/7, Fleishaker *et al, Clin Drug Investigat* 1999, **18**, 141–50).

Fluvoxamine + reboxetine
The manufacturers of reboxetine advise avoiding the combination (BNF).

Ketoconazole + reboxetine *
Ketoconazole decreases the clearance of the two enantiomers of reboxetine, with no adverse effects, but some caution may be advisable (n=11, open, Herman *et al, Clin Pharmacol Therapeut* 1999, **66**, 374–79).

Lidocaine + reboxetine
An interaction is possible (see above), and with other local anaesthetics. The manufacturers of reboxetine advise avoiding the combination (BNF).

MAOIs + reboxetine
This has not been evaluated so avoid until further notice, and leave a 2-week gap after an MAOI and one week after reboxetine before switching to the other.

Methadone + reboxetine
An interaction is possible (see above).

Potassium-losing diuretics + reboxetine
See diuretics (above).

Propafenone + reboxetine
The manufacturers of reboxetine advise avoiding the combination (BNF).

Propranolol + reboxetine
An interaction is possible (see above).

Tricyclics + reboxetine
An interaction is possible (see above).

Warfarin + reboxetine *
No interaction is known or suspected, but there is insufficient information to confirm this at present (Sayal *et al, Acta Psych Scand* 2000, **102**, 250–55).

4.3.3.6 TRAZODONE
Trazodone is metabolised by CYP2D6 and inhibits CYP3A4.

ALCOHOL + TRAZODONE
See alcohol (*4.7.1*).

Antipsychotics + trazodone
Enhanced hypotension may occur when trazodone was added to either chlorpromazine or trifluoperazine (n=2, *Can J Psych* 1986, **31**, 857–8). Thioridazine 40mg/d increased trazodone levels by about 25% in 11 elderly patients (Yasui *et al, Ther Drug Monit* 1995, **17**, 333–35).

Buspirone + trazodone
See buspirone (*4.1.2*).

Cocaine + trazodone
See antidepressants + cocaine (*4.7.3*).

Digoxin + trazodone
Two isolated cases of digoxin toxicity exist (*Psychosomatics* 1984, **25**, 334–35) with trazodone.

Fluoxetine + trazodone
See fluoxetine (*4.3.2.2*).

Interferon alpha + trazodone *
See paroxetine + interferon alpha (*4.3.2.4*).

MAOIs + trazodone
See MAOIs (*4.3.4*).

Phenytoin + trazodone
See phenytoin (*4.5.8*).

Warfarin + trazodone *
INR and PT fell when trazodone was added to warfarin, and rose when

trazodone was stopped, and so caution is necessary (adjust doses and/or monitor) if trazodone is used, especially if as a PRN (n=1, Small and Giamonna, *Ann Pharmacother* 2000, **34**, 734–36; previous case *Can Med Ass J* 1986, **135**, 1372).

4.3.3.7 TRYPTOPHAN

Fluoxetine + tryptophan

See fluoxetine (*4.3.2.2*).

Fluvoxamine + tryptophan

See fluvoxamine (*4.3.2.3*).

MAOIs + tryptophan

See MAOIs (*4.3.4*).

4.3.3.8 VENLAFAXINE

Venlafaxine is metabolised by CYP2D6 to o-desmethylvenlafaxine, a major active metabolite. Other, minor, metabolic pathways exist. Venlafaxine has low potential for CYP2D6 and 3A4 inhibition (Ball *et al, Br J Clin Pharmacol* 1997, **43**, 619–26) and does not appear to have a significant effect on other P450 enzymes.

Alcohol + venlafaxine

See alcohol (*4.7.1*).

Antipsychotics + venlafaxine *

Urinary retention has been reported with haloperidol (Benazzi, *Pharmacopsychiatry* 1997, **30**, 27) and the UK SPC notes that venlafaxine causes a 70% increase in **haloperidol** AUC and 88% increase in peak levels, so care is needed. Increased **clozapine** levels and adverse effects have also been reported.

Benzodiazepines + venlafaxine

A study showed that diazepam 10mg had no significant effect on venlafaxine or metabolite kinetics, but venlafaxine slightly increased diazepam clearance. No clinically significant interaction thus seems likely (n=17, Troy *et al, J Clin Pharmacol* 1995, **35**, 410–19).

Carbamazepine + venlafaxine

Lack of interaction has been shown in a manufacturers (Wyeth) study (n=17, Wiklander *et al*, poster presented at 8th meeting of ECNP, Venice 1995).

Cimetidine + venlafaxine

A 45% reduction in venlafaxine clearance via a reduced first-pass metabolism, can result in increased venlafaxine levels and patients should be monitored for dose-related side-effects,

eg. nausea, bp changes. The major metabolite, O-desmethylvenlafaxine, is unaffected.

Fluoxetine + venlafaxine

See fluoxetine (*4.3.2.2*).

Lithium + venlafaxine

Venlafaxine has been shown to have no significant effect on lithium kinetics in a single dose study (Troy *et al, J Clin Pharmacol* 1996, **36**, 175–81) but there are cases of raised lithium levels and of serotonin syndrome (eg. Mekler and Woggon, *Pharmacopsychiatry* 1997, **30**, 272–73). Lithium reduces the renal clearance of venlafaxine but without apparent clinical significance.

MAOIs + VENLAFAXINE

Wyeth state that venlafaxine and MAOIs should not be used together and recommend a 14-day gap after stopping an MAOI before starting venlafaxine, and a 7-day gap after venlafaxine before an MAOI is used. There are many reported cases of severe reactions, eg. extreme agitation, diaphoresis, rapid respiration and raised CPK levels (n=1, Phillips and Ringo, *Am J Psych* 1995, **152**, 1400–1), hypomania, heavy perspiration, shivering and dilated pupils (n=1, Klysner *et al, Lancet* 1995, **346**, 1298–99) and several of serotonin syndrome (Hodgman *et al, Human Toxicology* 1997, **16**, 14–17; n=1, Weiner *et al, Pharmacother* 1998, **18**, 399–403). The manufacturers' recommendations should thus be followed carefully.

Moclobemide + venlafaxine

The manufacturers of venlafaxine state very cautiously that venlafaxine and moclobemide should not be used together and that serious adverse reactions may occur. They recommend a 14-day gap after stopping moclobemide before starting venlafaxine, and a 7-day gap after venlafaxine before moclobemide is used. This seems overcautious.

Selegiline + venlafaxine

The manufacturers of venlafaxine state that venlafaxine and selegiline should not be used together and that serious adverse reactions may occur. They recommend a 14-day gap after stopping selegiline before starting venlafaxine, and a 7-day gap after venlafaxine before selegiline is used.

Sertraline + venlafaxine

See sertraline (*4.2.5*).

Verapamil + venlafaxine *

A fatality has been reported (n=1, Kusman *et al, J Forensic Sci* 2000, **45**, 926-28).

Warfarin + venlafaxine *

The UK SPC states that potentiation of anticoagulant effects of warfarin has been reported, including increased PT or INR.

4.3.3.9 St. John's wort *

Although not licensed for depression in the UK, this section has been included because concerns about its interactions are frequently raised. Minor serotonin, noradrenaline and dopamine reuptake inhibition activity has been detected from St. John's wort (SJW) and might thus potentiate any antidepressants, and so should in theory best be avoided, particularly at high dose. SJW, when taken at recommended doses for depression, is unlikely to inhibit CYP2D6 or 3A4 activity (n=7, open, Markowitz *et al, Life Sci* 2000, **66**, 133–39) and may induce CYP3A (n=2, Ruschitzka *et al, Lancet* 2000, **355**, 548). There are reports of serotonin syndrome with SJW and antidepressants in elderly patients (Lantz *et al, J Ger Psychiatry Neurol* 1999, **12**, 7–10). The UK CSM issued advice about potential interactions in February 2000 (*Pharm J* 2000, **264**, 358).

Reviews: * herbal medicine interactions (Cupp, *Am Fam Physician* 1999, **59**, 1239–45), general (Henney, *JAMA* 2000, **283**, 1679; *Curr Prob Pharmacovig* 2000, **26**, 6–7).

Anticonvulsants + St. John's wort *

SJW may induce the metabolism of carbamazepine, phenobarbital and phenytoin, increasing the risk of seizures, and so should not be taken together (CSM warning, 2000), although suddenly stopping SJW may require dose adjustment of any anticonvulsant. Check anticonvulsant levels before and after stopping SJW.

Anti-HIV drugs + St. John's wort *

SJW may induce the metabolism of anti-HIV drugs, reducing efficacy, and so should not be taken together (CSM warning, 2000), although suddenly stopping SJW may require dose adjustment of any anti-HIV drug.

Ciclosporin + St. John's wort *

SJW may induce the metabolism of ciclosporin, reducing plasma levels significantly, and so should not be taken together (CSM warning, 2000). Heart transplant rejection due to SJW has been reported (n=2, Ruschitzka *et al, Lancet* 2000, **355**, 548; Breidenbach *et al, Lancet* 2000, **355**, 1912).

Digoxin + St. John's wort *

SJW may induce the metabolism of digoxin, reducing AUC by up to 25%, and so should not be taken together (n=25, 10/7, s/b, p/c, Johne *et al, Clin Pharmacol & Therapeut* 1999, **66**, 338–45; Cheng, *Arch Int Med* 2000, **160**, 2548). Suddenly stopping SJW may also require dose adjustment of digoxin.

Indinavir + St. John's wort *

SJW may reduce the levels of indinavir (AUC reduced by 57%), reducing efficacy, and so should not be taken together (n=8, Piscitelli *et al, Lancet* 2000, **355**, 547) and SJW should be avoided in patients receiving indinavir as their sole protease inhibitor. The same would probably be true for other protease inhibitors, eg. ritonavir and saquinavir.

MAOIs + St. John's wort *

Minor MAOI activity has been detected from SJW and might thus potentiate existing MAOI therapy, and should be avoided, particularly at high dose.

Oral contraceptives + St. John's wort *

The UK CSM has recommended that, since SJW reduces the effectiveness of oral contraceptives, the two should not be taken together.

SSRIs + St. John's wort *

Minor serotonin reuptake inhibition activity has been detected from SJW and might thus potentiate existing SSRI therapy and so should, in theory, be avoided, particularly at high dose.

Theophylline + St. John's wort *

SJW may induce the metabolism of theophylline, reducing efficacy, and so should not be taken together (CSM warning, 2000), although suddenly stopping SJW may require dose adjustment of theophylline (Nebel *et al,*

Ann Pharmacother 1999, **33**, 502, letter). Check theophylline levels before and after stopping SJW.

Tricyclics + St. John's wort *

Minor serotonin and noradrenaline reuptake inhibition activity has been detected from SJW and might thus potentiate existing tricyclic therapy, and so should, in theory, be avoided, particularly at high dose.

Triptans + St. John's wort *

The CSM has warned that SJW may increase the serotonergic effects of sumatriptan, naratriptan, rizatriptan and zolmitriptan, with increased adverse effects and so the two should not be used together.

Tyramine + St. John's wort *

There is not thought to be an interaction (mentioned by Cupp, *Am Fam Physician* 1999, **59**, 1239–45).

Warfarin + St. John's wort *

SJW may induce the metabolism of warfarin, reducing efficacy, and so should not be taken together (CSM warning, 2000). Suddenly stopping SJW may require dose adjustment of warfarin so check INR before and after stopping SJW and adjust doses as necessary.

4.3.4 MONO-AMINE OXIDASE INHIBITORS (MAOIs)

Review of MAOI interactions; Berlin and Lecrubier, *CNS Drugs* 1996, **5**, 403–13.

Adrenaline + MAOIs

See noradrenaline + MAOIs.

ALCOHOL + MAOIs

See alcohol (*4.7.1*).

Amantadine + MAOIs

Hypertension occurred in one patient taking amantadine, 48 hours after starting phenelzine (*Arch Gen Psych* 1984, **41**, 726) with one case of safe use of both (*Am J Psych* 1985, **142**, 273).

AMFETAMINE + MAOIs

See dexamfetamine + MAOIs.

Anaesthetics + MAOIs

With proper monitoring, general and local anaesthesia can be given safely with MAOIs (*Anesth Analg* 1985, **64**, 592–96) although occasional cases of reactions have been reported (eg. *Anaesthesia* 1987, **42**, 633–35). Generally considered safe although care with analgesics and sympathomimetics is needed.

Anticholinergics + MAOIs

Enhanced anticholinergic effects have been postulated.

Anticoagulants + MAOIs

An enhanced anticoagulant effect has been shown in animals (*Thromb Diath Haemorrh* 1965, **14**, 83).

Antipsychotics + MAOIs

Unexplained deaths with levomepromazine (methotrimeprazine) exist (eg. *NZ Med J* 1980, **91**, 226), probably are not related to a drug interaction. The combination is a risk factor for NMS and may enhance anticholinergic and extrapyramidal side-effects. See also clozapine (*4.2.2*).

Aspartane + MAOIs

A single case of recurrent headaches following aspartane ingestion exists (*Am J Psych* 1985, **142**, 271).

Atracurium + MAOIs

A single case report of atracurium-induced hypertension exists (*Anaesthesia* 1987, **42**, 633).

Barbiturates + MAOIs

Barbiturate sedation may be prolonged. Although little human data exists, be aware of the potential toxicity as one fatality has been reported (*BMJ* 1965, **i**, 1554).

Benzodiazepines + MAOIs

Although there are isolated cases of MAOI toxicity, oedema and hepatotoxicity (eg. *Lancet* 1983, **ii**, 787; Young and Walpole, *Med J Aust* 1986, **144**, 166–67), this is normally considered a safe combination.

Beta-blockers + MAOIs

Propranolol used with MAOIs has caused severe hypertension (*J Clin Psych* 1982, **43**, 16) and slight bradycardia (*Psychosomatics* 1989, **30**, 106–8) although not invariably so (*J Clin Psych* 1984, **45**, 81). Best to monitor bp carefully, especially in the elderly.

Bretylium + MAOIs

Bretylium may increase the heart rate with MAOIs but it is only dangerous if other sympathomimetics are present. There are no case reports.

Bupropion + MAOIs *

See bupropion (*4.6.4*).

BUSPIRONE + MAOIs

There are four unpublished reports of increased bp and possible CVA although the combination has been used safely.

Caffeine + MAOIs

Case reports exist of increased jitteriness with caffeine taken while on MAOIs (*Eur J Pharmacol* 1971, **16**, 315).

Carbamazepine + MAOIs

Carbamazepine is structurally related to the tricyclics and so an interaction is postulated with case reports of raised carbamazepine levels but a lack of interaction with tranylcypromine (*J Clin Psych* 1987, **7**, 360) and phenelzine (Yatham *et al*, *Am J Psych* 1990, **147**, 367).

Chloral + MAOIs

There are two poorly documented case reports of fatal hyperpyrexia and hypertension with chloral and phenelzine. Not thought to be important.

Citalopram + MAOIs

There are many reported cases of sero-tonin syndrome (see *1.32*) with other SSRIs and MAOIs and so care is needed if this combination is used (Graber *et al*, *Ann Pharmacother* 1994, **28**, 732–35).

Clozapine + MAOIs

See clozapine (*4.2.2*).

Cyproheptadine + MAOIs

An isolated case of hallucinations with cyproheptadine and phenelzine exists (*Am J Psych* 1987, **144**, 1242).

DEXAMFETAMINE + MAOIs

There is a case report of a death with phenelzine and dexamfetamine (*BMJ* 1965, **ii**, 168) and one with amfetamine (*Lancet* 1963, **i**, 1323).

Dextromethorphan + MAOIs

Although this is mainly extrapolation from pethidine, case reports exist with cough mixtures containing dextro-methorphan but since all also contained sympathomimetics, these are questionable. Two were fatal so care is advised. Dizziness and muscle spasms with dextromethorphan have been reported (*J Clin Psych* 1989, **50**, 64), as has a serotonin syndrome (Nierenberg *et al*, *Clin Pharmacol & Ther* 1993, **53**, 84–88).

Dextropropoxyphene + MAOIs

Dextropropoxyphene sedation has been enhanced by phenelzine (n=1, *Am J Psych* 1987, **144**, 251–52) as has severe hypotension, ataxia and impaired coordination when propoxyphene was added to phenelzine (n=1, Zornberg & Hegarty, *Am J Psych* 1993, **150**, 1270).

Disulfiram + MAOIs

See disulfiram (*4.6.6*).

DOPAMINE/DOXAPRAM + MAOIs

Animal studies show a clear interaction, with side-effects enhanced by MAOIs. The manufacturers recommend that dopamine or doxapram can be used if their initial dose is reduced to one tenth the normal dose and great care is taken.

Droperidol/hyoscine + MAOIs

There is an isolated questionable case of hypotension when droperidol and hyoscine were given as a pre-med (*BMJ* 1966, **i**, 483).

Ecstasy/MDMA + MAOIs

There is a case of a hypertensive crisis with MDMA/Ecstasy and phenelzine (*Clin Toxicol* 1987, **25**, 149–59) and two of muscle tension, coma and delirium with raised blood pressure (*Am J Psych* 1992, **192**, 412).

FLUOXETINE + MAOIs

There are several reported interactions (eg. *Lancet* 1988, **ii**, 850–51), including 4 deaths. A gap must be also be left when switching from one to the other (see *2.2.5*).

FLUVOXAMINE + MAOIs

There is an SPC recommendation to allow a 2-week gap between therapies. There are many reported cases of serotonin syndrome with other SSRIs and MAOIs and so care is needed with this combination.

Ginseng + MAOIs *

There are cases of headache, tremor (Shader and Greenblatt, *J Clin Psychopharmacol* 1985, **5**, 65) and mania (Jones and Runikis, *J Clin Psychopharmacol* 1987, **7**, 201–2) with Ginseng and phenelzine.

GUANETHIDINE + MAOIs

MAOI reversal of hypotension has been seen in a single-dose study (n=5, *Clin Pharmacol Ther* 1966, **7**, 510).

Hypoglycaemics + MAOIs

An enhanced hypoglycaemic effect with insulin (*Lancet* 1964, **i**, 1133) and sulphonylureas (eg. *Diabetes* 1968, **17**, 628) has been noted.

Indoramin + MAOIs

The SPC for indoramin states this to be a contraindication, as indoramin antagonises alpha-receptors, thus competing with noradrenaline for post-synaptic alpha-receptors. With increased noradrenaline activity, combination of the two drugs could cause vaso-constriction and raised blood pressure. No case reports are known.

Isoprenaline + MAOIs

This is a postulated interaction with some evidence that no interaction occurs. No case reports exist.

LEVODOPA + MAOIs

Low dose levodopa with carbidopa or benserazide seems safe but higher doses should be avoided, as should levodopa on its own (*Clin Pharmacol Ther* 1975, **18**, 273).

Lithium + MAOIs

Lack of an interaction has been reported (*Am J Psych* 1988, **145**, 249–50).

MAOIs + MAOIs

There is some evidence that different MAOIs may interact with each other especially if abruptly changed, eg. isocarboxazid to tranylcypromine (Bazire, *Drug Intell Clin Pharm* 1986, **20**, 954–55) and phenelzine to isocarboxazid (*Ann Pharmacother* 1992, **26**, 337–38). Tranylcypromine is metabolised to an amfetamine and an internal autoreaction (ie. interacts with itself) has been postulated (*BMJ* 1989, **298**, 964).

Methadone + MAOIs

Lack of an interaction has been reported (*Med J Aust* 1979, **1**, 400).

METHOXAMINE + MAOIs

There is evidence of enhanced bp with methoxamine and MAOIs (*J Lab Clin Med* 1960, **56**, 747).

Methyldopa + MAOIs

There is a single-case report of hallucinations with methyldopa and pargyline (*BMJ* 1966, **i**, 803).

METHYLPHENIDATE + MAOIs

A less severe interaction than with amfetamines would be expected. A single case of headaches and hyperventilation has been reported (*Am J Psych* 1964, **120**, 1019).

Mirtazapine + MAOIs

See mirtazapine (*4.3.3.2*).

Morphine + MAOIs

This is mainly extrapolation from pethidine. Two cases exist of hypotension and loss of consciousness with IV morphine (*Anaesth Intens Care* 1979, **7**, 194), responsive to naloxone. Low dose morphine and other narcotics, eg. codeine and fentanyl are probably safe. Methadone may be a suitable alternative. If opiates are used, it is best to start at a third or half the normal dose of opiate and titrate carefully, noting blood pressure and levels of consciousness. See also pethidine.

Nefazodone + MAOIs

A slow dose introduction is recommended if MAOIs are stopped shortly before nefazodone is started. The BNF recommends a 2-week gap between an MAOI and nefazodone, and a 1-week gap between nefazodone and starting an MAOI.

NEFOPAM + MAOIs

The manufacturers of nefopam recommend avoiding this combination.

Noradrenaline + MAOIs

Noradrenaline is potentially dangerous by injection and/or if other sympathomimetics are present (*BMJ* 1967, **ii**, 75) but is unlikely to cause problems if used with care.

Orciprenaline + MAOIs

The manufacturers recommend caution if the two are used together.

Oxcarbazepine + MAOIs *

See oxcarbazepine (*4.5.6*).

Oxymetazoline/xylometazoline + MAOIs

There is thought to be little systemic effect when these drugs are used nasally, but use in nose drops and sprays has not been studied.

OXYPERTINE + MAOIs

CNS excitation and hypertension can occur (MI).

Paraldehyde + MAOIs

Enhanced CNS sedation and respiratory depression have been suggested.

PAROXETINE + MAOIs

Nothing has been reported but see other SSRIs in this MAOI section.

PETHIDINE + MAOIs

A well-documented, rapid, severe and potentially fatal interaction, although it is not inevitable (*Br J Anest* 1968, **40**, 279). It may not be well known amongst junior medical staff (*BMJ* 1989, **298**, 671).

Reboxetine + MAOIs

See reboxetine (*4.3.3.5*).

RIZATRIPTAN + MAOIs

This is an SPC contraindication.

Salbutamol + MAOIs

No interaction occurs.

SERTRALINE + MAOIs

The manufacturers suggest a one-week washout period after sertraline before an MAOI is used. Several cases of suspected serotonergic syndrome have been reported, so care is essential (eg. Cases and review, Graber *et al, Ann Pharmacother* 1994, **28**, 732–35, including a review of the subject).

St. John's wort + MAOIs

See St. John's wort (*4.3.3.9*).

Sulphonamides + MAOIs

An isolated case exists of adverse effects with sulphafurazole and phenelzine (Boyer and Lake, *Am J Psych* 1983, **140**, 264–65).

SUMATRIPTAN + MAOIs

The SPC recommends sumatriptan is not used with MAOIs, or for two weeks after an MAOI has stopped.

Suxamethonium + MAOIs

There are three cases of enhancement of suxamethonium by phenelzine (Bodley *et al, BMJ* 1969, **3**, 510–12).

SYMPATHOMIMETICS + MAOIs

Hypertension has been reported with many indirectly acting sympatho-mimetic amines, eg. ephedrine, metaraminol, pseudoephedrine and phenylpropanolamine. Phenylephrine is found in many O-T-C cough and cold remedies and can cause a massive rise in blood pressure with MAOIs. Use in nasal sprays and drops is not recommended although there are no case reports.

Tetrabenazine + MAOIs

Reports exist of a central excitation and hypertension with tetrabenazine (*Ann NY Acad Sci* 1959, **80**, 680).

Trazodone + MAOIs

There are many reported cases of serotonin syndrome with SSRIs and MAOIs and so care may be needed if this combination is used (Graber *et al, Ann Pharmacother* 1994, **28**, 732–35).

TRICYCLICS + MAOIs

The combination of tranylcypromine and clomipramine has caused death in four cases but other MAOI/tricyclic combinations have been used with extreme care (*Lancet* 1982, **ii**, 440). There are cases of excitation, seizures and hyperpyrexia (eg. Spiker and Pugh, *Arch Gen Psych* 1976, **33**, 828) and a serotonin syndrome after a clomipramine overdose (325–750mg) with phenelzine (Nierenberg *et al, Clin Pharmacol and Ther* 1993, **53**, 84–88). The dangers could have been exaggerated and the combination may be relatively event-free if the following precautions are taken:

Avoid imipramine, desipramine, clomipramine and tranylcypromine.
Prefer amitriptyline, trimipramine and nortriptyline.
Use oral doses only.
Monitor patient closely.
Start both drugs simultaneously at low dose.
Keep doses in check.

See also combinations in depression (*1.14*) for a review of the potentially beneficial effects.

Tryptophan + MAOIs

There are cases of behavioural and neurological toxicity with high doses of tryptophan, mostly with tranyl-cypromine (*Am J Psych* 1985, **142**, 491–92), which may respond to pro-pranolol (*J Clin Psychopharmacol* 1986, **6**, 119–20). Potentiation of the therapeutic effect is well known. If used together it is best to monitor carefully.

TYRAMINE + MAOIs

Ingestion of dietary tyramine or levo-dopa or a sympathomimetic drug by a patient on an MAOI can produce a hypertensive crisis, eg. headache, rapid and prolonged rise in blood pressure, intracranial haemorrhage, acute cardiac failure and death. The effect is probably only seen with slow acetylators, as fast acetylators seem able to handle tyramine and other monoamines etc (60% of the UK population are slow acetylators). The effect is hugely variable, but 8mg tyramine can produce a 30mm Hg rise in bp in 50% people, and 25mg and above is potentially dangerous (Blackwell and Mabbitt, *Lancet* 1965, **1**, 938–40). 20–50mg tyramine produces hypertension with tranylcypromine (Berlin *et al, Clin Pharmacol Ther* 1989, **46**, 344–51). In a normal person, BP rises within 10–20 minutes (range 0–60) of tyramine ingestion, peaking at 20–110 minutes, prolonged if an MAOI is taken. The actual incidence of interaction is low (*BMJ* 1989, **298**, 345–46) if care is taken. For advice on dietary tyramine see the following section.

VENLAFAXINE + MAOIs

See venlafaxine (*4.3.3.8*).

Warfarin + MAOIs *

No interaction is known, although tranylcypromine is known to inhibit 2C19 and so some potential exists (Sayal *et al, Acta Psych Scand* 2000, **102**, 250–55).

Xanthines + MAOIs

There is a single case report of possible hypertension with phenelzine and oxtriphylline, a theophylline derivative (*J Clin Psychopharmacol* 1985, **5**, A17).

Xylometazoline + MAOIs

See oxymetazoline + MAOIs.

FOODS

Compliance with the MAOI diet is often very poor (Neil *et al, J Clin Psych* 1979, **40**, 3–37).

Reviews: Cheese and drink tyramine contents (Berlin and Lecrubier, *CNS Drugs* 1996, **5**, 403–13), 'The making of a user-friendly MAOI diet' (Gardner *et al, J Clin Psych* 1996, **57**, 99–104).

1. General Principles

Freshness of food is vital. If there is any sign of spoilage then omit. Avoid foods which are matured or might be 'spoiling'. Avoid tyramine-containing foods. Generally, the more 'convenience' the food, the safer it is, eg. packet soups are generally safe. Although many foods

Treatments for MAOI hypertensive crisis:

1. Phentolamine 2–10mg by slow IV infusion (adults), repeated if necessary.
2. If no phentolamine, chlorpromazine 50–100mg IM can be used, as can diazoxide (50–100mg by IV injection). Repeat after 10 minutes if necessary.
3. Alternative advice might be to bite open a 10mg capsule of nifedipine, swallow the contents with water (*Am J Psych* 1991, **148**, 1616) then go immediately to a hospital casualty department. This produces a consistent and prompt fall in arterial blood pressure (*Am Heart J* 1986, **111**, 963–9) but due to serious adverse events (stroke, hypotension etc), s/l nifedipine should only be used with care (Marwick, *JAMA* 1996, **275**, 423–4; Grossman *et al, JAMA* 1996, **276**, 1328–31). **NB**. nifedipine is light-sensitive and should not be left in bright light. Safer alternatives include sublingual captopril, clonidine and labetolol (review Matuschka, *J Pharm Tech* 1999, **15**, 199–203)
4. Cool any fever with external cooling.

• **Blood pressure should be monitored frequently.**

PATIENT INFORMATION: WARNING SIGNS OF A REACTION

If a patient experiences any of the following symptoms, especially after eating, taking drugs of any type or if unexpected or severe, a reaction should be suspected and appropriate medical attention sought immediately: *Headache (especially at the back of the head), lightheadedness or dizziness, flushing of the face, pounding of the heart, numbness or tingling of the hands or feet, pain or stiffness in the neck, photophobia, chest pain or nausea and vomiting. It usually occurs about two hours after ingestion of the compound.*

have only small amounts of tyramine, it is possible to have local concentrations which might give a reaction.

2. Tyramine-containing foods to avoid

The following may be of use as general guidelines:

● Dairy products:

Hard cheeses, soft cheeses and cheese spreads (eg. Philadelphia) must be avoided. Special care is needed with salty, bitter tasting, refrigerated cheese. Foods containing cheese (eg. pizzas, pies, etc, see below) must also be avoided and are a known cause of inadvertent ingestion and death. Cottage cheese, 'Dairylea' cream cheese, Ricotta and processed cheese contain only minute amounts of tyramine and large quantities would be needed to produce a reaction.

● Fruit and vegetables:

Broad bean pods (but not the beans) and banana skins (occasionally cooked as part of whole unripe bananas in a stew) must be avoided. Avocado has been reported to produce a reaction and should be avoided if possible.

● Game, meat and fish:

Pickled or salted dried herrings and any hung or badly stored game, poultry or other meat which might be 'spoiling' must be avoided. NB. The original reports with pickled herrings may have been due to spoilage in the brine surrounding the fish, and are probably safe.

● Meat products:

Avoid chicken liver pâté, liver pâté and any other liver which is not fresh. Avoid aged and cured meats (eg. salami, mortadella, pastrami). **Fresh** chicken liver, **fresh** beef liver and **fresh** pâté, however, should be safe.

● Pizzas: *

Commercially available pizzas from large chain outlets seem safe (analysis by Shulman and Walker, *J Clin Psych* 1999, **60**, 191–93; comment by Feinberg and Holzer, reply by Shulman and Walker, *J Clin Psych* 2000, **61**, 145–46), and even those with double orders of cheese appeared safe. Gourmet pizzas from smaller outlets had higher tyramine contents, especially if mature cheeses were used.

● Soy and Soybean:

Some samples of Soy sauce and soybean preparations may have very high tyramine levels. Either avoiding entirely or a 10ml maximum is recommended. **Soy sauce** (Pearl River etc) — some have high quantities, ie. up to 3.4mg/15ml, and so double or triple helpings could be well above thresholds for a reaction (Shulman and Walker, *J Clin Psych* 1999, **60**, 191–93)

Soybean curd (eg. Tofu) — some have high quantities, especially if kept refrigerated for 7 days or longer, ie. up to 5mg/300mg helping, and so double or triple helpings could be well above thresholds for reactions (Shulman and Walker, *J Clin Psych* 1999, **60**, 191–93).

● Yeast and meat extracts:

'Oxo', 'Marmite', 'Bovril' and other meat or yeast extracts must be avoided. Gravy made with UK 'Bisto' is safe (all contain less than 0.0022mg/g tyramine and a full half pint of gravy would contain less than 0.05mg tyramine). Gravy made from juices of the roast or fresh meat should be safe. Brewers yeast (Shulman *et al*, *J Clin Psychopharmacol* 1989, **9**, 397–402) and bread are safe.

3. Foods known to contain some tyramine where excessive consumption is not advisable, albeit unlikely:

Plums, matured pork, sauerkraut, spinach.

4. Foods thought to contain only minute amounts of tyramine :

Banana pulp (skins unsafe), chocolate (one anecdotal report of headache), cottage cheese, cream cheese, dairylea cheese, aubergine, fruit juices, octopus, peanuts, raspberries (some minor reports of raised tyramine content), sausages, soy milk, tomato, vinegar, yoghurt (commercial), Worcester sauce, eg. Lee and Perrins and others (very low, Shulman and Walker, *J Clin Psych* 1999, **60**, 191–93).

5. Other foods with isolated reports:

Chicken nuggets, chapatti, protein dietary supplement, sea kale.

6. Alcoholic drinks:

Patient instructions usually state that all alcoholic and some non-alcoholic drinks must be avoided. Real ales may contain up to 110mg/L, with reports of hypertensive crisis after 0.6pint (Tailor *et al, J Clin Psychopharmacol* 1994, **14**, 5–14). There is some evidence that low or non-alcoholic beers contain significant amounts of tyramine (*Lancet* 1988, **i**, 1167–68), shown by three reactions to less than 2/3 pint of alcohol-free and 'de-alcoholised' beer (*Int Clin Psychopharmacol* 1992, **7**, 59, mentioned in *Pharm J* 1993, **250**, 174). There is a large variation in other beers, so use in moderation (ie. 1–2 bottles a day maximum), prefer canned beers from major brewers and take care with de-alcoholised beers. The maximum reported level in Chianti wine is 12mg/l, likely to be dangerous only in overdose. The following may, however, be of use where a particular patient wishes to drink:

1. **Avoid**:
   Chianti
   Home-made beers and wines
   Real ales
   Red wines*

2. **True moderation** (eg. 1 unit):
   White wines
   Non-alcoholic beers and lagers

3. **Safest**:
   Gin, vodka
   Other clear spirits

* Red wines contain phenolic flavanoids which inhibit the enzymes which metabolise catecholamines, including tyramine (*BMJ* 1990, **301**, 544).

OVER THE COUNTER MEDICINES

Each patient should be warned about the possibility of interactions with over-the-counter medicines. The general advice for patients is:

1. Only buy medicines from a Pharmacy.

Do not use supermarket shelves, drug stores, newsagents etc. Do not take medicines given to you by friends or relatives. Do not take medicines taken before the MAOI was prescribed until advice has been sought.

2. Carry an MAOI card and show it to any doctor, dentist or pharmacist who may treat you.

3. Take special care over any medicines for coughs, colds, flu, hay fever, asthma and catarrh.

4.4 LITHIUM

Lithium may interact with other drugs particularly via changes in renal excretion.

Review: clinical relevance of lithium interactions (Finley *et al, Clin Pharmacokinetics* 1995, **29**, 172–91, 147 refs).

ACE INHIBITORS + LITHIUM *

There are many cases of lithium toxicity with ACE inhibitors (n=9, open, DasGupta *et al, J Clin Psych* 1992, **53**, 398-400). Elderly people may be particularly susceptible to this interaction (n=20, Finley *et al, J Clin Psychopharmacol* 1996, **16**, 68-71), so either monitor very carefully (Lehmann and Ritz, *Am J Kidney Dis* 1995, **25**, 82-87) or use, eg. beta-blockers.

Acetazolamide + lithium

Lithium excretion may be increased or, less likely, possibly decreased by acetazolamide (*L'Encephale* 1985, **11**, 261–62). This is inadequately studied and probably of minimal importance.

Alcohol + lithium

See alcohol (*4.7.1*).

AMINOPHYLLINE + LITHIUM

See theophylline + lithium.

Amiodarone + lithium

The BNF notes an increased risk of hypothyroidism with the combination.

Amfetamines + lithium

Lithium may suppress amfetamine 'highs' (*Am J Psych* 1974, **131**, 820).

Antacids + lithium

See sodium + lithium.

Antipsychotics + lithium *

This is generally considered a useful combination but cases of mostly reversible neurotoxicity have been reported, particularly with haloperidol (although these may have been undiagnosed NMS). Reports of encephalopathy, neurotoxicity or irreversible brain damage have been reviewed (*Human Psychopharmacol* 1990, **5**, 263–97) but without being able to demonstrate the interaction. The main risk factors seem to be if high doses of both drugs are used and signs of impending toxicity are ignored. Extrapyramidal side-effects may be enhanced. There are a number of reports for individual drugs. **Chlorpromazine** levels may be lowered by up to 40% by lithium (*Clin Pharmacol Ther* 1978, **78**, 451). Enhanced EPSEs (*Am J Psych* 1986, **143**, 942) and rarely neurotoxicity (especially with phenothiazines) have been reported, as has delirium after **risperidone** was added to a stable lithium regimen in an elderly woman (n=1, Chen and Cardasis, *Am J Psych* 1996, **153**, 1233–34), and possible NMS when risperidone replaced chlorpromazine in a man also taking lithium (n=1, Swanson *et al, Am J Psych* 1995, **152**, 1096). No interaction has been noted with **olanzapine** (MI). With **clozapine** there is an increased risk of developing NMS (MI) and reversible neurotoxicity (n=1, Blake *et al, J Clin Psychopharmacol* 1992, **12**, 297–99), and one despite lithium levels below 0.5mEq/l (n=1, Lee and Yang, *Chung Hua I Hsueh Tsa Chih (Taipei)* 1999, **62**, 184–87). Cases of diabetic ketoacidosis have been reported (eg. n=1, Peterson and Byrd, *Am J Psych* 1996, **153**, 737–38), and so glucose monitoring might be indicated with this particular combination. For a review of reported cases, with the suggestion that all symptoms are consistent with lithium toxicity alone, with the antipsychotic affecting fluid balance mechanisms and intracellular concentrations, see Knorring (*Hum Psychopharmacol* 1990, **5**, 287–92).

Baclofen + lithium

Two cases of aggravation of movement disorder in Huntington's disease exist (*Lancet* 1973, **ii**, 93).

Beta-blockers + lithium

A case of bradycardia with propranolol and lithium has been reported (Becker, *J Clin Psych* 1989, **50**, 473), although propranolol and nadolol (n=1, Dave and Langbart, *Ann Clin Psych* 1994, **6**, 51–52) have been used uneventfully for lithium-induced tremor.

Benzodiazepines + lithium

There have been several anecdotal reports of reactions, eg. hypothermia (Naylor *et al, BMJ* 1977, **2**, 22) and, although a neurotoxic syndrome in combination with lithium has been reported (Koczerginski *et al, Int Clin Psycho-*

pharm 1989, **4**, 195–99), extensive use of this usually beneficial combination suggests it to be safe.

Bumetanide + lithium

Although studies have shown a minimal effect (eg. *J Aff Dis* 1983, **5**, 289–92), bumetanide may cause lithium toxicity (*BMJ* 1980, **281**, 371).

Calcium-channel blockers + lithium

Cases of enhanced effect and toxicity with unchanged plasma levels have been reported with verapamil (*J Clin Pharmacol* 1986, **26**, 717–19), as have reduced lithium levels (*Am Heart J* 1984, **108**, 1378–79). Acute EPSEs and bradycardia have been reported with diltiazem (Binder *et al, Arch Int Med* 1991, **151**, 373).

Cannabis + lithium

See cannabis (*4.7.2*).

Carbamazepine + lithium

See carbamazepine (*4.5.1*), plus 'combinations' in bipolar disorder (*1.10*) for a review of some beneficial effects.

Cisplatin + lithium *

Reports exist of lithium levels decreased by up to 64% (eg. Vincent *et al, Cancer Chemother Pharmacol* 1995, **35**, 533–34; n=1, Beijnen *et al, Cancer Chemother Pharmacol* 1994, **33**, 523–26).

Citalopram + lithium

No pharmacokinetic interaction was noted in one study (n=24, open, Gram *et al, Ther Drug Monit* 1993, **15**, 18–24).

Clonidine + lithium

Lithium may reduce the hypotensive effect of clonidine (*Biol Psych* 1984, **19**, 883). Monitor carefully.

Cocaine + lithium

See cocaine (*4.7.3*).

Corticosteroids + lithium

An isolated case of lithium reducing the effect of corticosteroids on the kidneys exists (Stewart *et al, Clin Endocrinol* 1987, **27**, 63).

Co-trimoxazole + lithium

Two cases exist of enhanced toxicity with reduced levels (*NZ Med J* 1984, **97**, 729–32).

Digoxin + lithium

Lack of interaction has been shown (n=6, open, Cooper *et al, Br J Clin Pharmac* 1984, **18**, 21–25) but one isolated case of toxicity on the combination does exist.

Dipyridamole + lithium

Lack of interaction has been shown (Wood *et al, B J Clin Pharmacol* 1989, **27**, 749–56).

Disulfiram + lithium

See disulfiram (*4.6.6*).

Domperidone + lithium

An enhanced risk of EPSEs exists.

Fluoxetine + lithium *

Lack of significant pharmacokinetic interaction has been shown (n=10, open, Breuel *et al, Int J Clin Pharmacol Ther* 1995, **33**, 415–19), although the combination may be poorly tolerated (n=14, open, Hawley *et al, Int Clin Psychopharmacol* 1994, **9**, 31–33), with serotonin syndrome (Muly *et al, Am J Psych* 1993, **150**, 1565), absence seizures (Sacristan *et al, Am J Psych* 1991, **148**, 146–47) and acute confusion or lithium toxicity reported (*Int J Ger Psych* 1992, **7**, 687–88, reviewed by Levinson *et al, DICP Ann Pharmacother* 1991, **25**, 657–61). The incidence may, however, actually be low (n=110, open, Bauer *et al, J Clin Psychopharmacol* 1996, **16**, 130–34).

Fluvoxamine + lithium

See fluvoxamine (*4.3.2.3*).

Furosemide (frusemide) + lithium

Although studies have shown a minimal effect and furosemide to be the safest diuretic with lithium (eg. n=13, RCT, Crabtree *et al, Am J Psych* 1991, **148**, 1060–63), isolated cases of toxicity have been reported (eg. *JAMA* 1979, **241**, 1134–36).

Gabapentin + lithium

Although both are exclusively eliminated by renal excretion, a single-dose study showed that the pharmacokinetics of lithium are not altered by gabapentin (n=13, Frye *et al, J Clin Psychopharmacol* 1998, **18**, 461–64).

Hypoglycaemics + lithium *

Lithium has been used to improve glucose metabolism and assist the effects of oral hypoglycaemics and insulin (n=38, Hu *et al, Biol Trace Elem Res* 1997, **60**, 131–37).

Iodides + lithium

Enhanced antithyroid and goitre effects of lithium have been reported.

Ispaghula husk + lithium

A single case exists of reduced lithium levels (Perlman, *Lancet* 1990, **335**, 416).

Levodopa + lithium *

Lithium has been used to treat levodopa-induced psychiatric side-effects, eg. psychosis, mania etc (*Am J Psych* 1977, **134**, 808). Reversible Creutzfeldt-Jakob like syndrome has been reported (n=1, Broussolle *et al, J Neurol Neurosurg Psychiatry* 1989, **52**, 686–87).

Losartan + lithium

A case has been reported of marked lithium toxicity five weeks after losartan 50mg/d was added to stable therapy (n=1, Blanche *et al, Eur J Clin Pharmacol* 1999, **52**, 501).

MAOIs + lithium

See MAOIs (*4.3.4*).

METHYLDOPA + LITHIUM

Many cases of rapidly appearing lithium toxicity with normal plasma levels have been reported (eg. *Drug Intell Clin Pharm* 1980, **14**, 638).

METOCLOPRAMIDE + LITHIUM

An enhanced risk of EPSEs and of neurotoxicity exists.

Metronidazole + lithium

Cases of toxic lithium levels induced by metronidazole exist (*JAMA* 1987, **257**, 365–66).

Mirtazapine + lithium

See mirtazapine (*4.3.3.2*).

Nefazodone + lithium

See nefazodone (*4.3.3.4*).

Neostigmine + lithium

The effect may be antagonised by lithium.

Neuromuscular blocking agents + lithium

A few cases of enhanced blockade have been reported with neostigmine (eg. *Am J Psych* 1982, **139**, 1326–28). Animal studies indicate the possibility of an interaction and so the last dose or two before the use of an NMBA could be omitted.

NON-STEROIDAL ANTI-INFLAMMATORY DRUGS+LITHIUM*

This is a well known interaction, probably due to inhibition of renal prostoglandin PGE2 and reduced blood flow. Lithium levels should be monitored frequently if the combination is to be used. The BNF also notes the possibility of raised lithium levels with azapropazone. For a review, see Brouwers and de Smet, *Clin Pharmacokinet* 1994, **27**, 462–85.

Avoid:

Indometacin: 61% increases in lithium levels have been reported (eg. *Arch Gen Psych* 1983, **40**, 283–86).

Extra care:

Ibuprofen: Studies show a variable effect, with a 25% increase in lithium levels possible (eg. Ragheb, *J Clin Psych* 1987, **48**, 161–63; Bailey *et al, South Med J* 1989, **82**, 1197). As ibuprofen is available over the counter in the UK this interaction should be considered carefully.

Diclofenac: Lithium levels may rise by up to 23% (n=5, Reimann and Frolich, *Clin Pharmacol Ther* 1981, **30**, 348–52).

Piroxicam: Several cases exist of a slow-onset (eg. several months) lithium toxicity (eg *B J Psych* 1986, **147**, 343).

Care:

Ketoprofen: raised lithium levels have been reported (n=1, *Therapie* 1981, **36**, 323–26).

Ketorolac: lithium levels nearly doubled by ketorolac have been reported (n=1, Langlois and Paquette, *Can Med Ass J* 1994, **150**, 1455–56; n=5, Cold *et al, J Clin Psychopharmacol* 1998, **18**, 33–37).

Mefenamic acid: acute lithium toxicity, possibly with renal damage, has been reported (n=2, MacDonald and Neale, *BMJ* 1988, **297**, 1339).

Naproxen: short-term naproxen has little effect on lithium levels (n=12, Levin *et al, J Clin Psychophamacol* 1998, **18**, 237–40) although one study showed some increased lithium levels (n=7, Ragheb and Powell, *J Clin Psychopharmacol* 1986, **6**, 150–54).

Phenylbutazone: doubled lithium levels have been reported (n=1, Singer et al, *L'Encephale* 1978, **4**, 33–40; see also Ragheb, *J Clin Psychopharmacol* 1990, **10**, 149–50).

Tiaprofenic acid: increased serum lithium concentration (requiring a dose reduction) occurred in a woman taking fosinopril and lithium to which tiaprofenic acid was added (Alderman and Lindsay, *Ann Pharmacother* 1996, **30**, 1411–13).

Least risk:

Aspirin: 4g/d for seven days had no effect on lithium levels in one study (n=10, Reimann *et al, Arch Gen Psych* 1983, **40**, 283–86), and other studies have shown a mildly variable effect (eg. Ragheb, *J Clin Psych* 1987, **48**, 425; Bendz and Feinberg, *Arch Gen Psych* 1984, **41**, 310–11).

Sulindac:* Reports show either a slightly reduced level of lithium (*Drug Intell Clin Pharm* 1986, **19**, 374–76), no effect (*J Clin Psych* 1986, **47**, 33–34) or raised levels (n=2, Jones and Stoner, *J Clin Psych* 2000, **61**, 527–28).

Oxcarbazepine + lithium *

See oxcarbazepine (*4.5.6*).

Phenytoin + lithium

Three cases of lithium neurotoxicity occurred without increased lithium levels (eg. *BMJ* 1980, **280**, 610). With such few cases reported it would seem that with care both drugs can be used together safely.

Potassium iodide + lithium

An additive effect may cause hypothyroidism.

Psyllium + lithium

See Ispaghula husk + lithium.

Pyridostigmine + lithium

The effects may be antagonised by lithium.

Quetiapine + lithium

See quetiapine (*4.2.4*).

Smoking + lithium

See smoking (*4.7.4*).

Sodium + lithium

Excess sodium (eg. as bicarbonate in antacids) can reduce lithium levels (eg. *Med J Aust* 1978, **1**, 38) and sodium restriction can lead to lithium intoxication (eg. *J Psych Res* 1971, **8**, 91–105).

Spironolactone + lithium

A rise in lithium levels has been reported (*J Psych Res* 1971, **8**, 91–105), as has synergism (see combinations, *1.10*).

SSRIs + lithium

See fluoxetine (*4.3.2.2*) and fluvoxamine (*4.3.2.3*). No interaction has been seen yet with citalopram, paroxetine or sertraline.

Sumatriptan + lithium

The BNF notes an increased risk of CNS toxicity with the combination.

Tetracyclines + lithium

Cases of lithium intoxication (eg. *BMJ* 1978, **2**, 1183) have been reported so monitor lithium regularly.

THEOPHYLLINE + LITHIUM

Theophylline may reduce lithium levels by 20–30% (*J Clin Psych* 1985, **46**, 278–79) as may aminophylline, probably by increased excretion. An increased lithium dose can counteract this so monitoring of levels is essential, especially if theophylline is then stopped. The interaction has been made use of to treat lithium toxicity.

THIAZIDE DIURETICS + LITHIUM *

Thiazides reduce the renal clearance of lithium and levels rise within a few days, with potentially serious consequences. Thiazides should only be used where unavoidable and where strict monitoring is used. The combination has occasionally been used in patients where large doses of lithium do not produce therapeutic levels and a thiazide can thus reduce intake.

Chlorothiazide: A 50% rise in lithium levels has been reported (*Am J Psych* 1973, **130**, 1014).

Bendroflumethiazide (bendroflu-azide): a 24% reduction in lithium excretion has been shown, (*BMJ* 1974, **2**, 143), as has lithium toxicity (n=1, Vipond *et al, Anaesthesia* 1996, **51**, 1156–58).

Co-amilozide: Single case report (*Am J Psych* 1986, **143**, 257–58).

Hydroflumethiazide: One study showed a 24% reduction in lithium excretion (*BMJ* 1974, **2**, 143).

Hydrochlorthiazide (n=13, RCT, Crabtree *et al, Am J Psych* 1991, **148**, 1060–63)

Hydrochlorthiazide + spironolactone: Mentioned in *J Med Soc New Jersey* 1975, **72**, 439.

Triamterene + hydrochlorthiazide: Case report in *Postgrad Med J* 1980, **56**, 783.

Triamterene; Two cases of increased lithium clearance exist.

Tricyclics + lithium

See tricyclics (*4.3.1*).

Venlafaxine + lithium

See venlafaxine (*4.3.3.8*).

Warfarin + lithium *

No interaction is suspected nor reported (mentioned in Sayal *et al, Acta Psych Scand* 2000, **102**, 250–55).

4.5 ANTICONVULSANTS

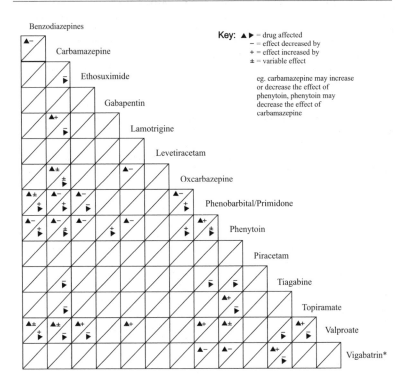

Key: ▲ ▶ = drug affected
− = effect decreased by
+ = effect increased by
± = variable effect

eg. carbamazepine may increase or decrease the effect of phenytoin, phenytoin may decrease the effect of carbamazepine

The above table shows the effect of adding one anticonvulsant to a therapy including another. The opposite effect to the above will usually occur when a drug is discontinued from a regimen.

Reviews: detailed reviews of pharmacokinetic interactions between anticonvulsants (Riva *et al, Clin Pharmacokinetics* 1996, **31**, 470–93, 260 refs, and Anderson, *Ann Pharmacother* 1998, **32**, 554–63; Tanaka, *J Clin Pharm & Ther* 1999, **24**, 87).

4.5.1 CARBAMAZEPINE

Carbamazepine is principally metabolised by the CYP3A4 enzyme but is also a potent inducer of CYP3A4 and other oxidative mechanisms in the liver. This auto-induction takes 1–4 weeks to occur, although is virtually complete after a week. Carbamazepine (CBZ) is metabolised to carbamazepine-epoxide (CBZ-E), which may be more toxic than carbamazepine itself and so alteration of the CBZ:CBZ-E ratio by another drug would alter toxicity. Carbamazepine is extensively plasma protein-bound. Major diurnal variations in plasma levels occur, which can be as much as 90% during polytherapy compared to monotherapy (Hoppener *et al, Epilepsia* 1980, **21**, 341–50).

Review: significant interactions (Spina *et al, Clin Pharmacokinet* 1996, **31**, 198–214).

Acetazolamide + carbamazepine

CYP3A4 inhibition may raise carbamazepine levels (mentioned in Spina *et al, Clin Pharmacokinet* 1996, **31**, 198–214).

Alcohol + carbamazepine

See alcohol (*4.7.1*).

ANTIPSYCHOTICS + CARBAMAZEPINE *

There are a variety of well documented interactions. Carbamazepine very significantly reduces **haloperidol** levels, resulting in worsening symptoms and worsening outcome (eg. n=27, 4/52,

Hesslinger *et al, J Clin Psycho- pharmacol* 1999, **19**, 310–15). More importantly, a significantly extended QT interval has been shown, probably by increased haloperidol metabolite concentrations. Care is thus needed (n=2, Iwahashi *et al, Am J Psych* 1996, **153**, 135). **Loxapine** may induce CBZ metabolism to CBZ-E or inhibit CBZ-E metabolism (Collins *et al, Ann Pharmacother* 1993, **27**, 1180–83), which may enhance toxicity, even with normal carbamazepine levels (n=1, Collins *et al, Ann Pharmacother* 1993, **27**, 1180–83). There are cases of **clozapine** levels increasing by up to 100% after carbamazepine was stopped (*Am J Psych* 1993, **150**, 169) and of neurotoxicity (*Am J Psych* 1985, **142**, 785–86). There is also the very real enhanced risk of agranulocytosis (mandatory precaution in UK SPC), so carbamazepine and clozapine should not be used together (Gerson, *Lancet* 1991, **338**, 262–63). Carbamazepine markedly reduces plasma levels of **risperidone** and 9-hydroxyrisperidone, probably via 3A4 induction (n=34, Spina *et al, Ther Drug Monit* 2000, **22**, 481–85; Lane and Chang, *J Clin Psych* 1998, **59**, 430–31). The Japanese SPC notes that carbamazepine may reduce **zotepine** levels, via CYP3A4 induction. Antipsychotics lower the seizure threshold, antagonising the anti-convulsant effects.

Benzodiazepines+carbamazepine

Carbamazepine mildly induces clonaze-pam metabolism via CYP3A4, reducing its half-life (*Clin Pharmacol Ther* 1978, **24**, 316). Slightly higher benzodiaze-pine doses may be needed (Baba *et al, B J Clin Pharmacol* 1990, **29**, 766–69). Carbamazepine toxicity has occurred after the addition of clobazam (Genton *et al, Epilepsia* 1998, **39**, 1115–18), probably related to progressive increases in norclobazam.

Bupropion + carbamazepine *

See bupropion (*4.6.4*).

Caffeine + carbamazepine

Carbamazepine induces the metabolism of caffeine via CYP1A2 (Parker *et al, Br J Clin Pharmacol* 1998, **45**, 176–78).

CALCIUM-CHANNEL BLOCKERS + CARBAMAZEPINE

One study showed that verapamil increases carbamazepine plasma levels by 50%, via CYP3A4 inhibition (*Lancet* 1986, **i**, 700–7; *Neurology* 1991, **41**, 740–42). Other evidence, eg. cases with diltiazem (*Drug Intell Clin Pharm* 1987, **21**, 340–42), and verapamil suggests a substantial risk of toxicity. Since no interaction occurs with nifedipine (*Neurology* 1991, **41**, 740–42; Brodie and MacPhee, *BMJ* 1986, **292**, 1170–71), it is the calcium-channel blocker of choice with carbamazepine, although the BNF notes the efficacy of nifedipine may be reduced, so care is needed.

Charcoal, activated + carbamazepine

Carbamazepine absorption may be almost completely stopped if activated charcoal is given five minutes after ingestion, with a lesser affect if given after an hour (Neuvonen *et al, Eur J Clin Pharmacol* 1980, **17**, 51).

Cocaine + carbamazepine

See cocaine (*4.7.3*).

CORTICOSTEROIDS + CARBAMAZEPINE

Corticosteroid CYP3A4 metabolism is accelerated by carbamazepine, giving a reduced effect (*Clin Pharmacol Ther* 1987, **42**, 424–32).

Clarithromycin + carbamazepine

See erythromycin + carbamazepine.

CYCLOSPORIN + CARBAMAZEPINE

Cyclosporin metabolism is accelerated by carbamazepine, to give reduced plasma levels.

DANAZOL + CARBAMAZEPINE

Danazol inhibits carbamazepine meta-bolism to give an increased effect (*Ther Drug Monit* 1987, **9**, 24–27) so monitor levels and observe for side-effects.

DEXTROPROPOXYPHENE + CARBAMAZEPINE

Dextropropoxyphene enhances carba-mazepine toxicity via CYP3A4 inhibition (eg. *Neurology* 1987, **37** [Suppl 1], 87) and levels may rise by 44–77%. In one case, carbamazepine levels increased 4-fold over 24 hours and led to cerebellar dysfunction, which resolved over 48 hours (n=1, Allen, *Postgrad Med J* 1994, **70**, 764). Monitor closely if used together.

Digoxin + carbamazepine

An isolated case exists of bradycardia with digitalis and carbamazepine (*Arch Neurol* 1968, **19**, 129), but this has not been reported with digoxin.

Disulfiram + carbamazepine *

See disulfiram (*4.6.6*).

Diuretics + carbamazepine

Hyponatraemia may uncommonly occur with frusemide or hydrochlorothiazide (*J Clin Psych* 1987, **48**, 281–83).

DOXYCYCLINE + CARBAMAZEPINE

Doxycycline metabolism is accelerated by carbamazepine, reducing efficacy and halving half-life (*BMJ,* 1974, **2**, 470). Other tetracyclines appear not to interact.

Enteral feeds + carbamazepine

Carbamazepine suspension absorption has been shown to be slightly slowed and reduced during nasogastric feeding (Bass *et al, Epilepsia* 1989, **30**, 364) so take care with dosing after enteral feeding is stopped.

Ethosuximide + carbamazepine

See ethosuximide (*4.5.2*).

Etretinate + carbamazepine

A girl treated with the combination only responded to etretinate when carbamazepine was withdrawn (n=1, Mohammed, *Dermatology* 1992, **185**, 79).

ERYTHROMYCIN + CARBAMAZEPINE

A rapid 100–200% rise in carbamazepine levels has been reported (n=4, *JAMA* 1986, **255**, 1165–67; n=1, Tatum and Gonzalez, *Hosp Pharm* 1994, **29**, 45) and with IV erythromycin use (*Drug Intell Clin Pharm* 1989, **23**, 878–79), probably via CYP3A4 inhibition. Other reports show that the combination should only be used with great care. Monitor levels or use an alternative antibiotic.

Fluconazole + carbamazepine *

Potential fluconazole-induced carbamazepine toxicity has been reported (Nair and Morris, *Ann Pharmacother* 1999, **33**, 790–92).

Fluoxetine + carbamazepine

See fluoxetine (*4.3.2.2*).

Fluvoxamine + carbamazepine

See fluvoxamine (*4.3.2.3*).

Gabapentin + carbamazepine

See gabapentin (*4.5.3*).

Grapefruit juice + carbamazepine

300ml grapefruit juice increased peak carbamazepine levels by 40%, trough levels by 39% and AUC by 41%, probably by CYP3A4 inhibition in the gut wall and liver (n=10, RCT, Garg *et al, Clin Pharmacol Ther* 1998, **64**, 286–88).

Griseofulvin + carbamazepine

A reduced griseofulvin level by enzyme induction (*Am J Hosp Pharm* 1986, **16**, 52) has been postulated.

H2-BLOCKERS + CARBAMAZEPINE

Studies have shown a transient 20% rise in carbamazepine levels with cimetidine (n=8, open, 7/7, Dalton *et al, Epilepsia* 1986, **27,** 553–58), reduced clearance, prolonged half-life (*E J Clin Pharmacol* 1986, **27,** 325–28) and inhibition of non-renal elimination (*Epilepsia* 1985, **26**, 127–30) via CYP3A4 inhibition. Studies show no interaction with ranitidine (eg. n=8, RCT, Dalton *et al, Drug Intell Clin Pharm* 1985, **19**, 941–44; *E J Clin Pharmacol* 1986, **27**, 325–28), which would thus appear a safer option.

Indinavir + carbamazepine

The BNF notes the possibility of reduced plasma indinavir levels with the combination.

Influenza vaccine + carbamazepine

A transient 10% increase in carbamazepine levels occurred in one study (*Clin Pharm* 1986, **5**, 817–20).

ISONIAZID + CARBAMAZEPINE

Rapid carbamazepine toxicity may occur via 3A4 inhibition by isoniazid, in this potentially serious interaction (*BMJ* 1982, **285**, 261–62). It may be potentiated by cimetidine (n=1, *Ann Pharmacother* 1992, **26**, 841–42). Monitor carefully for toxicity.

Isotretinoin + carbamazepine

Isotretinoin may slightly reduce carbamazepine plasma levels and alter the CBZ:CBZ-E ratio (n=1, Marsden *et al, Br J Derm* 1988, **119**, 403).

Isradipine + carbamazepine

Carbamazepine may reduce the effect of isradipine.

Itraconazole + carbamazepine

Sub-therapeutic itraconazole levels may occur with carbamazepine so monitor for lack of efficacy (Tucker *et al, Clin Infect Dis* 1992, **14**, 165–74).

Lamotrigine + carbamazepine

See lamotrigine (*4.5.4*).

Levetiracetam + carbamazepine *

See levetiracetam (*4.5.5*).

Levothyroxine (thyroxine) + carbamazepine

Levothyroxine metabolism is accelerated by carbamazepine, increasing the thyroxine requirements in hypo-thyroidism.

Lithium + carbamazepine

Although this combination is often used in rapid-cycling bipolar disorder, neurotoxicity may occur without increased plasma levels (*Am J Psych* 1984, **141**, 1604; Marcoux, *Ann Pharmacother* 1996, **30**, 547). Risk factors include a history of lithium neurotoxicity or concurrent medical or neurological illness. Occasional neurotoxic reactions have been reported, but mostly in patients with pre-existing brain damage (*Am J Psych* 1984, **141**, 1604–6), although there is some evidence of minor cognitive impairment on the combination (*Human Psychopharmacology* 1990, **5**, 41–45). An additive anti-thyroid effect can occur, lowering T4 and free T4 levels (*Am J Psych* 1990, **147**, 615–20). Monitor carefully and regularly for signs of toxicity.

MAOIs + carbamazepine

See MAOIs (*4.3.4*).

Methadone + carbamazepine

Carbamazepine may reduce methadone levels (Bell *et al, Clin Pharmacol Ther* 1988, **43**, 623–29).

Metoclopramide + carbamazepine

There is a single case of apparent carbamazepine neurotoxicity occurring three days after metoclopramide 30mg/d was added, which resolved when metoclopramide was discontinued (Sandyk, *BMJ* 1984, **288**, 830).

Metronidazole + carbamazepine

Plasma carbamazepine levels rose by 60% in a woman when metronidazole was added, resulting in symptoms of toxicity (Patterson, *Ann Pharmacother* 1994, **28**, 1304).

Mianserin + carbamazepine *

See mianserin (*4.3.3.1*).

Miconazole + carbamazepine

An isolated case report of an adverse response has appeared (*Therapie* 1982, **37**, 437–41).

Mirtazapine + carbamazepine

See mirtazapine (*4.3.3.2*).

NEFAZODONE + CARBAMAZEPINE

See nefazodone (*4.3.3.4*).

Neuromuscular blocking agents + carbamazepine

Studies show reduced responses and recovery times to NMBAs (*Anaesthesiology* 1989, **71**, A784), eg. vecuronium doses need to be significantly higher in patients on maintenance carbamazepine (Whalley and Ebrahim, *B J Anaesth* 1994, **72**, 125–26) and recovery times can be 40–60% faster with atracurium and pancuronium (Tempelhoff *et al, Anesth Analg* 1990, **71**, 665–69).

NICOUMALONE+CARBAMAZEPINE

The metabolism of nicoumalone is accelerated by carbamazepine to give a reduced effect.

Olanzapine + carbamazepine

See olanzapine (*4.2.3*).

ORAL CONTRACEPTIVES + CARBAMAZEPINE

The CYP3A4 metabolism of OCs is accelerated by carbamazepine to give a **reduced contraceptive effect** (*JAMA* 1986, **256**, 238–40; *B J Clin Pharmacol* 1990, **30**, 892–96). Use higher dose OCs (equivalent to 50–100mcg ethinyl-oestradiol, eg. Eugynon-50) and adjust the dose if necessary or use alternative methods.

Oxcarbazepine + carbamazepine *

See oxcarbazepine (*4.5.6*).

Paroxetine + carbamazepine

See paroxetine (*4.3.2.4*).

Phenobarbital + carbamazepine

Phenobarbital induces carbamazepine CYP3A4 metabolism, slightly reducing plasma levels (Christianssen *et al, Acta Neurol Scand* 1973, **49**, 543–46). Carbamazepine may raise phenobarbital levels but not to a clinically significant amount (Cereghino *et al Clin Pharmacol Ther* 1975, **18**, 733).

PHENYTOIN + CARBAMAZEPINE

Phenytoin induces carbamazepine CYP3A4 metabolism, reducing levels, often dramatically (eg. *Drug Intell Clin Pharm* 1993, **27**, 708–11) but with some evidence of increased carbamazepine metabolites in the CSF (discussion in *Neurology* 1987, **37**, 1111–18). Monitoring of CBZ levels is useful, although seizure control may not be affected. Raised carbamazepine levels may result from withdrawal of phenytoin via removal of enzyme induction (Chapron *et al, Ann Pharmacother* 1993, **27**, 708–11). Thus, if stopping phenytoin, carbamazepine levels must be monitored during the deinduction stage to prevent toxicity developing. Carbamazepine may induce phenytoin metabolism, reducing plasma concentrations (*Clin Pharmacol Ther* 1971, **12**, 539) although competitive inhibition of the common oxidase pathways increased phenytoin half-life and increased mean serum levels by 35% (some studies by up to 100%), producing neurotoxicity (*Neurology* 1988, **38**, 1146–50). The clinical effect may be limited but best to monitor the levels of both drugs.

Progabide + carbamazepine

Progabide has no effect on carbamazepine levels (*Epilepsia* 1987, **28**, 68–73) but may slightly increase CBZ-E levels.

PROTON-PUMP INHIBITORS + CARBAMAZEPINE *

Carbamazepine induces the CYP3A4 catalysed sulphoxidation of **omeprazole**, but has little or no effect on hydroxylation via CYP2C19 (Bertilsson *et al, Br J Clin Pharmacol* 1997, **44**, 186). Multiple dose omeprazole may decrease carbamazepine clearance by 40% and thus increase levels (Naidu *et al, Drug Invest* 1994, **7**, 8–12). **Pantoprazole** appears to have no effect on carbamazepine (n=20, RCT, Huber *et al, Int J Clin Pharmacol Ther* 1998, **36**, 521–24; Steinijans *et al, Int J Clin Pharmacol Ther* 1996, **34**, S31– S50).

Quetiapine + carbamazepine

See quetiapine (*4.2.4*).

Rifampicin + carbamazepine

Rapid CYP3A4 induction may lower carbamazepine levels.

Ritonavir + carbamazepine *

Raised carbamazepine levels and toxicity (including hepatic) have been reported with ritonavir, a protease inhibitor, probably by CYP3A4 inhibition (n=1, Kato *et al, Pharmacother* 2000, **20**, 851–54).

Sertraline + carbamazepine *

See sertraline (*4.3.2.5*).

Terfenadine + carbamazepine

Terfenadine may displace carbamazepine from plasma protein binding sites, resulting in raised free levels and toxicity (n=1, Hirschfeld and Jarosinski, *Ann Int Med* 1993, **118**, 907–8).

Theophylline + carbamazepine

Theophylline metabolism is accelerated by carbamazepine to give a reduced effect (*NEJM* 1983, **308,** 724–25).

Tiagabine + carbamazepine

See tiagabine (*4.5.10*).

Topiramate + carbamazepine

See topiramate (*4.5.11*).

TRICYCLICS + CARBAMAZEPINE

The CYP3A4 metabolism of imipramine, doxepin and amitriptyline may be accelerated by carbamazepine to give plasma levels reduced by 42–50% (eg. *Pharmacotherapy* 1988, **8**, 135, Leinonen *et al, J Clin Psychopharmacol* 1991, **11**, 313–18). This is a common combination and other evidence supports this to be a clinically significant interaction but not well recognised. Carbamazepine toxicity with desipramine has also been reported (n=1, *J Clin Psych* 1984, **45,** 360).

VALPROATE + CARBAMAZEPINE

Valproate seems to inhibit several carbamazepine metabolic pathways, resulting in raised CBZ-10,11-epoxide concentrations (which has led to CBZ-E-induced psychosis, McKee *et al, Lancet* 1989, **i**, 167, and so watch closely for toxicity) but sometimes unchanged carbamazepine levels (n=27, Bernus *et al, Br J Clin Pharmacol* 1997, **44**, 21). In one study, carbamazepine levels fell by about 25% when valproate was added (n=7, *Epilepsia* 1984, **25**, 338–45). Valproate may also displace carbamazepine from binding sites on plasma proteins (*B J Clin Pharmacol* 1988, **25,** 59–66). Conversely, carbamazepine induces valproate metabolism, reducing plasma levels by about 20% (Bowdle *et al, Clin Pharmacol Ther* 1979, **26**, 629–34; Larkin *et al, B J Clin Pharmacol* 1989, **27**, 313–22). This is probably minor **but** a mean 59% increase in valproate levels can occur on carbamazepine withdrawal (*Epilepsia* 1988, **29**, 578–81). Overall, no adjustments in carbamazepine doses are generally necessary but beware of the altered metabolite ratio and monitor if clinical symptoms change.

Venlafaxine + carbamazepine
See venlafaxine (*4.3.3.8*).

Vigabatrin + carbamazepine
See vigabatrin (*4.5.13*).

Vincristine + carbamazepine *
Carbamazepine significantly increases the clearance of vincristine, probably by CYP3A4 induction (n=15, open, Villikka *et al, Clin Pharmacol & Therapeut* 1999, **66**, 589–93).

WARFARIN + CARBAMAZEPINE *
The metabolism of warfarin is accelerated by carbamazepine to produce a reduced efficacy. Warfarin doses may need to be increased by up to 100% (Kendall and Boivin, *Ann Int Med* 1981, **94**, 280) and then reduced carefully if carbamazepine is discontinued (Denbow and Fraser, *South Med J* 1990, **83**, 981).

Zaleplon + carbamazepine
See zaleplon (*4.1.4*).

Zotepine + carbamazepine
See zotepine (*4.2.6*).

4.5.2 ETHOSUXIMIDE

Barbiturates + ethosuximide
See phenobarbital (*4.5.7*).

Carbamazepine + ethosuximide
Carbamazepine induces ethosuximide metabolism, reducing plasma levels by about 17% (Warren *et al, Clin Pharmacol Ther* 1980, **28**, 646–51) although this is probably of minor significance.

Phenytoin + ethosuximide
A study showed that phenytoin reduces ethosuximide plasma levels (n=198, *Clin Pharmacokinet* 1982, **7**, 176–80).

Valproate + ethosuximide
Valproate may increase ethosuximide plasma levels by up to 50% via enzyme inhibition, although this may only be a

transient effect (*Epilepsia* 1984, **25**, 229–33), and standard regular monitoring will probably suffice. Monitor ethosuximide levels if the patient becomes sedated. Conversely, adding ethosuximide to valproate may reduce valproate levels by 28% (n=4) and stopping ethosuximide from an ethosuximide/valproate combination has led to valproate levels rising by 36% (n=9). The mechanism is unknown (open, Salke-Kellermann *et al, Epilepsy Res* 1997, **26**, 345–49).

Zotepine + ethosuximide
See zotepine (*4.2.6*).

4.5.3 GABAPENTIN
Gabapentin is not protein bound so there is little chance of interaction via this mechanism. Excretion is almost completely via the kidney.

Antacids + gabapentin
The antacid 'Maalox' reduces gabapentin levels by 20% when given concurrently. Separating the doses by 2 hours resulted in only a 5% reduction in levels (Busch *et al, Epilepsia* 1993, **34**[Suppl 2], 158).

Carbamazepine + gabapentin
No significant interaction has been noted (eg. Radulovic *et al, Epilepsia* 1994, **35**, 155–61).

Cimetidine + gabapentin
1200mg/d of cimetidine reduces gabapentin clearance by about 10%, which requires no dosage adjustment (Busch *et al, Epilepsia* 1993, **34**[Suppl 2], 158).

Clonazepam + gabapentin
No significant interaction has been noted (*Lancet* 1990, **335**, 1114–17).

Levetiracetam + gabapentin *
See levetiracetam (*4.5.5*).

Lithium + gabapentin
See lithium (*4.4*).

Oral contraceptives + gabapentin
No change in the kinetics of nore-thisterone and ethinyloestradiol were seen with gabapentin (Busch *et al, Epilepsia* 1993, **34**[Suppl 2], 158).

Phenobarbital + gabapentin
One study showed no significant interaction (n=12, Hooper *et al, B J Clin Pharmacol* 1991, **31**, 171–74).

Phenytoin + gabapentin

Only a slight trend towards an increase in phenytoin levels has been observed (eg. Graves *et al, Pharmacotherapy* 1989, **9**, 196) although toxic phenytoin levels have occurred with gabapentin 600mg/d (n=1, Tyndel, *Lancet* 1994, **343**, 1363–64).

Valproate + gabapentin

No significant interaction has been noted (*Lancet* 1990, **335**, 1114–47).

Zotepine + gabapentin

See zotepine (*4.2.6*).

4.5.4 LAMOTRIGINE

Barbiturates + lamotrigine

Lamotrigine has no significant effect on primidone and phenobarbital (*Epilepsia* 1991, **32**[Suppl 1], 96).

Benzodiazepines + lamotrigine

Lamotrigine has no significant effect on clonazepam (*Epilepsia* 1991, **32**[Suppl 1], 96).

Carbamazepine + lamotrigine

A higher incidence of CNS side-effects with the combination has been noted (Gilman, *Ann Pharmacother* 1995, **29**, 144–51). Toxicity appears more likely to occur when lamotrigine is added to CBZ if the initial CBZ level is high, eg. greater than 8mg/L. This appears to be the result of a pharmacodynamic interaction (n=47, Besag *et al, Epilepsia* 1998, **39**, 183–87). However, lamotrigine does not seem to raise the levels of CBZ-E and, in fact, may reduce the levels of this active but toxic metabolite (n=14, Eriksson and Boreus, *Ther Drug Monit* 1997, **19**, 499–501). Carbamazepine reduces the half-life of lamotrigine from 29 hours to about 15 hours via enzyme induction (*Epilepsia Res* 1987, **1**, 194–201).

Fosphenytoin + lamotrigine

See phenytoin + lamotrigine.

Levetiracetam + lamotrigine *

See levetiracetam (*4.5.5*).

Oral contraceptives + lamotrigine

No interaction occurs (*Epilepsia* 1991, **32**[Suppl 1], 96).

Oxcarbazepine + lamotrigine *

See oxcarbazepine (*4.5.6*).

Phenytoin + lamotrigine

Lamotrigine has no effect on phenytoin but phenytoin reduces the half-life of lamotrigine from 29 hours to about 15 hours via enzyme induction (*Epilepsia Res* 1987, **1**, 194–201).

Sertraline + lamotrigine

Sertraline may increase lamotrigine levels. A case of sertraline 25mg/d doubling lamotrigine levels and another of a 25mg/d dose reduction halving levels (despite a 33% lamotrigine dose increase) has been reported (Kaufman and Gerner, *Seizure* 1998, **7**, 163–65).

VALPROATE + LAMOTRIGINE *

Lamotrigine has no effect *on* valproate but valproate inhibits lamotrigine glucuronidation resulting in reduced clearance (by 21%), and half-life lengthening from 29 hours to about 59 hours (eg. Panay *et al, Lancet* 1993, **341**, 445), probably a dose-dependent effect (n=28, Kanner and Frey, *Neurology* 2000, **55**, 588–91) rather than concentration-dependent (n=62, Gidal *et al, Epilepsy Res* 2000, **42**, 23–31). Doses of lamotrigine should start at half the usual dose when used with valproate. The interaction has been used to enhance the effect of both drugs with striking responses in adults and children with intractible epilepsy (Pisani *et al, Lancet* 1993, **341**, 1224), although disabling postural and action tremor has been reported (n=3, Reutens *et al, Lancet* 1993, **342**, 185–86), as has a raised incidence of rash. In one study, adding lamotrigine to valproate was without incident in 76%, but with an increased incidence of rash and other adverse effects in the remainder (n=112, Faught *et al, Epilepsia* 1999, **40**, 1135–40). There is a case of lupus anticoagulant induced by the combination of valproate and lamotrigine in a 5-year-old boy (n=1, Echaniz-Laguna *et al, Epilepsia* 1999, **40**, 1661–63).

Zotepine + lamotrigine

See zotepine (*4.2.6*).

4.5.5 LEVETIRACETAM *

Levetiracetam has, as yet, no demonstrable drug interactions. It is not bound to plasma proteins, is not extensively metabolised and does not inhibit nor induce P450 (1A2, 2A6, 2C8/9/10, 2C19, 2D6, 2E1 and 3A4) nor UGT enzymes.

Alcohol + levetiracetam *

No data is available (MI).

Carbamazepine + levetiracetam *

Lack of pharmacokinetic interaction has been demonstrated (MI).

Digoxin + levetiracetam *

Lack of pharmacokinetic interaction has been demonstrated (MI).

Food + levetiracetam *

Levetiracetam absorption is slightly slowed by food, but total absorption remains unchanged.

Gabapentin + levetiracetam *

Lack of pharmacokinetic interaction has been demonstrated (MI).

Lamotrigine + levetiracetam *

Lack of pharmacokinetic interaction has been demonstrated (MI).

Oral contraceptives+levetiracetam *

Lack of pharmacokinetic interaction has been demonstrated (MI).

Phenobarbital + levetiracetam *

Lack of pharmacokinetic interaction has been demonstrated (MI).

Phenytoin + levetiracetam *

Levetiracetam has no effect on the kinetics of phenytoin (n=6, Browne *et al, J Clin Pharmacol* 2000, **40**, 590–95).

Primidone + levetiracetam *

Lack of pharmacokinetic interaction has been demonstrated (MI).

Probenecid + levetiracetam *

Probenecid may inhibit the clearance of the primary (inactive) metabolite of levetiracetam, but not of the parent drug (MI).

Valproate + levetiracetam *

Lack of pharmacokinetic interaction has been demonstrated (MI).

Warfarin + levetiracetam *

Lack of pharmacokinetic interaction has been demonstrated (MI).

Zotepine + levetiracetam*

See zotepine (*4.2.6*).

4.5.6 OXCARBAZEPINE *

Some enzyme induction has been suggested at higher doses (Patsalos *et al, Eur J Clin Pharmacol* 1990, **39**, 187–88), but not lower doses (n=8, Larkin *et al, Br J Clin Pharmacol* 1991, **31**, 65–71). Oxcarbazepine and MHD inhibit cytochrome CYP2C19 and induce CYP3A4 and CYP3A5

Alcohol + oxcarbazepine *

Caution should be exercised if alcohol is taken (SPC) as additive sedation can occur.

Antipsychotics + oxcarbazepine *

It should be well known that carbamazepine reduces the plasma levels of many antipsychotics. As oxcarbazepine seems to have little enzyme-inducing activity, when substituted for carbamazepine, it can lead to plasma levels of antipsychotics increasing by 50–200% over 2–4 weeks (Raitasuo *et al, Psychopharmacology* [*Berl*] 1994, **116**, 115–16).

Carbamazepine + oxcarbazepine *

Addition of oxcarbazepine to carbamazepine has resulted in a less than 10% change in carbamazepine plasma levels (US SPC).

Cimetidine + oxcarbazepine *

Cimetidine has no effect on the kinetics of oxcarbazepine (n=8, c/o, Keranen *et al, Acta Neurol Scand* 1992, **85**, 239–42).

Citalopram + oxcarbazepine *

Carbamazepine may induce the plasma levels of citalopram, and when oxcarbazepine is substituted, citalopram plasma levels may rise (n=2, Leinonen *et al, Pharmacopsychiatry* 1996, **29**, 156–58).

Erythromycin + oxcarbazepine *

Erythromycin has no effect on the kinetics of oxcarbazepine (n=8, c/o, Keranen *et al, Acta Neurol Scand* 1992, **86**, 120–23).

Felodipine + oxcarbazepine *

Repeated doses of oxcarbazepine reduced felodipine AUC and plasma levels by 28% and 34% respectively, which might slightly reduce its clinical effect (n=8, open, Zaccara *et al, Ther Drug Monit* 1993, **15**, 39–42).

Fosphenytoin + oxcarbazepine *

See phenytoin + oxcarbazepine.

Lamotrigine + oxcarbazepine *

Oxcarbazepine induces the metabolism of lamotrigine, and so plasma levels fall by 29%. Reduced doses may be necessary if oxcarbazepine is discontinued (n=222, May *et al, Therap Drug Monit* 1999, **21**, 175–81).

Lithium + oxcarbazepine *

The combination of lithium and oxcarbazepine might theoretically cause enhanced neurotoxicity (SPC).

MAOIs + oxcarbazepine *

A theoretical risk of interaction exists (SPC).

ORAL CONTRACEPTIVES + OXCARBAZEPINE *

Oxcarbazepine can produce significant reductions in some OC plasma levels, with some breakthrough bleeping (n=10, Klosterskov-Jensen *et al, Epilepsia* 1992, **33**, 1149–52; RCT, n=16, Fattore *et al, Epilepsia* 1999, **40**, 783–87). Increased doses of ethinyl-estradiol and levonorgestrel or additional non-hormonal contraception are recommended with oxcarbazepine.

Phenobarbital + oxcarbazepine *

Phenobarbital levels raised by 14% and reduced oxcarbazepine/MHD levels by 25% have been observed with the combination (US SPC). The clinical significance has not been quantified.

Phenytoin + oxcarbazepine *

Doses of oxcarbazepine above 1200mg/d have been reported to increase phenytoin levels by up to 40% (less than 10% for doses below 1200mg/d) and so close monitoring of phenytoin is essential, especially at higher doses (Patsalos *et al, Eur J Clin Pharmacol* 1990, **39**, 187–88).

Propoxyphene + oxcarbazepine *

Unlike carbamazepine, propoxyphene has no significant effect on oxcarbazepine kinetics (n=8, Morgensen *et al, Acta Neurol Scand* 1992, **85**, 14–17).

Valproate + oxcarbazepine *

Valproate levels may rise if oxcarbazepine replaces carbamazepine (n=4, Patsalos *et al, Eur J Clin Pharmacol* 1990, **39**, 187–88). There is a theoretical increase in the risk of teratogenicity with the combination, due to the presence of increased levels of metabolites.

Verapamil + oxcarbazepine *

Verapamil can produce a 20% reduction in MHD levels, which could be clinically significant (US SPC).

Warfarin + oxcarbazepine *

Oxcarbazepine does not appear to affect the anticoagulant activity of warfarin (n=10, Kramer *et al, Epilepsia* 1992, **33**, 1145–48).

Zotepine + oxcarbazepine *

See zotepine (*4.2.6*).

4.5.7 PHENOBARBITAL (phenobarbitone) AND PRIMIDONE

ALCOHOL + BARBITURATES

See alcohol (*4.7.1*).

ANTICOAGULANTS + BARBITURATES

A well-documented and clinically significant reduction in anticoagulant levels and effects with barbiturates occurs. Doses of the anticoagulant may need to be raised by up to 60% if a barbiturate is started.

ANTIPSYCHOTICS + BARBITURATES

See antipsychotics (*4.2.1*).

Benzodiazepines + barbiturates

See benzodiazepines (*4.1.1*).

Beta-blockers + barbiturates

Blood levels of metoprolol and propranolol are reduced by barbiturates (Seideman *et al, B J Clin Pharmacol* 1987, **23**, 267). Those of timolol (Mantyla *et al, Eur J Clin Pharmacol* 1983, **24**, 227), atenolol and nadolol do not appear to be altered.

Bupropion + phenobarbital *

See bupropion (*4.6.4*).

CALCIUM-CHANNEL BLOCKERS + BARBITURATES

Phenobarbital may induce the CYP3A4 metabolism of verapamil (Rutledge *et al, J Pharmacol Exp Therap* 1988, **7**, 246), diltiazem, isradipine, nicardipine and nifedipine, reducing efficacy and so some care may be needed.

Carbamazepine + phenobarbital

See carbamazepine (*4.5.1*).

Charcoal, activated + barbiturates

If given within 5 minutes, activated charcoal can almost completely prevent barbiturate absorption and can be an effective adjunct in overdose treatment (Neuvonen *et al, Eur J Clin Pharmacol* 1980, **17**, 51).

Chloramphenicol + barbiturates

Chloramphenicol metabolism is accelerated by barbiturates to reduce oral chloramphenicol efficacy (*Clin Pharmacol Ther* 1978, **24**, 571).

Cimetidine + phenobarbital
Reduced actions of both can occur but this is of very limited significance (*Eur J Clin Pharmacol* 1981, **19**, 343).

Clozapine + phenobarbital
See clozapine (*4.2.2*).

CORTICOSTEROIDS + PHENOBARBITAL
CYP3A4 induction reduces the effect of some corticosteroids (*NEJM* 1972, **286**, 1125).

CYCLOSPORIN + PHENOBARBITAL
Even low dose phenobarbital induces the CYP3A4 metabolism of cyclosporin (Brooks *et al, B J Clin Pharmacol* 1986, **21**, 550–51).

Digitoxin + phenobarbital
Digitoxin (but not digoxin) levels can be reduced by up to 50% by phenobarbital, probably via enzyme induction (*Int J Clin Pharmacol* 1975, **12**, 403).

Disopyramide + phenobarbital
Disopyramide CYP3A4 metabolism is accelerated by barbiturates, reducing plasma levels (*Br J Clin Pharmac* 1987, **24**, 781–91).

Doxorubicin + phenobarbital
Indirect results from one study showed that doxorubicin clearance may be increased by barbiturates and so doses may need to be increased (Riggs *et al, Clin Pharmacol Ther* 1982, **31**, 263).

Doxycycline + phenobarbital
Doxycycline metabolism is accelerated by barbiturates, reducing its effect, with a halved half-life (Neuvonen and Penttila, *BMJ* 1974, **2**, 470). Other tetracyclines appear not to interact.

Ethosuximide + phenobarbital
A possible interaction may lead to reduced phenobarbital effectiveness. A study showed that ethosuximide levels may fall if primidone is used (n=198, *Clin Pharmacokinet* 1982, **7**, 176–80).

Fenoprofen + phenobarbital
Phenobarbital may slightly increase fenoprofen elimination and reduce its efficacy (Helleberg *et al, B J Clin Pharmacol* 1974, **1**, 371).

Furosemide (frusemide) + phenobarbital
One study showed no effect of barbiturates on furosemide diuresis (Lambert *et al, Clin Pharmacol Ther* 1983, **34**, 170).

Gabapentin + phenobarbital
See gabapentin (*4.5.3*).

Glyceryl trinitrate + phenobarbital
A reduced nitrate effect via enzyme induction may occur.

Griseofulvin + phenobarbital
Cases of griseofulvin levels reduced by up to 45% by phenobarbital, either by enzyme induction, eg. (*Am J Hosp Pharm* 1986, **16**, 52) or reduced absorption have been reported.

Indinavir + barbiturates
The BNF notes that the plasma levels of indinavir may be reduced by barbiturates via CYP3A4 induction.

Influenza vaccine + phenobarbital
A transient 20% rise in barbiturate levels occurred in one study (*Clin Pharm* 1986, **5**, 817–20).

Isoniazid + primidone
Steady state primidone levels rose by 80% in a patient given isoniazid 300mg/d (n=1, *Neurology* 1975, **25**, 1179). Blood levels should be monitored.

Ketoconazole + phenobarbital
A single case exists of reduced ketoconazole levels in a man taking phenobarbital (*Antimicrob Ag Chemother* 1982, **21**, 151–58).

Lamotrigine + barbiturates
See lamotrigine (*4.5.4*).

Levetiracetam + phenobarbital *
See levetiracetam (*4.5.5*).

Levonorgestrel + phenobarbital
There is a case of levonorgestrel implant (Norplant) failing twice in a woman also taking phenobarbital (Shane-McWhorter *et al, Pharmacotherapy* 1998, **18**, 1360–64).

Levothyroxine (thyroxine) + barbiturates
Levothyroxine metabolism is accelerated by barbiturates to give a reduced effect and this may increase requirements in hypothyroidism.

Lidocaine + barbiturates
Serum lidocaine levels may be lower in people taking barbiturates than in those not (*Toxicol Appl Pharmacol* 1978, **44**, 657), via CYP3A4 induction.

MAOIs + barbiturates
See MAOIs (*4.3.4*).

Methadone + phenobarbital
Reduced methadone levels have been

reported (eg. *Clin Pharmacol Ther* 1988, **43**, 623–29, n=1, Liu and Wang, *Am J Psych* 1984, **141**, 1287–88).

Methyldopa + phenobarbital

Methyldopa levels are not reduced by phenobarbital (eg. Kristensen *et al, BMJ* 1973, **1**, 49).

Metronidazole + phenobarbital

One study showed metronidazole metabolism to be accelerated by barbiturates, giving levels reduced by a third (*Clin Pharmacol Ther* 1987, **41**, 235).

Nicotinamide + primidone

There is one reported case of interaction (*Neurology* 1982, **32**, 1122).

NICOUMALONE + BARBITURATES

Nicoumalone metabolism is accelerated by barbiturates, giving a reduced anti-coagulant effect.

ORAL CONTRACEPTIVES + PHENOBARBITAL

Contraceptive failure via CYP3A4 enzyme induction has been reported many times (reviewed in *B J Clin Pharmacol* 1990, **30**, 892–96). Use higher dose OC (equivalent to 50–100mcg ethinyl-estradiol, eg. Eugynon-50) and adjust the dose if necessary or use alternative contraceptive methods. See also levonorgestrel.

Oxcarbazepine + phenobarbital *

See oxcarbazepine (*4.5.6*).

Paracetamol + phenobarbital

An isolated case of enhanced hepato-toxicity exists (*Ann Int Med* 1984, **101**, 403).

Paroxetine + phenobarbital

See paroxetine (*4.3.2.4*).

Pethidine + phenobarbital

A single case of severe CNS sedation on the combination has been reported (*J Clin Pharmacol* 1978, **18**, 482).

Phenylbutazone + phenobarbital

Reduced levels of phenylbutazone may occur (*Lancet* 1968, **i**, 1275).

Phenytoin + phenobarbital

See barbiturates + phenytoin (*4.5.8*).

Pyridoxine + phenobarbital

Large doses of pyridoxine (eg. 200mg/d) can reduce phenobarbital levels by up to 40–50% (*Lancet* 1976 **i**, 256).

Quetiapine + barbiturates

See quetiapine (*4.2.4*).

Quinidine + phenobarbital

CYP3A4 induction may reduce quinidine levels by up to 50% (*Drug Intell Clin Pharm* 1983, **17**, 819–20).

Rifampicin + barbiturates

Rifampicin has been shown to induce barbiturate metabolism and so a decreased efficacy might be predicted (for effect on hexobarbital, see Richter *et al, Eur J Clin Pharmacol* 1980, **17**, 197).

Smoking + phenobarbital

See smoking (*4.7.3*).

Sulphonamides + barbiturates

No reports of interaction exist.

Testosterone + phenobarbital

A reduced steroid effect via CYP3A4 induction can occur.

THEOPHYLLINE + BARBITURATES

Theophylline metabolism is accelerated by barbiturates, giving a reduced effect (*Ther Drug Monit* 1990, **12**, 139–43).

Tiagabine + barbiturate

See tiagabine (*4.5.10*).

Topiramate + phenobarbital

See topiramate (*4.5.11*).

TRICYCLICS + BARBITURATES

See tricyclics (*4.3.1*).

Tropisetron + barbiturates

Phenobarbital reduces the plasma levels of tropisetron (BNF).

WARFARIN + PHENOBARBITAL

See anticoagulants + barbiturates in this section.

VALPROATE + PHENOBARBITAL

Valproate may reduce glucuronidation and increase phenobarbital plasma concentrations by up to 25% (mean of 5.87mg/L, n=20, Bernus *et al, B J Clin Pharmacol* 1994, **38**, 411–16), increasing sedation and other side-effects (eg. Kapetanovic *et al, Clin Pharmacol Ther* 1981, **99**, 314), although this may only be transient (*Drug Intell Clin Pharm* 1982, **16**, 737–39). Thus, reduce the pheno-barbital dosage if sedation occurs and monitor blood levels regularly. Indeed, phenobarbital dose reduction by a third or a half may be possible without loss of seizure control (Wilder *et al, Neurology* 1978, **28**, 892).

Vigabatrin + phenobarbital

See vigabatrin (*4.5.13*).

Zaleplon + phenobarbital

See zaleplon (*4.1.6*).

Zotepine + phenobarbital

See zotepine (*4.2.6*).

4.5.8 PHENYTOIN

Phenytoin is prone to drug-drug interactions via several mechanisms, eg. its narrow therapeutic index, extensive binding to plasma proteins, CYP3A4 induction and saturable metabolism. It can be displaced, giving an increased proportion of free active phenytoin, significant where TDM just measures **total** phenytoin rather than the proportion of free (hence active) phenytoin. Measuring free phenytoin levels may be more appropriate in certain circumstances, eg. interaction with drugs displacing it from binding sites, as well as hypoalbuminaemia and renal failure, eg. total plasma levels may be within the alleged therapeutic range. Decreased protein binding produces a decline in total concentration, but no change in free levels (Wilkinson, *Pharmacol Rev* 1987, **39**, 1–47). Thus, low concentrations may appear below the normal therapeutic range, but free (active) levels are appropriate, prompting inappropriately increased doses or discontinuation. More usual concentrations could have toxic (seizure-inducing) free levels, which might then provoke a disastrous increase in dosage to bring it into the 'optimum' range (see Toler, *Ann Pharmacother* 1994, **28**, 808–9).

Review: pharmacokinetic interactions (Nation *et al, Clin Pharmacokinet* 1990, **18**, 37–60).

Acetazolamide + phenytoin

Case reports indicate that acetazolamide may enhance the osteomalacia secondary to phenytoin use in a few patients (*Arch Int Med* 1977, **137**, 1013).

ALCOHOL + PHENYTOIN

See alcohol (*4.7.1*).

Allopurinol + phenytoin *

Phenytoin toxicity may occur with repeated high-dose allopurinol (Ogiso et al, *et al, J Pharmacobiodyn* 1990, **13**, 36–43).

AMIODARONE + PHENYTOIN

Amiodarone reduces phenytoin metabolism, toxicity developing over 2 weeks (n=7, *Am J Cardiol* 1990, **65**,

1252–57). Reduce the phenytoin dose by at least 25%.

Anaesthetics + phenytoin

Documentation of an interaction is limited but case reports of phenytoin toxicity following halothane exist (*J Pediat* 1970, **76**, 941) and so caution should be used.

Antacids + phenytoin

Antacids probably reduce phenytoin levels, shown in several studies (eg. *Br J Clin Pharmacol* 1982, **13**, 501) and seizure control could be impaired. It is thus best to separate doses by about three hours or use ranitidine (see also cimetidine).

ANTIPSYCHOTICS + PHENYTOIN

See antipsychotics (*4.2.1*) and risperidone (*4.2.5*).

Ayurvedic herbal mixtures + phenytoin *

See shankhapushpi + phenytoin.

Barbiturates + phenytoin

At normal doses it is thought that the tendency is for phenobarbital to enhance the metabolism of phenytoin, reducing levels. The clinical effect may be minimal (*Neurology* 1988, **38**, 639–42). Phenytoin serum levels are increased by very high dose barbiturates and the effect may be dose-dependent with a curvilinear relationship (Kuranari *et al, Ann Pharmacother* 1995, **29**, 83–84). Care may also be needed if phenobarbital is stopped, as phenytoin levels may rise. Conversely, one study showed that phenytoin may raise phenobarbital levels by up to 100%, producing increased sedation. This is probably of minor clinical significance (*B J Clin Pharmacol* 1982, **14**, 294) but regular monitoring should still be done. As a case of fatal agranulocytosis in an epileptic taking primidone and phenytoin has been reported regular monitoring of longer-term therapy would thus be wise (Letter by Laurenson et al, *Lancet* 1994, **344**, 332–33).

Benzodiazepines + phenytoin

Diazepam, clonazepam and chlordiazepoxide have been reported to potentiate phenytoin leading to possible intoxication although some studies have not shown this effect. It is best to monitor phenytoin plasma levels regularly.

Conversely, phenytoin induces the metabolism of clonazepam, reducing levels by up to 50% (*Eur J Clin Pharmacol* 1975, **8**, 249).

Bupropion + phenytoin *

See bupropion (*4.6.4*).

Buspirone + phenytoin

See buspirone (*4.1.2*).

Calcium-channel blockers + phenytoin *

High dose **diltiazem** (240mg 8hourly) increases phenytoin levels and toxicity and in one patient a 40% reduction in phenytoin dose was needed to stabilise levels (Clarke *et al, Pharmacotherapy* 1993, **13**, 402–5; *Neurology* 1991, **41**, 740–42). Lack of interaction between **nifedipine** and phenytoin has been noted in several studies (eg. Schellens *et al, B J Clin Pharmacol* 1991, **31**, 175–78; *Neurology* 1991, **41**, 740–42), although tremor, headache and restlessness with phenytoin levels tripled has been reported, which fell to normal after the nifedipine was discontinued (n=1, Ahmad *et al, J Am Coll Cardiol* 1984, **3**, 1581). **Verapamil** may inhibit phenytoin metabolism (*Lancet* 1986, **i**, 700–7; *Neurology* 1991, **41**, 740–42). Almost complete lack of verapamil absorption (at up to 400mg/d) has been reported (n=1, *NEJM* 1991, **325**, 1179). The effects of **isradipine** and **nicardipine** may be reduced by phenytoin.

CARBAMAZEPINE + PHENYTOIN

See carbamazepine (*4.5.1*).

Charcoal, activated + phenytoin

Phenytoin absorption is almost completely (98%) prevented if activated charcoal is taken within 5 minutes. Phenytoin absorption is reduced by about 80% if the charcoal is given after one hour (Neuvonen *et al, Eur J Clin Pharmacol* 1978, **13**, 213). Multiple-dose activated charcoal has been used successfully over several days for phenytoin toxicity secondary to hepatitis and thus, extraordinarily, may have some use even up to a week after phenytoin ingestion (Howard *et al, Ann Pharmacother* 1994, **28**, 201–3).

Chinese medicines + phenytoin *

Phenytoin poisoning after using Chinese proprietary medicines has been reported (Lau *et al, Hum & Experimental Toxicol* 2000, **19**, 385–86).

Chloral + phenytoin

Dichloralphenazone has been shown to decrease phenytoin levels in a five-patient study (Riddell *et al, B J Clin Pharmacol* 1980, **9**, 118P), although whether the chloral part of the molecule was responsible for this is not known.

CHLORAMPHENICOL + PHENYTOIN

Phenytoin toxicity may occur with oral chloramphenicol via enzyme inhibition (*Aust J Hosp Pharm* 1987, **17**, 51–53). This is an uncommon combination but a well-documented and serious interaction. Monitor very carefully if the combination has to be used.

Chlorphenamine (chlorpheniramine) + phenytoin

Two isolated cases exist of phenytoin intoxication (*Br J Clin Pharmac* 1975, **2,** 173) and so care may be needed.

Ciprofloxacin + phenytoin

Phenytoin toxicity would be expected to occur via P450 enzyme inhibition, and raised phenytoin levels from oral ciprofloxacin has been reported (n=1, Hull, *Ann Pharmacother* 1993, **27**, 1283). Several cases exist, however, of reduced phenytoin levels, dropping by a half (n=1, *Int Pharm J* 1992, **6**, 109), and resulting in sub-therapeutic levels, seizures and increased phenytoin dose requirements with IV ciprofloxacin (*Ann Pharmacother* 1992, **26**, 263; n=1, Brouwers and de Boer, *Ann Pharmacother* 1997, **31**, 498). There is a case of phenytoin dose increased during ciprofloxacin therapy, only for toxic levels to appear when the antibiotic course was completed (n=1, Pollak and Slayter, *Ann Pharmacother* 1997, **31**, 61–64). More frequent phenytoin plasma level monitoring would be wise.

Clinafloxacin + phenytoin *

A slight decrease in phenytoin clearance but a 20% higher steady state plasma level has been reported, and so additional monitoring and dosage adjustments are recommended (Randinitis *et al, Drugs* 1999, **58**[Suppl 2], 254–55).

CLOZAPINE + PHENYTOIN

See clozapine (*4.2.2*).

CORTICOSTEROIDS + PHENYTOIN

Steroid metabolism is accelerated by phenytoin to give a reduced effect (*Lancet* 1978, **i**, 1096) and so higher doses may be needed. Hydrocortisone may be less affected than other steroids. Phenytoin levels may also be changed.

Co-trimoxazole + phenytoin

A single case exists of phenytoin intoxication caused by increased plasma phenytoin levels and an enhanced antifolate effect (*Arch Int Med* 1985, **102**, 509).

CYCLOSPORIN + PHENYTOIN

Cyclosporin levels can be reduced by 80% by phenytoin, via increased metabolism (*B J Clin Pharmacol* 1984, **18**, 887–93).

Cytotoxics + phenytoin

Increased phenytoin clearance has occurred (n=1, *J Paediatrics* 1988, **112**, 996–99).

DEXAMETHASONE + PHENYTOIN *

Variable phenytoin levels have been reported with dexamethasone. Phenytoin levels may be halved by dexamethasone (eg. Wong *et al, JAMA* 1985, **254**, 2062–63; Lackner, *Pharmacother* 1991, **11**, 344–47; n=1, Griffiths and Taylor, *Can J Hosp Pharm* 1999, **52**, 96–98) and very high doses of phenytoin may be necessary (eg. 900mg/d) to maintain levels if dexamethasone is used concomitantly (case and review by Recueno *et al, Ann Pharmacother* 1995, **29**, 935). Regular and frequent monitoring of phenytoin levels is thus essential.

Dextropropoxyphene + phenytoin

See propoxyphene + phenytoin.

DIAZOXIDE + PHENYTOIN

Reduced phenytoin levels occur via increased metabolism (*J Pediatr* 1976, **89**, 331; Turck *et al, Presse Med* 1986, **15**, 31) so monitor carefully.

DICOUMAROL + PHENYTOIN

Phenytoin levels may rise rapidly by over 100% (*Lancet* 1966, **ii**, 265; Hansen *et al, Acta Med Scand* 1971, **189**, 15–19) via enzyme inhibition. Avoid the combination if at all possible or monitor very carefully.

Digoxin + phenytoin

Phenytoin reduces digoxin half-life by 30% (*E J Clin Pharmacol* 1985, **29**,

49–53) and also that of digitoxin, so monitor levels of both.

DISOPYRAMIDE + PHENYTOIN

Phenytoin reduces the plasma levels of disopyramide, possibly to below therapeutic levels (*Clin Pharm* 1982, **1**, 263–64).

Disulfiram + phenytoin

Phenytoin toxicity and delirium may occur via enzyme inhibition (n=1, Taylor *et al, Am J Hosp Pharm* 1981, **38**, 93–95; n=1, Brown *et al, Ann Emerg Med* 1983, **12**, 310–13).

Dopamine + phenytoin

A report has appeared of five cases of hypotension in patients on dopamine when phenytoin was added (Bivins *et al, Arch Surg* 1978, **113**, 245) although lack of interaction has been reported in a well studied single case (Torres *et al, Ann Pharmacother* 1995, **29**, 1300–1).

DOXYCYCLINE + PHENYTOIN

Doxycycline metabolism is accelerated by phenytoin to give a reduced effect, with a halved half-life (*BMJ* 1974, **ii**, 470). Other tetracyclines appear not to interact, so make dosage adjustments or use an alternative.

Enteral feeds + phenytoin

See nasogastric feeds + phenytoin.

Ethosuximide + phenytoin

See ethosuximide (*4.5.2*).

Famotidine + phenytoin

No significant interaction occurs (*Clin Pharmacol Ther* 1986, **39**, 225).

FLUCONAZOLE + PHENYTOIN

Oral fluconazole inhibits phenytoin metabolism producing rapid and severe toxicity (*BMJ* 1989, **298**, 1315; reviewed by Cadle *et al, Ann Pharmacother* 1994, **28**, 191–95). Continuous phenytoin plasma monitoring is recommended with doses of fluconazole at 200mg/d or above (study by Hutabarat *et al, Clin Pharmacol & Ther* 1991, **49**, 402–9).

FLUOXETINE + PHENYTOIN *

Phenytoin levels raised by 66% were seen in a woman taking phenytoin 370mg/d, 13 days after fluoxetine 20mg/d was added, with levels falling back to nearly normal within a week of stopping fluoxetine (Woods *et al, N Z Med J* 1994, **107**, 19). Conversely, loss of phenytoin efficacy as a result of fluoxetine discontinuation has been reported (n=1, Shad and Preskorn, *J Clin Psychopharmacol* 1999, **19**, 471).

Folic acid + phenytoin

Serum folate decreases when phenytoin is started and folic acid supplementation is usually used to counteract this folate deficiency. However, folic acid supplementation in folate-deficient patients changes the kinetics of phenytoin and plasma phenytoin levels are then reduced (Berg *et al, Ther Drug Monit* 1983, **5**, 389–99). Folate supplementation should thus be started with phenytoin. If started later, phenytoin levels should be monitored and changes in seizure activity looked for (extensive review by Lewis *et al, Ann Pharmacother* 1995, **29**, 726–35).

Furosemide (frusemide) + phenytoin *

The diuretic effect may be reduced by up to 50% by phenytoin (*Colloids and Surfaces* 1986, **19**, 83–88; Bissoli *et al, Recenti Prog Med* 1996, **87**, 227–28) so larger doses may be needed.

Gabapentin + phenytoin

See gabapentin (*4.5.3*).

Glucagon + phenytoin

Patients on phenytoin may get false negatives with glucagon stimulation tests (*Ann Int Med* 1974, **80**, 697).

Glucocorticoids + phenytoin

A reduced steroid effect via enzyme induction is possible.

Griseofulvin + phenytoin

It is postulated that reduced griseofulvin levels may occur, via enzyme induction (*Am J Hosp Pharm* 1986, **16**, 52).

H2-blockers + phenytoin *

Phenytoin toxicity has occurred with **cimetidine** (n=1, *Med J Aus* 1984, **141**, 602), with a 30% increase in phenytoin levels in other reports (*Pharm International* 1985, **6**, 223–24; *Epilepsia* 1983, **24**, 284–88) and so toxicity may occur, even with OTC cimetidine (n=9, Rafi *et al, Ann Pharmacother* 1999, **33**, 769–74), although this open study showed little overall detectable effect from cimetidine on phenytoin levels. The effect is rapid and can occur within two days. An alternative is ranitidine, where lack of interaction has been shown (*Aust*

NZ J Med 1983, **13**, 324, Watts *et al, B J Clin Pharmacol* 1983, **15**, 499–500). There have, however, been several cases of elevated phenytoin levels (eg. Tse *et al, Ann Pharmacother* 1993, **27**, 1448–51; Bramhall *et al, Drug Intell Clin Pharm* 1988, **22**, 979), including where oral ranitidine induced toxic phenytoin levels, remaining high for a week even though the phenytoin was stopped, and only dropping when the ranitidine was also stopped (Tse and Iagmin, *Ann Int Med* 1994, **120**, 892–93). Best to monitor phenytoin levels.

Indinavir + phenytoin

The BNF notes the possibility of reduced plasma indinavir level with phenytoin.

Influenza vaccine + phenytoin

This is reported to reduce total and free phenytoin levels (*Clin Pharm,* 1988, **7**, 828–32), although one study showed a transient 60% increase in levels (*Clin Pharm* 1986, **5**, 817–20).

ISONIAZID + PHENYTOIN

Phenytoin toxicity may occur via enzyme induction (*Drug Intell Clin Pharm* 1984, **18**, 483–86) so observe for toxicity and reduce phenytoin doses if necessary.

KETOCONAZOLE + PHENYTOIN

Phenytoin toxicity may occur via enzyme inhibition. Ketoconazole may also have a reduced effect.

Lamotrigine + phenytoin

See lamotrigine (*4.5.4*).

Levetiracetam + phenytoin *

See levetiracetam (*4.5.5*).

Levodopa + phenytoin

Levodopa can be completely antagonised by phenytoin (Mendez *et al, Arch Neurol* 1975, **32**, 44–46) and so increased levodopa doses may be necessary.

Levothyroxine (thyroxine) + phenytoin

Levothyroxine metabolism is accelerated by phenytoin, increasing requirements (*Ann Int Med* 1983, **99**, 341).

Lidocaine (lignocaine) + phenytoin

CNS effects may be enhanced if used concurrently (*Eur J Clin Pharmacol* 1974, **7**, 455). Sinoatrial arrest has been reported (Wood, *BMJ* 1971, **i**, 645) which was reversed by isoproterenol. The mechanism is probably enhanced cardiac depression so beware of possible toxicity.

Lithium + phenytoin

See lithium (*4.4*).

Methadone + phenytoin

Phenytoin may reduce methadone levels (*Clin Pharmacol Ther* 1988, **43,** 623–29). Dosage adjustment may be needed.

Methotrexate + phenytoin

An increased antifolate effect with phenytoin may occur.

Methylphenidate + phenytoin

Phenytoin toxicity has been reported (n=3, Ghofrani, *Dev Med Child Neurol* 1988, **30,** 267–68).

METRONIDAZOLE + PHENYTOIN

Mild phenytoin toxicity via enzyme inhibition is possible (*Clin Pharmacol Ther* 1988, **28,** 240–45) but the combination does not usually cause problems.

MEXILITINE + PHENYTOIN

Mexilitine levels are reduced by up to 50% via enzyme induction and so dosage adjustment may be necessary (*Br J Clin Pharmac* 1982, **14,** 219–23).

MICONAZOLE + PHENYTOIN

Two cases of phenytoin toxicity via enzyme inhibition have been reported (*BMJ* 1983, **287,** 1760).

Nasogastric feeds + phenytoin *

Reduced phenytoin levels have been reported with nasogastric feeds (eg. Fortison, Isocal, Osmolite, Ensure) and other enteral feeds (*Pharm J* 1989, **243,** 181; *Hosp Pharm* 1989, **24,** 562). One study showed that the absolute bioavailability of phenytoin acid and phenytoin sodium was unaffected by enteral feeds but that the absorption patterns were significantly different, with the sodium solution more rapidly absorbed (n=10, RCT, Doak *et al, Pharmacother* 1998, **18,** 637–45). Phenytoin dosage should be spaced to one hour before feeding or two hours after feeding (tube may need to be clamped). Monitor plasma levels frequently (see comment by Au Yeung and Ensom, *Ann Pharmacother* 2000, **34,** 896–905, 32 refs).

Nefazodone + phenytoin

Single doses of nefazodone have no effect on phenytoin kinetics (n=18,

Marino *et al, J Clin Psychopharmacol* 1997, **17,** 27–33), but multiple doses might.

Neuromuscular blocking agents + phenytoin

Phenytoin reduces the effects of most NMBAs, eg. pancuronium (*Anaesthesia* 1988, **43,** 757–59) and vecuronium (n=100, Ornstein *et al, Anesthesiology* 1987, **67,** 191–96), although atracurium appears not affected (*Anesthesiology* 1987, **67,** A607).

NICOUMALONE + PHENYTOIN

The metabolism of nicoumalone is accelerated by phenytoin reducing its effect, although enhancement has also been reported.

Nitrofurantoin + phenytoin

There is a single case report of a stable epileptic developing seizures when nitrofurantoin was added, requiring increased phenytoin dosage (Heipertz and Pilz, *J Neurol* 1978, **218,** 297–301).

Nizatidine + phenytoin

A lack of effect of nizatidine on phenytoin kinetics has been reported (Bachmann *et al, B J Clin Pharmacol* 1993, **36,** 380–82).

NSAIDs + phenytoin *

One study shows no interaction to occur with **ibuprofen** (*B J Clin Pharmacol* 1986, **21,** 165–69) but a single case of toxicity has been reported (Sandyk, *S Afr Med J* 1982, **62,** 592). There is a case report of plasma phenytoin levels increased by **aspirin** via binding displacement (*Clin Pharmacol Ther* 1981, **29,** 260), free levels seeming to remain constant. Transient toxicity may be the only effect and then only at high (900mg 4hrly) aspirin doses. Plasma phenytoin levels may be increased by **azapropazone** via enzyme inhibition (*Br J Clin Pharmac* 1983, **15,** 727–34).

ORAL CONTRACEPTIVES + PHENYTOIN

Contraceptive failure via enzyme induction has been reported many times (eg. *JAMA* 1986, **256,** 238–40) so use higher dose OCs or alternative contraceptive methods.

Oxcarbazepine + phenytoin *

See oxcarbazepine (*4.5.6*).

Paroxetine + phenytoin

See paroxetine (*4.3.2.4*).

Pethidine + phenytoin

Attenuation of pethidine's effect via enzyme induction, with increased metabolite levels, is possible (*Clin Pharmacol Ther* 1981, **29**, 273).

Phenindione + phenytoin

No interaction is thought to occur (*Acta Med Scand* 1976, **199**, 513).

PHENYLBUTAZONE + PHENYTOIN

Phenytoin toxicity may occur via enzyme inhibition and plasma protein displacement (*Eur J Clin Pharmacol* 1979, **15**, 263). Dosage adjustment may be necessary.

PROGABIDE + PHENYTOIN

Phenytoin levels may rise by up to 40% (*Epilepsia* 1987, **28**, 68–73).

Propoxyphene + phenytoin

Large doses of propoxyphene may raise phenytoin levels (Kutt *et al, Ann NY Acad Sci* 1971, **179**, 704) but normal doses have little or no effect (Hansen *et al, Acta Neurol Scand* 1980, **61**, 357).

Proton pump inhibitors + phenytoin

A lack of effect of **omeprazole** on phenytoin kinetics has been reported (Bachmann *et al, Br J Clin Pharmacol* 1993, **36**, 380–82), as has a mild rise in phenytoin levels (*Br J Clin Pharmac* 1987, **24**, 534–35). The SPC for omeprazole states that patients should be monitored on this combination and doses adjusted if necessary. Lack of interaction has been reported with **pantoprazole** (Middle *et al, Int J Clin Pharmacol Ther* 1996, **34**, S72–S75).

Pyrimethamine + phenytoin

There is an increased risk of an antifolate effect.

Pyridoxine + phenytoin

Large doses of pyridoxine (eg. 200mg/d) can reduce phenytoin levels by up to 40–50% (*Lancet* 1976, **i**, 256). Monitoring levels would thus be wise.

Quetiapine + phenytoin

See quetiapine (*4.2.4*).

QUINIDINE + PHENYTOIN

A reduced quinidine effect may occur via enzyme induction (*NEJM* 1983, **308**, 725) so monitoring of quinidine levels/effect may be necessary.

RIFAMPICIN + PHENYTOIN

Significant reductions in phenytoin levels may occur via enzyme induction (*BMJ* 1988, **297**, 1048).

Sertraline + phenytoin

See sertraline (*4.3.2.5*).

Shankhapushpi + phenytoin *

It has been recommended to avoid the Ayurvedic herbal mixture shankhapushpi, as decreased plasma phenytoin levels may occur, although no reference is quoted (mentioned by Fugh-Berman, *Lancet* 2000, **355**, 134–38).

Statins + phenytoin *

There is a case of phenytoin reducing the therapeutic effect of simvastatin and atorvastatin, probably via 3A4 induction (n=1, Murphy and Dominiczak, *Postgrad Med J* 1999, **75**, 359–60).

SUCRALFATE + PHENYTOIN

One study showed a small reduction in phenytoin bioavailability (*Drug Intell Clin Pharm* 1986, **20**, 607–11) by decreased absorption. This can be avoided by giving phenytoin two hours or more after sucralfate.

SULPHINPYRAZONE + PHENYTOIN

Raised phenytoin levels can occur (*Clin Pharmacokinet* 1982, **7**, 42–56) via P450 inhibition.

Sulphonamides + phenytoin

Phenytoin toxicity is known to be possible via P450 inhibition with co-trimoxazole (*Ann Int Med* 1985, **102**, 559; Paxton, *NZ Med J* 1981, **94**, 396–97) and other sulphonamides so monitor plasma levels and reduce phenytoin doses if necessary.

Terfenadine + phenytoin

No interaction occurs (Coniglio *et al, Epilepsia* 1989, **30**, 611–16).

Theophylline + phenytoin

Phenytoin produces a 45% increase in clearance of theophylline so higher doses may be needed (*Clin Pharmacol Ther* 1984, **35**, 666–69). Phenytoin absorption may also be reduced (*Int Pharm J* 1989, **3**, 98–101). Separating the doses by 1–2 hours may reduce the effect.

Tiagabine + phenytoin

See tiagabine (*4.5.10*).

Ticlodipine + phenytoin *

Ticlodipine 500mg/d inhibits phenytoin clearance so dose adjustment and careful monitoring should be considered (n=6, Donahue *et al, Clin Pharmacol & Therapeut* 1999, **66**, 563–68; n=1, Privitera and Welty, *Arch Neurology* 1996, **53**, 1191–92).

Tolbutamide + phenytoin *

Mild phenytoin toxicity may occur via increased free levels (Beech *et al, BMJ* 1988, **297**, 1613–14; n=18, Tassaneeyakul *et al, B J Clin Pharmacol* 1992, **34**, 494–98).

Topiramate + phenytoin

See topiramate (*4.5.11*).

Trazodone + phenytoin

There is an isolated case of phenytoin toxicity developing when relatively high dose trazodone was added to therapy (Dorn, *J Clin Psych* 1986, **47**, 89).

TRIMETHOPRIM + PHENYTOIN

Plasma phenytoin levels and the anti-folate effect may be increased by trimethoprim.

TRICYCLICS + PHENYTOIN

Phenytoin levels may be raised by imipramine (Perucca & Richens, *Br J Clin Pharmac* 1977, **4**, 485), but not nortriptyline (*Int J Clin Pharmacol* 1975, **12**, 210) nor amitriptyline (*Clin Pharmacol Ther* 1975, **18**, 191). Phenytoin levels may need to be monitored frequently. Tricyclics may lower the seizure threshold.

VALPROATE + PHENYTOIN

Valproate inhibits phenytoin metabolism and competes for its binding sites. If enzyme saturation has not occurred then this displacement of phenytoin leads to decreased bound but increased free phenytoin. More phenytoin is then metabolised so the net result is reduced total and bound concentrations. The free concentration will remain about the same and **lower** plasma levels will still contain about the same amount of active/free drug. Thus, beware of raising the dose of phenytoin to bring the total plasma concentration into the 'therapeutic range' as it would then be toxic (*Drug Intell Clin Pharm* 1982, **16,** 737–39). If the enzyme is saturated, then displacement may lead to a stable total concentration but decreased bound and increased free phenytoin (Johnson *et al B J Clin Pharmacol* 1989, **27**, 843–49). This could lead to toxic effects within the therapeutic range. In practice, phenytoin levels tend to fall initially by up to 50%, then return to normal over about five weeks. Toxicity is possible if levels were higher at the start. Reports of a toxic interaction are not common but monitoring is essential. Of the two main methods for calculating the unbound phenytoin concentrations in patients also receiving valproate, the Haidukewych method (*Ther Drug Monit* 1989, **11**, 134–39) has been shown to be more accurate (n=88, Kerrick *et al, Ann Pharmacother* 1995, **29**, 470–74). Finally, changing valproate from a standard tablet to a slow-release tablet has been shown to result in a 30% rise in phenytoin levels and toxicity (n=11, Suzuki *et al, Eur J Clin Pharmacol* 1995, **48**, 61–63).

VIGABATRIN + PHENYTOIN

Vigabatrin produces a 20–30% reduction in phenytoin levels, not due to plasma protein binding changes nor enzyme induction (*B J Clin Pharmacol* 1989, **27**, 27S–33S) and this has been thought to compromise seizure control (eg. *Neurology* 1987, **37**, 184–89).

Vincristine + phenytoin *

Phenytoin significantly increases the clearance of vincristine, probably by CYP3A4 induction (n=15, open, Villikka *et al, Clin Pharmacol & Therapeut* 1999, **66**, 589–93).

WARFARIN + PHENYTOIN *

Warfarin metabolism is accelerated by phenytoin, reducing its effect, although enhanced levels of both and death have been reported (n=1, Panegyres and Rischbieth, *Postgrad Med J* 1991, 67, **98**; Meisheri, *J Ass Physicians India* 1996, **44**, 661–62).

Zinc + phenytoin

One case exists of reduced phenytoin levels probably caused by zinc (*Am J Hosp Pharm* 1988, **18**, 297–98).

Zotepine + phenytoin

See zotepine (*4.2.6*).

4.5.9 PIRACETAM
Warfarin + piracetam
Significantly prolonged prothrombin time has been reported with piracetam and warfarin in a single patient (Pan and Ng, *Eur J Clin Pharmacol* 1983, **24**, 711).

4.5.10 TIAGABINE
Tiagabine is relatively new and most information comes from the manufacturers. It appears to be metabolised by CYP3A4.
Alcohol + tiagabine *
Lack of interaction has been shown (n=20, Kastberg *et al, Drug Metabol Drug Interact* 1998, **14**, 259–73), although some caution is still advised.
Benzodiazepines + tiagabine *
No interaction with triazolam has been detected (n=12, RCT, Richens *et al, Drug Metabol Drug Interact* 1998, **14**, 159–77).
Carbamazepine + tiagabine
Tiagabine clearance is 60% greater in people also taking carbamazepine, with plasma levels reduced by a factor of 1.5–3, probably by CYP3A4 induction (MI). There is no effect on carbamazepine.
Cimetidine + tiagabine
No interaction has been detected (MI).
Digoxin + tiagabine
There was no effect by tiagabine on digoxin kinetics (n=13, open, Snel *et al, Eur J Clin Pharmacol* 1998, **54**, 355–57).
Erythromycin + tiagabine *
Lack of significant interaction has been shown (n=13, open, c/o, Thomsen *et al, J Clin Pharmacol* 1998, **38**, 1051–56).
Fosphenytoin + tiagabine
See phenytoin + tiagabine.
Oral contraceptives + tiagabine
No interaction has been detected (MI).
Phenobarbital + tiagabine
Tiagabine clearance is 60% greater in people also taking phenobarbital, with plasma levels reduced by a factor of 1.5–3, probably by CYP3A4 induction (MI). There is no effect on phenobarbital.
Phenytoin + tiagabine
Tiagabine clearance is 60% greater in people also taking phenytoin and plasma levels are reduced by a factor of

1.5–3, probably by CYP3A4 induction (MI). There is no effect on phenytoin.
Primidone + tiagabine
See phenobarbital above.
Theophylline + tiagabine
No interaction has been detected (MI).
Valproate + tiagabine *
Tiagabine causes a 10–12% reduction in steady-state valproate levels whilst valproate increases free tiagabine levels by about 40% (n=12, open, Gustavson *et al, Am J Ther* 1998, **5**, 73–79).
Warfarin + tiagabine
No interaction has been detected (MI).
Zotepine + tiagabine
See zotepine (*4.2.6*).

4.5.11 TOPIRAMATE
Data on topiramate remains limited. It is poorly bound to plasma proteins (and thus unlikely to interact with highly bound drugs) and not extensively metabolised. Excretion is mainly via the kidneys. *In vitro* data suggests that effects on hepatic enzyme metabolism are small and interactions with antipsychotics, tricyclics, antidepressants, caffeine, theophylline and coumarin are unlikely via this mechanism.

Concomitant use is not recommended with drugs predisposing to nephrolithiasis (renal stone formation) is not recommended, and might imply drugs such as allopurinol, megadose ascorbic acid, furosemide (frusemide), methyl-dopa, phenolphthalein abuse, steroids and Worcester Sauce overdose. Most information is currently via the manufacturers.
Reviews: Johannessen, *Epilepsia* 1997, **38**[Suppl 1], S18–S23, Bourgeois, *Epilepsia* 1996, **37**[Suppl 2], S14–S17).
Acetazolamide + topiramate
There may be an increased risk of renal stone formation in susceptible patients.
Carbamazepine + topiramate
Topiramate has been shown to have no effect on the plasma levels of CBZ or CBZ-E. Conversely, topiramate plasma levels are reduced by about 40% by carbamazepine, which could be important if carbamazepine is withdrawn (Wilensky *et al, Epilepsia* 1989, **30**, 645).

Digoxin + topiramate

Topiramate may decrease the plasma concentration of digoxin, with peak levels reduced by 16%, possibly by reduced bioavailability. Routine digoxin blood levels might be considered.

ORAL CONTRACEPTIVES + TOPIRAMATE

Serum estrogen levels are reduced by topiramate in patients taking combined estrogen/progesterone oral contraceptives. An oral contraceptive containing not less than 35–50mcg of estrogen is recommended, or the use of alternative methods (n=12, Rosenfeld *et al, Epilepsia* 1997, **38**, 317–23). Any changes in bleeding patterns should be reported. There were no contraceptive failures reported in 52 patients in early clinical trials.

Phenobarbital + topiramate

Topiramate has been shown to have no effect on the plasma levels of phenobarbital or primidone (Floren *et al, Epilepsia* 1989, **30**, 646). The effect of the barbiturates on topiramate has not been studied.

Phenytoin + topiramate

Decreases in phenytoin clearance may occur with topiramate, probably via CYP2C inhibition. Conversely, topiramate plasma levels are reduced by about 40% by phenytoin, which could be important if phenytoin is withdrawn (Floren *et al, Epilepsia* 1989, **30**, 646).

Triamterene + topiramate

There may be an increased risk of renal stone formation in susceptible patients.

Valproate + topiramate

Topiramate has been shown to produce a small but significant increase in valproate clearance, reducing plasma levels. Topiramate plasma levels are increased by about 15% by valproate, which could be important if valproate is withdrawn (MI).

Zotepine + topiramate

See zotepine (*4.2.6*).

4.5.12 VALPROATE (sodium valproate, valproic acid, valproate semisodium, divalproex sodium etc)

Antacids + valproate

A small, insignificant decrease in valproate absorption with antacids has

been noted (May *et al, Clin Pharm* 1982, **1**, 244).

ANTIDEPRESSANTS+VALPROATE*

Antidepressants lower the seizure threshold and may antagonise valproate's anticonvulsant effect. Tricyclic levels may be raised by 19% by valproate (n=15, open, amitriptyline and nortriptyline, Wong *et al, Clin Pharmacol Ther* 1996, **60**, 48–53).

Antipsychotics + valproate

See antipsychotics (*4.2.1*).

Aspirin + valproate

Valproate's effect and toxicity may be enhanced by repeated high-dose aspirin (*Neurology* 1987, **37**, 1392–94), and levels may rise by 12–43% (*Clin Pharmacol Ther* 1982, **31**, 642), so the potential for interaction should be noted.

Benzodiazepines + valproate

See benzodiazepines (*4.1.1*).

Bupropion + valproate *

See bupropion (*4.6.4*).

CARBAMAZEPINE + VALPROATE

See carbamazepine (*4.5.1*).

Charcoal, activated + valproate

Activated charcoal reduced the absorption of sodium valproate by 65% in one study (Neuvonen *et al, Eur J Clin Pharmacol* 1983, **24**, 243) but had no effect on valproate elimination in another study (n=8, Al-Shareef *et al, Br J Clin Pharmacol* 1997, **43**, 109–11).

Clozapine + valproate

See clozapine (*4.2.2*).

Erythromycin + valproate

There is a case of valproate levels rising three-fold when erythromycin was started, resulting in CNS toxicity (Redington *et al, Ann Int Med* 1992, **116**, 877–78).

Ethosuximide + valproate

See ethosuximide (*4.5.2*).

Fluoxetine + valproate

See fluoxetine (*4.3.2.2*).

Fluvoxamine + valproate

See fluvoxamine (*4.3.2.3*).

Gabapentin + valproate

See gabapentin (*4.5.3*).

H2-blockers + valproate

One study showed that **cimetidine** reduces the clearance and prolongs the half-life of valproate (*Eur J Clin*

Pharmacol 1986, **27**, 325–28), but another showed **ranitidine** to have no effect on the clearance or half-life of valproate (*Eur J Clin Pharmacol* 1986, **27**, 325–28).

Isoniazid + valproate

One case exists of enhanced hepatotoxicity in a younger girl (Dockweiler, *Lancet* 1987, **2**, 152).

LAMOTRIGINE + VALPROATE

See lamotrigine (*4.5.4*).

Levetiracetam + valproate *

See levetiracetam (*4.5.5*).

Oral contraceptives + valproate

A reduced contraceptive effect has not been reported with valproate (*JAMA* 1986, **256**, 238–40; n=6, Crawford *et al*, *Contraception* 1986, **33**, 23–29).

Oxcarbazepine + valproate *

See oxcarbazepine (*4.5.6*).

Paroxetine + valproate

See paroxetine (*4.3.2.4*).

PHENOBARBITAL + VALPROATE

See phenobarbital (*4.5.7*).

PHENYTOIN + VALPROATE

See phenytoin (*4.5.8*).

Risperidone + valproate

See risperidone (*4.2.5*) and antipsychotics (*4.2.1*).

Thiopental + valproate

An animal study suggested that the effects of thiopental may be slightly enhanced (Aguilera *et al*, *Br J Anaesth* 1986, **58**, 1380–83).

Tiagabine + valproate

See tiagabine (*4.5.10*).

Topiramate + valproate

See topiramate (*4.5.11*).

Tricyclics + valproate

A case of status epilepticus with the combination of valproic acid and clomipramine has been reported, with valproate possibly elevating clomipramine to toxic levels (DeToledo *et al*, *Ther Drug Monit* 1997, **19**, 71–73).

Verapamil + valproate

A single case exists of inhibition of valproate metabolism (*Lancet* 1986, **i**, 700–7).

Vigabatrin + valproate

See vigabatrin (*4.5.13*).

Warfarin + valproate *

Rapidly raised INR (to 3.9) has been reported after a single dose of valproate (Guthrie *et al, J Clin Psychopharmacol* 1995, **15**, 138–39). Care is thus needed.

Zidovudine + valproate

Valproate produces a dose-dependent inhibition of AZT glucuronidation, leading to raised zidovudine levels (Trapnell *et al, Antimicrob Agents Chemother* 1998, **42**, 1592–96), possibly by up to 3-fold (n=1, Akula *et al, Am J Med Sci* 1997, **31**, 244–46). This is a new UK SPC warning.

4.5.13 VIGABATRIN

Vigabatrin is not metabolised, does not induce enzymes and is not protein bound. It is renally excreted.

Carbamazepine + vigabatrin *

A 10% rise in carbamazepine levels has been reported with the addition of vigabatrin (n=66, Jedrzejczak *et al, Epilepsy Res* 2000, **39**, 115–20).

Oral contraceptives + vigabatrin

Vigabatrin 3g/d produced no significant difference in oral contraceptive kinetics in one study, although two subjects showed a 50% and 39% reduction in ethinylestradiol (but not levonorgestrel) AUC. The authors conclude that vigabatrin is unlikely to consistently affect the efficacy of these steroid oral contraceptives (n=113, Bartoli *et al, Epilepsia* 1997, **38**, 702–7).

Phenobarbital + vigabatrin

One study reported non-clinically significant 7–11% reductions in barbiturate levels (*Neurology* 1987, **37**, 184–89).

PHENYTOIN + VIGABATRIN

See phenytoin (*4.5.8*).

Valproate + vigabatrin

All double-blind prospective placebo-controlled trials have shown no interaction (eg. McKee *et al, Epilepsia* 1993, **34**, 937–43). A small retrospective study implied vigabatrin caused a rise in valproate levels (Lisart *et al, Eur Hosp Pharm* 1996, **2**, 33–36, disputed by Mumford, *Eur Hosp Pharm* 1996, **2**, 190–91).

Zotepine + vigabatrin

See zotepine (*4.2.6*).

4.6 OTHER DRUGS

4.6.1 ACAMPROSATE

Acamprosate is not protein bound, is excreted in the urine and is not significantly metabolised and so probably has a low liability for drug-drug interactions by these mechanisms.

Alcohol + acamprosate

See alcohol (*4.7.1*).

Benzodiazepines + acamprosate

Lack of interaction with diazepam has been shown (MI).

Disulfiram + acamprosate

Lack of interaction with disulfiram has been shown (n=118, Besson *et al, Alcohol Clin Exp Res* 1998, **22**, 573–79).

Food + acamprosate

Food reduces the oral absorption of acamprosate.

Tricyclics + acamprosate

Lack of interaction with imipramine has been shown (MI).

4.6.2 ANTICHOLINERGIC or ANTIMUSCARINIC AGENTS

Anticholinesterases + anticholinergics

Some antagonism would be expected.

Antipsychotics + anticholinergics

See antipsychotics (*4.2.1*).

Benzodiazepines + anticholinergics

See benzodiazepines (*4.1.1*).

Beta-blockers + anticholinergics

Propantheline increased atenolol bioavailability by 36%, increasing its effect (*Biopharm Drug Dispos* 1981, **2**, 79) but not metoprolol (*Eur J Clin Pharmacol* 1983, **25**, 353).

Betel nut + anticholinergics *

Heavy betel nut consumption has resulted in severe EPSEs, possibly by antagonising the effect of procyclidine (n=1, Deahl, *Mov Disord* 1989, **4**, 330–32).

H2-blockers + anticholinergics

A single-dose study showed possible reduced cimetidine absorption (*Br J Clin Pharmacol* 1981, **11**, 629) but not with ranitidine (*Pharmacother* 1984, **4**, 89) nor nizatidine (*Clin Pharmac Ther* 1988, **42**, 514).

Levodopa + anticholinergics

Anticholinergics may reduce the peak blood levels of levodopa and reduce total absorption (*Eur J Pharmacol* 1976, **35**, 293), possibly by slowed gut motility and increased gut metabolism.

MAOIs + anticholinergics

See MAOIs (*4.3.4*).

Nitrofurantoin + anticholinergics

Nitrofurantoin bioavailability may be increased by anticholinergics (*Int J Clin Pharmacol* 1978, **16**, 223).

Olanzapine + biperiden

See olanzapine (*4.2.3*).

Paracetamol + anticholinergics

Propantheline delays the absorption of paracetamol (*BMJ* 1973, **i**, 587).

Procarbazine + anticholinergics

Increased sedation could occur.

SSRIs + anticholinergics

There are several cases of the combination probably causing delirium, eg. sertraline and benztropine (n=1, Byerly *et al, Am J Psych* 1996, **153**, 965–66), paroxetine and benztropine (Armstrong and Schweitzer, *Am J Psych* 1997, **154**, 581–82, where paroxetine definitely raised benztropine levels) and a variety (n=5, Roth *et al, J Clin Psych* 1994, **55**, 491–95). CYP2D6 inhibition seems the likely mechanism.

Thiazide diuretics + anticholinergics

Thiazide bioavailability may be enhanced (*Eur J Clin Pharmacol* 1978, **13**, 385).

Tricyclics + anticholinergics

See tricyclics (*4.3.1*).

Zotepine + anticholinergics

See zotepine (*4.2.6*).

4.6.3 ANTICHOLINESTERASES

4.6.3.1 DONEPEZIL

Donepezil is metabolised slowly by a non-saturable P450 enzyme system to multiple metabolites, only one of which appears to be pharmacologically active.

Anticholinergics + donepezil

See anticholinergics (*4.6.2*).

Antipsychotics + donepezil

Lack of interaction reported (MI).

Cimetidine + donepezil *

Lack of significant pharmacokinetic interaction has been reported (n=19, open, Tiseo *et al, B J Clin Pharmacol* 1998, **46**[Suppl 1], 25–29).

Digoxin + donepezil *

Lack of significant pharmacokinetic interaction has been reported (n=12, open, Tiseo *et al, B J Clin Pharmacol* 1998, **46**[Suppl 1], 40–44).

Ketoconazole + donepezil *

Donepezil levels may rise by around 25% over a week (n=21, open, Tiseo *et al, B J Clin Pharmacol* 1998, **46**[Suppl 1], 30–34).

NMBAs + donepezil

A synergistic effect could be predicted (MI).

NSAIDs + donepezil

The manufacturers of donepezil recommend additional monitoring of patients at risk of developing ulcers, eg. if taking concomitant NSAIDs.

Risperidone + donepezil

See risperidone (*4.2.5*).

SSRIs + donepezil *

Lack of interaction has been reported, although case reports exist with paroxetine (Carrier, *J Am Geriatr Soc* 1999, **47**, 1037).

Succinylcholine + donepezil

Donepezil is a cholinesterase inhibitor and would be likely to enhance the effect of succinylcholine-type muscle relaxants during ECT.

Theophylline + donepezil *

Lack of significant pharmacokinetic interaction has been reported (n=12, open, Tiseo *et al, B J Clin Pharmacol* 1998, **46**[Suppl 1], 35–39).

Warfarin + donepezil *

Lack of significant pharmacokinetic interaction has been reported (n=12, open, Tiseo *et al, B J Clin Pharmacol* 1998, **46**[Suppl 1], 45–50).

4.6.3.2 GALANTAMINE *

Galantamine is metabolised by CYP2D6 and CYP3A4, and any interaction with potent inhibitors may result in increased side-effects initially, eg. nausea and vomiting. Reduced maintenance doses might be appropriate (SPC). Galantamine has minimal effect on P450 enzymes.

Anticholinergics + galantamine *

See anticholinergics (*4.6.2*).

Beta-blockers + galantamine *

As galantamine may cause bradycardia, the UK SPC recommends care with drugs that significantly reduce heart rate, eg. beta-blockers.

Digoxin + galantamine *

As galantamine may cause bradycardia, the UK SPC recommends care with drugs that significantly reduce heart rate, eg. digoxin. Galantamine has been shown to have no effect on the kinetics of digoxin (SPC).

Erythromycin + galantamine *

A 12% increase in galantamine plasma levels has been reported (SPC), probably by CYP3A4 inhibition.

Ketoconazole + galantamine *

A 30% increase in galantamine plasma levels has been reported (SPC), probably by CYP3A4 inhibition, and so a reduced maintenance dosage might be appropriate.

Paroxetine + galantamine *

A 40% increase in galantamine plasma levels has been reported (SPC), probably by CYP2D6 inhibition, and so a reduced maintenance dosage might be appropriate.

Succinylcholine + galantamine *

Galantamine is likely to enhance the effect of succinylcholine-type muscle relaxants (SPC).

Warfarin + galantamine *

Galantamine has been shown to have no effect on the kinetics of warfarin (SPC).

4.6.3.3 RIVASTIGMINE

Rivastigmine has minimal protein binding, a short half-life and little effect on P450 enzymes and lack of significant interaction has been shown with 22 different therapeutic classes (Grossberg *et al, Int J Ger Psychiatry* 2000, **15**, 242–47).

Anticholinergics + rivastigmine

See anticholinergics (*4.6.2*).

Benzodiazepines + rivastigmine

No interaction in healthy volunteers has been seen (MI).

Digoxin + rivastigmine

No interaction in healthy volunteers has been seen (MI).

Fluoxetine + rivastigmine

No interaction in healthy volunteers has been seen (MI).

Succinylcholine + rivastigmine

Rivastigmine may enhance the effect of succinylcholine-type muscle relaxants during anaesthesia (MI).

Warfarin + rivastigmine

No interaction in healthy volunteers has been seen (MI).

4.6.4 BUPROPION *

Bupropion is primarily metabolised by CYP2B6, with a significant first-pass metabolism, although poor metabolisers may accumulate hydroxybupropion, leading to reduced efficacy (n=12, Pollock *et al, Ther Drug Monit* 1996, **18**, 581–85).
Review: interactions with anticonvulsants (Popli *et al, Ann Clin Psychiatry* 1995, **7**, 99–101).

Alcohol + bupropion *

There is an increased risk of seizures, so alcohol should be avoided or minimised. Extreme care is needed in overdose, chronic use and in alcohol withdrawal states.

Carbamazepine + bupropion *

Carbamazepine induces bupropion metabolism, markedly decreasing bupropion plasma levels (n=17, RCT, Ketter *et al, J Clin Psychopharmacol* 1995, **15**, 327–33).

Cimetidine + bupropion *

Cimetidine may inhibit the metabolism of bupropion, and increase adverse effects, although no effect on bupropion SR was seen in one study (n=24, open, RCT, Kustra *et al, J Clin Pharmacol* 1999, **39**, 1184–88).

Clonidine + bupropion *

Lack of interaction has been reported (Cubeddu *et al, Clin Pharmacol Ther* 1984, **35**, 576–84).

Fluoxetine + bupropion *

Panic disorder has been reported with the combination (Young, *J Clin Psych* 1996, **57**, 177–78)

Fosphenytoin + bupropion *

See phenytoin + bupropion.

Guanfacine + bupropion *

There is a single case of a grand mal seizure with the combination (Tilton, *J*

Am Acad Child Adolesc Psych 1998, **37**, 682–83).

MAOIs + bupropion *

Animal studies have indicated that acute bupropion toxicity might occur, and the combination is contraindicated.

Levodopa + bupropion *

An increased incidence of side-effects has been reported with the combination.

Moclobemide + bupropion *

See MAOIs + bupropion.

Phenobarbital + bupropion *

Phenobarbital may induce the metabolism of bupropion, which would reduce bupropion efficacy.

Phenytoin + bupropion *

Phenytoin may induce the metabolism of bupropion, which would reduce bupropion efficacy.

Ritonavir + bupropion *

Ritonavir may decrease the metabolism of bupropion, which would increase side-effects.

Selegiline + bupropion *

See MAOIs + bupropion.

Smoking + bupropion *

In a single-dose study, cigarettes had no detectable effect on bupropion kinetics (Hsyu *et al, J Clin Pharmacol* 1997, **37**, 737–43).

Tricyclics + bupropion *

Bupropion has been reported to increase imipramine and desipramine levels, through decreased clearance (n=1, Shad and Preskorn, *J Clin Psychopharmacol* 1997, **17**, 118–19).

Valproate + bupropion *

Valproate does not seem to induce bupropion metabolism, but raised metabolite levels are possible (n=17, RCT, Ketter *et al, J Clin Psychopharmacol* 1995, **15**, 327–33).

Zolpidem + bupropion *

There are some reported cases of antidepressants and zolpidem causing short-lived hallucinations (eg. Elko *et al, Clin Toxicol* 1998, **36**, 195–203).

4.6.5 CLOMETHIAZOLE
(chlormethiazole)

Alcohol + clomethiazole

See alcohol (*4.7.1*).

Cimetidine + clomethiazole

Cimetidine inhibits the metabolism of clomethiazole, raising plasma levels.

4.6.6 DISULFIRAM

Disulfiram is a potent inhibitor of CYP2E1, the enzyme responsible for the metabolism of ethanol. Review of disulfiram interactions: *Acta Psych Scand* 1992, **86**[Suppl 369], 59–66.

Acamprosate + disulfiram

See acamprosate (*4.6.1*).

ALCOHOL + DISULFIRAM

See disulfiram under 'Alcohol abuse and dependence' treatment options (*1.4*) and alcohol (*4.7.1*).

Antipsychotics + disulfiram

There is a single case of psychotic symptoms reappearing when disulfiram was started and an increased first-pass metabolism of perphenazine has been noted (Hansen *et al, Lancet* 1982, **2**, 1472).

Benzodiazepines + disulfiram

Disulfiram may inhibit the metabolism of diazepam, chlordiazepoxide and temazepam (n=1, Hardman *et al, Lancet* 1994, **344**, 1231–32), leading to lengthened half-lives (*Clin Pharmacol Ther* 1978, **24**, 583) but not with alprazolam (*Eur J Clin Pharmacol* 1990, **38**, 157–60) nor oxazepam (*Clin Pharmacol Ther* 1978, **24**, 583–89).

Caffeine + disulfiram

Disulfiram may reduce caffeine clearance from the body by a half (*Clin Pharmacol Ther* 1986, **39**, 265–70).

Cannabis + disulfiram

See cannabis (*4.7.2*).

Carbamazepine + disulfiram *

Lack of significant interaction has been shown (n=7, Krag *et al, Acta Neurol* 1981, **63**, 395–98).

Isoniazid + disulfiram

CNS toxicity has been reported in patients taking isoniazid who then took disulfiram (*JAMA* 1972, **219**, 1216).

Lithium + disulfiram

These appear compatible, with no theoretical or clinical reasons why an interaction should occur.

MAOIs + disulfiram

Delirium has been reported with the combination (n=1, Blansjaar and Egberts, *Am J Psych* 1995, **152**, 296;

n=1, Circulo, *J Clin Psychopharmacol* 1989, **9**, 315–16).

Methadone + disulfiram

No interaction occurs (*J Clin Pharmacol* 1980, **20**, 507).

Methyldopa + disulfiram

A risk of reduced hypotensive effect exists (n=1, *Clin Res* 1984, **32**, 923A).

Metronidazole + disulfiram

Psychotic reactions have been reported (Hotson *et al, Arch Neurol* 1976, **33**, 141).

NICOUMALONE + DISULFIRAM

An enhanced anticoagulant effect is possible.

Omeprazole + disulfiram

An isolated case of confusion, disorientation and catatonia on the combination has been reported (Hajela *et al, Can Med Assoc J* 1990, **143**, 1207).

Paraldehyde + disulfiram

In this theoretical interaction, an enhanced disulfiram-reaction could be expected (mentioned in Hadden and Metzner, *Am J Med* 1969, **47**, 642).

Phenytoin + disulfiram

See phenytoin (*4.5.8*).

Theophylline + disulfiram

Theophylline levels may be increased by disulfiram via enzyme inhibition. Monitor and reduce the theophylline dose if necessary (Loi *et al, Clin Pharmacol Ther* 1989, **45**, 476–86).

Tricyclics + disulfiram

See tricyclics (*4.3.1*).

WARFARIN + DISULFIRAM

Prothrombin time can fall by about 10% (Rothstein, *JAMA* 1972, **221**, 1051–52), with one study showing a marked effect with reduced warfarin doses sometimes necessary (n=7, open, O'Reilly, *Clin Pharmacol Ther* 1981, **29**, 332). The BNF notes this to be a significant effect.

4.6.7 MODAFINIL

Modafinil is moderately bound to plasma proteins (62%), essentially to albumin. Renal excretion is the main route of elimination.

Methylphenidate + modafinil *

Lack of significant interaction has been shown, although methylphenidate may slightly slow the absorption of modafinil (RCT, Wong *et al, J Clin Pharmacol* 1998, **38**, 276–82).

Oral contraceptives + modafinil

Higher dose oral contraceptives containing 50mcg ethinylestradiol should be used (MI).

Tricyclics + modafinil

A single dose study showed a clinically important interaction with clomipramine 50mg/d (n=1, Grozinger *et al, Clin Neuropharmacol* 1998, **21**, 127–29).

4.7 NON-PRESCRIBED DRUGS (alcohol, cannabis and smoking)

4.7.1 ALCOHOL

Alcohol/ethanol-psychotropic drug interactions can occur frequently and with varied outcome, depending upon:

Alcohol usage (eg. chronic and/or acute, leading to altered enzymes etc)
Consumption (amount, time span)
Type of interaction (eg. additive sedation, antagonism or cross-tolerance)
What the individual then tries to do (eg. sleep, drive etc.)
Comorbidity (eg. asthma etc).

These variables need to be taken into consideration when assessing the effect or potential effect of the interaction.

Alcohol distribution is wide, with the direct central depressant effect impairing all central functions (eg. cognition, respiration etc), and contributing to many of the drug-drug interactions. Alcohol also promotes the action of GABA and may release other amines such as dopamine and endorphins.

Reviews: pharmacokinetic interactions (Fraser, *Clin Pharmacokinet* 1997, **33**, 79–90, 151 refs), interactions between alcohol and drugs (Ferner, *Adv Drug React Bull* 1998, **189**, 719–22, 40 refs).

Acamprosate + alcohol

Continued alcohol consumption may negate the therapeutic effect of acamprosate. There is no detectable pharmacokinetic interaction (review by Nalpas *et al, Encephale* 1990, **16**, 175–79).

ANTIPSYCHOTICS + ALCOHOL

Enhanced CNS depression is well-documented, particularly with the phenothiazines, resulting in impaired concentration, co-ordination and judgement, drowsiness and lethargy, as well as hypotension and respiratory depression. Alcohol-related drowsiness is significant with **phenothiazines** and **flupentixol**. EPSEs may also be enhanced (Freed, *Med J Aust* 1981, **2**, 44–45), as can hepatotoxicity with, eg. chlorpromazine (Strubelt, *Biochem Pharmacol* 1980, **29**, 1445–49). Single oral doses of **amisulpride** do not seem to enhance the effects of alcohol on the performance and memory of healthy subjects (n=18, RCT, Mattila *et al, Eur J Clin Pharmacol* 1996, **51**, 161). There is no published evidence that alcohol reduces antipsychotic efficacy (Chetty *et al, Eur J Clin Pharmacol* 1994, **46**, 523–26). Overall, this is a potentially important interaction, especially in the community. Accidental alcohol overdosage, especially in people with asthma, respiratory depression or chest infections, could prove fatal if combined with antipsychotics.

BARBITURATES + ALCOHOL

Enhanced or prolonged CNS and respiratory depression can occur, seriously impairing concentration and performance. *Acute* alcohol ingestion may *increase* barbiturate levels but *chronic* alcohol use may *decrease* barbiturate levels (Mezey and Robles, *Gastroenterology* 1974, **66**, 248–53). The lethal dose of barbiturates is up to 50% lower when alcohol is also present (Bogan and Smith, *J Forensic Sci* 1967, **7**, 37–45), mainly due to additive respiratory depression.

BENZODIAZEPINES + ALCOHOL

Alcohol can enhance the sedation caused by benzodiazepines by 20–30%. This is a well established, documented and predictable interaction. Synergistic sedation has been reported with lorazepam (Lister and File, *J Clin Psychopharmacol* 1983, **3**, 66–71), clorazepate and diazepam. Larger quantities of alcohol may inhibit benzodiazepine metabolism, especially in those with impaired or borderline hepatic function (review by Guthrie and Lane, *Alcoholism* 1986, **10**, 686–90), and diazepam, where acute ethanol decreases diazepam clearance by up to 50%, (Laisi *et al, Eur J Clin Pharmacol* 1979, **16**, 263–70).

Beta-blockers + alcohol

Alcohol may slightly reduce pro-pranolol absorption and increase excretion (Grabowski *et al, Int J Clin Pharmacol Ther Toxicol* 1980, **18**, 317–19; Sotaniemi *et al, Clin Pharmacol Ther* 1981, **29**, 705–10).

Bupropion + alcohol *

See bupropion (*4.6.4*).

Buspirone + alcohol *

A minimal interaction and slightly increased sedation has been reported (Erwin *et al, J Clin Psychopharmacol* 1986, **6**, 199–209).

Cannabis + alcohol

See cannabis (*4.7.2*).

Carbamazepine + alcohol

There is virtually nothing published but additive sedation would be expected.

CHLORAL + ALCOHOL

Additive (or more) CNS depressant effects occur when alcohol is taken with chloral. Tachycardia, impaired con-centration, disulfiram-like effects and profound vasodilation may also occur (Owen and Taberner, *B J Pharmacol* 1978, **64**, 400).

Clomethiazole + alcohol

Alcohol increases the bioavailability of oral clomethiazole, probably via inhibition of first pass metabolism (Neuvonen *et al, Int J Clin Pharmacol Ther Toxicol* 1981, **19**, 552–60).

Citalopram + alcohol

There is little published at present on this. The manufacturers state that citalopram does not enhance the sedation caused by alcohol.

Cocaine + alcohol

See cocaine (*4.7.3*).

DISULFIRAM + ALCOHOL

Disulfiram inhibits the aldehyde dehy-drogenase enzyme, leading to accumu-lation of acetaldehyde from incomplete alcohol metabolism. The main symp-toms of the 'Antabuse reaction' are flushing, sweating, palpitations, hyper-ventilation, increased pulse, hypo-tension, nausea and vomiting (often in that order). Arrhythmias and shock can follow. The reaction occurs within 5–15 minutes and can be fatal. Factors affecting the severity of the reaction include the dose of disulfiram, rate and

dose of alcohol ingestion, sensitivity, individual aldehyde dehydrogenase activity, concurrent medication (see disulfiram interactions, *4.6.4*) and co-existing pulmonary or cardiac disease. Patients should be warned that reactions can occur with disguised sources of alcohol, eg. 'Listerine' mouthwash, sauces, pharmaceuticals (eg. cough mixtures), topical preparations (eg. shampoo; Stoll and King, *JAMA* 1980, **244**, 2045) etc.

Fluoxetine + alcohol

Alcohol has no additional significant effect on drowsiness, sedation or task performance tests with fluoxetine 40mg/d, compared with fluoxetine alone (eg. Shaw *et al, Human Psycho-pharmacol* 1989, **4**, 113–20).

Fluvoxamine + alcohol

Moderately enhanced sedation has been reported (*J Clin Pharmacol* 1989, **29**, 91–95), but a later study showed no significant potentiation of the cognitive effects of 40g IV alcohol by single and multiple doses of 50mg fluvoxamine (n=24, van Harten *et al, Clin Pharmacol Ther* 1992, **52**, 427–35).

Levetiracetam + alcohol *

See levetiracetam (*4.5.5*).

Lithium + alcohol

Impaired driving skills has been reported (*Eur J Clin Pharmacol* 1974, **7**, 337), although no clinically significant adverse interactions have actually been reported. Alcohol may produce a slight (12%) increase in peak lithium levels (Anton *et al, Clin Pharmacol Ther* 1985, **38**, 52).

MAOIs + ALCOHOL

As well as an interaction occurring with alcoholic and low alcoholic drinks (see MAOIs, *4.3.4*), alcohol may increase central catecholamine synthesis and release, and MAOIs may inhibit alcohol dehydrogenase, potentiating alcohols effect (comprehensive review in *Psycho-somatics* 1984, **25**, 301).

Methadone + alcohol

Predictably, increased sedation occurs with the combination (Bellville *et al, Clin Pharmacol Ther* 1971, **12**, 607–12).

MIANSERIN + ALCOHOL

Mianserin causes drowsiness which is enhanced considerably by alcohol (n=13, RCT, Seppala *et al, Eur J Clin Pharmacol* 1984, **27**, 181–89).

Mirtazapine + alcohol *

Lack of pharmacokinetic interaction has been shown, but additive sedation was noted (Mercer, mentioned in Timmer *et al, Clin Pharmacokinet* 2000, **38**, 461–74).

Moclobemide + alcohol

Some degree of potentiation of the effects of alcohol has been noted, albeit less than with trazodone and clomipramine (*Acta Psych Scand* 1990, **360**[Suppl], 84–6).

Nefazodone + alcohol

The SPC states that alcohol-induced psychomotor and cognitive impairment is unaffected by nefazodone (n=12, 8/7, RCT, Frewer and Lader, *Int Clin Psychopharmacol* 1993, **8**, 13–20).

Olanzapine + alcohol

Enhanced CNS sedation would be expected. Raised heart rate and increased postural hypotension have been reported (MI).

Oxcarbazepine + alcohol *

See oxcarbazepine (*4.5.6*).

Paraldehyde + alcohol

An enhanced sedative effect can be expected (BNF).

Paroxetine + alcohol

Lack of interaction has been shown (review by Boyer and Blumhardt, *J Clin Psych* 1992, **53**[Suppl 2], 132–34).

PHENYTOIN + ALCOHOL *

Alcohol usually decreases phenytoin levels but increases them via enzyme induction if alcohol intake is heavy, and so higher doses may be needed initially in alcoholics. The half-life of phenytoin can be up to 50% shorter in an abstaining alcoholic than in a non-drinker (Kater *et al, Gastroenterology* 1969, **56**, 412; see also n=1, Bellibas and Tuglular, *Therapie* 1995, **50**, 487–88).

Quetiapine + alcohol

Additive sedation would be expected.

Reboxetine + alcohol

No potentiation of alcohol's cognitive effects has been reported (UK SPC), and up to 4mg/d showed no interaction with alcohol in a small trial (n= 10, d/b, Kerr *et al, B J Clin Pharmacol* 1996, **42**, 239–41).

Sertraline + alcohol

The evidence for a lack of interaction has been reviewed by Warrington (*Int Clin Psychopharmacol* 1991, **6**[Suppl 2], 11–21).

Tiagabine + alcohol

See tiagabine (*4.5.10*).

TRAZODONE + ALCOHOL

Alcohol enhances the sedation caused by trazodone (*Neuropsychobiology* 1986, **15**[Suppl 1], 31–37).

TRICYCLICS + ALCOHOL

Enhanced sedation with most tricyclics is known, but surprisingly little has actually been published and most studies refer to the effect on driving performance. Sedation caused by amitriptyline (Shaw *et al, Human Psychopharmacol* 1989, **4**, 113–20) and doxepin is enhanced by alcohol, but less, or minimally so, with nortriptyline, clomipramine, desipramine and amoxapine, which are less sedating. With maprotiline, increased drowsiness was reported in a small study (*Arch Int Pharmacodyn* 1988, **291**, 217–28). Both alcohol and tricyclics lower the seizure threshold and care is needed in patients susceptible to seizures. Concurrent alcohol may also increase the oral bioavailability of tricyclics by reducing the first pass effect (Dorian *et al, Eur J Clin Pharmacol* 1983, **25**, 325–31).

Venlafaxine + alcohol

There appears to be no significant additive effect between alcohol and venlafaxine (n=16, Troy *et al, J Clin Pharmacol* 1997, **37**, 1073–81).

Zaleplon + alcohol

See zaleplon (*4.1.4*).

Zolpidem + alcohol

There is no published information available indicating an interaction.

Zopiclone + alcohol

There appears to be no significant interaction (*Int Clin Psychopharmcol* 1990, **5**[Suppl 2], 105–13).

Zotepine + alcohol

See zotepine (*4.2.6*).

4.7.2 CANNABIS
(Tetrahydrocannabinol)

Cannabis/marijuana is a frequently (and usually secretively) used drug but with the exception of perhaps tricyclics, has few known important adverse drug interactions.

Alcohol + cannabis

Decreased ethanol metabolism may occur, with enhanced CNS depression (Consroe *et al, Psychopharmacol* 1979, **66**, 45–50). Cannabis may also reduce peak alcohol levels (Lukas *et al, Neuropsychopharmacology* 1992, **7**, 77–81).

Antidepressants + cannabis

Mental state changes consistent with delirium and tachycardia and other clinically significant adverse events have been reported following use of marijuana and tricyclic antidepressants (n=4, Wilens *et al, J Am Acad Child Adolesc Psychiatry* 1997, **36**, 45–48; *Lancet* 1997, **349**, 106). Increased heart rate has been reported, eg. marked sinus tachycardia, possibly via a combined beta-adrenergic effect (eg. n=2, Hillard and Vieweg, *Am J Psych* 1983, **140**, 626–27).

Antipsychotics + cannabis

Chlorpromazine clearance has been shown to be increased by cannabis smoking, although the clinical significance is not known (Chetty *et al, Eur J Clin Pharmacol* 1994, **46**, 523–26). Additive drowsiness has been reported (review by Benowitz and Jones, *Clin Pharmacol Ther* 1977, **22**, 259–68).

Benzodiazepines + cannabis

Additive drowsiness with benzodiazepines and hypnotics has been reported (review by Benowitz and Jones, *Clin Pharmacol Ther* 1977, **22**, 259–68).

Cocaine + cannabis

See cocaine (*4.7.3*).

CNS depressants + cannabis

The combination has resulted in additive drowsiness (review by Benowitz and Jones, *Clin Pharmacol Ther* 1977, **22**, 259–68), eg. antidepressants, anticholinergics, benzodiazepines.

Disulfiram + cannabis

There have been two reported reactions; a hypomanic episode in an alcoholic on disulfiram taking marijuana (Lacoursiere and Swatek, *Am J Psych* 1983, **140**, 242–44) and an acute confusional state (Mackie and Clark, *B J Psych* 1994, **164**, 421).

Fluoxetine + cannabis

Mania has been reported with this combination (n=1, Stoll *et al, J Clin Psych* 1991, **52**, 280–81).

Lithium + cannabis

A single case exists of lithium levels raised into the toxic range by secretive use of cannabis (*J Clin Psychopharmcol* 1981, **1**, 32) and additive drowsiness has been reported (review by Benowitz and Jones, *Clin Pharmacol Ther* 1977, **22**, 259–68).

4.7.3 COCAINE

Review: Ciraulo, *J Clin Psychopharmacol* 1992, **12**, 49–55 (73 refs).

Alcohol + cocaine

Simultaneous cocaine and alcohol may produce changes in heart rate and blood pressure, increasing the risk of cardiovascular toxicity (Farre *et al, J Pharmacol Exp Ther* 1993, **166**, 1364–73). Combined use has led to enhanced cocaine-induced hepatotoxicity.

Antidepressants + cocaine

In combination with cocaine, desipramine may reduce the effect, fluoxetine has no significant effect (n=5, Walsh *et al, J Clin Psychopharmacol* 1994, **14**, 396–407), trazodone has minor physiological effects and MAOIs probably augment the pressor effect.

Antipsychotics + cocaine *

Flupentixol may reduce cocaine craving and haloperidol may moderate the stimulant effects. Clozapine increases cocaine levels but reduced cocaine 'high', and some cardiac events (near-syncopal episode) have been reported, so caution is necessary (n=8, Farren *et al, Drug Alcohol Depend* 2000, **59**, 153–63).

Cannabis + cocaine

Enhanced cardiotoxicity (eg. increased heart rate) may occur.

Carbamazepine + cocaine

Cocaine may enhance the cardiac effects of carbamazepine.

Lithium + cocaine

Lithium probably has little effect.

4.7.4 SMOKING

Many people with mental health problems smoke. There are over 3000 different known chemicals in cigarette smoke, but which ones are significant is not fully known. Only a few smoking-drug interactions are significant, and only brief details of the more significant psychotropic ones are included here (review by Schein, *Ann Pharmacother* 1995, **29**, 1139–48). The major enzyme metabolising nicotine is probably CYP2A6, with CYP2B6 and CYP2D6 playing lesser, but still substantial, roles. Cigarette smoke contains polycyclic aromatic hydrocarbons, which are potent inducers of CYP1A2.

Reviews *: general (Zevin and Benowitz, *Clin Pharmacokinet* 1999, **36**, 425–38, 128 refs).

Antipsychotics + smoking *

Evidence supporting a significant interaction is that schizophrenics who smoke tend to receive higher doses of antipsychotics than non-smokers (n=78, Goff *et al, Am J Psych* 1992, **149**, 1189–94), possibly via increased hepatic metabolism and renal excretion (d/b, p/c, Salokangas *et al, Schizophren Res* 1997, **23**, 55–60). Plasma levels of haloperidol are around 23% lower in smoking than in non-smoking schizo-phrenic patients, probably by enzyme induction (Shimoda *et al, Ther Drug Monit* 1999, **21**, 293–96; confirmed by another study, n=63, Pan *et al, Ther Drug Monit* 1999, **21**, 489). **Chlorpromazine** clearance may be increased by cigarette smoking, but the clinical significance is unclear (n=31, Chetty *et al, Eur J Clin Pharmacol* 1994, **46**, 523–26). **Clozapine** levels are lowered by smoking (Haring *et al, Am J Psych* 1990, **147**, 1471–75), the 1A2 induction leading to clozapine non-response, with fluvoxamine occasionally used to inhibit CYP1A2 to raise clozapine levels (n=3, Bender and Eap, *Arch Gen Psych* 1998, **55**, 1048–50), so stopping

smoking could be dangerous for someone taking clozapine (n=1, Skogh *et al, Ther Drug Monit* 1999, **21**, 580). **Olanzapine** clearance may be higher and half-life 21% shorter in smokers compared to non-smokers (MI), probably via CYP1A2 induction. Smoking seems to have no effect on zotepine plasma levels (n=14, Kondo *et al, Psychopharmacol [Berl]* 1996, **127**, 311–14). Many schizophrenics may smoke to relieve subjective distress from the illness and treatment (review, McEvoy, *Curr Opin Psych* 2000, **113**, 115–19).

Benzodiazepines + smoking

Early studies suggested an increased clearance of benzodiazepines in smokers (review by Schein, *Ann Pharmacother* 1995, **29**, 1139–48). One study concluded that higher doses are not needed (*Clin Pharmacol Ther* 1978, **87**, 223).

Bupropion + smoking *

See bupropion (*4.6.4*).

Lithium + smoking

Smoking induces CYP1A2 and caffeine is metabolised by CYP1A2. Theoretically, ceasing smoking could raise xanthine levels, which could increase lithium excretion (as with theophylline), lowering levels.

Phenobarbital + smoking

Smoking has been shown not to effect the drowsiness caused by phenobarbital (BCDSP, *NEJM* 1973, **288**, 277–80).

Propranolol + smoking

Steady-state propranolol levels may be reduced in smokers, via 1A2 induction.

Tricyclics + smoking

Although serum levels of tricyclics fall in smokers, free levels rise, minimising the clinical significance (*Ther Drug Monit* 1986, **8**, 279–84).

Cytochrome P450 Drug Metabolism/Inhibition

The knowledge of the role of the P450 enzyme system is rapidly developing. These tables may be of use in determining actual or potential interactions. There are, however, many discrepancies in the published literature and so these tables may inadvertently perpetuate some inaccuracies or incomplete knowledge.

Some points about P450 interactions include:

1. Some drugs are metabolised by several enzymes, so if one enzyme is inhibited, another may compensate. There are over 40 known human P450 enzymes.

2. A drug may inhibit or induce an enzyme, but be metabolised by another.

3. Onset and offset of inhibition is dependent on the half-life and time to steady state of the inhibitory drug (may be 24 hours or several months) and the drug to be metabolised.

4. Onset and offset of induction may take hours or several weeks to become apparent, dependent on the inducing drugs half-life, enzyme turnover, age (induction reduces with age) and concurrent liver disease (reduced induction ability).

5. Also important are the **UGT** (uridine diphosphate glucuronosyltransferase) enzymes (de Wildt *et al, Clin Pharmacokinet* 1999, **36**, 439–52). Phenytoin, valproate, phenobarbital and CBZ are UGT inducers, lamotrigine a weak UGT inducer. The Flavin Mono-oxygenase (FMO) system is also important. Humans have FMO1, FMO3, FM04 and FM05 enzymes in the liver, intestine and kidney. Imipramine, chlopromazine and orphenadrine are known to be metabolised by this enzyme system.

The general rules for avoiding P450 interactions are:

1. Avoid reported and predictable interactions.

2. With potential interactions, use reduced doses where possible (ie. start low and go slow).

3. Measure plasma levels of drugs with narrow therapeutic indices.

CYP1A2

Substrates, ie drugs metabolised by this enzyme	Significant enzyme inducers	Significant enzyme inhibitors
Caffeine Clozapine (most) Diazepam Fluvoxamine (partly) Haloperidol (partly) Mirtazapine (partly) Olanzapine (partly) Ondansetron Paracetamol Pimozide (possibly) Propranolol? Tacrine Tamoxifen Theophylline Tricyclics — tertiary (eg. amitriptyline, clomipramine, desipramine, imipramine) Verapamil Warfarin-R (major) Zotepine Ziprasidone (minor)	Cabbage Caffeine Charcoal-broiled food Cigarette smoke Omeprazole Phenobarbital (weak) Phenytoin (weak) Rifampicin Ritonavir	Celery Cimetidine Ciprofloxacin Clarithromycin Diet (low protein/high carbohydrate) Enoxacin Erythromycin Fluoroquinolones (eg. ciprofloxacin and norfloxacin) (strong) Fluvoxamine (potent — other SSRIs only very weakly) Grapefruit juice Griseofulvin? Isoniazid Ketoconazole Mirtazapine (very weak) Moclobemide Nefazodone (very weak/nil) Norfloxacin Omeprazole Parsley Parsnip Sertraline (weak)

CYP2C family

2C is a sub-family, containing many closely related enzymes, eg. 2C9, 2C10, 2C19 etc. About 20% Asians and 3–5% Caucasians are poor CYP2C19 metabolisers.

Substrates, ie drugs metabolised by this enzyme	Significant enzyme inducers	Significant enzyme inhibitors
Amitriptyline Clomipramine Diazepam Imipramine Moclobemide Omeprazole NSAIDs (some) Phenytoin Tolbutamide Warfarin	Carbamazepine (weak) Phenobarbital (weak) Phenyton (weak) Rifampicin (weak)	Fluoxetine? Fluvoxamine? Sertraline?

CYP2C9/10/19

(9 and 19 are closely related)

Substrates, ie. drugs metabolised by this enzyme	Significant enzyme inducers	Significant enzyme inhibitors
Barbiturates (19) Bupropion (8/9) Citalopram (19, major 60%) Diazepam (19) Fluoxetine (9) Losartan (9) Mephenytoin (19) Moclobemide (19) NSAIDs (8/9) Omeprazole (19) Phenytoin (8/9/19) Propranolol (part)(19) Tricyclics — tertiary (eg. amitriptyline, clomipramine, imipramine) (19) Tolbutamide (8/9) Topiramate (19) Warfarin (part) (8/9) R-Warfarin (19) (minor) S-Warfarin (9) (major)	Rifampicin (9)	Amiodarone (9) Carbamazepine (9) Chloramphenicol (9) Cimetidine (9) Fluconazole Fluoxetine? (9,weak?) Fluoxetine (19, moderate) Fluvoxamine? (9/19) Ketoconazole Moclobemide (19) Omeprazole (9/19) Oxcarbazepine (19) Phenylbutazone (9) Sertraline (9, moderate) Ticlopidine (19) Topiclone (19) potent Topiramate Tranylcypromine (19) Venlafaxine (weak)

CYP2D6

CYP2D6 metabolism occurs both in the liver and in the brain. An individual's CYP2D6 status can be determined by giving the person debrisoquine or dextromethorphan and measuring the ratios of drug and metabolite. 5–8% whites, 8.5% African-Americans and 2–10% Asians are slow metabolisers. All CYP2D6 inhibition is probably concentration-dependent and so inclusion in this list only predicts that an interaction could occur, not that it will occur.

Substrates, ie. drugs metabolised by this enzyme	Significant enzyme inducers	Significant enzyme inhibitors
Amfetamines	Carbamazepine (weak)	Amiodarone
Antiarrhythmics Type 1c (encainide, flecainide etc.)	Phenobarbital (weak)	Chloroquine
	Phenytoin (weak)	Chlorpromazine
Beta-blockers (especially lipophilic)	Rifampicin (weak)	Cimetidine
Chlorphenamine	Ritonavir (weak)	Citalopram (very weak/nil)
Chlorpromazine		Dextromethorphan
Citalopram (minor)		Dextropropoxyphene
Clozapine (minor and unproven)		Diltiazem (weak)
Codeine (to morphine)		Diphenhydramine
Desipramine (weak)		Fenfluramine?
Dexfenfluramine		Flecainide
Dextromethorphan		Fluoxetine (strong)
Donepezil		Fluphenazine
Encainide		Fluvoxamine (very weak)
Fenfluramine		Haloperidol
Flecainide		Methadone
Fluoxetine (partly)		Metoclopramide
Fluphenazine		Metoprolol
Fluvoxamine (very weakly)		Mexiletine
Galantamine		Mibefradil
Haloperidol		Mirtazapine (very weak/nil)
Hydrocodone		Moclobemide
Loratadine		Nefazodone (very weak/nil)
m-CPP		Nicardipine
Methadone		Norfluoxetine (strong)
Methamphetamine		Paroxetine (strong, dose-related)
Metoprolol		Perphenazine
Mexiletine		Pindolol
Mirtazapine (minor)		Primaquine
Morphine derivatives		Propafenone
Nefazodone		Propranolol
Nicotine (partly)		Quinidine (strong)
Olanzapine (partly)		Quinine
Oxycodone		Sertraline (weak, dose-related, moderate at ≥150mg/d))
Paroxetine		Thioridazine
Perphenazine		Timolol
Phenothiazines		Topiclone (potent)
Propafenone		Tricyclics (all, strong)
Propranolol		Trifluoperidol
Risperidone		Venlafaxine (very weak/nil)
Sertindole (partly)		Yohimbine
Thioridazine		
Timolol		
Tramadol		
Trazodone		
Tricyclics — secondary and tertiary tricyclics (eg. nortriptyline, imipramine, maprotiline, amitriptyline (weak), desipramine (weak), clomipramine (weak))		
Venlafaxine (partly)		

CYP3A3/4 (very similar structures, so are often grouped together)

CYP3A4 is a most important P450 enzyme, and may acount for up to 50–60% of the total liver P450. There is little genetic polymorphism so little inter-individual variation exists. CYP3A4 occurs in the liver, gut and, possibly, the brain.

Substrates, ie. drugs metabolised by this enzyme	
Alfentanil	Lovastatin
Amiodarone	Macrolides (eg. erythromycin and clarithromycin)
Amlodipine	Mianserin
Antihistamines (eg. astemizole)	Mibefradil
Astemizole	Miconazole
Benzodiazepines (eg. alprazolam, clonazepam, diazepam, midazolam, temazepam, triazolam, but not lorazepam)	Mirtazapine (partly)
	Nefazodone
	Nicardipine
Buspirone	Nifedipine
Busulfan	Omeprazole
Calcium Channel Blockers	Ondansetron
Cannabinoids	Orphenadrine
Carbamazepine	Paclitaxol
Cisapride	Paracetamol
Citalopram (minor, 30%)	Pimozide (mostly)
Clindamycin	Pravastatin
Clozapine (partly)	Prednisone
Cocaine	Progesterone
Codeine	Propafenone
Cortisol	Quetiapine
Cyclophosphamide	Quinine
Cyclosporin	Reboxetine
Dapsone	Rifampicin
Desamethasone	Risperidone
Dextromethorphan	Ritonavir
Diltiazem	Saquinavir
Disopyramide	Sertindole (partly)
Donepezil	Sertraline
Doxorubicin	Sodium valproate
Estradiol (oestradiol)	Steroids, eg. dexamethasone
Ethosuximide	Tacrolimus
Ethinylestradiol	Tamoxifen
Felodipine	Terfenadine
Fentanyl	Testosterone
Fexofenadine	Tiagabine
Fluoxetine	Tricyclics – tertiary (eg. imipramine, amitriptyline,
Galantamine	clomipramine
Glyburide	Venlafaxine
Indinavir	Verapamil
Itraconazole	Vinblastine
Isradipine	Vincristine
Ketoconazole	R-Warfarin (minor)
Lansoprazole (weak)	Zaleplon (secondary route)
Lidocaine (lignocaine)	Ziprasidone
Loratadine	Zolpidem (mainly)
Losartan	Zotepine
	Zopiclone

Significant enzyme inducers (decrease levels of substrates)	Significant enzyme inhibitors (increase levels of substrates)	
Barbiturates (all)	Acetazolamide	Mibofradil
Carbamazepine	Amiodarone	Miconazole (strong)
Cortisol	Cannabinoids	Mirtazpine (very weak/nil)
Dexamethasone	Cimetidine (moderate)	Nefazodone (strong)
Ethosuximide	Citalopram (weak)	Nelfinavir
Oxcarbazepine	Clarithromycin	Norfluoxetine (moderate)
Phenobarbital	Clotrimazole	Omeprazole (weak)
Phenytoin	Danazol	Paroxetine (weak)
Prednisone	Diltiazem (weaker)	Quinine
Primidone	Fluconazole (strong)	Ritonavir (moderate)
Rifampicin (rapid)	Fluoxetine (weak)	Sertindole (weak)
Troglitazone	Fluvoxamine (moderate)	Sertraline (minor/mod)
	Grapefruit juice (weaker)	Trazodone
	Indinavir (moderate)	Tricyclics (moderate)
	Itraconazole (strong)	Troleandomycin (strong)
	Ketoconazole (strong)	Venlafaxine (weak)
	Macrolides (some, eg. erythromycin) (strong)	Verapamil (weak)
	Metronidazole	Zafirlukast

References used include: Meyer *et al*, *Acta Psych Scand* 1996, **93**, 71–79; Slaughter and Edwards, *Ann Pharmacother* 1995, **29**, 619–24; Nemeroff *et al*, *Am J Psych* 1996, **153**, 311–20; Callahan *et al*, *Harvard Rev Psych* 1996, **4**, 153–58; Centorinno *et al*, *Am J Psych* 1996, **153**, 820–82; Cohen and De Vane, *Ann Pharmacother* 1996, **30**, 1471–80.

CHAPTER FIVE
DRUG-INDUCED PSYCHIATRIC DISORDERS

The drugs listed in each section have been reported to cause that condition in some context (eg. standard dose, high dose, prolonged courses etc). The main references at the end of this section and others (where known or where they exist) next to the drug should be consulted to ascertain the circumstances of reports. The references are offered without qualification and no indication of frequency or status of reports can be given as this information is not really available, except where a side-effect is well-recognised. The UK CSM requests reports of all side-effects of new drugs and severe reactions to established drugs. **Review**: psychiatric adverse effects of anticonvulsant drugs (Wong *et al, CNS Drugs* 1997, **8**, 492–509), general (Bishop and Lee, *Pharm J* 1998, **261**, 935–39).

5.1 AGITATION, ANXIETY and NERVOUSNESS

● Psychotropics etc *
Benzodiazepine withdrawal (eg. *Am J Psych* 1984, **141**, 848–52)
Bromocriptine
Bupropion (9.7%, MI)
Carbamazepine (*J Am Acad Child Adolesc Psych* 1988, **27**, 500–3)
Clomethiazole
Citalopram (cases in *Eur J Clin Pharmacol* 1986, **31**, 18–22)
Dexamfetamine (*Curr Ther Res* 1973, **15**, 358–66)
Fluoxetine (9% incidence? eg. *J Clin Psych* 1985, **46** (3 Pt 2), 32–37)
Moclobemide (5–10% incidence, eg. *J Neural Transm* 1989, **28** [Suppl], 77–89)
Olanzapine (*Can J Psych* 1998, **43**, 1054)
Paroxetine (11%? incidence, *Acta Psych Scand* 1989, **80**[Suppl 350], 117–37)
Phenobarbital and other barbiturates
Risperidone (n=1, *Am J Psych* 1995, **152**, 1096–97)
Rivastigmine (<5%, MI)
Temazepam
Triazolam (*Pharmacopsychiatry* 1989, **22**, 115–19)

Tricyclics (eg. amitriptyline, lofepramine at <2%, review in *Drugs* 1989, **37**, 123–40)

● Anticonvulsants
Carbamazepine
Clonazepam
Ethosuximide
Gabapentin
Gabapentin withdrawal (n=1, *et al, J Clin Psych* 1998, **59**, 131)
Lamotrigine
Vigabatrin

● Anti-Parkinsonian drugs
Atropine eye drops (n=1, *J Ped Ophthal Strabis* 1985, **22**, 38–39)
Levodopa (common, eg. *Arch Neurol* 1970, **23**, 193–200)

● Gastrointestinal
Famotidine (mentioned in *Digestion* 1985, **32**[Suppl 1] 24–31)
Mesalazine (MI)
Nizatidine (MI)
Omeprazole (MI)

● Cardiovascular
Doxazosin (2.4% incidence)
Hydralazine
Methyldopa (rare, *JAMA* 1974, **230**, 1428)
Nicardipine (rare, *B J Clin Pharmacol* 1985, **20**[Suppl], 178S–186S)

● NSAIDs and analgesics
Ibuprofen (several cases, eg. *Arthritis Rheum* 1982, **25,** 1013)
Indometacin (n=1, *South Med J* 1983, **76**, 679–80)
Mefenamic Acid
Naproxen
Naproxen + chloroquine (*Ann Pharmacother* 1993, **27**, 1058–59)
Nefopam
Pentazocine (eg. *BMJ* 1974, **2**, 224)

● Miscellaneous
Amantadine (MI)
Aminophylline
Baclofen (n=2, *Lancet* 1977, **2**, 44)
Bismuth Intoxication (*Postgrad Med J* 1988, **64**, 308–10)
Botulinum toxin A injection (*South Med J* 1999, **92**, 738)
Caffeine OD

Co-trimoxazole (n=1, *J Clin
Psychopharmacol* 1991, **11**, 144–5)

Dexamethasone and other
glucocorticoids (eg. *Arch Gen Psych*
1981, **38**, 471–77)

Fentanyl transdermal

Flumazenil (MI)

Flunisolide (MI)

Gancyclovir (*NEJM* 1990, **322**, 933–34)

Ginseng (see *Arch Gen Psych* 1998, **55**,
1033–44)

Granisetron (unconfirmed, eg. *Eur J
Cancer* 1990, **26** (Supp 1), S19–23)

Isoniazid (*Lancet* 1989, **ii**, 735–36)

Levamisole (rare, *NEJM* 1990, **322**,
352–58)

Levothyroxine

Mefloquine (*Pharm J* 1989, **243**, 561)

Methoxamine (MI)

Methyltestosterone

Misoprostol (MI)

Morphine

Naltrexone

Neostigmine (cases in *Deutsch Med
Wschr* 1966, **91**, 699)

Octreotide (MI)

Phenylephrine (rare, eg. *JAMA* 1982,
247, 1859–60)

Phenylpropanolamine OD (*Lancet*
1979, **ii**, 1367)

Piperazine (see *Trans Roy Soc Trop
Med Hyg* 1976, **70**, 358)

Prednisone (esp. in children, cases in
Clin Paediatr 1990, **29**, 382–88)

Pseudoephedrine (n=1, *Eur J Clin
Pharmacol* 1978, **14**, 253–59)

Pyridostigmine (obscure case in
Deutsch Med Wschr 1966, **9**, 699)

Salbutamol

Streptokinase (reported in *Drugs* 1973,
5, 357)

Theophylline

Yohimbine (see *Arch Gen Psych* 1998,
55, 1033–44)

5.2 AGGRESSION * *including
hostility and violence*

Review - Shaw and Fletcher, *Adv Drug
React & Toxicolog Rev* 2000, **19**, 35-45,
64 refs.

Alcohol withdrawal

Amantadine (cases in *BMJ* 1972, **3**, 50)

Amphetamine withdrawal

Anabolic steroid withdrawal

Barbiturate withdrawal

Benzodiazepines (alprazolam study, *J
Aff Dis* 1995, **35**, 117–23)

Carbamazepine

Chlordiazepoxide (increased hostility,
eg. *Psychosomatics* 1969, **10**)

Dapsone (*BMJ* 1991, **4**, 300)

Donepezil (n=1, *Am J Psych* 1998, **155**,
1626–27; n=7, *Am J Psych* 1998, **155**,
1632–33)

Lamotrigine (survey, n=19, *Epilepsia*
1998, **39**, 280–82)

Naloxone IV (n=2, *Ann Pharmacother*
1992, **26,** 196–98)

Omeprazole (MI)

Olanzapine (*Can J Psych* 1998, **43**,
1054)

Oxandrolone (and other anabolic
steroids)

Paroxetine withdrawal (*Lancet* 1995,
346, 57)

Tricyclics (rare, eg. *Am J Psych* 1986,
143, 1603–5)

Vigabatrin (eg. *Drugs* 1991, **41**,
889–926)

5.3 BEHAVIOURAL CHANGES

Anabolic steroids (*Am J Psych* 1992,
149, 271–72)

Barbiturates

Benzodiazepines

Clonazepam (*Develop Med & Child
Neurol* 1991, **33**, 362–65)

Bismuth (*Acta Neurologica Belgica*
1979, **79**, 73)

Carbamazepine (*J Paediatrics* 1982,
101, 785–87)

Donepezil (n=1, *Am J Psych* 1998, **155**,
1626–27; n=7, *Am J Psych* 1998, **155**,
1632–33)

Levodopa

Levodopa + carbidopa

Lithium + antipsychotics

Methyldopa + haloperidol

Prednisone withdrawal (*JAMA* 1989,
261, 1731)

Theophylline (disputed — not in
children, *JAMA* 1992, **267**, 2621–24)

5.4 DELIRIUM (*acute organic
psychosis*) and CONFUSION *

Drug-induced delirium is usually an
acute reaction and always with
fluctuating levels of awareness of self
and environment. It is most frequent in
frail or dementing elderly, drug misusers
and with pre-existing organic brain

disease and strongly associated with anticholinergic activity:

- High risk drug groups are TCAs and typical antipsychotics
- Medium risk drugs include benzo-diazepines, sedatives, dopamine-activating drugs, anti-epileptics, histamine H2 receptor blockers, digoxin, beta-blockers and analgesics. Most of these do not have direct anticholinergic effects but *in vitro* have shown to bind to muscarinic receptors.

Reviews*: drug-induced delirium, including management (Francis, *CNS Drugs* 1995, **5**, 103–14), short review (Jacoby, *Pres J* 1998, **38**, 242–48), general review (Karlsson, *Dement Geriatr Cogn Disord* 1999, **10**, 412–15; Brown, *Semin Clin Neuropsychiatry* 2000, **5**, 113–24), in the elderly (Moore and O'Keeffe, *Drugs & Aging* 1999, **15**, 15–28; Inouye, *Demen & Geri Cog Disord* 1999, **10**, 393–400).

● **Psychotropics etc ***

Amfetamines
Anticholinergic drugs (particular association, *J Am Geriatr Soc* 1988, **36**, 525)
Barbiturates
Benzodiazepines (commonest cause)
Bromides
Bupropion (cases, eg. *J Clin Psych* 1990, **51**, 307–8)
Butyrophenones
Cannabis
Chloral and derivatives
Clomethiazole
Clozapine withdrawal (n=3, *et al, J Clin Psych* 1997, **58**, 252–55)
Cocaine (*Am J Forensic Med Pathol* 1999, **20**, 120–27)
Disulfiram (*Am J Psych* 1974, **131**, 1281)
Fluoxetine (n=1, *Am J Psych* 1995, **152**, 295–96)
Lithium (eg. *Am J Psych* 1983, **140**, 1612)
MAOIs
Meprobamate
Mianserin (*BMJ* 1988, **296**, 137)
Mirtazapine (n=3, *Int Clin Psychopharmacol* 2000, **15**, 239–43)
Paroxetine and benztropine (*Am J Psych* 1997, **154**, 581–82)
Phenelzine (*J Clin Psych* 1987, **48**, 340–41)

Phenothiazines (esp. sedative ones)
Risperidone (n=1, *Can J Psych* 1998, **43**, 194)
Rivastigmine (<5%, MI)
Trazodone (n=3, *Int Clin Psychopharmacol* 1998, **13**, 225–28)
Tricyclics (*J Clin Psych* 1983, **44**, 173–76)

● **Drug withdrawal etc**

Alcohol cessation (*Am J Psych* 1997, **154**, 846–51)
Barbiturates
Benzodiazepines
Clomethiazole
Dextropropoxyphene
Nicotine withdrawal (*J Pain & Symptom Manage* 1998, **15**, S18)
Solvent intoxication

● **Anticonvulsants**

Barbiturates (dose-related)
Carbamazepine (especially early in therapy)
Ethosuximide
Phenytoin (dose-related)
Primidone
Valproate (high dose)

● **Anti-parkinsonian drugs**

Amantadine (case in *Am J Psych* 1980, **137**, 240–42)
Anticholinergics (esp. longer-acting ones, eg. benzhexol)
Bromocriptine
Levodopa (*Lancet* 1973, **ii**, 929)
Lysuride
Methixene
Pergolide withdrawal (*Clin Neuro-pharmacology* 1988, **11**, 545–48)
Selegiline

● **Cardiovascular drugs**

Amiodarone (n=1, *Am J Psych* 1999, **156**, 1119)
Amiloride
Beta-blockers (eg. *Postgrad Med J* 1990, **66**, 1050–52)
Atenolol (n=1, *BMJ* 1988, **297**, 1048)
Clonidine (*Curr Med Res Opin* 1977, **4**, 630)
Digoxin (*Am Heart J* 1983, **106**, 419; *J Clin Pharmac* 1979, **19**, 747)
Disopyramide
Diuretics (via severe K+ loss)
Hydralazine
Lidocaine
Methyldopa
Mexilitine

Procainamide
Spironolactone

● **NSAIDs and analgesics**
Aspirin toxicity (*Lancet* 1971, **2**, 242)
Fenoprofen
Ibuprofen (*Arthritis Rheumat* 1982, **25**, 1013)
Indometacin (*Curr Med Research Opin* 1974, **2**, 600–10)
Indometacin OD (*Drugs* 1980, **19**, 220–42)
Nalbuphine
Naproxen (*Arthritis Rheumat* 1982, **25**, 1013)
Narcotics
Papaveretum
Salicylate OD (*Arch Int Med* 1976, **85**, 745–48)
Sulindac (*JAMA* 1980, **243**, 1630)
Tramadol (n=11, *Curr Problems* 1995, **21**, 2)

● **Anticholinergics**
Anti-parkinsonian drugs (separate section)
Atropine and homatropine eye drops
Scopolamine (transdermal) (*JAMA* 1988, **260**, 478)

● **Anti-infection**
These may indirectly cause delirium if inducing diarrhoea and dehydration.
Acyclovir (n=1, *Clin Infect Dis* 1995, **21**, 435–36; *Nervenarzt* 1998, **69**, 1015–18)
Cephalosporins (*BMJ* 1989, **299**, 393)
Chloramphenicol (*Clin Pharmac Therap* 1970, **11**, 194)
Chloroquine
Ciprofloxacin (*Arch Int Med* 1989, **110**, 170–71; n=1, *Ann Pharmacother* 1997, **31**, 252, letter)
Clarithromycin (*Psychosomatics* 1998, **39**, 540–42)
Cycloserine
Isoniazid (*BMJ* 1969, **i**, 461)
Mefloquine (*Pharm J* 1989, **243**, 561)
Penicillin
Rifampicin
Streptomycin
Sulphadiazine
Sulphonamides

● **Miscellaneous**
Adrenocorticotrophin
Aminophylline
Baclofen

Caffeine (*Am J Psych* 1978, **135**, 855–56)
Cimetidine (eg. *Ann Int Med* 1992, **115**, 658–59)
Corticosteroids (11% incidence? review by Ismail and Wessely, *B J Hosp Pharm* 1995, **53**, 495–99)
Cycloserine
Doxapram
Famotidine (n=1, *Pharmacother* 1998, **18**, 404–7)
Gancyclovir (*NEJM* 1990, **322**, 933–34)
Hydroxychloroquine
Hypoglycaemics (oral)
Iodoform gauze (n=1, *Lancet* 1997, **350**, 1294)
Interferon Alfa (*Arch Int Med* 1987, **147**, 1557–80)
Methylprednisolone
Misoprostol (*Drug Intell Clin Pharm* 1991, **25**, 133–44)
Nabilone
Nalbuphine
Phenylpropanolamine O/D (*Br Heart J* 1982, **47**, 51–54)
Piperazine
Ranitidine (*Ann Int Med* 1992, **115**, 658–59; *BMJ* 1987, **294**, 1616)
Theophylline (*BMJ* 1982, **284**, 939)
Triamcinolone

5.5 DEPRESSION

Occurs mainly in patients with a history of depression.
Reviews*: general (Patten and Love, *Psychother Psychosom* 1997, **66**, 63–73), in elderly (Dhondt *et al*, *Int J Ger Psych* 1996, **11**, 141–48).

● **Psychotropics etc ***
Benzodiazepines (especially resistant depression):
  Alprazolam (*Am J Psych* 1987, **144**, 664–65)
  Bromazepam (*Acta Psych Scand* 1989, **74**, 451–58)
  Clorazepate
  Lorazepam (*Am J Psych* 1989, **146**, 1230)
Benzodiazepine withdrawal (*Psychol Med* 1984, **14**, 937–40)
Buspirone (3% incidence? *J Clin Psych* 1982, **43**[sect 2], 100–2)
Disulfiram (case in *Arch Neurol* 1976, **33**, 141)
Flumazenil (<1% incidence, MI)

Fluoxetine (intense suicidal ideation) (*Am J Psych* 1990, **147**, 570–72 etc), disproven (*BMJ* 1991, **303**, 685–92), as fluoxetine shows a slight reduction in suicidal behaviour (n=185, Leon *et al, Am J Psych* 1999, **156**, 195–201)

Fluphenazine depot (n=1, *BMJ* 1969, **3**, 564–67)

MDMA ('Ecstasy') (case in *Lancet* 1991, **338**, 1520, letter, *Lancet* 1996, **347**, 833)

Nortriptyline (n=2, *BMJ* 1964, **2**, 1593)

Smoking cessation (n=1, *Acta Psych Scand* 1998, **98**, 507–8; n=304, *Am J Psych* 2000, **157**, 368–74)

Tetrabenazine

Zuclopenthixol

● **Anticonvulsants**

Carbamazepine

Clobazam (n=1, *BMJ* 1983, **286**, 1246–47)

Clonazepam

Ethosuximide

Lamotrigine (rare, *Epilepsia* 1991, **32** [Suppl 2], S17–21)

Levetiracetam (MI)

Phenobarbital (*Pediatrics* 1990, **85**, 1086–91)

Vigabatrin (<10%, *Neurology* 1991, **41**, 363–64; *Lancet* 1990, **335**, 970)

● **Anti-parkinsonian drugs**

Amantadine (mentioned in *JAMA* 1972, **222**, 792–95)

Anticholinergics

Levodopa (well known, review in *NEJM* 1976, **295**, 814–18)

● **Cardiovascular drugs ***

Amiodarone (n=1, *B J Psych* 1999, **174**, 366–67; n=1, *J Pharm Tech* 1999, **15**, 50–53)

Beta-blockers (*Drug Intell Clin Pharm* 1984, **18**, 741–42). Lipophilic drugs may be more likely: atenolol, nadolol (low lipid solubility), labetalol, oxprenolol, timolol, acebutol (low/moderate), pindolol (moderate), metoprolol (moderate/high), propranolol (high). Theory disputed in *JAMA* 1992, **267**, 1783–87;1826–27).

Acebutol (mentioned in *Am J Med* 1987, **83**, 223–26)

Atenolol (*J Hum Hypertens* 1987, **1**, 87–93)

Metoprolol (5% incidence? review in *Drugs* 1977, **14**, 321–48)

Nadolol (*Lancet* 1982, **i**, 1286)

Propranolol (*Am J Psych* 1982, **139**, 1187–88)

Timolol

Calcium-channel blockers (no increased risk of suicide with use of calcium channel blockers compared to other antihypertensives, n=153,458, Gasse *et al, BMJ* 2000, **320**, 1251)

Felodipine (cases in *Br Heart J* 1987, **58**, 122–28)

Nicardipine (cases mentioned in *B J Clin Pharmacol* 1985, **20**[Suppl], 178–86)

Nifedipine (*B J Psych* 1991, **159**, 447–48)

Clonidine (1% incidence, case study in *Postgrad Med J* 1993, **150**, 1750)

Diltiazem (*BMJ* 1989, **299**, 796)

Enalapril (n=1, *South Med J* 1989, **82**, 402–3)

Hydralazine

Inositol (n=3, *Am J Psych* 1996, **153**, 839)

Lisinopril (rare, MI)

Methyldopa (review in *Am J Psych* 1983, **140**, 534–38)

Prazosin

Procainamide

Quinapril (n=1, *Am J Psych* 1999, **156**, 1115)

Quinidine (several cases eg. *J Am Geriatr Soc* 1985, **33**, 504–6)

Streptokinase (cases, eg. *Drugs* 1973, **5**, 357–445)

● **Gastrointestinal**

Cimetidine (several cases, eg. *Can J Psych* 1981, **26**, 260–61; *Am J Psych* 1979, **136**, 346)

Famotidine (rare reports, MI)

Metoclopramide (cases, eg. *Am J Gastroenterology* 1989, **84**, 1589–90)

Omeprazole (unproven reports)

Ranitidine (n=3, *Am J Psych* 1986, **143**, 915–16)

Sulphasalazine (MI)

● **NSAIDs and analgesics**

Diflunisal (<1% incidence, MI)

Etodolac (rare, MI)

Flurbiprofen (>1% incidence? MI)

Ibuprofen (uncommon, *Arthritis Rheumat* 1982, **25**, 1013)

Indometacin (4% incidence? *BMJ* 1972, **4**, 398)

Nabilone

Nalbuphine
Naproxen (rare)
Pentazocine (*Southern Med J* 1975, **68**, 808)
Sulindac
Tramadol (n=1, *Am J Psych* 1996, **153**, 843–44)

● **Anti-infection ***

Anti-TB drugs (*Lancet* 1989, **ii**, 735–36)
Cephradine (n=1, *Med J Aus* 1973, **2**, 742)
Chloramphenicol (rare mild cases)
Ciprofloxacin (very rare)
Clotrimazole – oral (review in *Drugs* 1975, **9**, 424)
Co-trimoxazole (rare, but severe cases, eg. *Drug Intell Clin Pharm* 1988, **22**, 267)
Dapsone (*BMJ* 1989, **298**, 1524)
Griseofulvin (as part of psychosis, case in *JAMA* 1974, **229**, 1420)
Mefloquine (*Am J Psych* 1992, **149**, 712; CSM warning, *Curr Prob Pharmacovig* 1999, **25**, 15)
Metronidazole (n=1, *Am J Psych* 1977, **134**, 329–30)
Piperazine (cases, eg. *J Indian Med Assoc* 1976, **66**, 33)
Primaquine (n=1, *Ann Int Med* 1980, **92**, 435)
Sulphonamides/sulfonamides

● **Respiratory**

Aminophylline (*BMJ* 1980, **281**, 1322)
Ephedrine (as part of a psychosis, *BMJ* 1968, **2**, 160)
Flunisolide (inhaled, 1–3% incidence, MI)
Theophylline (*BMJ* 1980, **281**, 1322)

● **Cytotoxics etc**

Interferon alfa (review in *Arch Int Med* 1987, **147**, 1577–80)
Mesna
Mithramycin
Octreotide (rare, MI)
Plicamycin
Tamoxifen (n=1, *Ann Int Med* 1984, **101**, 652)
Triamcinolone (up to 8%, see *BMJ* 1969, **i**, 682)

● **Steroids**

Review: Ismail and Wessely, *B J Hosp Med* 1995, **53**, 495–99.
Dexamethasone (up to 40% incidence, *Arch Gen Psych* 1981, **38**, 471–77)

Methyltestosterone (rare)
Prednisolone (*J Ass Physicians India* 1973, **21**, 909)
Prednisone (review in *Clin Paediatr* 1990, **29**, 382–88)
Stanozolol

● **Miscellaneous ***

Allopurinol
Astemizole (debatable – *Drugs* 1984, **28**, 38–61)
Baclofen (rare cases eg. *Arch Int Med* 1985, **145**, 1717–18)
Botulinum toxin A injection (*South Med J* 1999, **92**, 738)
Caffeine withdrawal (review in *NEJM* 1992, **327**, 1160–61)
Cinnarizine (*BMJ* 1988, **297**, 722)
Clomiphene
Codeine – long-term use (community survey, *J Clin Psychopharmacol* 1999, **19**, 373–76)
Danazol (rare cases, *Am J Obstet* 1977, **127**, 130)
Diphenoxylate (MI)
Etretinate (*BMJ* 1989, **298**, 964)
Fentanyl (transdermal)
Hydroxyzine (some reports)
Interferon (n=1, *Am J Psych* 1999, **156**, 1120)
Isotretinoin (v. rare, *J Am Dermatol* 1988, **18**, 543–52; summary — *Pharm J* 1998, **260**, 547; case of suicide – *JAMA* 1998, **279**, 1057)
Ondansetron (n=1, *Am J Psych* 1995, **152**, 1101)
Oral contraceptives combined (16–56% incidence, review in *J Adolescent Health Care* 1981, **2**, 53–64)
Phenylpropanolamine (*Am J Psych* 1990, **147**, 367–68)
Pravastatin (n=4, *Lancet* 1993, **341**, 910)
Progestogens (*Drug Treatment Psych* 1982, **12**, 234–35)
Roaccutane (SPC)
Simvastatin (*Curr Prob* 1992, **33**, n=4, *Lancet* 1993, **341**, 14. Low cholesterol is a high risk factor for attempted suicide – *Am J Psych* 1995, **152**, 419–23)
Trimeprazine/alimemazine
Xylometazoline (case in child in *JAMA* 1970, **211**, 123–24)

5.6 HALLUCINATIONS (including visual disturbances, see also psychosis)

● **Psychotropics etc ***

Alcohol

Amfetamines (*Biol Psych* 1980, **15**, 749)

Benzodiazepines

Carbamazepine

Fluoxetine (case in *Am J Psych* 1993, **150**, 1750)

Gabapentin

Imipramine

LSD (*J Nerv Mental Dis* 1991, **179**, 173–74)

Maprotiline (n=1, *Acta Psych Scand* 2000, **101**, 476–77)

Methadone (*J Am Acad Child Adolesc Psych* 1999, **38**, 355–56)

Midazolam IV (*Drug Intell Clin Pharm* 1989, **23**, 671–72)

Nefazodone (visual field shimmering, n=2, *J Clin Psych* 1999, **60**, 124)

Phenelzine (n=1, *Am J Psych* 1994, **151**, 450)

Tricyclics

Valproate

Zolpidem (n=5, *J Toxicol Clin Toxicol* 1998, **36**, 195–203)

Zopiclone (*Pharm J* 1990, **245**, 210)

● **Anti-parkinson drugs**

Amantadine (n=1, *Med J Aus* 1973, **1**, 444)

Anticholinergics

Bromocriptine (<1% incidence – *Ann Int Med* 1984, **101**, 149)

Levodopa (<26% incidence in elderly, eg. *Postgrad Med J* 1989, **65**, 358–61)

Pergolide (in up to 13% eg. *Neurology* 1982, **32**, 1181–84)

Pergolide withdrawal (*Clin Neuro-pharmacology* 1988, **11**, 545–48)

● **Cardiovascular drugs**

Beta-blockers (*Postgrad Med J* 1987, **63**, 57–58)

Clonidine (n=3, *Ann Int Med* 1980, **93**, 456)

Digoxin *(Ann Int Med* 1979, **91**, 865).

Diltiazem (*Psychiatr Prax* 1998, **25**, 91–92)

Disopyramide

Procainamide

Streptokinase (reported in *Drugs* 1973, **5**, 357–445)

Timolol (*JAMA* 1980, **244**, 768)

● **NSAIDs and analgesics**

Buprenorphine (rare <1%, eg. *BMJ* 1988, **296**, 214)

Buprenorphine – epidural (*BMJ* 1989, **298**, 928)

Fenbufen (*BMJ* 1985, **290**, 822)

Indometacin (rare, eg. *BMJ* 1966, **1**, 80; OD in *Drugs* 1980, **19**, 220–42)

Nefopam (*Curr Problems*, **24**, *1.89*)

Pentazocine

Salicylates

Tramadol (n=6, *Curr Probs* 1995, **21**, 2)

● **Anti-infections**

Amoxycillin/amoxicillin (*Practitioner* 1984, **228**, 884)

Ciprofloxacin (*Arch Int Med* 1989, **110**, 170–71)

Gentamicin (*JAMA* 1977, **238**, 53)

Itraconazole, oral (n=1, *Clin Infect Dis* 1995, **21**, 456)

● **Miscellaneous ***

Cimetidine (*Arch Int Med* 1983, **98**, 677)

Corticosteroids

Decongestants (*BMJ* 1984, **288**, 1688)

Erythropoetin (n=5, *NEJM* 1991, **325**, 285; *J Neurol* 1999, **246**, 614–16)

Famotidine (n=1, *Pharmacother* 1998, **18**, 404–7)

Hydroxyurea

Khat chewing (n=4, *B J Hosp Med* 1995, **54**, 322–26)

Ketamine (*Anaesthesia* 1990, **45**, 422)

Mefloquine (*NEJM* 1990, **322**, 1752–53)

Phenylephrine (*JAMA* 1982, **247**, 1859)

Phenylpropanolamine (*JAMA* 1981, **245**, 601–2)

Promethazine (*Acta Paediatrica Scand* 1989, **78**, 131–32)

Pseudoephedrine

Radiocontrast media (n=2, review, *Br J Clin Pharmacol* 1999, **47**, 226–27)

Ranitidine (*E J Clin Pharm* 1985, **29**, 375–76)

Salbutamol (nebulised) (*BMJ* 1986, **292**, 1430)

Sulphasalazine

Tolterodine (n=1, *B J Urol* 1999, **84**, 1109)

5.7 MANIA, HYPOMANIA or EUPHORIA

Antidepressant-induced mania may be a marker for increased vulnerability to

antidepressant-induced cycle acceleration. The most common symptoms of drug-induced mania are increased activity, rapid speech, elevated mood and insomnia. The main risk factors are prior history, family history or concurrent mood disorder. Steroids, levodopa, triazolo-benzodiazepines and hallucinogens are most commonly associated. A sudden switch to mania or hypomania may be indicative of the diagnosis of Bipolar III.
Reviews: antidepressant-induced mania (Altshuler *et al, Am J Psych* 1995, **152**, 1130–38), drug induced mania (Peet and Peters, *Drug Safety* 1995, **12**, 146–53).

● **Hallucinogens**
LSD (*Am J Psych* 1981, **138**, 1508–9)

● **CNS stimulants**
Amfetamine withdrawal (*J Clin Psych* 1980, **41**, 33–34)
Dexamfetamine (*Am J Psych* 1976, **133**, 1177–80)
Ephedrine (*J Clin Psychopharmacol* 1983, **3**, 97–100; and in a Herbal Diet Supplement, case in *Am J Psych* 1995, **152**, 647)
Methylphenidate (*J Clin Psych* 1986, **47**, 566–67)
Pemoline (possible case in *Biol Psych* 1981, **16**, 987–89)
Phenylephrine (*Am J Psych* 1981, **138**, 837–38)
Phenylpropanolamine (*Am J Psych* 1981, **138**, 392)
Pseudoephedrine (*Psych J of Uni Ottawa* 1987, **12**, 47–48)

● **Antidepressants ***
Antidepressant-induced switching to mania is well known (especially in Bipolar III), as is the spontaneous swing to hypomania from depression in bipolars. SSRIs and bupropion are generally considered less likely to switch. The incidence of switch from depression to mania is in the order of 25% with placebo and 50% with tricyclics (Post *et al, CNS Drugs* 1997, **8**, 352–65, 80 refs)
Reviews: Peet, *B J Psych* 1995, **164**, 549–50; Benazzi, *J Aff Dis* 1997, **46**, 73–77.
Amitriptyline (*BMJ* 1991, **303**, 331–32, 720, 1200; *Neurology* 1989, **39**, 305)
Amitriptyline withdrawal (*J Clin Psych* 1980, **41**, 33–34)

Amoxapine (*Compr Psych* 1982, **23**, 590–92)
Clomipramine (*Arch Gen Psych* 1979, **36**, 560–65)
Desipramine (*Am J Psych* 1985, **142**, 386)
Desipramine withdrawal (*Am J Psych* 1983, **140**, 624–25)
Fluoxetine (cases in *Ann Pharmacother* 1991, **25**, 1395–96; *Am J Psych* 1991, **148**, 1403–4; n=3, *J Child Adolesc Psychopharmacol* 1998, **8**, 73–80)
Fluvoxamine (*Am J Psych* 1991, **148**, 1263–64; case series in *Ann Pharmacother* 1993, **27**, 1455–57)
Imipramine (eg. *J Clin Psychopharmacol* 1985, **5**, 342–43)
Imipramine withdrawal (*Am J Psych* 1986, **143**, 260)
Isocarboxazid (n=3, *J Clin Psych* 1986, **47**, 40–41)
Isocarboxazid withdrawal (n=2, *J Clin Psychopharmacol* 1985, **5**, 340–42)
Maprotiline (cases in *Curr Ther Res* 1976, **19**, 463–68)
Mianserin
Mirtazapine (n=1, *J Neuropsychiatry Clin Neurosci* 1999, **11**, 115–16; n=1, *B J Psych* 1999, **175**, 390)
Mirtazapine withdrawal (n=1, *B J Psych* 1999, **175**, 390)
Mirtazapine + sertraline (n=1, *J Clin Psychiatry* 1998, **59**, 320)
Nefazodone (n=1, *Am J Psych* 1997, **154**, 578–79)
Paroxetine (case of psychotic mania, *Am J Psych* 1995, **152**, 1399–440)
Phenelzine (eg. *Biol Psych* 1985, **20**, 1009–14)
Sertraline (cases in *Am J Psych* 1987, **144**, 1513–14; *Am J Psych* 1994, **343**, 606–7)
St. John's wort (n=1, *J Clin Psych* 1998, **59**, 689; n=2, *Biol Psych* 1999, **46**, 1707–8)
Trazodone (eg. *B J Psych* 1991, **158**, 275–78)
Trazodone withdrawal (*B J Psych* 1987, **151**, 274)
Tryptophan + MAOI (*Am J Psych* 1985, **142**, 1487–88)
Venlafaxine (*J Clin Psychopharmacol* 1999, **19**, 184–85)

● **Other Psychotropics etc ***

Alprazolam (*J Clin Psych* 1987, **48**, 117–18)

Benzodiazepine withdrawal (*Acta Psych Scand* 1989, **79**, 406–7)

Bupropion (rare, *Am J Psych* 1991, **148**, 541)

Buspirone (*B J Psych* 1991, **158**, 136–37)

Disulfiram (*J Clin Psychopharmacol* 1986, **6**, 178–80; *J Am Acad Child Adolesc Psych* 1988, **27**, 500–3)

Fenfluramine (eg. *Med J Aus* 1976, **2**, 537; *Am J Psych* 1997, **154**, 711)

Lithium + TCA (*B J Psych* 1988, **153**, 828–30)

Lithium toxicity (*Drug Intell Clin Pharm* 1987, **21**, 979)

Lorazepam withdrawal (*J Aff Dis* 1989, **17**, 93–95)

Midazolam (euphoria possible)

Olanzapine (review, concludes half of reports are poorly documented but in the others mood elevating effects were prominent, n=26, *J Clin Psych* 2000, **61**, 649–55).

Risperidone (review, concludes half of reports are poorly documented but in the others mood elevating effects were prominent, n=26, *J Clin Psych* 2000, **61**, 649–55; eg. *Ann Pharmacother* 1999, **33**, 380–81).

Risperidone withdrawal (n=1, *J Clin Psych* 1998, **59**, 620–21)

● **Anticonvulsants**

Carbamazepine (*J Clin Psych* 1984, **45**, 272–74)

Carbamazepine withdrawal (n=1, *B J Psych* 1995, **167**, 698)

Clonazepam (*Drug Intell Clin Pharm* 1991, **25**, 938–39)

Ethosuximide (MI)

Gabapentin (n=1, *B J Psych* 1995, **166**, 679–80; review in *B J Psych* 1995, **167**, 549–54; n=1, *B J Psych* 1999, **175**, 291)

Phenobarbital (*Paediatrics* 1984, **74**, 1133)

Valproate

Vigabatrin (n=1, *Lancet* 1994, **343**, 606–7)

● **Anti-Parkinsonian drugs**

Amantadine (n=1, *J Clin Psych* 1989, **50**, 143–44)

Bromocriptine (*BMJ* 1984, **289**, 1101–3)

Levodopa (cases in, eg. *NEJM* 1971, **285**, 1326 etc)

Levodopa + carbidopa (*J Clin Psychopharmacol* 1985, **5**, 338–39)

Procyclidine (eg. *B J Psych* 1982, **141**, 81–84)

● **Cardiovascular drugs**

Captopril (*Am J Psych* 1985, **142**, 759–60; case in *Am J Psych* 1993, **150**, 1429–30)

Clonidine (*Am J Psych* 1982, **139**, 1083)

Clonidine withdrawal (*J Clin Psychopharmacol* 1981, **1**, 93–95)

Digoxin (*Medical Journal & Record* 1929, **130**, 381–82)

Diltiazem (*Clin Cardiology* 1984, **7**, 611–12)

Hydralazine

Methyldopa withdrawal (*Am J Psych* 1989, **146**, 1075–76)

Procainamide (*Am J Psych* 1988, **145**, 129–30)

Propranolol (*Southern Med J* 1984, **77**, 1603)

Propranolol withdrawal (*Am J Psych* 1986, **143**, 1633)

Reserpine (*J Nerv Mental Dis* 1982, **170**, 502–4)

● **NSAIDs and analgesics**

Buprenorphine (up to 1%, *B J Clin Pract* 1980, **34**, 144–46)

Codeine + paracetamol (n=1, *Aust N Z J Psych* 1998, **32**, 586–88)

Indometacin (*J Clin Psychopharmacol* 1987, **7**, 203–4)

Nefopam IM (euphoria reported — *B J Anaesth* 1979, **51**, 691–95)

Pentazocine (*Southern Med J* 1975, **68**, 808)

● **Gastrointestinal**

Cimetidine (*J Clin Psych* 1983, **44**, 267–68)

Metoclopramide (case in *J Clin Psych* 1984, **45**, 180)

Ranitidine IV (case in *Southern Med J* 1987, **80**, 1467)

● **Steroids**

ACTH (*Psychosomatic Med* 1953, **15**, 280–91)

Beclometasone/beclomethasone aerosol (*Am J Psych* 1989, **146**, 1076–77)

Beclometasone/beclomethasone nasal spray (*B J Psych* 1989, **155**, 871–72)

Corticosteroids (*Clin Pharm* 1987, **6**,
186; n=1, *Anesthesiology* 1996, **85**,
1194–96)
Cortisone (*Psychosomat Med* 1953, **15**,
589–97)
Dexamethasone (up to 31% incidence,
Arch Gen Psych 1981, **38**, 471–77)
Hydrocortisone (*J Nerv Mental Dis*
1979, **167**, 229–36; *Postgrad Med J*
1992, **68**, 41–43)
Prednisone (*J Aff Dis* 1983, **5**, 319–24)
Testosterone-patches (n=1, *Am J Psych*
1999, **156**, 969)
Triamcinolone (rare cases)

● **Anti-infection**
Anti-TB drugs (*Lancet* 1989, **ii**,
735–36)
Chloroquine (*B J Psych* 1991, **159**,
164–65 + 735)
Clarithromycin (n=1, *Am J Psych* 1998,
155, 1626)
Dapsone (*BMJ* 1989, **298**, 1524)
Isoniazid (*BMJ* 1957, **ii**, 743–46)
Mepacrine (*Mayo Clin Proceed* 1989,
64, 129)
Zidovudine (*JAMA* 1988, **259**, 3406)

● **Miscellaneous ***
Alimemazine/trimeprazine (rare cases)
Aminophylline
Baclofen (eg. *Biol Psych* 1982, **17**,
757–59)
Baclofen withdrawal (*Am J Psych* 1980,
137, 1466–67)
Bromide (*Am J Psych* 1976, **133**,
228–29)
Calcium IV (*J Nerv Mental Dis* 1980,
168, 562–63)
Cyclizine (MI)
Cyclosporin (*Biol Psych* 1984, **19**,
1161–62)
Cyproheptadine (rare, eg. *Am J Psych*
1980, **137**, 378–79)
Decongestants
Dextromethorphan abuse (cases in *BMJ*
1986, **293**, 597 & *BMJ* 1993, **306**,
896)
Dihydroepiandrosterone (*Biol Psych*
1999, **45**, 241–42)
Herbal remedies (n=1, *Am J Psych*
1998, **155**, 1627)
Interferon-alpha (n=1, *Postgrad Med J*
1997, **73**, 834–35)
Mazindol (not reported — *B J Addict*
1972, **67**, 39–44)
Nicotine withdrawal (*Am J Psych* 1990,

147, 1254–55; *Am J Psych* 1992, **149**,
708)
Omega-3 fatty acids (n=1, *Arch Gen
Psych* 2000, **57**, 715–16)
Procarbazine (*BMJ* 1982, **284**, 82)
Salbutamol
Terfenadine (cases of euphoria, eg.
Lancet 1989, **2**, 615–16)
Thyroid (*Am J Psych* 1970, **126**,
1667–69)
Tramadol (n=1, *Am J Psych* 1997, **154**,
1624)
Triptorelin (n=1, *B J Psych* 1999, **175**,
290–91),
Triiodothyronine (*J Clin Psych* 1986,
47, 521–32)
Yohimbine? (see *Arch Gen Psych* 1998,
55, 1033–44)

5.8 MOVEMENT DISORDERS

EXTRA-PYRAMIDAL DISORDERS
Four distinct types of drug-induced extra-
pyramidal or movement disorders are
common, especially by antipsychotics.
These are dystonia, akathisia, pseudoparkinsonism and dyskinesia. All can occur
acutely or be delayed (tardive). Acute
reactions are usually at the start of
treatment or after a dose increase and are
usually reversible. The tardive forms are
not invariably reversible on discontinuation of the drug or on dose
reduction and can be aggravated by
anticholinergics.
Reviews*: calcium channel blockers as
cause of EPSEs (*Ann Pharmacother* 1995,
29, 73–75), general (Jimenez-Jimenez *et
al, Drug Safety* 1997, **16**, 180–204, 643
refs; n=1559, Muscettola *et al, J Clin
Psychopharmacol* 1999, **19**, 203–8),
SSRI-induced movement disorders
(Gerber and Lynd, *Ann Pharmacother*
1998, **32**, 692–98), management of acute
antipsychotic-induced EPSEs (Remington
and Bezchlibnyk-Butler, *CNS Drugs* 1996,
5[Suppl 1], 21–35), tardive EPSEs
(Marsalek, *Pharmacopsychiatry* 2000,
33[Suppl 1], 14–33).

5.8.1 Pseudoparkinsonism
This is characterised by akinesia, tremor
and rigidity, and generally occurs within
a month of the start of treatment.
● **Psychotropics etc ***
Amoxapine (*Am J Psych* 1983, **140**,
1233–35)

Antipsychotics (see *2.1.5*).
Bromocriptine
Bupropion (n=1, *J Clin Psych* 1992, **53**, 157–59)
Clozapine (n=1, *Ann Pharmacother* 2000, **34**, 615–18)
Cocaine abuse (*Arch Int Med* 1997, **157**, 241)
Dexamfetamine
Donepezil (n=1, *Ann Pharmacother* 1998, **32**, 610–11)
Fluoxetine (*Am J Psych* 1989, **146**, 1352–53; case in *Neurology* 1993, **43**, 211–13)
Fluoxetine withdrawal (*Am J Psych* 1991, **148**, 1263)
Fluvoxamine (*Am J Psych* 1989, **146**, 1352–53)
Lithium
  long-term (eg. *B J Psych* 1980, **136**, 191)
  short-term (*J Neurol Sci* 2000, **176**, 78–79)
MAOIs
Olanzapine overdose (n=1, *Am J Psych* 1998, **155**, 1630–31)
Paroxetine (cases reported in *Current Problems* 1993, **19**, 1; incidence as with other SSRIs – *Lancet* 1993, **341**, 624)
Prochlorperazine
Risperidone (case with 2mg/d, Mahmood, *Lancet* 1995, **346**, 1226; probable case, *Am J Psych* 1996, **153**, 843)
Sertraline (n=1, *Am J Psych* 1994, **151**, 288)
Trazodone (*Clin Neuropharmacol* 1988, **11**, 180–82)
Tricyclics

● **Anticonvulsants**
Carbamazepine (tremor may occur in 22% of pts, *NEJM* 1992, **327**, 765–71)
Valproate

● **NSAIDs and analgesics**
Fenoprofen
Flurbiprofen (*BMJ* 1990, **300**, 549)
Ibuprofen (case in *Postgrad Med J* 1987, **63**, 593–94)
Indometacin
Mefenamic acid (n=1, *J Roy Soc Med* 1983, **76**, 435)
Nabilone
Pethidine and other opioids
Sulindac (single case in *Ann Neurol* 1985, **17**, 104–5)

● **Cardiovascular drugs**
Amiodarone (*Annals Neurol* 1989, **25**, 630–32)
Diazoxide (n=6, *BMJ* 1973, **3**, 474–75)
Diltiazem (*Am J Med* 1989, **87**, 95–96)
Methyldopa (cases in *Can Med Assoc J* 1966, **95**, 928)
Metirosine
Mexilitine
Nifedipine (*BMJ* 1978, **i**, 1619)
Tocainide

● **Gastrointestinal**
Cimetidine (possible case in *Postgrad Med J* 1982, **58**, 527–28)
Domperidone (rare, case in *Helv Paediat Acta* 1984, **39**, 285–88)
Metoclopramide (2–30% incidence, see *Drugs* 1983, **25**, 451–54; cases in, eg. *Ann Int Med* 1989, **149**, 2486–92; *Am J Gastroent* 1989, **84**, 1589–90)
Prochlorperazine (common, eg. *Lancet* 1984, **2**, 1082–83)

● **Anti-infection**
Acyclovir
Cephaloridine
Chloroquine

● **Respiratory drugs**
Antihistamines
Brompheniramine (*NEJM* 1975, **293**, 486)
Cinnarizine (*Lancet* 1987, **i**, 1324)
Diphenhydramine (*NEJM* 1977, **296**, 111)
Orciprenaline
Promethazine (*Clin Pharm* 1984, **3**, 83)
Salbutamol
Terbutaline

● **Hormones**
Medroxyprogesterone

● **Cytotoxics**
Cyclosporin
Interferons

● **Miscellaneous**
Cyclizine
Levodopa
Ondansetron (cases in *Ann Pharmacother* 1994, **28**, 280 and *Ann Pharmacother* 1996, **30**, 196)
Prednisolone (increases incidence with neuroleptics, review in *JAMA* 1973, **224**, 889)
Tetrabenazine

5.8.2 Akathisia

Characterised by motor restlessness, with an inability to stay still. Onset is around 6–60 days and has been implicated with all antipsychotics, but especially with the high potency ones.

Review: symptoms, classification, drug effects, classification, treatment etc (Gattera *et al, Aus J Hosp Pharm* 1994, **24**, 480–89).

● Psychotropics etc *

Alprazolam (MI)

Amoxapine (*Curr Ther Res* 1972, **14**, 381–89)

Antipsychotics (*Psychopharmacol* 1989, **97**, 1–11. Trifluoperazine and haloperidol more likely than less potent drugs, eg. chlorpromazine or thioridazine)

Buspirone (case in *Ann Int Med* 1983, **99**, 794–95).

Citalopram (case in *J Clin Psych* 1988, **49**[Suppl], 18–22)

Clozapine (6% incidence claimed by Kutz *et al, Psychopharmacology* 1995, **118**, 52–56; but may be rarer, see *Biol Psych* 1991, **29**, 1215–19)

Fluoxetine (*J Clin Psych* 1991, **52**, 491–93; *J Clin Psych* 1989, **50**, 339–42)

Fluvoxamine (n=1, resulting in suicide attempt, *J Clin Psych* 1999, **60**, 869)

Haloperidol (review in *Psychopharmacol* 1985, **21**, 69–72)

Imipramine (n=1, *J Clin Psychopharmacol* 1987, **7**, 254–57)

Lithium (*J Neurol Sci* 2000, **176**, 78–79)

Lorazepam (n=1, *Oncology* 1990, **47**, 415–17)

Mianserin (*B J Psych* 1989, **155**, 415–17)

Olanzapine (6% incidence)

Paroxetine (*Can J Psych* 2000, **45**, 398)

Pipothiazine (study in *Curr Ther Res* 1981, **29**, 903–14)

Prochlorperazine (44% incidence with IV, n=140, *Ann Emerg Med* 1999, **34**, 469–75)

Promazine (MI)

Risperidone (Shulman *et al, Neurology* 1995, **45**, 1419)

Risperidone withdrawal (*Am J Psych* 1997, **154**, 437–38)

Sertraline (n=1, *Am J Psych* 1993, **150**, 986–87; *J Clin Psych* 1993, **54**, 321)

Tricyclics (*BMJ* 1986, **282**, 1529)

Trimeprazine/alimemazine (MI)

Venlafaxine withdrawal (n=1, *Am Fam Physician* 1997, **56**, 455–62)

Zuclopenthixol (study in *Pharmatherapeutica* 1989, **5**, 380–86)

● Others

Diltiazem (n=1, *Ann Int Med* 1983, **99**, 794)

Interferon-alpha (*Gen Hosp Psychiatry* 1999, **21**, 134–35)

Levodopa (review in *Neurology* 1990, **40**, 340–45)

Melotonin withdrawal (*Mov Disord* 1999, **14**, 381–82)

Metoclopramide (n=1, *Milit Med* 1987, **152**, 585–86)

Ondansetron (n=1, *Cancer* 1992, **69**, 1275)

Prochlorperazine (n=1, *JAMA* 1985, **253**, 635)

Verapamil (*Lancet* 1991, **338**, 893)

5.8.3 Dystonias *

Includes oculogyric crisis, trismus and torticollis. May occur within 72 hours of start of therapy. Occurs more frequently with high-potency antipsychotics, where the incidence may be as high as 10% (*Applied Therapeutics*, Koda-Kimble, 1988).

Review: van Harten *et al, BMJ* 1999, **319**, 623–26, 34 refs.

● Psychotropics etc *

Amoxapine (*Psychosomatics* 1984, **25**, 66–69)

Benztropine (case in child in *Ann Emerg Med* 1986, **15**, 594–96)

Bupropion (n=1, *J Clin Psych* 1997, **58**, 218)

Buspirone (possible case in *Neurology* 1990, **40**, 1904; discussion in *Neurology* 1991, **41**, 1850)

Carbamazepine (n=1, *Postgrad Med J* 1994, **70**, 54; n=1, *NZ Med J* 1994, **107**, 360–61)

Clozapine (rare, n=1, *Am J Psych* 1995, **152**, 647–48)

Clozapine withdrawal, abrupt (cases, *J Clin Psych* 1998, **59**, 472–77)

Cocaine (risk factor for neuroleptic-induced acute dystonia, van Harten *et al, J Clin Psych* 1998, **59**, 128–30)

Cocaine withdrawal (*Neurology* 1989, **39**, 996)

Disulfiram (n=1, *Mov Disord* 1991, **6**, 166–70)

Fluoxetine (*Am J Psych* 1994, **151**, 149)

Flupentixol decanoate (n=1, *BMJ* 1981, **282**, 1756)

Loxapine (MI)

Midazolam (*BMJ* 1990, **300**, 614)

Olanzapine (n=1, *Am J Psych* 1999, **156**, 1662)

Paroxetine (cases reviewed in *Current Problems* 1993, **19**, 1)

Phenelzine (n=1, *J Clin Psychopharmacol* 1990, **10**, 144–45)

Prochlorperazine

Risperidone (n=1, *Am J Psych* 1996, **153**, 577; *Can J Psych* 1999, **44**, 507–8; n=1, *Lancet* 1999, **353**, 981, letter)

Sertraline (n=1, *J Clin Psychopharmacol* 1999, **19**, 98–100)

Tricyclics

Zuclopenthixol (study in *Acta Psych Scand* 1991, **84**, 14–16)

● **Others**

Alimemazine/trimeprazine (MI).

Amiodarone (isolated case in *Lancet* 1979, **1**, 981–82)

Azapropazone (n=1, *J Neurol Neurosurg Psych* 1988, **51**, 731–32)

Diphenhydramine oral (*Clin Pharm* 1989, **8**, 471)

Diphenhydramine IV (*Ann Int Med* 1989, **111**, 92–93)

Domperidone

Ergotamine (*Mov Disord* 1991, **6**, 263–64)

Indometacin (n=1, *J Neurol Neurosurg Psych* 1988, **51**, 731–32)

Metoclopramide (3% incidence, see *NEJM* 1983, **309**, 433; cases in, eg. *Ann Int Med* 1989, **149**, 2486–92)

Nifedipine (*Ann Int Med* 1985, **104**, 125)

Penicillamine (review in *Arch Neurol* 1987, **44**, 490–93)

Prochlorperazine (many cases)

Promethazine (n=1, *Clin Pharm* 1984, **3**, 83–85)

Propranolol

Sumatriptan (possible case in *Ann Pharmacother* 1994, **28**, 1199)

Amoxapine (mentioned in *J Clin Psychopharmacol* 1987, **7**, 243–46)

Benztropine (study showed worsening TD — *Neuropsychobiology* 1980, **6**, 109)

Bupropion (*J Clin Psych* 1997, **58**, 218)

Buspirone? (*Pharm J* 1989, **243**, 480)

Clomipramine (*Am J Psych* 1993, **150**, 165–66)

Clozapine (n=1, *Biol Psych* 1994, **35**, 886–87)

Clozapine withdrawal, abrupt (cases, *J Clin Psychiatry* 1998, **59**, 472–77)

Doxepin (10% incidence in study in *J Clin Psychopharmacol* 1987, **7**, 243–46)

Diphenhydramine (n=1, *Can J Psych* 1985, **30**, 370–71)

Fluoxetine (*Am J Psych* 1991, **148**, 1403; *Am J Psych* 1995, **152**, 122–25)

Fluvoxamine (n=1, *J Clin Psychopharmacol* 1993, **13**, 365–66)

Fluoxetine + low dose neuroleptics (*Am J Psych* 1991, **148**, 683)

Flupentixol decanoate (*Psychopharmacol* 1983, **81**, 359–62)

Haloperidol (many cases)

Lithium (*Am J Psych* 1979, **136**, 1229–30; *B J Psych* 1990, **156**, 128–29)

Loxapine (MI)

Metoclopramide (BNF, many cases, eg. *Neurology* 1984, **34**, 238–39)

Olanzapine (n=2, *Ann Int Med* 1999, **131**, 72; n=1, *J Clin Psych* 1999, **60**, 870)

Phenytoin (n=1, *NEJM* 1978, **298**, 457)

Pimozide (35% incidence reported, probably rarer – see *Neurology* 1982, **32**, 1335–46)

Quetiapine (n=1, *Am J Psych* 1999, **156**, 796–97)

Risperidone (n=2, *Am J Psych* 1996, **153**, 734–35; case, Silberbauer, *Pharmacopsychiatry* 1998, **31**, 68–69; clear case, *Am J Psych* 1999, *156*, 1290; n=1, *J Clin Psych* 1999, **60**, 485–87)

Sulpiride (*Clin Neuropharmacology* 1990, **13**, 248–52)

5.8.4 Tardive Dyskinesia *

A potentially irreversible movement disorder with some relationship to drug, dose and duration (see *1.20.3*).

5.8.5 OTHER MOVEMENT DISORDERS

5.8.5.1 Catatonia *

Review: in young people (Cohen *et al, J Am Acad Child Adolesc Psych* 1999, **38**, 1040–46)

Allopurinol (n=1, *BMJ* 1991, **302**, 970)

Baclofen (cases, *Clin Neuropharmacol* 1992, **15**, 56–62)

Benzodiazepine withdrawal (n=5, Rosebush and Mazurek, *J Clin Psychopharmacol* 1996, **16**, 315–19)

Bupropion (n=1, *J Clin Psych* 1992, **53**, 210)

Cycloserine

Cocaine (n=1, *Am J Psych* 1998, **155**, 1629)

Disulfiram (n=1, *Arch Neurol* 1989, **46**, 798–804; pos. case in *Am J Psych* 1992, **149**, 1279–80)

Fluphenazine (n=1, *B J Psych* 1973, **122**, 240)

Loxapine (n=1, *J Clin Psych* 1983, **44**, 310–12)

Morphine epidural (n=1, *Lancet* 1980, **2**, 984)

Phenelzine + haloperidol (n=1, *Can J Psych* 1988, **33**, 633–34)

Piperazine (mentioned in *Trans Roy Soc Trop Med Hyg* 1976, **70**, 358)

Prochlorperazine (n=1, *Postgrad Med* 1976, **60**, 171–73)

5.8.5.2 Choreas

● **Psychotropics etc ***

Amoxapine

Amfetamines/amphetamines (chronic abuse, eg. *J Clin Psychopharmacol* 1988, **8**, 146)

Benzhexol/trihexyphenidyl

Chlorpromazine (n=1, *Postgrad Med J* 1970, **540**, 633–34)

Cocaine (cases in *Am J Emerg Med* 1991, **9**, 618–20)

Fluoxetine (n=1, *J Clin Psych* 1999, **60**, 868–69)

Haloperidol (many cases)

Methadone

Methylphenidate

Mianserin (case in *B J Psych* 1989, **154**, 113–14)

Oral contraceptives (n=2, *Rev Med Chil* 1999, **127**, 468–71)

Paroxetine (n=1, after a single dose, *B J Psych* 1997, **170**, 193–94)

Phenytoin (review in *Pediatr* 1983, **72**, 831–34)

Risperidone (n=1, *J Clin Psych* 1999, **60**, 485–87)

Sulpiride (n=1, *J Psychopharmacol* 1993, **7**, 290–92; n=6, *Clin Neuropharmacol* 1990, **13**, 248–52)

Valproate (n=3, *Arch Neurol* 1994, **51**, 702–4)

● **Others**

Anabolic steroids

Cimetidine (pos. case in *Ann Int Med* 1982, **96**, 531)

Cyclizine (n=1, *J Neurol Sci* 1977, **31**, 237–44)

Dienoestrol/dienestrol (MI)

Metoclopramide (n=1, *Lancet* 1982, **2**, 1153)

Oral Contraceptives (cases in *Drugs* 1983, **26**, 124)

Ranitidine (n=1, *Lancet* 1988, **2**, 158)

5.8.5.3 Tics (inc. Tourette's Syndrome)

Amfetamines (*JAMA* 1982, **247**, 1729–31)

Androgenic steroids (eg. stanozolol, methandrostenolol, testosterone) (*NEJM* 1990, **322**, 1674)

Carbamazepine (*Clin Neuropharmacol* 1989, **12**, 298–302)

Clozapine (n=1, *Am J Psych* 1995, **152**, 649)

Cocaine (*NEJM* 1986, **315**, 398; n=1, *Am J Psych* 1996, **153**, 965)

Dexamfetamine (see amfetamine)

Fluoxetine (cases in *Drug Intell & Clin Pharm* 1993, **27**, 725–26; *Am J Psych* 1994, **151**, 946–47)

Haloperidol (*Am J Psych* 1986, **143**, 1176–77)

Lamotrigine (n=3, *Neurology* 1999, **52**, 1191–94; n=5, *Epilepsia* 2000, **41**, 862–67)

Methylphenidate (*JAMA* 1982, **247**, 1729–31)

Ofloxacin (n=1, *Ann Pharmacother* 1996, **30**, 138–41)

Pemoline (*JAMA* 1982, **247**, 1729–31)

Risperidone withdrawal (n=1, *J Am Acad Child Adolesc Psych* 1997, **36**, 162–63)

Thioridazine + methylphenidate (n=1, *J Clin Psych* 1986, **47**, 44–45)

5.9 NEUROLEPTIC MALIGNANT SYNDROME

NMS is mostly related to the use of therapeutic or high doses of neuroleptics, particularly phenothiazines and high potency drugs. It frequently occurs within 4–11 days of initiation, or alteration of dosages, of neuroleptic therapy (*Am J Psych* 1989, **146**, 717–25). NMS may be due to a sudden and profound reduction in dopaminergic function, caused by dopamine blocking drugs. See *Chapter 1.22* for treatments.

Review: NMS with risperidone, clozapine and other novel antipsychotics (Hasan and Buckley, *Am J Psych* 1998, **155**, 1113–16).

● **Antidepressants**

Amoxapine (pos. cases in *B J Psych* 1991, **159**, 889; *Drug Intell Clin Pharm* 1989, **23**, 50–51)

Clomipramine (MI)

Desipramine (n=1, *Neurology* 1990, **40**, 1797–98)

Phenelzine (many cases, eg. *Can Med Assoc J* 1991, **145**, 817–19)

Trimipramine (n=1, *J Clin Psych* 1989, **50**, 144–45)

● **Antipsychotics** *

Clozapine (rare, but cases exist, eg. *Ann Pharmacother* 1996, **30**, 248–50; n=1, *Am J Psych* 1997, **153**, 881–82; n=2 and review, *Ann Pharmacother* 1999, **33**, 623–30; review by Karagianis *et al, Ann Pharmacother* 1999, **33**, 623–30)

Chlorpromazine (eg. n=2, *Biol Psych* 1983, **18**, 1441–46)

Flupentixol (pos. case in *B J Psych* 1988, **152**, 558–59)

Fluphenazine (reviewed in *Compr Psych* 1985, **26**, 63–70)

Haloperidol (many cases, eg. *J Trauma* 1989, **29**, 1595–97)

Lithium + amoxapine (n=1, *Ann Clin Psychiatry* 2000, **12**, 107–9)

Lithium + risperidone (possible case in *Am J Psych* 1995, **152**, 1096)

Loxapine (*B J Psych* 1991, **159**, 572–73)

Olanzapine (n=1, *Arch Gen Psych* 1999, **56**, 101–2; case, n=1, *Am J Psych* 1999, **156**, 1115–16; n=1, *Ann Pharmacother* 1998, **32**, 1158–59;

Psychosomatics 1999, **40**, 267–68; n=1, *Am J Psych* 1999, **156**, 1836)

Promazine

Quetiapine (n=1, Stanley and Hunter, *B J Psych* 2000, **176**, 497)

Risperidone (many cases, eg. Gleason and Conigliaro, *Pharmacotherapy* 1997, **17**, 617–21; *Hosp Pharm* 1997, **32**, 42 and 512–18)

Thioridazine (several cases, eg. *Biol Psych* 1987, **22**, 1293–97)

Zuclopenthixol (n=1, *B J Psych* 1989, **154**, 562–63)

● **Others** *

Amantadine

Amantadine, abrupt withdrawal (n=1, *Am J Psych* 1994, **151**, 451–52)

Anticholinergic withdrawal (n=1, Spivak *et al, Int Clin Psychopharmacol* 1996, **11**, 207–9)

Carbamazepine (may also complicate symptoms, *B J Psych* 1990, **157**, 437–38; n=1, *B J Psych* 1994, **164**, 270)

Carbamazepine withdrawal (*Am J Psych* 1990, **147**, 1687)

Ganciclovir (n=1, *Pharmacother* 2000, **20**, 479–83)

Iron (low levels? *Am J Psych* 1991, **148**,148–49)

Levodopa

Levodopa withdrawal (n=3, *JAMA* 1985, **254**, 2792–95)

Lithium (pos. cases in *J Clin Psychopharmacol* 1987, **7**, 339–41)

Methylphenidate (n=1, *Pediatr Neurol* 1998, **19**, 299–301)

Metoclopramide (several cases eg. *Arch Int Med* 1987, **147**, 1495–97; *Ann Pharmacother* 1999, **33**, 644–45)

Oral contraceptives (possible case in *Drug Intell Clin Pharm* 1989, **23**, 811)

5.10 OBSESSIVE-COMPULSIVE SYMPTOMS

Clozapine (n=1, *Am J Psych* 1998, **155**, 1629–30; especially early in schizophrenia, n=121, *J Clin Psych* 1999, **60**, 364–65)

Gabapentin withdrawal (n=1, *J Clin Psych* 1998, **59**, 131)

Methamphetamine (*J Clin Psych* 1999, **60**, 337–38; n=1, *J Am Acad Child Adolesc Psych* 1998, **37**, 135)

Olanzapine (n=2, *Am J Psych* 1999, **156**, 799–800)

Risperidone (dose dependent case, *Aust NZ J Psychiatry* 1998, **32**, 299–301; n=1, *B J Psych* 1999, **174**, 559; see also *J Clin Psych* 1999, **60**, 261–63 for an obsessively pedantic discussion)

Stimulants (n=1, *Biol Psych* 1985, **20**, 1332–37)

5.11 PANIC DISORDER

● **Psychotropics etc ***

Amfetamines (n=3, *Biol Psych* 1992, **32**, 91–95)

Buspirone (case + correspondence in *Lancet* 1989, **2**, 46–47, 615, 682–83)

Clobazam (withdrawal, eg. *BMJ* 1981, **282**, 1931)

Cocaine (review in *J Addict Dis* 1992, **11**, 47–58)

Flumazenil (mentioned in *Psych Res* 1991, **36**, 115)

Fluoxetine (unless initial doses kept very low, eg. *J Clin Psychopharmacol* 1987, **7**, 329–32)

Fluoxetine + bupropion (*J Clin Psych* 1996, **57**, 177–78)

Marijuana (n=1, *Acta Psych Scand* 1998, **98**, 254–55)

Naltrexone (*Am J Psych* 1998, **155**, 447)

Trazodone

● **Others**

Aspartame (unproven case with high doses in *Lancet* 1986, **12**, 631)

Co-trimoxazole (n=1, *J Clin Psychopharmacol* 1991, **11**, 144–45)

Lactate oral (eg. in calcium lactate tablets, case in *Ann Pharmacother* 1995, **29**, 539–40)

Oxymetazoline (case in abuse, *J Clin Psych* 1987, **48**, 293)

Phenylephrine (n=1, *B J Psych* 1980, **136**, 297–99)

Sodium lactate (study in *Arch Gen Psych* 1989, **46**, 135–40)

Steroids (mentioned in *J Psychiatry Neurosci* 1997, **22**, 346–47)

Sumatriptan (7%, panic being interpretation of side-effects such as chest pain, palpitations etc, Loi *et al*, *Am J Psych* 1996, **153**, 1505)

Yohimbine (see *Arch Gen Psych* 1998, **55**, 1033–44)

5.12 PARANOID or SCHIZOPHRE-NIC-LIKE PSYCHOSES *(see also hallucinations, 5.6)*

Characterised by paranoid delusions and hallucinations in a person with little clouding of consciousness.

The literature on drug-induced psychosis is extensive but mainly case reports and short uncontrolled studies. A classification has been proposed:

Intoxication mimicking functional: (ie. drug-induced), eg. stimulants and cannabis. Persists for several days until the drug has cleared.

Psychoactive drugs altering the clinical presentation of an existing psychosis: eg. cannabis or amphetamines etc. creating a more aggressive and disturbed schizophrenic patient (Davison and Roth, *B J Psych* 1996, **168**, 651).

Chronic hallucinations induced by substance abuse: insight usually present, no clouding of consciousness, continue despite long-term abstinence, eg. alcoholic hallucinosis, LSD or cannabis flashbacks.

Drug-induced relapse of functional psychosis: eg. schizophrenia.

Withdrawal states: eg. delirium tremens, benzodiazepine or barbiturate withdrawal.

Others: acute intoxication/confusion with clouding of consciousness, post-intoxication depression, eg. post-amphetamine crash, panic/anxiety attacks, eg. from hallucinogens such as LSD.

True drug-induced psychosis: any psychotic symptoms which occur with drug intoxication and then persist after elimination of the causing drug, ie. one to two drug-free weeks.

There is, surprisingly, little, if any proof that such causal link can be made firmly between drug use and later psychosis, eg. there is no direct proof that cannabis causes schizophrenia rather than schizo-phrenics trying to self-medicate before symptoms become clear to others (extensive and thoughtful review by Poole and Brabbins, *B J Psych* 1996, **168**, 135–38, plus correspondence *B J Psych* 1996, **168**, 651–52).

● **Hallucinogens** (Major cause)

Cannabis (*Acta Psych Scand* 1991, **83**, 34–36; reviews in *B J Psych* 1990, **157**, 25–33; *ibid* 1992, **161**, 648–53)

Dimethoxy-methylamphetamine (DOM)

Lysergic acid diethylamide (LSD)

Khat chewing (n=4, *B J Hosp Med* 1995, **54**, 322–26)

Mescaline

MDMA/Ecstasy (*BMJ* 1991, **302**, 1150, *B J Psych* 1991, **159**, 713–15; *Arch Gen Psych* 1993, **50**, 75)

Petrol (*Am J Psych* 1964, **126**, 757)

Phencyclidine (angel dust)

Psilocybin (magic mushrooms). (*B J Psych* 1978, **132**, 602)

Volatiles (*BMJ* 1962, **ii**, 1448)

● **CNS stimulants** (Major cause)

Amfetamines/amphetamines (eg. *Biol Psych* 1980, **15**, 749; treatment/review in *Topic Emerg Med* 1985, **7**, 18–32)

Cocaine (*Am J Psych*, 1991, **148**, 495–98)

Ephedrine (review in (*B J Psych* 1987, **150**, 252–55)

Methamphetamine (n=1, *Am J Psych* 1999, **4**, 662)

Phenylephrine (eg. *JAMA* 1982, **247**, 1859–60)

Phenylpropanolamine (*Am J Psych* 1990, **147**, 367–68)

Pseudoephedrine (many cases, eg. *South Med J* 1990, **83**, 64–65)

Solvent abuse (*B J Psych* 1989, **152**, 132)

● **CNS depressants**

Alcohol (*Schizophrenia Today,* 1976, Pergamon Press, Oxford)

Antihistamines

Barbiturates

Benzodiazepines:

Alprazolam

Lorazepam (*B J Psych* 1985, **147**, 211)

Midazolam (pos. case in *Drug Intell Clin Pharm* 1989, **23**, 671–72)

Triazolam (eg. *Pharmacopsychiat* 1989, **22**, 115–19)

Benzodiazepine withdrawal (*Int J Ger Psych* 1995, **10**, 901–2)

Buspirone (*Am J Psych* 1991, **148**, 1606; *J Psychopharmacol* 1993, **7**, 295–300)

Cannabis (acute onset, usually resolves in 2–7 days, *Acta Psych Scand* 1991, **83**, 134–36)

Chloral

Chlorpromazine (n=1, *Can Med Assoc J* 1970, **102**, 642; n=1, *Brain Inj* 1993, **7**, 77–83)

Clozapine withdrawal (ie. rebound psychosis, study in *Psychopharmacol* 1988, **24**, 260–63; n=3, *J Clin Psych* 1997, **58**, 252–55)

Codeine OD (n=1, *Neurobehavioral Toxicol Teratol* 1985, **7**, 193–94)

Disulfiram (n=1, *BMJ* 1992, **305**, 763)

Fluoxetine (*J Nerv Mental Dis* 1990, **178**, 55–58)

Haloperidol (*Drug Intell Clin Pharm* 1981, **15**, 209)

Imipramine (eg. *Am J Psych* 1974, **131**, 21)

Methadone withdrawal (eg. *J Clin Psych* 1995, **56**, 73–76)

Morphine (rare, *B J Psych* 1990, **157**, 758–59)

Paroxetine (case of psychotic mania, *Am J Psych* 1995, **152**, 1399–440)

Phenelzine – eg. *B J Psych* 1991, **159**, 716–17)

Promethazine (rare but possible, eg. *NEJM* 1960, **263**, 747)

Zolpidem (*Lancet* 1992, **339**, 813)

Zopiclone (some cases reported —*WHO Drug Information*, 1990, **4**, 179)

● **Anticonvulsants** *

Psychosis induced by anticonvulsants may be the result of 'forced normal-isation'. Risk factors include TLE, treatment resistance, past history of psychosis or affective disorder, and becoming suddenly seizure-free (best to do this gradually). Drug regimens should be changed gradually and compliance should be maintained to prevent epileptic psychoses (n=44, Matsuura, *J Neurol, Neurosurg & Psych* 1999, **67**, 231–33).

Carbamazepine toxicity (*Lancet* 1989, **i**, 167)

Clonazepam (n=1, *J Nerv Ment Dis* 1982, **170**, 117)

Ethosuximide

Gabapentin

Phenytoin (*Arch Neurol* 1969, **21**, 631; *Drug Intell Clin Pharm* 1988, **22**, 1003–5)

Topiramate (n=5 and review, *Seizure* 1999, **8**, 235–37)

Valproate (isolated cases, eg. *Clin Electroencephalography* 1982, **13**, 50–53)

Vigabatrin (2% incidence, eg. *J Neurol Neurosurgery & Psychiatry* 1989, **52**, 467–71; cases in *Lancet* 1994, **343**, 606–7; *Ann Pharmacother* 1995, **29**, 1115–17)

Vigabatrin withdrawal (letter in *Lancet* 1990, **335**, 1279)

● **Anti-parkinsonian drugs** (excess DA)

Amantadine (mentioned in *Drugs* 1981, **21**, 341–53)

Anticholinergic withdrawal (*Am J Psych* 1980, **137**, 1613)

Benzhexol/trihexyphenidyl (see benztropine)

Benztropine (many cases, review in *J Psychoactive Drug* 1983, **15**, 319–21)

Bromocriptine (<1% chance, review in *Biol Psych* 1985, **20**, 326–28)

Levodopa (esp. hallucinations — *Arch Neurol* 1970, **23**, 193–200)

Lisuride/lysuride (a few cases, eg. *Lancet* 1986, **2**, 510)

Pergolide (esp. hallucinations, in up to 13%, eg. *Neurology* 1982, **32**, 1181–84)

Selegiline (a few cases, eg. *Neurology* 1981, **31**, 19–23)

● **NSAIDs and analgesics**

Aspirin (*JAMA* 1965, **193**, 555–58)

Ibuprofen (*J Clin Psych* 1982, **43**, 499–500)

Indometacin (rare, eg. *South Med J* 1983, **76**, 679–80; *BMJ* 1977, **2**, 994)

Pentazocine (esp. hallucinations, eg. *BMJ* 1974, **2**, 224)

Sulindac (*JAMA* 1980, **243**, 1420)

● **Cardiovascular drugs**

Amyl nitrate (Martindale 1993)

Beta-blockers (see under depression for differentials) eg:

 Atenolol (rare, n=1, *Am J Psych* 1983, **140**, 1382)

 Propranolol (well known, eg. *Biol Psych* 1989, **25**, 351–54)

Clonidine (n=1, *Prog NeuroPsychopharmacol* 1980, **4**, 21)

Clonidine withdrawal (*Am J Psych* 1982, **139**, 110–11)

Digoxin toxicity (rare, *J Nerv Mental Dis* 1978, **166**, 817)

Diltiazem (n=1, *Arch Int Med* 1991, **151**, 373–74)

Disopyramide (isolated cases, eg. *Lancet* 1978, **1**, 858 + 1152)

Doxazosin (n=1, *BMJ* 1997, **314**, 1869; n=1, *BMJ* 1997, **314**, 1869)

Enalapril (n=1, *Drug Intell Clin Pharm* 1991, **25**, 558–59)

Hydralazine

Lidocaine/lignocaine IV (n=6, *Ann Int Med* 1982, **97**, 149–50)

Methyldopa

Mexilitine (n=1, *Am Heart J* 1984, **107**, 1091–98)

Nifedipine (pos. case in *J Am Geriat Soc* 1984, **32**, 408)

Procainamide

Tocainide (*BMJ* 1984, **288**, 606–7)

● **Anti-infection** *

Amphotericin B IV (n=1, *Ariz Med* 1972, **29**, 322)

Antituberculous drugs (*Lancet* 1989, **ii**, 105 + 735–36)

Cefuroxime (*Lancet* 1984, **i**, 965)

Cephalexin (n=1, *Med J Aust* 1973, **i**, 497)

Cephalothin (*Drug Intell Clin Pharm* 1974, **8**, 71)

Chloroquine (cases in *Lancet* 1985, **2**, 37)

Ciprofloxacin (n=1, *Ann Pharmacother* 1992, **26**, 930–31; n=1, *Postgrad Med J* 1998, **74**, 189–90)

Clarithromycin (*Eur J Clin Microbiol Infect Dis* 1999, **18**, 70–71)

Colistin (esp. with large doses)

Dapsone (*BMJ* 1989, **299**, 324)

Erythromycin (*Arch Int Med* 1986, **146**, 897)

Ganciclovir (n=1, *Pharmacother* 2000, **20**, 479-83)

Isoniazid (rare — *Am J Psych* 1991, **148**, 1402; *Ann Pharmacother* 1998, **32**, 889–91)

Ketoconazole (*Am J Psych* 1990, **147**, 677)

Mefloquine (*Pharm J* 1989, **243**, 561)

Metronidazole (case in *Am J Psych* 1997, **154**, 1170–71)

Nalidixic acid (many cases, eg. *BMJ* 1965, **2**, 590)

Primaquine (n=1, *Ann Int Med* 1980, **92**, 435)

Procaine Penicillin G (several cases, eg. *B J Psych* 1990, **156**, 554)

Sulphonamides

Tobramycin (a few cases, eg. *Pediatr Pulmonol* 1988, **4**, 201–4)

● **Steroids** (*Postgrad Med J* 1984, **60**, 467–70)

Adrenocorticotrophin

Clomiphene (n=2, *Am J Psych* 1997, **154**, 1169–70)

Corticosteroids (11% incidence? Review by Ismail and Wessely, *B J Hosp Pharm* 1995, **53**, 495–99)

Cortisone

Methylprednisolone

Methyltestosterone (*Lancet* 1987, **i**, 863)

Prednisone (usually >40mg/d, eg. *J Clin Psych* 1982, **43**, 75–76 inc. brief overview, case and discussion in *B J Psych* 1993, **162**, 549–53)

Triamcinolone (possible but no specific reports)

● **Miscellaneous** *

Anti-diarrhoeals (OTC) (*B J Psych* 1990, **157**, 758–59)

Atropine (oral, IV, eye drops. Many cases, eg. *DICP Ann Pharmacother* 1990, **24**, 708–9)

Baclofen

Bupropion (many cases, eg. n=1, *Am J Psych* 1999, **156**, 2017–18)

Carbaryl (n=1, *Am J Psych* 1995, **152**, 646–47)

Carbimazole

Chlorphenamine OD (case in child in *Med J Aust* 1973, **1**, 382–86)

Cimetidine (*Am J Psych* 1980, **137**, 1112)

Desmopressin (n=1, *Lancet* 1981, **2**, 808)

Dextromethorphan (n=1, *Med J Aust* 1967, **2**, 231)

Dicyclomine (MI)

Diphenhydramine (n=1, *JAMA* 1968, **203**, 301)

Disulfiram

Hyoscine-transdermal (*Postgrad Med* 1988, **84**, 73–76)

Insulin abuse (*BMJ* 1971, **4**, 792–93)

Interferon alpha (*Drug Intell Clin Pharm* 1985, **19**, 887–93)

Isotretoin (possible case, *J Clin Psych* 1999, **60**, 407–8)

Ketamine (discussion, *Am J Psych* 1997, **154**, 805–11)

Lactate oral (eg. in calcium lactate tablets, case in *Ann Pharmacother* 1995, **29**, 539–40)

Lariam (severe is extremely low, eg 1 in 6000, *Pharm J* 1996, **256**, 184)

Melatonin (n=1, *Ann Pharmacother* 1997, **31**, 1408)

Nabilone

Nicotine, abrupt withdrawal of (*Am J Psych* 1994, **150**, 452)

Oxymetazoline (several cases, eg. *Scott Med J* 1982, **27**, 175–76)

Phenylephrine (*JAMA* 1982, **247**, 1859)

Pyridostigmine (case in German in *Deutsch Med Wschr* 1966, **9**, 699)

Quinine (*B J Psych* 1988, **153**, 575)

Quinidine (*BMJ* 1987, **294**, 1001–2; *Med J Aus* 1990, **153**, 47–49)

Salbutamol (*Biol Psych* 1989, **26**, 631–33)

Scopolamine (transient to transdermal, n=3, *Can J Hosp Pharm* 1994, **47**[2], 67–69)

Yohimbine (unproven, see *Arch Gen Psych* 1998, **55**, 1033–44)

5.13 SEIZURES

These are rare at normal doses and occur mostly where seizure threshold is reduced, in at-risk patients or in overdose. The list of drugs which could induce seizures is enormous and so a literature search would be needed to clarify the current situation for any one drug.

Reviews: drug-induced seizures: controversies in their identification and management (Alldredge, *Pharmacotherapy* 1997, **17**, 857–60, editorial, 26 refs), psychotropic drug-induced seizures (Stimmel and Dopheide, *CNS Drugs* 1996, **5**, 37–50).

● **Psychotropics etc** *

Alcohol (*NEJM* 1989, **320**, 596–97)

Amitriptyline (*Am J Psych* 1980, **137**, 1461–62)

Amoxapine (*J Clin Psych* 1981, **42**, 238–42)

Antipsychotics (esp phenothiazines)

Bupropion (see *3.4*)

Clozapine (*Neurology* 1991, **41**, 369–71; *CSM Current Problems* 1991, No 31; *Am J Psych* 1993, **150**, 1128. Higher incidence with rapid upward titration, recent ECT, head trauma with loss of consciousness and concurrent use of seizure threshold-lowering drugs. They may be due to hyponatremia *Lancet* 1992, **340**, 672)

Donepezil (*Curr Prob Pharmacovig* 1999, **25**, 7; *J Neurol, Neurosurg & Psych* 1999, **66**, 410)

Fluoxetine (*Clin Pharm* 1989, **8**, 296–98; *Am J Psych* 1992, **149**, 273; prolonged seizure reported in *Postgrad Med J* 1994, **70**, 383–84)

Fluvoxamine (*B J Psych* 1991, **159**, 433–25)

Imipramine

Levomepromazine + fluvoxamine (Grinshpoon *et al, Int Clin Psycho-pharmacol* 1993, **8**, 61–62)

Lithium (*Biol Psych* 1987, **22**, 1184–90)

MAOIs

Maprotiline (*J Clin Psych* 1982, **43**, 117–18)

Mianserin

Olanzapine (fatal case, *Ann Pharmacother* 1999, **33**, 787–89; non-fatal case *Ann Pharmacother* 1999, **33**, 554–56)

Sertraline (n=1, *Am J Psych* 1996, **153**, 732)

Tacrine (n=6, *Lancet* 1996, **347**, 1339–40)

Venlafaxine OD (*Ann Pharmacother* 1997, **31**, 178–80)

Zolpidem (review, *Lancet* 1998, **352**, 383–90)

● **Drug withdrawal**

Alcohol (*NEJM* 1989, **320**, 596–97)

Anticonvulsants (ie. *non-compliance*)

Barbiturates

Benzodiazepines: Alprazolam (*J Nerv Mental Dis* 1990, **178**, 208–9)

Carbamazepine (*J Clin Psych* 1988, **49**[Suppl], 410)

Zolpidem (abrupt high dose withdrawal, case report *JAMA* 1994, **272**, 1721–22)

● **CNS stimulants** *

Cocaine (*Neurology* 1990, **40**, 404–7)

Ephedrine (*Lancet* 1977, **1**, 587–88)

● **Anticonvulsants** *

Critical review: (Perucca *et al, Epilepsia* 1998, **39**, 5–17; 155 refs, editorial by Loiseau, *Epilepsia* 1998, **39**, 2–4, 43 refs), general review (Bauer, *Acta Neurol Scand* 1996, **94**, 367–77).

Carbamazepine

Ethosuximide

Phenobarbital

Phenytoin (*Epilepsia* 1989, **30**, 230–34)

Tiagabine (n=2, *Epilepsia* 1999, **40**, 1159–62)

Valproate

● **NSAIDs and analgesics** *

Dextroproxyphene (*Arch Inn Med* 1973, **132**, 191–94)

Fentanyl (*Anesth Anal [Cleve] 1982,* **61**, 1020–21)

Indometacin (rare, eg. *BMJ* 1966, **1**, 80)

Mefenamic Acid (*Drug Intell Clin Pharm* 1983, **17**, 204–5)

Penicillamine

Pentazocine (*Anesthesiology* 1971, **35**, 92–95; *Ann Emerg Med* 1983, **12**, 28–31)

Pethidine (*Ann Neurol* 1983, **13**, 180–85)

Propoxyphene (*Arch Intern Med* 1973, **132**, 191–94)

Salicylates OD (*Lancet* 1998, **352**, 383–90)

Sulindac

Tramadol (reviews in *JAMA* 1997, **278**, 1661 and *Pharmacother* 1998, **18**, 607–11; the latter concluding that seizures seem rarely attributable to tramadol)

● **Cardiovascular drugs** *

Beta-blockers, eg:

Oxprenolol (*Lancet* 1972, **i**, 587–88)

Propranolol (*Lancet* 1972, **i**, 587–88)

Digoxin toxicity (rare eg. *BMJ* 1982, **284**, 162–63)

Disopyramide

Enoximone Inf (*BMJ* 1990, **300**, 613)

Lidocaine (*Eur J Clin Pharmacol* 1989, **36**, 583–86)

— s/c (*Clin Pharm* 1989, **8**, 767–68)

Metolazone (*BMJ* 1976, **i**, 1381)

Mexilitine

Thiazide diuretics (review, *Lancet* 1998, **352**, 383–90)

Tocainide

● **Anti-infection** *

Ampicillin? (*Lancet* 1982, **ii**, 617)

Benzylpenicillin (*Lancet* 1977, **i**, 587)

Carbenicillin (*JAMA* 1971, **218**, 1942)

Cefazolin (*Am J Hosp Pharm* 1980, **37**, 271)

Ceftazidime (editorial in *Lancet* 1990, **340**, 400–1)

Cephalexin (n=1, *Med J Aust* 1973, **1**, 497)

Cephalosporins (high dose in renal failure)

Chloroquine (*BMJ* 1989, **299**, 1524)

Ciprofloxacin (*Pharm J* 1989, **242**, 340)

Cycloserine

Gentamicin (*J Neurol Orthop Med & Surg* 1985, **6**, 123)

Imipenem (*Ann Int Med* 1989, **149**, 1881–83)

Isoniazid (review in *J Clin Pharm Ther Toxicol* 1987, **25**, 259–61)

Mefloquine (*Pharm J* 1989, **243**, 561; CSM warning, *Curr Prob Pharmacovig* 1999, **25**, 15)

Metronidazole (*Drug Intell Clin Pharm* 1982, **16**, 409)

Nalidixic Acid (*BMJ* 1977, **2**, 1518)

Niridazole

Ofloxacin (n=1, *et al, Ann Pharmacother* 1997, **31**, 1475–77; *J Pharm Technol* 1997, **13**, 174)

Penicillins (reviewed in *Ann Pharmacother* 1992, **26**, 26–29, 30–31)

Piperazine

Piperacillin (*Clin Pediatr* 1997, **36**, 475–76)

Pyrimethamine

Zudovidine (case in *Lancet* 1995, **346**, 452)

● **Respiratory drugs**

Aminophylline (*Lancet* 1977, **i**, 587)

Doxapram

Phenylpropanolamine (*J Med Soc New Jersey* 1979, **76**, 591–92)

Terbutaline (*Am J Dis Child* 1982, **136**, 1091–92)

Theophylline (*Ann Int Med* 1975, **82**,784)

Theophylline toxicity (*J Toxicol Clin Toxicol* 1999, **37**, 99–101)

● **Hormones**

Glucocorticoids

Insulin

Oral contraceptives (exacerbate pre-existing)

Oxytocin

Prostaglandins

● **Cytotoxics** *

Alprostadil

Busulphan (*Ann Int Med* 1989, **111**, 543–44; *Ann Pharmacother* 1992, **26** 30–31)

Chlorambucil (*Postgrad Med J* 1979, **55**, 806–7)

Ciclosporin (*J Neurol Neurosurg Psych* 1989, **55**, 1068–71; *Psychosomatics* 1991, **32**, 94–102)

Cisplatin (*BMJ* 1991, **302**, 416)

Methotrexate

Vinblastine

Vincristine

● **Anaesthetics** *

Alfentanil (*Anaesthesia & Analgesia* 1989, **68**, 692–93)

Enflurane (*Anaesthesia* 1992, **47**, 79–80)

Ether

Etomidate (pre-ECT, n=1, *B J Psych* 2000, **177**, 373).

Halothane

Ketamine

Local Anesthetics

Bupivacaine (*Anesthesiology* 1979, **50**, 454–56)

Lidocaine (mentioned in *Drugs Aging* 1995, **7**, 38–48)

Etidocaine (*Anesthesiology* 1979, **50**, 51–53)

Procaine

Methohexital

Propofol (*Anaesthesia* 1990, **45**, 255–56, can be delayed by up to 6 days – *CSM Curr Prob* 1992, **35**, 2)

Propofol withdrawal (*Anaesthesia* 1990, **45**, 741–42)

● **Miscellaneous** *

Allopurinol withdrawal (*Ann Neurology* 1990, **27**, 691)

Aluminium toxicity (unproven, *Ann Int Med* 1989, **111**, 543–44)

Amantadine (unproven, *Ann Int Med* 1989, **110**, 323–24; *Drugs Aging* 1995, **7**, 38–48)

Baclofen IT (*Lancet* 1992, **339**, 373–74)

Baclofen withdrawal (*Neurology* 1992, **42**, 447–49)

Brompheniramine

Bupivacaine epidural (case 4yo in *Anaesthesia* 1995, **50**, 563–77)

Caffeine (*Acta Psych Scand* 1959, **15**, 331–34)

Camphor (*Clin Pediatr* [*Phila*] 1977, **16**, 901–2)

Clomiphene (n=1, *BMJ* 1994, **309**, 512)

Colchicine OD

Cyclopentolate eye drops (*J Paed & Child Health* 1990, **26**, 106–7)

Diphenhydramine (*J Pediat* 1977, **90**, 1017–18)

Diptheria-tetanus-pertussis vaccine (*JAMA* 1990, **263**, 1641–45)

Flumazenil (n=49, *Epilepsia* 2000, **41**, 186–92)

Fluorescin IV (*Annals Opthal* 1989, **21**, 89–90; *Acta Neurol Scand* 1999, **100**, 278–80)

Hepatitis B vaccine (*J Paed & Child Health* 1990, **26**, 65)

Interferon (n=1, *Pediatrics* 1994, **93**, 511–12)

Ketamine

Ketotifen (n=19, *Epilepsia* 1998, **39**[Suppl 5], 64)

Levodopa (mentioned in *Drugs Aging* 1995, **7**, 38–48)

Levothyroxine (n=1, *Ann Pharmacother* 1993, **27**, 1139)

Lindane, topical (*B J Dermatol* 1995, **133**, 1013)

Measles/Mumps/Rubella vaccine (review in *Pediatrics* 1991, **88**, 881–85)

Naftidrofuryl

Naloxone (rare)

Ondansetron (*Clin Pharm* 1993, **12**, 613–15)

Pertussis vaccine

Phenylpropanolamine (n=1, *J Pediatr* 1983, **102**, 143-45)

Pyrimethamine

Radiographic Contrast Media (eg. metrizamide)

Sodium bicarbonate (*JAMA* 1989, **262**, 1328–39)

Steroids, eg.
  Dexamethasone
  Hydrocortisone
  Prednisolone
  Prednisone (with hypocalcaemia) (mentioned in *Lancet* 1977, **1**, 587–88)

Sulphasalazine

Sulphonylureas

Terfenadine (*BMJ* 1993, **307**, 241)

Terfenadine OD (*BMJ* 1989, **298**, 325)

Yohimbe (unproven, see *Arch Gen Psych* 1998, **55**, 1033–44)

5.14 SEROTONIN SYNDROME *

Serotonin syndrome has been reported with a variety of antidepressants, buspirone, carbamazepine, pethidine, dextromethorphan and levodopa, usually in combination but can be single drugs or in overdose.

Reviews*: Lane and Baldwin, *J Clin Psychopharmacol* 1997, **17**, 208–21; Mir and Taylor, *Psych Bull* 1999, **23**, 742–47; Chan *et al*, *Med J Aust* 1998, **169**, 523–25.

● **Individual drugs ***

Amitriptyline (n=1, *Postgrad Med J* 2000, **76**, 254–56)

Clomipramine (*J Clin Psychopharmacol* 1999, **19**, 285–87)

Citalopram low dose (*J Clin Psychopharmacol* 2000, **20**, 713–14)

Dexfenfluramine (n=1, *JAMA* 1996, **276**, 1220–21)

Dothiepin overdose (*J Child Adolesc Psychopharmacol* 1998, **8**, 201–4)

Ecstasy (*JAMA* 1993, **269**, 869–70; review by Demirkiran *et al*, *Clin Neuropharmacol* 1996, **19**, 157–64)

Fluoxetine (n=1, *Psychiatr Pol* 1995, **29**, 529–38)

Fluvoxamine (*Ann Emerg Med* 1999, **33**, 457–59; after single dose n=1, *Ann Emerg Med* 1999, **34**, 806–7)

Nefazodone (n=8, *B J Gen Pract* 1999, **49**, 871–74)

Paroxetine (*Am J Emerg Med* 1995, **13**, 606–7)

Sertraline low dose (*J Clin Psychopharmacol* 2000, **20**, 713–14)

Sertraline overdose (n=1, *Arch Pediatr Adolesc Med* 1997, **151**, 1064–67)

Trazodone (*Int J Ger Psychiatry* 1997, **12**, 129–30)

Venlafaxine (n=1, *J Emerg Med* 1997, **15**, 491–93; n=1, *Postgrad Med J* 2000, **76**, 254–56)

Venlafaxine overdose (*J Accid Emerg Med* 1998, **15**, 333–34)

● **Combinations including SSRIs ***

SSRIs + MAOIs (overview, Henry, *Lancet* 1994, **343**, 607)

Citalopram + moclobemide (*Med Clin* [*Barc*] 1999, **113**, 677–78)

Citalopram overdose + moclobemide (*Lancet* 1993, **342**, 1419)

Citalpram + buspirone (n=1, *Int Clin Psychopharmacol* 1997, **12**, 61–63)

Fluoxetine/moclobemide/clomipramine overdose (fatal case in *Anaesth Intensive Care* 1995, **23**, 499–502)

Fluoxetine + buspirone (*Ann Pharmacother* 2000, **34**, 871–74)

Fluoxetine + carbamazepine (n=1, *Lancet* 1993, **342**, 442–43)

Fluoxetine + lithium (n=1, *Ugeskrift for Laeger* 1995, **157**, 1204–5)

Fluoxetine + mirtazapine (*Int J Geriatr Psychiatry* 1998, **13**, 495–96)

Fluoxetine + moclobemide (eg. Benazzi, *Pharmacopsychiatry* 1996, **29**, 162; n=1, *Can J Anaesth* 2000, **47**, 246–50)

Fluoxetine + nefazodone (n=1, *J Clin Psych* 2000, **61**, 146)

Fluoxetine + paroxetine (n=1, *Am Fam Physician* 1995, **52**, 1475–82)

Fluoxetine + sertraline (n=1, *Clin Pharmacol Ther* 1993, **1**, 84–88)

Fluoxetine + Parstelin (n=1, *Anaesthesia* 1991, **46**, 507–8)

Fluoxetine + tramadol (n=1, *J Royal Soc Med* 1999, **92**, 474–75)

Fluoxetine + trazodone (*Biol Psych* 1996, **39**, 384–85)

Fluoxetine + venlafaxine (*Ann Pharmacother* 1998, **32**, 432–36)

Paroxetine + lithium (n=1, *Pharmaco-psychiatry* 1997, **30**, 106–7)

Paroxetine + moclobemide (fatal case, *J Anal Toxicol* 1997, **21**, 518–20; *J Accid Emerg Med* 1999, **16**, 293–95)

Paroxetine + OTC cold remedy (*Am J Emerg Med* 1994, **12**, 642–44)

Paroxetine + risperidone (*J Clin Psychopharmacol* 2000, **20**, 103–5)

Paroxetine + tramadol (n=1l, Int Clin Psychopharmacol 1997, **12**, 181–82)

Paroxetine + trazodone (*Psychosomatics* 1995, **36**, 159–60)

Paroxetine + nefazodone (n=1, *Ann Emerg Med* 1997, **29**, 113–19)

Sertraline + amitriptyline (*Ann Pharmacother* 1996, **30**, 1499–500)

Sertraline + erythromycin (*Pharmacotherapy* 1999, **19**, 894–96)

Sertraline + phenelzine (n=1, *Ann Pharmacother* 1994, **28**, 732–35)

Sertraline + tramadol (n=1, *Ann Pharmacother* 1997, **31**, 175–77)

Sertraline + tranylcypromine (n=1, *Clin Pharm* 1993, **12**, 222–25)

● **Combinations including MAOIs**
  (see also above)

MAOIs + TCAs (overview, Henry, *Lancet* 1994, **343**, 607)

Phenelzine + clomipramine (n=1, *Clin Pharmacol Therap* 1993, **53**, 84–88)

Phenelzine + dextromethorphan (n=1, *Clin Pharmacol Therap* 1993, **53**, 84–88)

Phenelzine + venlafaxine (n=1, *Pharmacother* 1998, **18**, 399–403; n=1, *Ann Pharmacother* 1996, **30**, 84)

Tranylcypromine + venlafaxine (cases in *Vet Hum Toxicol* 1996, **38**, 358–61 and *Hum Exp Toxicol* 1997, **16**, 14–17)

● **Other combinations *** (see also above)

Moclobemide + clomipramine overdose (*Lancet* 1993, **342**, 1419 and *Intensive Care Med* 1997, **23**, 122–24; *J Toxicol Clin Toxicol* 1998, **36**, 31–32)

Moclobemide + clomipramine (n=1, *BMJ* 1993, **306**, 248)

Moclobemide + pethidine (possible case, *Med J Aust* 1995, **162**, 554)

Nortriptyline + selegiline (n=1, *J Neurol* 2000, **247**, 811)

Selegeline + venlafaxine (n=1, *J Clin Psychopharmacol* 1997, **17**, 66-67)

Trazodone + amitriptyline (n=1, *Int Clin Psychopharmacol* 1996, **11**, 289–90)

Venlafaxine + St John's wort? (*Presse Med* 2000, **29**, 1285–86)

5.15 SLEEP PROBLEMS

5.15.1 Sleep disturbances

Review of non-psychotropic causes: Novak and Shapiro, *Drug Safety* 1997, 16, 133–49.

● **Psychotropics etc ***

Benperidol

Bupropion (11%, MI)

Chlorpromazine

Donepezil (n=2, *J Am Geriatr Soc* 1998, **46**, 119–20)

Fluoxetine

Fluspirilene

Lamotrigine (dose dependent, n=7, *Epilepsia* 1999, **40**, 322–25)

Levetiracetam (MI)

Lorazepam

MAOIs (*Am J Psych* 1989, **146**, 1078)

Methysergide

Phentermine (*Practitioner* 1970, **24**, 423–25)

Phenytoin

Rivastigmine (<5%, MI)

SSRIs (somnambulism, n=1, *J Pharm Tech* 1999, **15**, 204–7)

Sulpiride

Stimulants (methylphenidate)

Trazodone

Tricyclics

● **Anti-parkinsonian drugs** *

Amantadine (4% incidence, see *J Clin Psych* 1981, **42**, 9)

Bromocriptine

Ropinirole and/or pramipexole (n=2, *Pharmacother* 2000, **20**, 724–26)

● **Cardiovascular drugs**

Amiodarone (frequent eg. *Am J Cardiol* 1983, **52**, 975–79)

Beta-blockers (very common, especially with propranolol)

Atenolol (see *Adv Psych Treat* 1999, **5**, 30–38)

Clonidine

Digoxin (see *Adv Psych Treat* 1999, **5**, 30–38)

Diltiazem (see *Adv Psych Treat* 1999, **5**, 30–38)

Isradipine (up to 3%, *Am J Med* 1989, **86**[Suppl 4A], 98–102)

Methyldopa

Nifedipine (see *Adv Psych Treat* 1999, **5**, 30–38)

● **NSAIDs and analgesics**

Diclofenac

Diflunisal

Fenoprofen

Indometacin

Naproxen (*Eur J Rheumatol Inflamm* 1981, **4**, 87–92)

Nefopam

Sulindac

● **Respiratory drugs**

Aminophylline

Brompheniramine

Clomiphene

Pseudoephedrine

Theophylline

● **Anti-infection**

Cinoxacin

Ciprofloxacin (n=1, *Lancet* 1986, **1**, 819–22)

● **Miscellaneous**

Bismuth toxicity (*Postgrad Med J* 1988, **64**, 308–10)

Dexamethasone

Ginseng (see *Arch Gen Psych* 1998, **55**, 1033–44)

Lovastatin (*Lancet* 1994, **343**, 973)

Propantheline

Ranitidine (see *Adv Psych Treat* 1999, **5**, 30–38)

Simvastatin (*Curr Prob* 1992, 33)

Sulphasalazine

Tolazamide

Triamcinolone

5.15.2 Vivid dreams and nightmares

Review: Thompson and Pierce, *Ann Pharmacother* 1999, **33**, 93–98

Baclofen

Beta-blockers:
Atenolol (*Clin Pharm Ther* 1979, **25**, 8)
Propranolol (*Adv Drug React Bull* 1983, **99**, 364)

Clonidine (*Adv Drug React Bull* 1983, **99**, 364)

Digoxin toxicity (*Ann Int Med* 1980, **93**, 639)

Famotidine (n=1, *Pharmacother* 1998, **18**, 404–7)

Indometacin (rare eg. *BMJ* 1965, **2**, 1281)

Methyldopa (*Adv Drug React Bull* 1983, **99**, 364)

Nalbumetone (*Pharm J* 1990, **244**, 764)

Pergolide (eg. *Clin Neuropharmacol* 1986, **9**, 160–64)

Nicotine patches (*Pharm J* 1992, **249**, 384)

Stanozolol (MI)

Verapamil (*NEJM* 1988, **318**, 929–30)

Withdrawal from barbiturates, benzodiazepines, narcotics etc.

6.1 SECTIONS OF THE MENTAL HEALTH ACT 1983

The England and Wales Mental Health Act came into effect on 30 September 1983 and comprises a series of 149 sections which modify, supplement and extend the 1959 Act. It is principally concerned with the grounds for detaining patients in hospital, aiming to improve patients' rights and protect staff, in a variety of ways. It is currently (2001) being reviewed.

6.1.1 COMPULSORY DETENTION ORDERS (non-offenders)

Section 2

- Admission for assessment, or assessment followed by treatment. It can include treatment as part of the assessment.
- Maximum of 28 days as you can be discharged before the end. Not renewable.
- Application made by nearest relative or Approved Social Worker, endorsed by two doctors (one a psychiatrist and the other, eg. a GP) and goes to a hospital manager.
- Can be appealed against or reviewed within 14 days.

Section 3

- Admission for treatment, but only where the patient's health or safety, or other's safety, is threatened.
- Maximum of six months, renewable after six months, then annually.
- Application made by a nearest relative or Approved Social Worker and endorsed by two medical recommendations.
- Can be appealed against or reviewed once every six months.
- Consent to treatment regulations refer to a professional person, other than a doctor or a nurse, who is involved with the case, so this can include a pharmacist (Branford, *Pharm J* 1988, **240**, 220–1).

Section 4 – Emergency admission

- Admission for assessment in cases of emergency. Used where the patient is incapable of giving consent, eg. unconscious, under age etc, and in areas where psychiatric resources are thinly spread.
- Maximum 72-hour holding order.
- Application made by a relative or Approved Social Worker and endorsed by one doctor (often the GP).

Section 5(2) – Emergency holding power by a doctor

- Detention of an informal patient already in hospital, on grounds of danger to self or others. Assessment should start as soon as possible. Usually proceeds to a Section 2.
- Maximum 72 hours.
- Application made by a doctor or a single nominated deputy.

Section 5(4) – Emergency holding power by a nurse

- Detention of an informal patient already in hospital and receiving psychiatric treatment, on grounds of danger to self or others.
- Nurses holding powers.
- Maximum six hours.
- Applied by a Registered Mental Nurse.

Section 57 – Consent to treatment

- For treatments which require consent AND a second opinion, ie. irreversible treatments, such as psychosurgery or hormonal implants.
- Informal or detained patients.

Section 58 – Consent to treatment

- For any treatment which requires consent OR a second opinion, eg. ECT or prolonged (more than three months) medication.
- There is no time limit but should be renewed annually.
- Detained patients only.

Section 59

- As for Section 58, but the person does not consent and thus requires a doctor appointed by the MHA Commission.

Section 117

- After-care co-ordination for long-term patients (post Sections 3, 37, 47, 48). Sets a planned programme, with a named responsible person. May include in-patients.

Section 136

- Removal from a public place to a place of safety by a police constable. Must then be assessed by an ASW and Doctor.
- Maximum 72 hours.

COMPULSORY DETENTION ORDERS (mentally abnormal offenders)

Section 35

- Remand to hospital for a medical report (on grounds of mental disorder).
- Made by Magistrates or Crown Court.
- 28 days duration, renewable every 28 days up to a maximum of 12 weeks.

Section 36

- Remand to hospital for treatment of a defendent awaiting trial, made by Crown Court.
- 28 days duration, renewable up to a maximum of 12 weeks.

Section 37 – Hospital treatment Order

- Hospital and guardianship order for convicted persons (Court equivalent of Section 3).
- Made by Crown (or exceptionally by Magistrates) Court.
- Six-month treatment order, renewable for 6 months, then yearly.
- Appeal allowed during the second 6 months, then yearly.

Section 38

- Interim Hospital order for assessment, allowing treatment for a convicted person (Hospitalisation appropriate).

- Made by Magistrates or Crown Court – no appeal allowed.
- 12 weeks duration, renewable at 28 day intervals up to a maximum of 6 months.

Section 41

- Restriction order for a convicted person (to protect public from serious harm).
- Imposed by Crown Court. Only dischargable by the Home Secretary.
- Not usually time limited.

Mental Health Review Tribunal:

Patients, or their nearest relatives, may appeal to the M.H.R.T., which has the power to grant leave and transfer or discharge patients.

6.2 NEW PSYCHOTROPIC DRUGS EXPECTED

This is a list of drugs which are known to have a product license application lodged in the UK or where it is thought to be planned soon. The time between application and approval can be as short as six months or as long as two or more years, depending upon the data presented and perceived risks. Accurate marketing dates are thus not available.

The author would be grateful for any additional information or corrections to help with this section, which relies to a large extent on 'randomly acquired' information.

Drugs or preparations possible in 2001–02

Adderall *

Adderall is a mixed amphetamine salt preparation, approved in USA for ADHD and possibly to be licensed in UK/Europe. In one study, 54% responded 'in a positive fashion' to Adderall. 38% were poor or non-responders. Acute anxiety occurred in 4 of 7 with co-morbid anxiety (n=24, open, Horrigan and Barnhill, *J Clin Psych* 2000, **61**, 414–17).

Aripiprazole (BMS) *

Aripiprazole is a presynaptic D2 autoreceptor antagonist, for schizophrenia, bipolar and psychosis in Alzheimer's disease. There is one published study comparing it with haloperidol in schizophrenia (n=400, 4/52, Kane *et al, Schizo Res* 2000, **41**, 39). It has a very low incidence of EPSE and no QTc prolongation. The main side-effects are sleepiness, headache and dizziness.

Dolasetron ('Anzemet', Hoechst Marion Roussel)

A once a day 5-HT$_3$ receptor antagonist to be licensed for emesis, migraine and possibly psychosis.

Escitalopram (Lundbeck) *

Lundbeck are developing the s-enantiomer of citalopram, which has been indicated to be the active enantiomer.

Fluoxetine (Prozac once-weekly) *

A 90mg once weekly oral form (slow-release to reduce peak levels) has been marketed in USA. Since fluoxetine and norfluoxetine have long half-lives and 5mg/d is the lowest effective dose, 90mg a week should be therapeutically active.

Gepirone ('Ariza', Organon) *

A 5HT1A partial agonist, with some alpha-2 activity, antidepressant, launch 2002/3 in USA. No dopamine blockade.

Iloperidone (Novartis) *

Iloperidone is a D2 and 5HT2 antagonist, with some alpha-1 blocking activity, currrently undergoing phase III trials for schizophrenia.

Melotonin (Genzyme)

This may be licensed for insomnia, as it produces a significant improvement in sleep (n=24, Dolberg *et al, Am J Psych* 1998, **155**, 1119–21), following 5–10mg at 9pm ('interesting, but not miraculous' review, Anon, *Prescrire Internat* 1998, **7**, 180–87, 83 refs).

Memantine (Lundbeck) *

Memantine is a non-competitive NMDA antagonist, currently licensed in Germany for dementia. It may be licensed for mild, moderate (n=531, Ruther *et al, Pharmacopsychiatry* 2000, **33**, 103–8) and severe dementia (RCT, n=151, Winblad and Poritis, *Int J Ger Psych* 1999, **14**, 135–46), as it appears to have a neuroprotective action (review, Jann, *Expert Opin Investig Drugs* 2000, **9**, 1397–406).

Metrifonate ('Memobay', Bayer. 2002?)

Metrifonate is an acetylcholine esterase inhibitor currently in use as a treatment for schistosomiasis (*Pharm J* 1997, **259**, 796), but being licensed for Alzheimer's disease. Studies have shown a modest reduction in the rate of decline (eg. 26-week RCT, n=408, Morris *et al, Neurology* 1998, **50**, 1222–30, reviewed by Luckman, *EBMH* 1998, **1**, 116). An older trial showed 40–80mg/d to be superior to placebo for cognitive and global function (n=605, McKeith, *Dem & Ger Cog Dis* 1988, **9**[Suppl 2], 2–7). Reports of a serious interaction with cimetidine have slowed development of this safe and established drug.

Milnacipran (Ixel) (Fabre)

SNRI, license currently on hold in UK, available in France (Peuch *et al, Int Clin Psychopharmacol* 1997, **12**, 99–108; study by Leinonen *et al, Acta Psych Scand* 1997, **96**, 497–504). Reviews by Lecrubier (*Hum Psychopharmacol* 1997, **12**, S127–S134) and Kasper (*Hum Psychopharmacol* 1997, **12**, S135–S141, Spencer and Wilde, *Drugs* 1998, **56**, 405–27), pharmacodynamics in young and elderly (Hindmarch *et al, B J Clin Pharmacology* 2000, **49**, 118–25).

Tianeptine ('Stablon', Servier)

'Novel tricyclic' (*B J Psych* 1992, **160** Suppl 15) which apparently works as a selective serotonin re-uptake enhancing properties, but decreases both serotonin transporter mRNA and binding sites, just like other SSRIs (Kuroda *et al, Eur J Pharmacol* 1993, **268**, R3–5). It may also increase extracellular dopamine (Sacchetti *et al, Eur J Pharmacol* 1993, **236**, 171–75), like bupropion. Available in France. Phase III trials in UK.

Ziprasidone ('Zeldox', Pfizer, late 2001–2002) *

D2-5HT2 antagonist antipsychotic with low EPSEs, weight gain and effect on prolactin. The main side-effects are transient somnolence and QT pro-longation. Produces minor inhibition of CYP2D6 (similar to risperidone), and minor inhibition of CYP3A. IM injection may be available, which has a rapid calming effect (eg. Meltzer, *CNS Drugs* 1997, **8**:160–61). A meta-analysis shows ziprasidone to be as effective as haloperidol with similar mild weight gain, but with different side effects (low EPSE but more nausea and vomiting) (n=1564, 7 trials, Bagnall *et al, Cochrane* review, comment by Gardner, *EBMH* 2000, **3**, 73). 2–10mg IM appears to have a dose-related, tolerable and rapid effect on acute agitation in psychotic patients (24hrs, RCT, n=117, Lesem *et al, J Clin Psych* 2001, **62**, 12–18).

Other drugs or preparations known to be under study and for which UK license applications may be made in due course:

Abecarnil (Schering)

Benzodiazepine receptor partial antagonist for anxiety, anxiety and alcohol withdrawal.

Alosetron (Glaxo)

5-HT$_3$ antagonist being investigated for schizophrenia and anxiety.

Amperozide (Novartis)

Has only a very weak dopamine-blocking activity but trials show it to be effective as an antipsychotic (*Pharm J* 1994, **253**, 638).

Eptastigmine *

Anticholinesterase for Alzheimer's disease (RCT, n=491, Imbimbo *et al, Neurology* 1999, **52**, 700–9), with good efficacy (6/12, d/b, p/c, n=349, Imbimbo *et al, Demen & Ger Cog Disord* 2000, **11**, 17–24) but potential adverse haematological effects.

Flesinoxan (Solvay)

5-HT$_{1A}$ receptor agonist being investigated for anxiety and depression.

Gepirone (Organon)

A buspirone analogue for anxiety.

Milameline (HMR)

M1 receptor agonist for Alzheimer's.

Nalmefene (Schering Plough)

More potent and longer-acting version of naloxone. Launched USA 1996.

Pramipexol (Mirapex, Pharmacia)

D2 agonist being investigated for depression and schizophrenia.

Raclopride (Astra)

D2 specific antipsychotic (*Inpharma* 1992, No **828**, 20).

Risperidone depot (2002/3?)

A microcrystalline injection, with a slow release characteristic.

Ritanserin (Janssen)

5-HT antagonist related to ketanserin, being investigated for depression, extra-pyramidal disorders and anxiety, plus drug abuse.

Roxindole (Merck)

SSRI, dopamine reuptake blocker, 5-HT$_{1A}$ agonist for depression or anxiety (*Am J Psych* 1994, **151**, 1499–502).

Rufinamide (Novartis)

GABA reuptake inhibitor for epilepsy.

Sabeluzole (Janssen)

Alzheimers Disease

Trandospirone (Pfizer)

5-HT$_1$ agonist being investigated for anxiety.

Zonisamide

GABA receptor antagonist anticonvulsant.

6.3 LABORATORY TEST INTERPRETATIONS

A guide to normal ranges, variations, causes and drug influences. Local ranges may differ slightly from these here.

UREA AND ELECTROLYTES (U&Es)

Check Maudsley 2001 and paper

Bicarbonate 22–30 mmol/l
Calcium 2.25–2.6 mmol/l
↑ malignancy (55%),
  hyperparathyroidism (35%),
  hyperthyroidism, Vit D excess.
↓ hypoparathyroidism, Vit D
  deficiency.
▲ OCs, lithium, thiazides.
▼ barbiturates, cimetidine,
  corticosteroids, phenytoin.
Chloride 9–105 mmol/l
Glucose 3.3–5.6 mmol/l
↑ >6.7 overnight = diabetes mellitus?
▲ cimetidine, OCs, furosemide,
  lithium, phenothiazines, thiazides,
  phenytoin.
(▲) ascorbic acid, levodopa, metronidazole.
▼ dextropropoxyphene.
(▼) ascorbic acid.
Magnesium 0.7–1.2 mmol/l
↑ renal failure
↓ severe diarrhoea
Phosphate 0.8–1.4 mmol/l (Adversely affects calcium metabolism)
↓ malnutrition (esp in alcoholics)

Potassium 3.5–5.3 mmol/l
↑ dangerous. Treat as emergency.
↓ produces muscle weakness.
▼ salbutamol, insulin.

Protein   Total 50–70 g/l
                   Albumin 35–55 g/l
↑ = haemoconcentration
↓ = haemodilution, neuropathy,
   cirrhosis, catabolism.

Sodium 133–149 mmol/l (Rate of change is as important as the actual level)
↑ excess fluid loss/poor intake, renal
   failure.
↓ cardiac or renal failure, D&V, chest
   disorders (infections or carcinoma),
   hypoalbuminaemia, bulimia?
▲ high dose sodium salt antibiotics,
   lithium.
▼ diuretics (esp thiazides), steroids,
   carbamazepine, oxcarbazepine,
   tricyclics, chlorpropamide,
   clofibrate.

Urea (2.5–8.0 mmol/l)
↑ renal failure, catabolism,
   haemorrhage
▲ salicylates, tetracyclines.

RENAL FUNCTION

Creatinine clearance
   M 97–140 ml/min,
   F 85–125 ml/min
(Best measure of GFR if collection of the
24-hour samples is accurate).

Creatinine conc
   M 50–120 mol/l
   F 40–100 mol/l
↑ Catabolism, pregnancy. Should
   decrease with age.
(▲) ascorbic acid, methyldopa.
▲ salicylates, captopril, cimetidine,
   co-trimoxazole.

Urea (BUN) 1–5 mmol/l
↑ renal failure, high protein food,
   catabolism.

LIVER FUNCTION TESTS (LFTs)

Ranges quoted by laboratories vary with
the method and conditions of the assay.

ALT (SGPT) 5–30 iu/l
↑ hepatocellular damage, cholestasis,
   occasionally cirrhosis.
▲ alcohol, OCs, levodopa, phenothiazines, phenytoin, valproate, antibiotics.
▼ vigabatrin.

(▼) metronidazole.

Albumin 35–55 g/l
↓ oedema, neuropathy, cirrhosis
(▲) penicillins.
▼ alcohol, phenytoin.

Alkaline Phosphatase (ALP) 20–100 iu/l
↑ cholestasis, hepatocellular damage,
   bone disease (eg. Pagets, carcinoma),
   pregnancy.
▲ alcohol, carbamazepine, disulfiram,
   phenothiazines, phenytoin.
(▼) nitrofurantoin, zinc.

Aspartate transaminase (AST or SGOT) 5–40 iu/l
↑ hepatocellular damage, cholestasis,
   cirrhosis, infarction, muscle trauma,
   respiratory failure.
▼ vigabatrin.

Bilirubin 2–20 mmol/l
↑ liver cell damage, cholestasis,
   haemolytic states.
(▲) beta-blockers, valproate, disulfiram, phenothiazines, alcohol,
   antibiotics.
(▼) ascorbic acid.

Gamma-Glutamyl transferase (GGT) 5–45 iu/l
↑ cholestasis, hepatitis, cirrhosis, cellular
   damage (eg. paracetamol or disulfiram
   OD), enzyme inducers (especially
   phenobarbital and phenytoin), excess
   alcohol, metastatic carcinoma
▲ alcohol, barbiturates, OCs, phenytoin,
   oxcarbazepine, simvastatin.

Prothrombin ratio 1–1.2
Prothrombin time 10–135
↑ severe, usually chronic, liver
   damage.

BLOOD

Blood pH 7.35–7.45
Outside range metabolic function is
impaired.

WBC/WCC 4.0–11.0 x10⁹/l
↑↑ malignancy.
↑ infection.
↓ many drugs, some infections.

RBC   M 4.5–6 x10¹²/l
              F 4.3–5.5 x10¹²/l
↑ fluid loss, polycythaemia.
↓ fluid overload, anaemia, marrow
   aplasia.

Hb   M 13–18 g/dl
         F 12–16 g/dl
↓ haemorrhage, Iron deficiency, marrow depression.

MCV (Mean Cell Volume) 80–95 fl
↑ folate or B12 deficiency, liver disease, alcohol.
↓ iron deficiency.

ESR   M 0–9 mm/h
         F 0–20 mm/h
(viscosities now more usually used).
↑ infections, inflammatory diseases.

Lymphocytes 1–4 x10⁹/l
↑ (lymphocytosis) mononucleosis, viral infections, TB, some leukemias, auto-immune diseases, toxoplasmosis.
↓ (lymphopenia) in marrow failure, plus treatment with corticosteroids and azathioprine.

Platelets 100–450 x10⁹/l
↓ marrow failure or toxicity, leukaemia, splenomegaly.

Neutrophils 1.8–8 x10⁹/l (45–75% of WBCs)
↑ infection, inflammation, carcinoma, leukaemia, gout.
↓ viral infections, autoimmune disease, marrow failure drugs
▼ chlorpromazine, phenytoin, chloramphenicol etc.

Monocytes 0.1–1.1 x10⁹/l
↑ (monocytosis) in TB, endocarditis, typhoid, leukaemia.

Eosinophils 0.04–0.8 x10⁹/l (1–4% of WBCs)
↑ eosinophilia) in atopic asthma, hay fever, worm infestations, lymphomas, skin disease.

Basophils 0.01–0.4 x10⁹/l
↑ (basophil leucocytosis) leukaemia, ulcerative colitis.

MISCELLANEOUS

Amylase (serum) 60–300 μ/l
↑ acute pancreatitis, abdominal trauma, renal failure.
▲ furosemide, morphine, valproate.

Blood pressure (Adult) ≤ 140/90
Systolic/Diastolic, the latter more important. Possibly higher limit allowed in elderly.

Cortisol/Dexamethasone Suppression Test 200nmol/l
↑ adrenal hyperplasia or tumour (or depression?)

CSF Protein 0.2–0.5 g/l
↑ infection, haemorrhage.

CSF glucose 2.8–4 mmol/l
↑ haemorrhage.
↓ infection.

Folate Serum 2.5–15 μg/l
↓ best guide to folate deficiency.

Folate RBC 150–750 μg/l
↓ guide to long term folate deficiency.
▼ chloramphenicol, erythromycin, penicillins
(▼) barbiturates, OCs, phenytoin, alcohol.

Iron Serum M 10–30 μmol/l
           F 7–25 μmol/l
↑ inflammation.
↓ iron deficiency, rheumatoid arthritis.

Iron Binding Capacity (serum) 45–72μmol/l
↑ iron deficiency.
↓ rheumatoid arthritis.

Lipids:
— cholesterol 4–7mmol/l
↑ hyperlipidaemia, diabetes, nephrotic syndrome, biliary obstruction.
▲ disulfiram, levodopa, OCs, phenytoin, oxcarbazepine.
▼ metronidazole, tetracyclines.
— **triglyceride** 0.6–1.8 mmol/l (post 12hr fasting)
↑ diabetes, nephrotic syndrome pancreatitis, alcohol abuse.
▲ alcohol, beta-blockers, clozapine, OCs.

Osmolality 285–295 mOsm/kg
↑ fluid depletion
↓ fluid excess.

pCO₂ 4.5–6kPa or 34–45 mmHg
Measure of respiratory function

Thyroxine-total 60–140nmol/l
↑ hyperthyroidism (Grave's Disease — confirm by TRH)— varies with age
↓ hypothyroidism
▲ beta-blockers, OCs.
▼ carbamazepine, lithium, phenytoin, salicylates.

T4/Thyroxine-Free 10–25pmol/l
↑ hypothyroidism (Myxodema)
↓ hyperthyroidism

T3 1.1–2.3nmol/l

↑ hypothyroidism
↓ hyperthyroidism

TSH 0.15–3.20mIU/l

↑ hypothyroidism
↓ hyperthyroidism

Urate 150–500 umol/l

↑ purine metabolic defect, carcinoma, diminished excretion (eg. acidosis, renal failure, diuretics)
▲ alcohol, furosemide, salicylates, thiazides.

Vitamin B12 160–900 ng/l

↓ diet deficiency, pernicious anaemia, ileitis or short bowel syndrome. May lead to macrocytic anaemia and peripheral neuropathy.

KEY

↑	increased level mainly caused by:
↓	decreased level mainly caused by:
▲	drugs which raise level include:
▼	drugs which lower level include:
(▲)	drugs which appear to raise levels by test interference:
(▼)	drugs which appear to lower levels by test interference:

All the main psychotropic drugs are indexed according to their BNF or other main indications in chapter one, but obviously may appear elsewhere. In order to keep the index down to a manageable size, you are then referred to the index listing for that drugs chemical or therapeutic group. Individual drugs should be looked up under their drug group.

Abbreviations used

* = new data added to the text since the 2000 edition

ACh = Acetylcholine

ADHD = Attention deficit hyperactivity disorder

ADD = Attention deficit disorder

ADME = Absorption, distribution, metabolism and excretion

ADR = Adverse drug reaction

AED = Anti-epileptic drug

AFP = Alpha-fetoprotein

AIMS = Abnormal involuntary movement scale

APE = Acute psychiatric emergency

APA = American Psychiatric Association

AWS = Alcohol withdrawal syndrome

BAP = British Association for Psychopharmacology

BDZ = Benzodiazepine(s)

BMA = British Medical Association

BMI = Body mass index

BNF = British National Formulary

BPD = Borderline psychiatric disorder

BPRS = Brief psychiatric rating scale

bp = blood pressure

BP = British Pharmacopoeia

CBT = Cognitive behavioural therapy

CBZ = Carbamazepine

CBZ-E = Carbamazepine-epoxide

CCK = Cholecystokinin

CDSR = Cochrane Database Systematic Reviews

CGI = Clinical global impression

CHD = coronary heart disease

CNS = Central nervous system

c/o = cross-over

CPK = Creatinine phosphokinase

CSM = Committee on the Safety of Medicines

D1 = Dopamine-1 (receptor)

D2 = Dopamine-2 (receptor)

DA = Dopamine

d/b = double-blind

DSM-IV = Diagnostic Statistical Manual IV

e/c = enteric-coated

ECG = Electrocardiogram

ECT = Electroconvulsive therapy

EBMH = Evidence-Based Mental Health (Journal)

EEG = Electro-encephalogram

EPO = Evening primrose oil

EPSE = Extra-pyramidal side-effects

FBC = Full blood count

GABA = Gamma-aminobutyric acid

GFR = Glomerular filtration rate

GTC = Generalised tonic-clonic (seizure)

5-HT = 5-hydroxytryptamine

HF = heart failure

IV = Intra-venous

IM = Intra-muscular

INR = International normalized ratio

ISE = Ion-selective electrode

L/A = Long-acting

LD = Low dose

LFT = Liver function tests

LTG = Lamotrigine

MAOI = Mono-amine oxidase inhibitor

MHA = Mental Health Act (1983)

MI = Manfacturers' information

MMSE = Mini-Mental State Examination

NE = Norepinephrine

NA = Noradrenaline

N/K = Not known

NMDA = N-methyl-D-aspartate receptor complex

NMS = Neuroleptic malignant syndrome

NNT = Numbers needed to treat

OCD = Obsessive-compulsive disorder

O/C = Oral contraceptive

OD = Overdose

OTC = Over-the-counter (medicine)

p/c = placebo-controlled

PD = Personality disorder, Pro-drug

PMH = Previous medical history

PMS = Pre-menstrual syndrome

PT= Prothrombin time

PTSD = Post-traumatic stress disorder

RCT = Randomised controlled trial

REM = Rapid eye movement

RIMA = Reversible Inhibitor of Monoamine-A

RPSGB= Royal Pharma-ceutical Society of Great Britain

RT = Rapid tranquillisation

SA = Short-acting

S/b = Single blind (trial)

s/c = sub-cutaneous

SF = Sugar-free

SIB = Self-injurious behaviour

SJW = St. John's wort

SPC = Summary of product characteristics

SSRI = Serotonin-selective reuptake inhibitor

$t_{1/2}$ = half-life

TCA = Tricyclic antidepressant

TD = Tardive dyskinesia

TDM = Therapeutic drug monitoring

U&E = Urea and electrolytes

UKPPG = United Kingdom Psychiatric Pharmacy Group

USP = United States Pharmacopoeia